Distraction of the Craniofacial Skeleton

Springer
New York
Berlin
Heidelberg
Barcelona
Budapest
Hong Kong
London
Milan
Paris
Singapore
Tokyo

Joseph G. McCarthy, MD
Institute of Reconstructive Plastic Surgery, New York University School of Medicine, New York University Medical Center, New York

Editor

Distraction of the Craniofacial Skeleton

Foreword by Paul Tessier, MD

With 224 Illustrations in 734 Parts

Springer

Joseph G. McCarthy, MD
Director
Institute of Reconstructive Plastic Surgery
New York University School of Medicine
New York University Medical Center
New York, NY 10016, USA

Library of Congress Cataloging-in-Publication Data

Distraction of the craniofacial skeleton / [edited by] Joseph G. McCarthy.
p. cm.
Includes bibliographical references and index.
ISBN 978-0-387-94912-3 ISBN 978-3-4612-2140-1 (eBook)
DOI 10.1007/978-3-4612-2140-1
1. Facial bones—Surgery. 2. Cranium—Surgery. 3. Bone regeneration. 4. Orthopedic surgery. I. McCarthy, Joseph G., 1938– .
[DNLM: 1. Facial Bones—surgery. 2. Bone Lengthening—methods. 3. Osteogenesis. 4. Craniotomy. WE 705 D614 1997]
RD763.D55 1997
617.5'2059—dc21
DNLM/DLC
for Library of Congress 97–13230

Printed on acid-free paper.

Production coordinated by Chernow Editorial Services, Inc., and managed by Bill Imbornoni; manufacturing supervised by Joe Quatela.
Typeset by Best-set Typesetter Ltd., Hong Kong.

9 8 7 6 5 4 3 2 1

ISBN 978-0-387-94912-3

This book is dedicated to two legendary surgeons, John M. Converse of New York and Paul Tessier of Paris. Their clinical skills, innovative talent, and concern for the patient with facial deformity attracted me as a young resident to the then emerging field of craniofacial surgery. Their spirit remains a part of my daily professional life.

FOREWORD

A revision may require an introduction for, as an example, taking the position of a ship at sea. But an original work is self-sufficient; it can stand by itself. It does not need a foreword, which is embarrassing for one to write who is ignorant in the matter.

New ideas—some often ridiculous—are daily occurrences in surgery, but successful clinical applications of them are rare. Moreover, when the applications of a new surgical concept extend rapidly to several areas, the fact deserves to be sharply emphasized. This is presently the case for Distraction Osteogenesis, called the "D.O.G." system by the writer. From the basic principles to animal experiments to quantitative evaluations and the wide spectrum of clinical applications, "D.O.G." is splendidly illustrated and its therapeutic appeals made convincing in this book.

MEMORIES

Ilizarov's concept (1952) for limb reconstruction was born in remote, deep-frozen Siberia. Then Snyder experimented (1973) with the canine mandible, but his work escaped the facial surgeon's vigilance. However, Joe McCarthy made subsequent canine experiments and presented the first applications on the human in Florence in 1989; the "D.O.G." method then exploded within only six years. The fact is so much more remarkable when one considers that, in general, it takes *one generation* from the infant's first steps to easy jogging; other examples are the transitions from Medawar's tissue compatibility to current kidney transplantation, from the chips to personal computers, and the development of safety in lens or total hip replacements.

PALEOCONCEPTS

It also took *one generation* for interceptive craniofacial surgery to be applied to the corrections of the deformities resulting from Crouzon syndrome, Apert syndrome, plagiocephaly, Franceschetti syndrome, hemifacial microsomia, "rare" facial clefts, and hypertelorbitism through the intracranial route. One generation of painful effort for all specialties, but only *six years* for McCarthy's performance in attracting facial and cranial surgical leaders.

JUBILATION

The writer of this foreword feels the situation so much more ironic because several of the surgical steps mentioned above have been dramatically short-circuited by a simple "jackscrew" device skillfully used. A mandibular endless screw has opened an unlimited adventure. This is a revolution that has spread to the maxilla in Mexico, then the midface and calvarium in France, Germany, the United States, and so on.

PANORAMIC PERSPECTIVES

Will an endless screw put an end to interceptive facial and cranial surgical procedures, which can still stand as landmarks and references for treatment goals? The D.O.G. system has been elaborated by Joe McCarthy for the child's mandible, which has a high potential for generating new bone. But D.O.G. has rapidly expanded to other young bones, and the method will probably remain a privilege for children. However, the principles have been already applied to nongrowing bones, such as those in craniosynostosis, and also to older posttraumatic mandibular deformities by the process of "bone transport," which might avoid the need for intraoral soft tissue transfers in adults.

Is it not amazing that the D.O.G. method has already attracted the orthodontists? Is it not encouraging that another gate of hope is now opened to the hopeless microphthalmic patients?

Further applications in the human will no longer be "human experiments," but sound applications of investigative surgeons who had either surrendered or had overwhelmed the problems by other means or other tools at different age groups.

THANK YOU

For the surgery of the human face, the year 1987 was a fabulous milestone. When Joe McCarthy uncorked the first bottle of "D.O.G." in Florence in 1989, he was continuing a half century NYU tradition for innovation and education.

PAUL TESSIER, MD

PREFACE

The development of distraction techniques represents only a time point in the historical evolution of reconstructive surgery of the craniofacial region. Joseph Murray, plastic surgeon and Nobel laureate, has described four periods in the development of modern surgery:

1. The period of resection or ablation of diseased tissue.
2. The period of reconstruction or rebuilding of an anatomic defect.
3. The period of transplantation or replacement of a missing part.
4. The period of regeneration or inductive surgery.

In the craniofacial region, early surgical efforts, dating back to the oldest historical reports, were directed at excising tumors or areas of osteomyelitis. The innovative efforts of military surgeons in World War I represented entry into the second (reconstructive) period by the skillful use of splints and the resurfacing of defects with local and other types of flaps. The use of autogenous bone grafts and microvascular free flaps represented the introduction of the transplantation period. The legendary accomplishments of Paul Tessier and others in the late 1960s and 1970s represented the high point of the second and third phases.

With the introduction of distraction osteogenesis, craniofacial surgery has entered the latest period—inductive surgery or the regeneration of missing anatomic parts. It also coincides with two other phenomena currently observed in all surgical disciplines: (1) the simplification or minimalization of surgery and (2) the recognition of the need for the delivery of health care services at a lower cost. With distraction techniques, the surgeon dealing with craniofacial deformity has available a treatment modality with unique properties: it can be simply applied with reduced hospital stays; it is highly effective with significantly lower morbidity and relapse rates; it eliminates the need for blood transfusion, bone grafts, and permanently implanted fixation devices; and it gives a superior result not only by augmenting the craniofacial skeleton but also the overlying soft tissue.

The craniofacial surgical community is indebted to Ilizarov of Russia for developing and pioneering the technique of distraction osteogenesis. It is ironic, however, that he spent his professional career developing the technique on the long bones (endochondral) of the extremities. Yet, the bones of the craniofacial skeleton are much more suited to surgical distraction. Membranous in embryologic origin, they are of a relatively smaller dimension, have a much richer blood supply, and are more accessible to surgical manipulation. These special attributes are reflected in the clinical experience which has evolved to date. The surgeon is not technically restricted, as in the long bones of the extremities, to a limited surgical exposure, but is able to employ wide subperiosteal dissection, a technical maneuver that greatly facilitates the procedure. He is able to reduce the latency period to only 4 to 5 days and occasionally distract at a rate that exceeds the classic 1.0 mm per day advocated by Ilizarov. There is also less morbidity than that experienced by the orthopedic surgeon involved in distraction of the long bones, and the patient also has less pain and discomfort during the period of distraction. Finally, the overall treatment program is completed within three months, a significantly shorter period than that of long bone distraction.

As the first decade of craniofacial distraction draws to a close, there have been enormous advances. It has been conclusively demonstrated that the hypoplastic mandible can be successfully augmented with concomitant distraction of the overlying soft tissue. Moreover, there has been sufficient clinical experience to demonstrate that mandibular reconstruction can be accomplished in multiple dimensions. The development of newer distraction devices has also shown that, in addition to multiplanar distraction, the lesser types of mandibular and maxillary hypoplasia are even amenable to distraction with intraoral devices, therefore obviating the need for cutaneous scars. Another remarkable finding has been an almost total absence of dental or skeletal relapse, and some patients have even demonstrated growth of the distracted mandible. In fact, most surgeons would agree that distraction is the treatment of choice for severe micrognathia with respiratory insufficiency and the Class IIa and IIb (Pruzansky) types of mandibular hypoplasia in craniofacial microsomia.

Maxillary, midface, and zygomatic distraction has already been successfully achieved in the animal model and, as shown in this text, clinical trials of maxillary and midface clinical distraction are already underway. Clinical zygomatic distraction has been accomplished in the Treacher Collins patient and cranial vault distraction has been reported in the patient with craniofacial synostosis.

Orbital distraction has a long history, when one considers serial enlargement of the conjunctional sac with ocular prostheses. Obviously, CT studies of the hypoplastic orbit and the development of newer types of devices will allow three-dimensional enlargement of the orbital cavity in patients with microphthalmos.

This book is an outgrowth of the first workshop on craniofacial distraction that was held at the Institute of Reconstructive Plastic Surgery at the New York University Medical Center in 1994. This conference, for the first time, assembled from many disciplines the clinicians who believed in the promise of distraction osteogenesis and appreciated the possibilities it offered for a simpler and more effective rehabilitation of the craniofacial skeleton.

I am indebted to all of the contributors, without whose cooperation the book would not have the comprehensive discussion of all aspects of craniofacial distraction. I recognize the effort required, especially in the midst of their busy clinical practices.

Since I arrived at New York University in 1971, I have been fortunate to work with and learn from a remarkable group of colleagues at the Institute of Reconstructive Plastic Surgery. Over the years my fellow members of the craniofacial surgery team have always stimulated me, aroused my curiosity, and, with wisdom, questioned my surgical dogma. They have also been invaluable in gathering critical clinical data and conducting the associated laboratory research. I especially want to express my gratitude to Lawrence Brecht, DDS, Court B. Cutting, MD, Mark Gianoutsis, MD, Paul M. Glat, MD, Arun Gosain, MD, Barry H. Grayson, DDS, Larry Hollier, MD, Nolan S. Karp, MD, Jamie Levine, MD, Michael T. Longaker, MD, Richard J. Mackool, MD, Susan McCormack, DDS, Douglas A. Roth, MD, Norman Rowe, MD, David Staffenberg, MD, Charles H. Thorne, MD, Andrew Turk, MD, Joseph K. Williams, MD, Robert Wood, MD, and Barry Zide, MD. Special thanks are due Marilyn Ostrow for typing the manuscripts, Patricia Chibbaro, RN, and Lynmarie Cipriano for coordinating clinical schedules, and Esther Gumpert, Jeff Sands, Barbara Chernow, and William Imbornoni of Springer-Verlag for providing editorial assistance and publishing equanimity.

I was fortunate as a young surgeon to be influenced and stimulated by two giants of the plastic surgery world—John M. Converse of New York and Paul Tessier of Paris. Broadly visioned, they based their surgical teachings on research, scholarship, and clinical experience. They also had a contagious way of imparting their passion for craniofacial surgery to their trainees. They left an indelible impression on me, and I continue to draw on their wisdom and teachings in my daily surgical endeavors. I dedicate this book to them—my teachers, my mentors, and my friends.

JOSEPH G. MCCARTHY, MD

CONTENTS

Contributors

Hans Anderl, MD
Department of Plastic and Reconstructive Surgery, University Hospital, Innsbruck, Austria

Hannu Aro, PhD
Department of Surgery, University of Turku, FIN-20520 Turku, Finland

James Aronson, MD
Department of Pediatric Orthopaedics, Arkansas Children's Hospital, University of Arkansas for Medical Sciences, Little Rock, AK 72202, USA

Constance M. Barone, MD
Division of Plastic Surgery, University of Missouri, Columbia, MO 65211, USA

William H. Bell, DDS
Dial and Maxillofacial Imaging Center, Paylor College of Dentistry, Dallas, TX 75266-0677, USA

Martin Chin, DDS
Pacific Presbyterian Professional Building, San Francisco, CA 94115, USA

Robert G. Colcleugh, MD, FACS, FRCS(C)
Department of Plastic and Reconstructive Surgery, University of Western Ontario, London, Ontario N6A 4G5, Canada

Barry L. Eppley, MD, DMD
Division of Plastic Surgery, Indiana University Medical Center, Indianapolis, IN 46202, USA

Jeffrey D. Fairley, MD
Krankenhaus München Bogenthausen, 81925 Munich, Germany

Alvaro A. Figueroa, DDS, MD
The Craniofacial Center, University of Illinois, Chicago, IL 60612, USA

Paul M. Glat, MD
Institute of Reconstructive Plastic Surgery, New York University School of Medicine, New York University Medical Center, New York, NY 10016, USA

Barry Grayson, DDS
Institute of Reconstructive Plastic Surgery, New York University School of Medicine, New York University Medical Center, New York, NY 10016, USA

Cesar A. Guerrero, MD
Cirujano Buco-Maxilo-Facial, Consultant, Catedra de Ortodoncia, Facultad de Ontologia, Universidad de Venezuala, Caracas, Venezuela

Jeffrey Hollinger, DDS, PhD
Division of Plastic and Reconstructive Surgery, Oregon Health Sciences University, Portland, OR 97201-3098, USA

Richard J. Mackool, MD
Institute of Reconstructive Plastic Surgery, New York University School of Medicine, New York University Medical Center, New York, NY 10016, USA

Michael H. Mayer, MD
Division of Plastic and Reconstructive Surgery, Oregon Health Sciences University, Portland, OR 97201-3098, USA

Joseph G. McCarthy, MD
Institute of Reconstructive Plastic Surgery, New York University School of Medicine, New York University Medical Center, New York, NY 10016, USA

Fernando Molina, MD
Hospital Angeles del Pedregal, Heroes De Padierna, Mexico DF 10700

Fernando Ortiz Monasterio, MD
Hospital Angeles del Pedregal, Heroes De Padierna, Mexico DF 10700

Wolfgang Muhlbauer, MD
Department of Plastic, Reconstructive, and Hand Surgery, Klinikum München-Bogenhausen, Akademisches Lehrkrankenhaus, 81925 Munich, Germany

John A. Persing, MD
Yale University School of Medicine, New Haven, CT 06520, USA

John W. Polley, MD
The Craniofacial Center, University of Illinois at Chicago, Chicago, IL 60612, USA

Douglas A. Roth, MD
Institute of Reconstructive Plastic Surgery, New York University School of Medicine, New York University Medical Center, New York, NY 10016, USA

A. Michael Sadove, MD
Division of Plastic Surgery, Indiana University Medical Center, Indianapolis, IN 46202, USA

Suzanne U. Stucki-McCormick, MS, DDS
New York Eye and Ear Infirmary, New York, NY 10013, USA

Bryant A. Toth, MD
Pacific Presbyterian Professional Building, San Francisco, CA 94115, USA

Andrew Turk, MD
Institute of Reconstructive Plastic Surgery, New York University School of Medicine, New York University Medical Center, New York, NY 10016, USA

Joseph K. Williams, MD
Institute of Reconstructive Plastic Surgery, New York University School of Medicine, New York University Medical Center, New York, NY 10016, USA

Part 1
Principles

CHAPTER 1

Bone Regeneration

Concepts and Update

Jeffrey Hollinger and Michael H. Mayer

Bone is a dynamic organ that can regenerate. Regeneration may be defined as restoration of form and function indistinguishable from that derived embryologically.

Developmental insufficiency, pathology, surgical resection, and traumatic avulsion can lead to osseous deficits. Exploitation of the regenerative capacity of bone has spawned a diverse spectrum of modalities to correct these deficits: including autogenous grafts, allogeneic bank bone, metals, ceramics, synthetics, electrical stimulation, recombinant therapeutics (eg, growth factors), and mechanical devices (such as distractors).

This chapter will use the classical fracture-healing model to integrate selected, recent information about growth factors that have clinical relevance to bone regeneration. Important concepts about these growth-modulating factors and cells will be highlighted.

CONCEPTS AND NOMENCLATURE

An increasing number of biological factors associated with bone homeostasis and regeneration are being identified. Attempts have been made to organize these factors into categories or classes, such as hormones, prostaglandins, cytokines, and growth factors. Classification according to physiological criteria may lead to controversy. This has been the case with two important groups of cell regulatory molecules: *growth factors* and *cytokines* (1). These two classes of molecules have been singled out because of intense interest in them for therapeutic applications to bone regeneration.

In general, growth factors and cytokines are mediators for normal cellular growth, embryogenesis, wound repair, and oncogenesis (2). In addition, a specific growth factor or cytokine may have either an inhibitory or stimulatory effect, or it may be both inhibitory and stimulatory, depending on the cellular interactions and gradients of local factors (3–5). Such schizophrenic behavior has led to confusion about categorizing biological regulatory molecules as either growth factors or cytokines. Therefore, restriction either to one category or to another may be artificial. Originally, the term *cytokine* included interleukins, lymphokines, monokines, colony-stimulating factors, and interferons, thus excluding growth factors (6). The review by Takaku neatly portrays several readily definable cytokines (7); however, the unique physiologic traits of certain cytokines have prompted a classification proposal according to receptors (8). A paradigm embracing this concept has been reviewed by Robertson and associates (6) and should provide additional standardization for cytokine nomenclature (6). (Typically, cytokine receptors lack tyrosine kinase activity; however, exceptions exist.) Unfortunately, the magnitude of complexities of some regulatory molecules defies attempts to file them neatly. However, for didactic reasons, simplicity should govern categorization. Consequently, growth factors usually exclude cytokines and hormones, even though there may be overlap in functional activities.

While cytokines, growth factors, and hormones are key interlocutory factors with indistinguishable roles during embryogenesis, immunologic phenomena, homeostasis, and wound healing, for the purpose of this review chapter, cytokines will be considered regulators for growth and differentiation of cells of the immune and hematopoietic systems. On this basis, biologic agents whose activities are exerted predominantly on mesenchymal lineage cells will be referred to as growth factors. Furthermore, the growth factors having the most commonly acknowledged influence on fracture repair and bone regeneration dynamics will be highlighted, and these include transforming growth factor beta (TGF-β), fibroblast growth factor (FGF), platelet derived growth factor (PDGF), and insulin-like growth factor (IGF).

FRACTURE HEALING

Classical studies have identified the cellular and molecular constituents of bone fracture repair, thereby providing a robust knowledge base chronicling the constellation of factors important in bone healing (9–21). The clan of regulatory molecules referred to as *growth factors* modulates bone regeneration at the fracture site almost from the moment of injury until the culmination of regeneration. Therefore, the dynamics of bone regeneration at the fracture wound provide an operational framework to discuss growth factors and establish a logical foundation that will lead to their applications as clinical therapies (Figure 1.1).

Within seconds after fracture, a series of events ensue to regenerate continuity and function. The first major event encompasses a cascade of factors for hemostasis known as the clotting cascade.

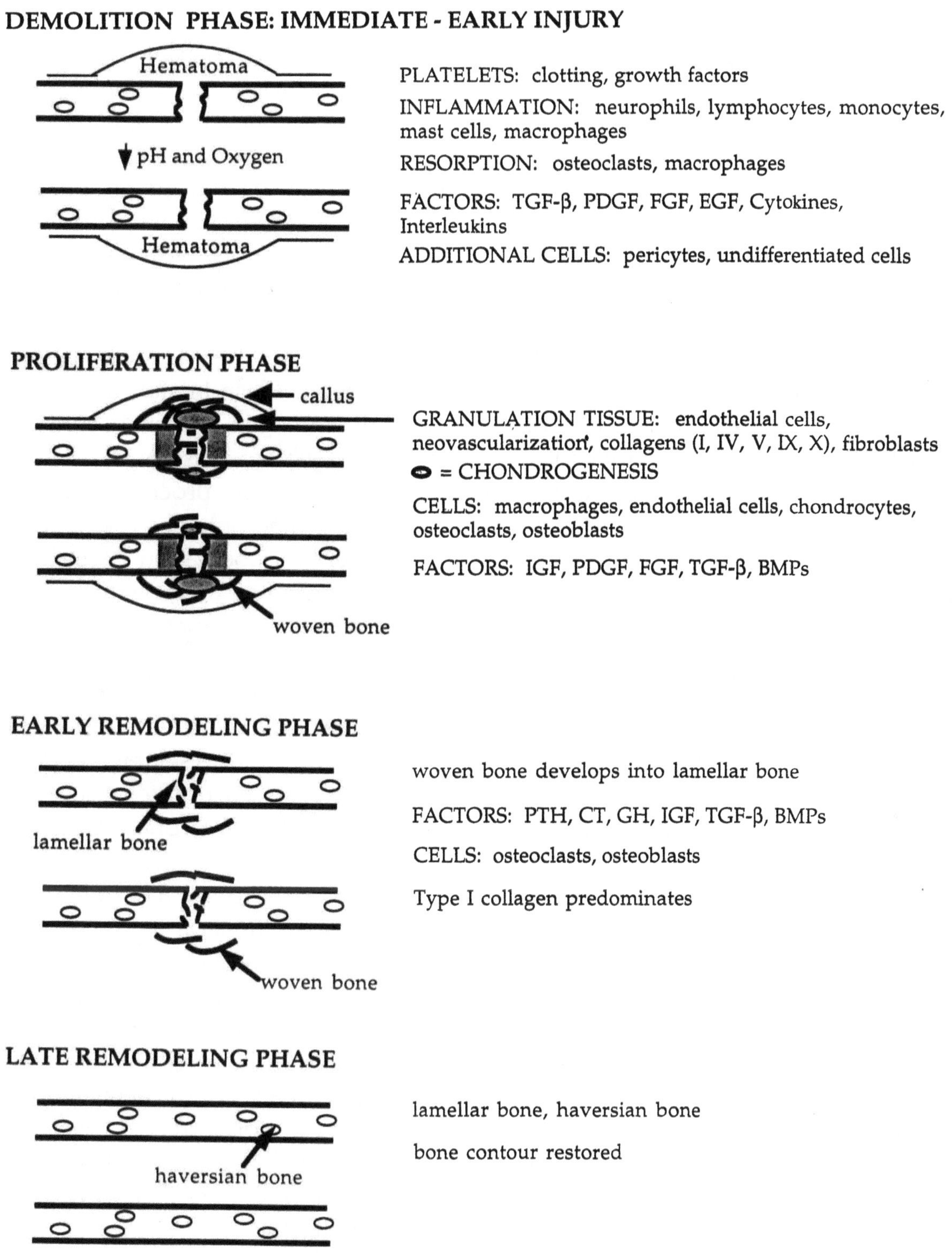

Figure 1.1. Schematic summary illustrating classic fracture repair.

The critical player is the platelet: a 2- to 4-micron diameter-sized remnant of a megakaryocyte, with a half-life of 8 to 12 days, that provides an indispensable role as a storehouse for growth factors. Growth factors expressed by the platelet (eg, PDGF, FGF, TGF-β) are mitogenic for vascular endothelial cells, vascular smooth muscle cells, and fibroblasts, thus promoting restoration of damaged vascularity, pivotal to bone regeneration. A component of hemostasis is hematoma formation, the localized collection of extravasated red blood cells and vascular elements. In addition to hematoma formation, disruption in blood vessel continuity incites a flurry of cells, predominantly undifferentiated, that surge to the fracture site, followed closely by macrophages, polymorphonuclear leukocytes, histiocytes, lymphocytes, and mast cells (13,22). Polymorphonuclear cells also are the hallmark of the acute inflammatory stage of bony repair.

The hematoma condenses through days 3 to 5, providing the physiologic role of a blood clot: the meshwork of fibrin, degenerating red blood cells, platelets, undifferentiated mesenchymal cells, and fibroblasts that form a physical plug and is a source of cell regulation factors (ie, growth and differentiating factors). These factors (eg, PDGF, FGF, TGF-β) are disgorged as the alpha granules of platelets degranulate, ushering endothelial cell migration, proliferation, capillary formation, and orchestrating cellular events. For example, PDGF promotes quiescent mesenchymal cells to react with modulating factors, a process referred to as competence: the stage when a cell is responsive to additional growth factor modulation (23). TGF-β is a mitogen; it directs differentiating cells to replicate (24,25). FGF induces new vessel formation (26).

Once the functional and physiologic imperatives of the clot (ie, hematoma) have been accomplished at the fracture site, there must be no delay in its removal. A lag in clot removal will detain the bone regeneration cascade. Controlled clot lysis is instigated by plasminogen activator expressed by local tissue such as vascular endothelium. Plasminogen activator converts plasminogen (which becomes trapped in the clot) to plasmin, leading to clot lysis and removal, processes augmented by resident macrophages and histiocytes. Concurrently, modulation of cell phenotypes is prompted by growth factors.

Trafficking of messages—communication—among cells by growth factors may be accomplished by three general paradigms: *autocrine*—the cell synthesizes a product that is secreted and acts on the same cell; *paracrine*—the synthesis product diffuses from one cell to another cell; and *endocrine*—the cell secretion transits the blood to a target cell. Cell products may function in more than one mode. For example, TGF-β is an autocrine and paracrine factor. As an autocrine factor, it is expressed by osteoblasts in a latent form and activated by osteoclast proteinases, and once activated, stimulates type I collagen expression from osteoblasts (25,27). Macrophages and osteoclasts also express TGF-β at the fracture and, functioning in a paracrine mode, recruit differentiated osteoblasts and enhance their activity (25,28,29).

Days 3 through 5 postfracture also are marked by fibroblast migration into the injury site and development of gossamery connective tissue speckled with proliferating capillary buds, the compendium referred to as granulation tissue. Isotypes of collagens localized to granulation tissue and the healing fracture include types I–V, IX, and X (30). Type I collagen is unique to bone, and type II is cartilage specific. Type IV collagen is associated with neovasculature endothelial cell matrix. Selective binding of growth factors to collagens ensures spatial localization for interaction with mesenchymal lineage cells that can differentiate into chondro-osteogenic phenotypes (31,32). Moreover, collagen isotypes and extracellular ground substances, such as proteoglycans, especially hyaluronic acid and chondroitin sulfate, form an interactive fabric: the extracellular matrix necessary for growth factor binding, cell attachment interactions (33), angiogenesis (the growth of branching capillary networks) (34), and conversion to chondro-osteogenic phenotypes (35,36).

Clot formation and granulation tissue usher in the next major event in bone regeneration at the fracture: callus. Callus, derived from the Latin for the word *hard*, has been applied inaccurately to include everything from granulation tissue to calcifying cartilage and woven bone forming periosteally and endosteally around fracture fragments (1). Traditional descriptive histology delimited "hard" and "soft" callus stages during endochondral bone healing. However, an admixture of tissues typically develops (Figure 1.2) (1).

Callus development and the quantity of callus are proportional to fracture fragment movement and bone embryogenesis (1).

Following open reduction for a rigid fixation prosthesis in the craniofacial complex, fracture fragments are reapproximated (that is, reduced), hardware is installed, and during healing, minimal movement should not stimulate callus. The healing process is called direct bone formation (also referred to as primary bone formation) and is promoted by osteoclast cutting cones followed by osteoblast-mediated osteoid deposition and calcification. Fracture callus at rigidly fixed locales in the craniofacial complex indicates failure of the fixation prosthesis (37). Healing in this region generally proceeds by direct, intramembranous bone formation, without a cartilaginous component. In contrast, cartilage and callus usually are identified at endochondrally derived bone healing sites. Therefore, to be inclusive in an embryologic sense, this discussion will continue through callus formation and its demise.

Vascular invasion of the callus increases oxygen tension, heralding chondrocyte death. Shortly thereafter, the cartilage matrix calcifies, and it is eroded by chondroclasts while providing a substratum for osteoblast attachment. Several lineage options are proposed for osteoblasts (38,39). Osteoprogenitor cells are lured to the fracture site in response to as yet unidentified chemoattractants (40). Osteoprogenitor cells may be either determined or inducible. Determined osteoprogenitor cells are derived from periosteum and bone marrow lineage cells, and binding with TGF-β leads to expression of an osteoblast phenotype. Inducible osteoprogenitors migrate to the fracture site by vascular highways and are referred to as pericytes (41). Allegedly, undifferentiated mesenchymal stem cells also may be inducible osteoprogenitors

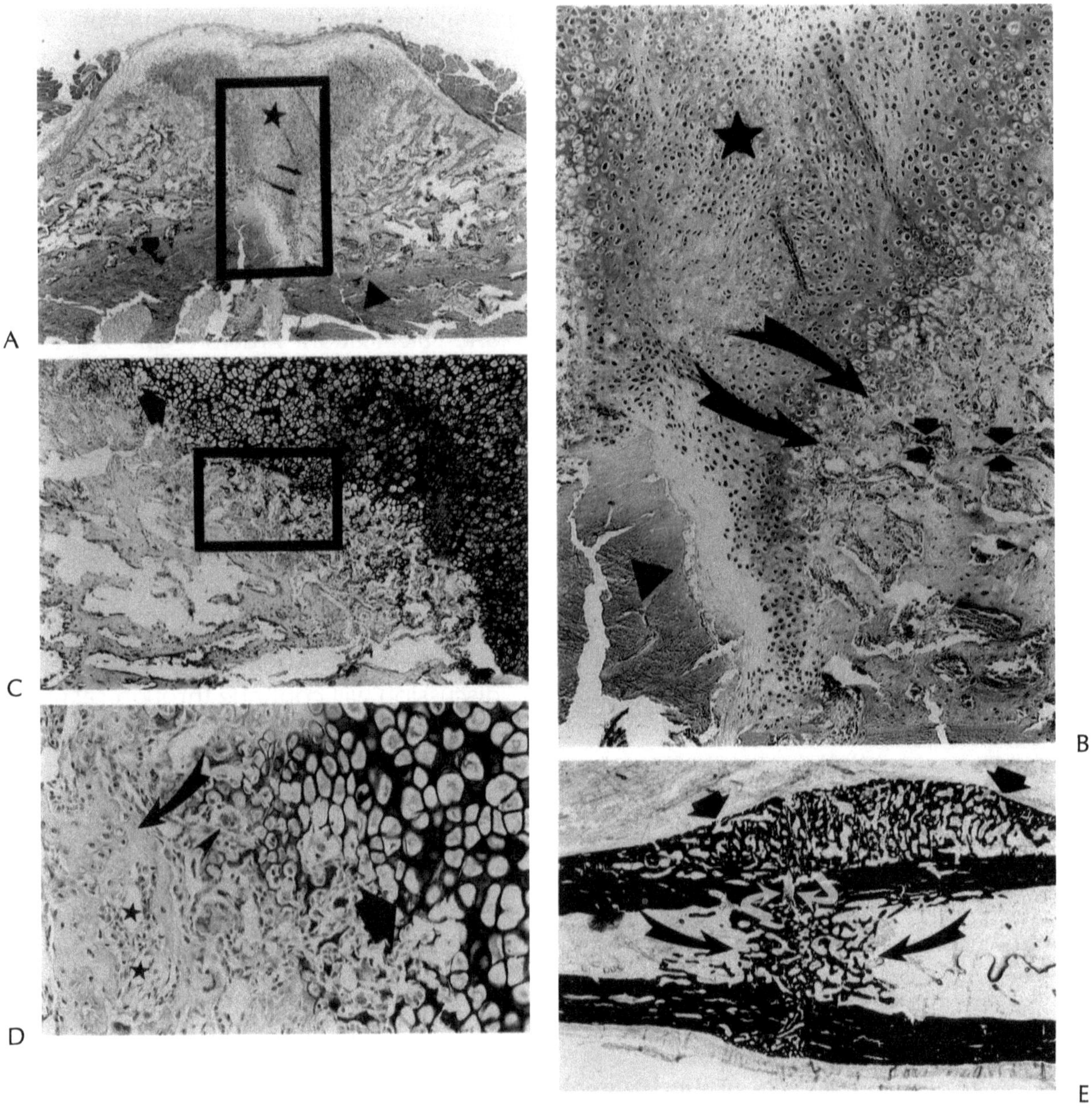

Figure 1.2. (A) Developing "soft" and "hard" callus approximately 14 days postfracture of the cortex (*triangle*) (rat tibia). The periosteal callus contains zones of cartilage (*star*) and woven bone (*arrow*). (Hematoxylin eosin stain; original magnification, ×1.25) (B) Higher magnification of section (A) with zone of cartilage (*star*), woven bone (*curved arrow*), and segment of fractured cortex (*triangle*). Between the small arrows are blood vessels found in areas of woven bone (hematoxylin and eosin stain; original magnification, ×5). (C) Callus approximately day 17 with heavily calcifying cartilage (*arrow*), darkly stained (uppermiddle right) and just inferior, woven bone (von Kossa stain; original magnification, ×1.25). (D) Higher magnification of section (C), with calcifying extracellular matrix of cartilage (*large arrow*), woven bone (*curved arrow*), new blood vessels (*star*), and multinucleated giant cell (osteoclast) (*arrow head*) (von Kossa stain; original magnification ×5). (E) Approximately 25 days postfracture, the periosteal callus is primarily woven bone (*large arrow*). Continuity gap in the cortex is present (*white curved arrows*), and the endosteal woven bone is evident (*curved black arrows*), (von Kossa stain; original magnification, ×1.25).

(42). (Undifferentiated mesenchymal stem cells may be inducible osteoprogenitors that become osteoblasts when exposed to bone morphogenetic protein (BMP), a subfamily of the TGF-β group.) The osteoprogenitor cells appear as early as the third day after fracture (43). A larger bank of committed osteoprogenitor cells probably exists in intramembranous bone than in endochondral bone, permitting intramembranous structures to progress directly from wounding to osseous consolidation without cartilage and callus.

At least 12 distinct BMPs have been reported (44–47). Furthermore, several BMP-like molecules known as growth/differentiation factors (GDFs) have been identified (46,48). GDF-5 (referred to as cartilage-derived morphogenetic protein-1, CDMP-1) is expressed during initial skeletal development and GDF-6 (CDMP-2) has been identified in later stages of skeletal embryogenesis (49). Additional molecules that have close genetic sequence identity to the BMPs include dpp (ie, the Drosophila gene, decapentaplegic), drosophila 60A, vegetal pole-derived gene, and the inhibins (inhibin-α, βA, βB, and Mullerian inhibiting substance) (50,51). Besides a unique osteoinductive capacity (52), the BMPs and BMP-like molecules have broad morphogenetic responsibilities. A morphogen is a substance that generates a unique developmental pattern expression, the effect being concentration gradient specific (53). Overall, BMPs are involved with proliferation, differentiation, and pattern formation of the developing limbs and teeth (5), and are expressed in such diverse tissues as the hair follicles, heart, kidney, oocytes, and central nervous system (54,55).

Specific functional roles for BMPs during fracture healing and continuity defect regeneration must be explored to harness their therapeutic potential. Currently, relatively little is known about the regulation of BMP expression in chondro-osteoblastic cells. Information about the BMPs is becoming gradually available. For example, Nakase and associates detected messenger RNA for BMP-4 between 12 to 72 hours after fracture (prior to cartilage and bone formation) (56). They determined that BMP-4 was produced by less-differentiated osteoprogenitor cells and not by differentiated osteoblasts. The authors concluded that BMP-4 is expressed prior to callus formation and, therefore, is one of the local modulators of early fracture healing. In addition to BMP-4, BMP-6 has been detected during early fracture healing (57).

It is increasingly evident that a suite of BMPs is operational during embryogenesis, limb formation, and bone regeneration (48,58–60). While the complex instructional outline for BMPs has not been elucidated, evidence supports their critical positions in morphodifferentiation. For example, BMP-2 induces differentiation of stem cells into osteoblasts; BMPs 3 and 4 may be involved with chondrogenesis; and BMP-7 induces formation of chondrogenic and osteogenic phenotypes from newborn rat calvaria (61).

In addition to BMPs, other fracture repair regulators have been identified (18,62). However, only a limited number offer immediate promise as therapeutics for bone healing, and they will be the focus for this chapter.

The bounty of literature derived from in vitro studies describing the effects of growth factors is intimidating and often contradictory. The curiously mercurial behavior of regulatory factors is evident in some in vivo reports (63,64). Moreover, the physiologic, mechanistic interactions among growth factors, resident cells, and the extracellular matrix are, in large part, still a mystery. Therefore, it is a challenge to define clearly mechanistic regulatory roles for growth factors. However, in controlled animal studies focusing on bone, compelling evidence validates their potential clinical benefits. Consequently, we have selected key preclinical studies to serve as references.

The therapeutic applications of recombinant human growth factors for restoring bone in several species have been completed, and for the BMPs these include: rat calvaria (65–67), rabbit ulna (68), rabbit radius (69), sheep long bone (70), mandibles in dogs (71), alveolar clefts (72) and long bone in dogs (73), and long bone in nonhuman primates (74). In the preclinical studies cited, recombinant human BMP-2 and 7 promoted regeneration of ablated segments of bone that ordinarily would not have healed by new bone formation. (These defects are called *critical-sized defects* [75,76].)

When TGF-β was injected onto and into the periosteum of intact bone, the responses were related to the dose and duration of application: A high dose promoted cartilage, and a low dose promoted bone formation (77–79). Bone formation abated and preapplication osseous contour returned when repetitive dosing was discontinued. A single administration of TGF-β to intraosseous wounds in rabbits' (80,81) and rats' (82) calvaria led to bone formation. In distinction to BMPs (exclusive of BMP-1), TGF-β is not osteoinductive (46,83,84). BMPs (eg, BMP-2, BMP-7) will induce heterotopic bone formation: conversion of mesenchymal stem cells within muscle to cells capable of producing bone and hematopoietic tissue (85). Growth factors such as TGF-β, PDGF, and insulin-like growth factors (IGF-I and II), either alone or combinatorially, may augment the bone healing cascade. For example, the activity of combinations of TGF-β_1 and FGF was enhanced in a dose-dependent manner by IGF-I in chondrocyte chick growth plate monolayers (86). These findings indicate IGF-I may function in chondrocyte mitogenesis and growth of long bones. This is significant in that activities at the healing fracture callus and during endochondral bone repair are homologous to the cartilaginous growth plate. Moreover, recent work has shown that IGF-I may substitute as a growth hormone to promote linear growth in children with growth hormone insensitivity (87). A study by O'Keefe and associates suggests that IGF-I might be a modulator for other bone growth factors (86).

Basic FGF is a potent chemoattractant and mitogen (88) found in endothelial cells that promotes new vessel formation (26). It is a mitogen for chondrocytes and a key regulator in their terminal differentiation at the growth plate (89). The duality of contradictory activities seems peculiar in that vascular invasion of cartilage portends death: calcification, removal, and replacement by bone. More work is needed to understand FGF's activities in fracture repair, cartilage formation and removal, and vascularity development.

Preliminary success with PDGF isoforms (BB, AA homodimers; AB heterodimer) for soft tissue repair (90,91) prompted study for applications to bone healing (63). Alveolar bone regeneration of periodontal lesions has been reported with PDGF combined with IGF-I in Beagle dogs (92,93), nonhuman primates (94), and in human patients (95). However, PDGF in combination with highly purified, native osteogenin (BMP-3) significantly reduced bone formation in calvarial critical-sized defects in rats (67). The authors suggested that the decrement in bone formation may have been due to receptor downregulation by PDGF, thereby abrogating cell-induced differentiation by BMP-3. Receptor interactions between PDGF and IGF-I at alveolar bone sites may have promoted a different sequence of cellular responses, thus stimulating bone regeneration.

There are many additional molecular modulators in bone aside from the growth factors that have been mentioned (18). The selection of factors to be discussed was based on preclinical data that appear to indicate potential therapeutic appeal. The reader of this review should not dismiss the notion that new preclinical data will become available, elucidating key roles for other biochemical modulators for fracture healing.

Over the approximately eight weeks required for fracture repair, biochemical mediators, cells, and biofunctionality restore the osseous unit and sculpt bone into a shape reminiscent of the prefractured form. The isotropic (ie, randomly oriented) trabecular pattern of immature bone, referred to as woven bone, will be transformed into lamellar bone. Biofunctional challenges and vascularity impact by centralizing lamellar architecture to an osteonal (haversian) format spatially oriented to respond to loading. The dynamic process to restore prefractured contour includes discrete events: cell activation, bone resorption, bone formation, cell quiescence, and apoptosis. Coupling of these events ensures restoration of osseous form and, therefore, function, and is the final phase of fracture healing known as remodeling (96).

REMODELING

The general concepts concerning remodeling have been organized in the classic works by Frost (97,98) that have been modified by others. Based on Frost's initiatives, investigators have shown that bone remodeling includes cellular activities and biomechanical events that restore form to damaged bone. Restorative events to maintain bone homeostasis in the mature individual (ie, skeletal maturity, meaning after closure of the epiphyseal plates) are known as remodeling. Remodeling has been confused with *modeling*. The latter process may be viewed as the events shaping maturing bone until epiphyseal plate closure.

Bone fracture repair requires remodeling of cortical and cancellous components, and each undergoes similar and dissimilar dynamic steps (99). Cortical bone remodeling (Figure 1.3) is accomplished by the basic multicellular unit (BMU): synchronized teams of osteoclasts and osteoblasts. The osteoclast cutting cone of the BMU burrows through cortical

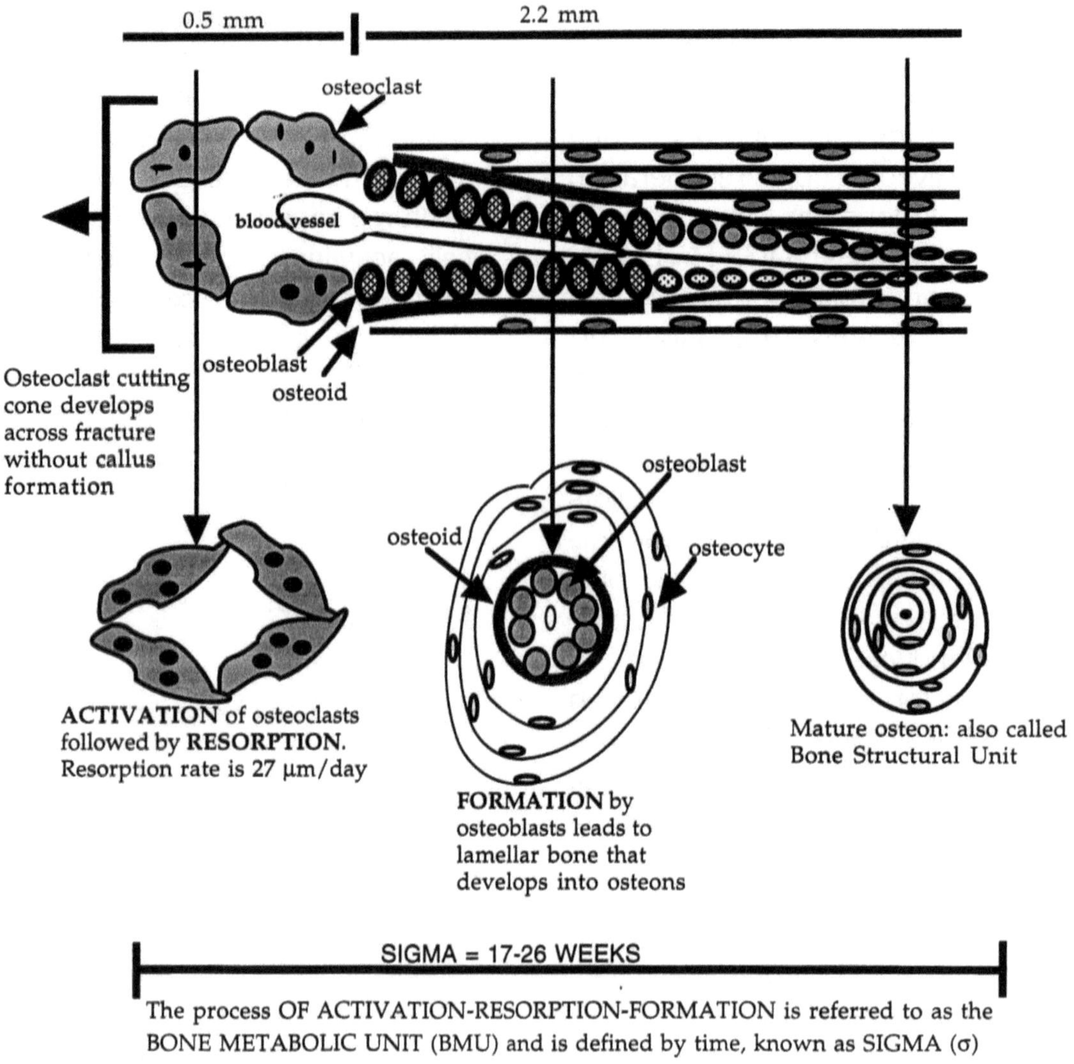

Figure 1.3. The cutting cone: remodeling in the cortical bone of humans.

plate. The burrows are filled sequentially with connective tissue, blood vessels, nerves, and new bone. A new osteon is restored, linking fractured cortical segments. Cancellous bone remodeling involves BMUs that form surface troughs, and contiguous, parallel troughs can develop, consuming bony spicules. In addition, adjacent spicules within the callus milieu may become surface-modified by advancing BMUs, and they condense through osteoblast-mediated bone matrix deposition.

The contemporary remodeling schema detailed for cortical bone has not been based on the fracture model, but rather, on a homeostatic paradigm (99,100). For this paradigm, Frost coined the term *intermediary organization* (ie, IO) to embrace the functional aspects of remodeling; he has postulated fracture healing to be a component of the IO

(97,98). However, cortical remodeling during fracture repair has not been detailed satisfactorily. Furthermore, there are insufficient data chronicling the remodeling dynamics for cancellous bone. These areas are relevant to clinical intervention with therapeutics in order to augment recalcitrant fracture healing for patients.

As noted briefly above, restoring contour to fractured bone involves callus consolidation—the osseous callus component is trabecular spicules of cancellous bone. Cancellous remodeling under the aegis of the BMU includes packets of surface eroding osteoclasts and packets of surface eroding osteoclasts functioning concurrently with osteoblastic deposition, thus leading to coalescence of osseous architecture. The molecular signaling to coordinate simultaneous activities between osteoclasts and osteoblasts and between packets of teams of these cells has not been elucidated. The term *coupling* has been proposed to emphasize the interrelationship between osteoblastic and osteoclastic activities. Communication links for coupling events are cell products, that is, growth factors and cytokines, functioning through hormonal, paracrine, and autocrine modes that enable cells to manage their local environment during remodeling. Moreover, it is hypothesized that an additional cell regulatory control is invoked by stress-strain transductive mechanisms across cells, and, by modifying cell shape, they may act as morphogenetic switches to control phenotype expression (101). The cells are the ultimate microcraftsmen chiseling and building fracture architecture to the prefracture contour; therefore, a few comments are warranted about these remodeling masters.

Osteoblast ontogeny and expression products were described earlier in this review. Osteoblast activity produces the osseous struts to stabilize and buttress structurally inadequate bone to withstand functional challenges; however, the outcome of this effort is the production of an overabundance of bone: the callus. Consequently, the excess structure must be honed to an appropriate contour. Osteoclasts provide that functional role.

Osteoclasts are believed to originate from circulating mononuclear precursor cells resident in the vasculature. Molecular signals, perhaps from osteoblasts and mesenchymal cells populating the healing callus (eg, macrophages), prompt a homing-in of mononuclear osteoclast precursor cells. For example, osteoblasts respond to parathyroid hormone by moving from their attachment site, leaving the site exposed. Following this type of motility, it is speculated that osteoblasts express a factor or factors and stimulate preosteoclast-like cell attachment to the exposed bone surface. Either prior to attachment of the mononuclear cells or following attachment, poikilocarynosis yields the classically appearing multinucleated giant cell: the osteoclast.

The short residence time and high turnover of osteoclasts (approximately 16 days life expectancy) attest to the dispatch with which osteoclasts perform their role (102). Sustenance of osteoclastic resorption in light of the high turnover rate of these cells must likely be accomplished by autocrine-paracrine loops to recruit new precursor cells and enhance the activity of the osteoclasts. Two regulatory molecules that may be candidates for these functions are interleukin-6 and annexin-II. In human bone marrow cultures, it has been demonstrated that interleukin-6 and annexin-II increase osteoclast quantity and expression products (103,104).

It has not been proven what cue (or cues) instructs termination of osteoclast activity. It may be speculated that, when "extra bony spicules" of the callus are removed by the osteoclasts, subtle biomechanical alterations due to structural modification of the substratum prompt activity to cease and attachment abandonment, followed by apoptosis (ie, cell death). (An osteocyte-mediated homeostatic mechanism associated with mechano-sensory transduction has been proposed that is similar in concept to the above noted osteoclast paradigm [105].) It has been shown in vitro that osteoclast apoptosis is promoted by TGF-β (106). Perhaps, osteoclast activity terminates with an increase in local TGF-β concentration as it is released from the osteoclast-eroding matrix. Moreover, additional modulation of osteoclastic-osteoblastic functional activities during fracture callus remodeling may be coordinated through IGF-I. A model proposed for this coordination suggests that IGFs are released from bone during resorption, and, functioning as chemoattractants and mitogens, they increase the number and activity of preosteoblasts and osteoblasts (107). The latter elaborate bone matrix among contiguous spicules causing condensation, consolidation, and restoration of the osseous unit.

The traditional approach to describe fracture repair by chronicling discrete morphological events is no longer satisfactory by itself. In light of the remarkable progress in the cloning and expressing of human factors, it is prudent to detail the temporal and spatial expression of molecular regulators trafficking among cells during the fracture remodeling continuum. This accomplishment will facilitate therapeutic intervention with recombinantly engineered molecules such as the BMPs.

There is ample opportunity for investigations to explore the myriad of factors operational during fracture remodeling, cell "cross-talk," and the "on" and "off" switches for cell activation, activity abatement, senescence, and apoptosis. These areas represent an expanse with many unknowns. They are critical areas for applied research leading to clinical therapies.

References

1. Hollinger JO, Wong MEK. The integrated processes of hard tissue regeneration with special emphasis on fracture healing. *Oral Surg, Oral Med, Oral Path, Oral Radiol* 82:594–606, 1996.
2. Herndon DN, Nguyen TT, Gilpin DA. Growth factors, Local and Systemic. *Arch Surg* 128:1227–1233, 1993.
3. Riddle RD, Johnson R, Laufer E et al. Sonic hedgehog mediates the polarizing activity of the ZPA. *Cell* 75:1401–1416, 1993.
4. Robinson CJ. Growth factors: therapeutic advances in wound healing. *Ann Med* 25:535–538, 1993.
5. Kaplan FS, Shore EM. Bone morphogenetic proteins and c-fos: early signals in endchondral bone formation. *Bone* 19 Supp:13s–21s, 1996.
6. Robertson SA, Seamark RF, Guilbert LJ et al. The role of cytokins in gestation. *Crit Rev Immunol* 14:239–292, 1994.
7. Takaku F. Clinical applications of cytokines for cancer treatment. *Oncology* 51:123–128, 1994.

8. Sato N, Miyajima A. Multimeric cytokine receptors: common versus specific functions. *Curr Opin Cell Biol* 6:174–184, 1994.
9. Enneking WF, Burchardt H, Fume JJ et al. Physical and biological aspects of repair in dog cortical-bone transplants. *J Bone Joint Surg* 57-A:237–252, 1975.
10. Burchardt H, Glowczewskie BS, Enneking WF. Allogeneic segmental fibular transplants in azathioprine-immunosuppressed dogs. *J Bone Joint Surg* 59-A:881–893, 1977.
11. Burchardt H, Enneking WF. Transplantation of bone. Surg Clin North Am 58:403–427, 1978.
12. Burchardt H. The biology of bone graft repair. *Clin Orthop* 174:28–42, 1983.
13. Simmons DJ. Fracture healing perspectives. *Clin Orthop* 200:100–113, 1985.
14. Hauschka PV, Mavrakos AE, Iafrati MD et al. Growth factors in bone matrix. Isolation of multiple types with affinity chromatography and heparin sepharose. *J Biol Chem* 261:12665–12674, 1986.
15. Albrektsson T, Albrektsson B. Osseointegration of bone implants. A review of an alternative mode of fixation. *Acta Orthop Scand* 58:567–577, 1987.
16. Burchardt H. Biology of bone transplantation. *Orthop Clin North Am* 18:187–196, 1987.
17. Goldberg VM, Stevenson S. Natural history of autografts and allografts. *Clin Orthop* 225:7–16, 1987.
18. Hauschka PV. Growth factor effects in bone. In: Hall BK, ed. *The Osteoblast and Osteocyte*. Telfor Press; 1990:103–170.
19. Enneking WF, Mindell ER. Observations on massive retrieved human allografts. *J Bone Joint Surg* 73-A:1123–1142, 1991.
20. Stevenson S, Li XQ, Martin B. The fate of cancellous and cortical bone after transplantation of fresh and frozen tissue antigen-matched and mismatched osteochondral allografts in dogs. *J Bone Joint Surg* 73-A: 1143–1156, 1991.
21. Bolander ME. Regulation of fracture repair by growth factors. *Proc Soc Exp Biol Med* 200:165–170, 1992.
22. Pierce GF. Macrophages: Important physiologic and pathologic sources of polypeptide growth factors. *Am J Respir Cell Mol Biol* 2:233–234, 1992.
23. Pierce GF, Mustoe TA, Altrock BW et al. Role of platelet-derived growth factor in wound healing. *J Cell Biochem* 45:319–326, 1991.
24. Massagué J. The transforming growth factor-beta family. *Annu Rev Cell Biol* 6:597–641, 1990.
25. Centrella M, McCarthy TL, Canalis E. Current concepts review. Transforming growth factor beta and remodeling of bone. *J Bone Joint Surg* 73-A:1418–1428, 1991.
26. Davidson J, Buckley A, Woodward S et al. Mechanisms of accelerated wound repair using epidermal growth factor and basic fibroblast growth factor. In: Barbul A, Pines E, Caldwell M, Hunt T, eds. *Growth Factors and Other Aspects of Wound Healing. Biological and Clinical Implications. Proceedings of the Second International Symposium on Tissue Repair, Tarpon Springs, Florida, May 13–17, 1987*. New York: Alan R. Liss; 1988:63–75.
27. Oursler MJ. Osteoclast synthesis and secretion and activation of latent transforming growth factor beta. *J Bone Miner Res* 9:443–452, 1994.
28. Baylink D, Finkelman RD, Mohan S. Growth factors to stimulate bone formation. *J Bone Miner Res* 8:565–572, 1993.
29. Mundy GR. Cytokines and growth factors in the regulation of bone remodeling. *J Bone Miner Res* 8:505–510, 1993.
30. Pan WT, Einhorn TA. The biochemistry of fracture healing. *Curr Orthop* 6:207–213, 1992.
31. Paralkar VM, Nandedkar AKN, Pointer RH et al. Interaction of osteogenin, a heparin binding bone morphogenetic protein, with type IV collagen. *J Biol Chem* 265:17281–17284, 1990.
32. Paralkar VM, Vukicevic S, Reddi AH. Transforming growth factor β type I binds to collagen IV of basement membrane matrix: Implications for development. *Dev Biol* 143:303–308, 1991.

33. Raghow R. The role of extracellualr matrix in postinflammatory wound healing and fibrosis. *FASEB J* 8:823–831, 1994.

34. Ingber DE, Deepa P, Sun Z et al. Cell shape, cytoskeletal mechanics, and cell cycle control in angiogenesis. *J Biomech* 28:1471–1484, 1995.

35. Reddi AH. Regulation of bone differentiation by local and systemic factors. In: Peck WA, ed. *Bone and Mineral Research/3*. Amsterdam: Elsevier Science; 1985:27–47.

36. Reddi AH. Bone and cartilage morphogenesis: Cell biology to clinical applications. *Curr Opin Gen Dev* 4:737–744, 1994.

37. Spiessl B. New concepts in maxillofacial bone surgery. In: Spiessl B, ed. *New Concepts in Maxillofacial Bone Surgery*. Berlin: Springer-Verlag; 1976:1–179.

38. Friedenstein AJ. Determined and inducible osteogenic precursor cells. In: *Hard Tissue Growth, Repair, and Remineralization. Ciba Foundation, Symposium 11*. Amsterdam: Associated Scientific; 1973: 169–185.

39. Owen M. Lineage of osteogenic cells and their relationship to the stromal system. In: Peck W, ed. *Lineage of Osteogenic Cells and Their Relationship to the Stromal System*. Amsterdam: Elsevier Science; 1985:1–25.

40. Brighton CT, Lorich DG, Kupcha R et al. The pericyte as a possible osteoblast progenitor cell. *Clin Orthop* 275:287–299, 1992.

41. Owen M. The origin of bone cells in the postnatal organism. *Arthritis Rheum* 23: 1073–1080, 1980.

42. Wakitani S, Tatsuhiko G, Pineda SJ et al. Mesenchymal cell-based repair of large, full-thickness defects of articular cartilage. *J Bone Joint Surg* 76A:579–592, 1994.

43. Brighton CT, Hunt RM. Early histological and ultrastructural changes in medullary fracture callus. *J Bone Joint Surg* 73-A:832–847, 1991.

44. Wozney JM. The bone morphogenetic protein family and osteogenesis. *Mol Reprod Dev* 32:160–167, 1992.

45. Celeste AJ, Song JJ, Cox K et al. Bone morphogenetic protein-9, a new member of the TGF-β superfamily. *J Bone Miner Res* 9:S137, 1994.

46. Kingsley DM. The TGF-beta superfamily: New members, new receptors, and new genetic tests of function in different organisms. *Genes Dev* 8:133–146, 1994.

47. Nguyen AM, Tran M, Oates T et al. Mitogenic responses of human PDL cells to tissue growth factors. *J Dent Res* 74:251, 1995.

48. Storm EE, Huynh TV, Copeland NG et al. Limb alterations in brachypodism mice due to mutations in a new member of the TGF-beta superfamily. *Nature* 368:639–643, 1994.

49. Chang SC, Hoang B, Thomas JT et al. Cartilage-derived morphogenetic proteins. *J Biol Chem* 269:28227–28234, 1994.

50. Einhorn TA. Enhancement of fracture healing by molecular or physical means: An overview. In: Brighton CT, Freidlander GE, Lane JM, eds. *Bone Formation and Repair*. Rosemont, IL: AAOS; 1994:223–238.

51. Ishidou Y, Kitajima I, Obama H et al. Enhanced expression of type I receptors for bone morphogenetic proteins during bone formation. *J Bone Miner Res* 10:1651–1659, 1995.

52. Urist MR. The search for and discovery of bone morphogenetic protein. In: Urist MR, O'Conner BT, Burwell RG, eds. *Bone Grafts, Derivatives and Substitutes*. London: Butterworth; 1994:315–362.

53. Wolpert L. Positional information revisited. *Development* 107:3–12, 1989.

54. Elima K. Osteoinductive proteins. *Ann Med* 25:395–402, 1993.

55. Harris SE, Harris MA, Mahy P et al. Expression of bone morphogenetic protein messenger RNAs by normal rat and human prostate and prostate cancer cells. *Prostate* 24:204–211, 1994.

56. Nakase T, Nomura S, Yoshikawa H et al. Transient and localized expression of bone morphogenetic protein 4 messenger RNA during fracture healing. *J Bone Miner Res* 9:651–659, 1994.

57. Bostrom MG, Lane J, Berberian WS et al. Immunolocalization and expression of bone morphogenetic proteins 2 and 4 in

fracture healing. *J Orthop Res* 13:357–367, 1995.

58. Duboule D. How to make a limb? *Science* 266:575–576, 1994.
59. Laufer E, Nelson CE, Johnson RL et al. Sonic hedgehog and Fgf-4 act through a signaling cascade and feedback loop to integrate growth and patterning of the developing limb bud. *Cell* 79:993–1003, 1994.
60. Tickle C. On making a skeleton. *Nature* 368:587–588, 1994.
61. Carey D, Liu X. Expression of bone morphogenetic protein-6 messenger RNA in bovine gowth plate chondrocytes of different size. *J Bone Miner Res* 10:401–405, 1995.
62. Hollinger JO. Factors for osseous repair and delivery: Part 1. *J Craniofac Surg* 4:115–121, 1993.
63. Goodkin DA, Pierce GF. The role platelet-derived growth factor in osteoblast function and bone synthesis: Conflicting evidence. *Wound Rep Regen* 1:203–212, 1993.
64. Pierce GF, Mustoe TA. Pharmacologic enhancement of wound healing. *Annu Rev Med* 46:467–481, 1995.
65. Kenley R, Yim K, Abrams J et al. Biotechnology and bone graft substitutes. *Pharm Res* 10:1393–1401, 1993.
66. Kenley R, Marden L, Turek T et al. Osseous regeneration in the rat calvarium using novel delivery systems for recombinant human bone morphogenetic protein-2 (rhBMP-2). *J Biomed Mater Res* 28:1139–1147, 1994.
67. Marden LJ, Hollinger JO, Chaudhari A. et al. Recombinant bone morphogenetic protein-2 is superior to demineralized bone matrix in repairing craniotomies defects in rat. *J Biomed Mater Res* 28:1127–1138, 1994.
68. Cook SD, Baffes GC, Wolfe MW et al. The effect of human recombinant osteogenic protein-1 on healing of large segmental bone defects. *J Bone Joint Surg* 76A:827–838, 1994.
69. Zegzula HD, Hollinger JO, Brekke J et al. Bone formation with use of rh BMP-2 (Recombinant Human Bone Morphogenetic Protein-2). *J Bone Joint Surg* 79-A:1778–1790, 1997.
70. Gerhart TN, Kirker-Head CA, Kriz MJ et al. Healing segmental femoral defects in sheep using recombinant human bone morphogenetic protein (rhBMP-2). *Clin Orthop* 293:317–326, 1993.
71. Toriumi DM, Kotler HS, Luxunberg DP et al. Mandibular reconstruction with a recombinant bone-inducing factor. Functional, histologic, and biomechanical evaluation. *Arch Otolaryngol Head Neck Surg* 117:1101–1112, 1991.
72. Mayer MH, Hollinger JO, Ron E et al. Repair of alveolar clefts in dogs with recombinant bone morphogenetic protein and poly (α-hydroxy acid). *Plastic Reconstr Surg* 98:247–259, 1996.
73. Cook SD, Baffes GC, Wolfe MW et al. Recombinant human bone morphogentic protein-7 induces healing in a canine long-bone segmental defect model. *Clin Orthop* 301:302–312, 1994.
74. Cook SD, Wolfe MW, Salkeld SL et al. Effect of recombinant human osteogenic protein-1 on healing of segmental defects in non-human primates. *J Bone Joint Surg* 77-A: 734–750, 1995.
75. Schmitz JP, Hollinger JO. The critical sized defect as an experimental model for craniomandibulofacial nonunions. *Clin Orthop* 205:299–308, 1986.
76. Hollinger JO, Kleinschmidt J. The critical size defect as an experimental model to test bone repair materials. *J Craniofac Surg* 1:60–68, 1990.
77. Noda M, Camilliere JJ. In vivo stimulation of bone formation by transforming growth factor-β. *Endocrinology* 124:2991–2994, 1989.
78. Joyce ME, Roberts AB, Sporn MB et al. Transforming growth factor-beta and the initiation of chondrogenesis and osteogenesis in the rat femur. *J Cell Biol* 110:2195–2207, 1990.
79. Tanaka T, Taniguchi Y, Gotoh K et al. Morphological study of recombinant human transforming growth factor β1-induced intramembranous ossification in neonatal rat parietal bone. *Bone* 14:117–123, 1993.

80. Beck LS, Deguzman L, Lee WP et al. TGF-β1 induces bone closure of skull defects. *J Bone Miner Res* 6:1257–1265, 1991.

81. Beck LS, Ammann AJ, Aufdemorte TB et al. In vivo induction of bone by recombinant human transforming growth factor beta 1. *J Bone Miner Res* 6:961–968, 1991.

82. Gombotz WR, Pankey SC, Bouchard LS et al. Stimulation of bone healing by transforming growth factor beta-1 released from polymeric or ceramic implants. *J Appl Biomater* 5:141–150, 1994.

83. Wozney JM, Rosen V, Byrne M et al. Growth factors influencing bone development. *J Cell Sci Suppl* 13:149–156, 1990.

84. Kingsley D. What do BMPs do in mammals? Clues from the mouse short-ear mutation. *Trends Genet* 10:16–21, 1994.

85. Urist MR. Bone: Formation by autoinduction. *Science* 150:893–899, 1965.

86. O'Keefe RJ, Crabb ID, Puzas JE et al. Effects of transforming growth factor beta-a and fibroblast growth factor on DNA synthesis in growth plate chondrocytes are enhanced by insulin-like growth factor-I. *J Orthop Res* 12:299–310, 1994.

87. Bondy C. Clinical uses of insulin-like growth factor I. *Ann Intern Med* 120:593–601, 1994.

88. Klagsbrun M, Vlodavsky I. Biosynthesis and storage of basic fibroblast growth factor (BFGF) by endothelial cells: implication for the mechanism of angiogenesis. In: Barbul A, Pines E, Caldwell M, Hunt T, eds. *Growth Factors and Other Aspects of Wound Healing. Biological and Clinical Implications. Proceedings of the Second International Symposium on Tissue Repair, Tarpon Springs, Florida, May 13–17, 1987.* New York: Alan R Liss; 1988:55–61.

89. Chintala SK, Miller RR, McDevitt CA. Basic fibroblast growth factor binds to heparin sulfate in the extracellular matrix of rat growth plate chondrocytes. *Arch Biochem Biophys* 310:180–186, 1994.

90. Mustoe TA, Pierce GF, Morishima C et al. Growth factor-induced acceleration of tissue repair through direct and inductive activities in a rabbit dermal ulcer model. *J Clin Invest* 87:694–703, 1991.

91. Pierce G, Tarpley J, Yanagihara D et al. Platelet-derived growth factor (BB homodimer), transforming growth factor-β, and basic fibroblast growth factor in dermal wound healing. *Am J Pathol* 140:1375–1388, 1992.

92. Lynch SE, Ruiz G, Williams RC et al. The effects of short-term application of a combination of platelet-derived growth factor and insulin-like growth factors on periodontal wound healing. *J Periodontol* 62:458–467, 1991.

93. Giannobile WV. Periodontal tissue engineering by growth factors. *Bone* 19 Supp:23s–37s, 1996.

94. Giannobile WV, Finkelman RD, Lynch SE. Comparison of canine and non-human primate animal models for periodontal regenerative therapy: Results following a single administration of PDGF/IGF-I. *J Periodontol* 65:1158–1168, 1994.

95. Howell TH, Fiorellini JP, Paquette DW et al. Evaluation of a combination of recombinant human platelet-derived growth factor-BB and recombinant human insulin-like growth factor-I in patients with periodontal disease. *J Dent Res* 74:253, 1995.

96. Parfitt MA. The cellular basis of bone remodeling: The quantum concept reexamined in light of recent advances in the cell biology of bone. *Calcif Tissue Int* 36:37–45, 1984.

97. Frost HM. *Intermediary Organization of the Skeleton*. Vol. I. Boca Raton, FL: CRC Press; 1986.

98. Frost HM. *Intermediary Organization of the Skeleton*. Vol. II. Boca Raton, FL: CRC Press; 1986.

99. Parfitt AM, Roodman GD, Hughes DE et al. A new model for the regulation of bone resorption, with particular reference to the effects of bisphosphonates. *J Bone Miner Res* 11:150–159, 1996.

100. Parfitt AM. Osteonal and hemi-osteonal remodeling: The spatial and temporal framework for signal traffic in adult human bone. *J Cell Biochem* 55:273–286, 1994.

101. Bussey H. Cell shape determination: A pivotal role for Rho. *Science* 272:224–225, 1996.

102. Heersche JN. Bone cells and bone turnover—the basis for pathogenesis. In: Tam CS, Heersche JN, Murray TM, eds. *Metabolic Bone Disease: Cellular and Tissue Mechanisms*. Boca Raton: CRC Press; 1989:1–17.

103. Roodman GD, Kurihara N, Ohashi Y et al. Interleukin-6: A potential autocrine/paracrine factor in Paget's dieseas of bone. *J Clin Invest* 89:46–52, 1992.

104. Takahashi S, Reddy SV, Chirgwin JM et al. Cloning and identification of annexin II as an autocrine/paracrine factor that increases osteoclast formation and bone resorption. *J Biol Chem* 269:28696–28701, 1994.

105. Kimmel D. A paradigm for skeletal strength homeostasis. *J Bone Joint Miner Res* 8: 515–522, 1993.

106. Hughes DE, Wright KR, Mundy GR et al. TGF-beta 1 induces osteoclast apoptosis *in vitro*. *J Bone Miner Res* 9:S138, 1994.

107. Linkhart TA, Mohan S, Baylink DJ. Growth factors for bone growth and repair: IGF, TGF beta, and BMP. *Bone* 19 Supp:1s–12s, 1996.

CHAPTER 2

BIOMECHANICS OF DISTRACTION

Hannu Aro

Distraction osteogenesis presents a unique form of clinical tissue engineering (Table 2.1). Using easily controlled mechanical conditions (ie, slow gradual distraction of the corticotomized or osteotomized bone fragments), a clinician is able to guide the formation of new bone and its spatial orientation to form a structural part of the distracted bone. This happens without application of any growth factor or other controlling agents. There is no question about the biologic feasibility of the distraction method in promotion of human bone regeneration. The technique also works during gradual transportation of a bone segment.

The critical factors of the process appear to be the stability of fixation, the rate of daily distraction, and the preservation of the local soft-tissue envelope and vascular supply (1,2). The mechanical window for distraction osteogenesis seems to be fairly wide. In fact, the primary target of the applied tensile stress may be not only the osteoblasts but also the endothelial cells in the induction of angiogenesis. The angiogenic mechanism of action would explain the reported efficiency of the distraction treatment both in infected (3,4) and irradiated bones (5).

The distraction techniques are demanding and time consuming but relatively reliable in achieving the original goals of surgery (6,7). Bone healing problems are not infrequent, but they usually respond to modification of the treatment strategy. Biomechanical and surgical principles are important since delayed consolidation not uncommonly reflects technical errors such as an overly traumatic corticotomy, an initial diastasis, instability (lack of fixation), or overly rapid distraction.

The distraction technique was originally applied in limb-lengthening procedures and in salvage of congenital, posttraumatic, or other acquired limb deformities. In these procedures, the muscle has proved to be the single largest limiting factor (6). For anatomical reasons, selected craniofacial reconstruction may be the most amenable to application of the distraction techniques. The main disadvantages of gradual mechanical distraction

Table 2.1. Biomechanical steps in the clinical application of distraction osteogenesis.

- Detailed preoperative planning, including determination of precise correction of angular deformities
- Selection of an appropriate distraction device with known stiffness properties under different loading conditions
- Selection of pins of optimal design and diameter
- Creation of an atraumatic bone discontinuity (corticotomy) at an optimal site
- Careful creation of a pin-bone interface and subsequent prevention of pin loosening
- Construction of a stable external fixation configuration, followed by regular tightening of the critical components
- Selection of a rate and rhythm of the distraction matched with the biologic process of distraction osteogenesis
- Intermittent halt or even reverse motion (compression) in the case of delayed osteogenesis
- Maintenance of the protective fixation after cessation of the distraction, supplemented by dynamization (gradual disassembly of the fixator frame) if necessary
- Inductive bone grafting in selected cases of delayed consolidation
- Removal of the distraction device after sufficient maturation of the distraction new bone (remodeling)
- Protection of the distracted bone from undue stresses during the final remodeling period

Table 2.2. Shortcomings or needs in biomechanical knowledge and methodology for application of distraction osteogenesis.

- Molecular mechanisms of distraction osteogenesis
- Biologic significance of intermittent shear and compressive stresses during distraction osteogenesis
- Optimal fixation stiffnesses (structural properties of the fixation device systems) before, during, and after the distraction period
- Sophisticated devices designed for precise multiplanar distraction
- Advanced methodology for noninvasive imaging and mechanical monitoring of the progress of distraction osteogenesis
- Role of bioactive pin coating in prevention of mechanical pin loosening
- Need for computer-assisted preoperative planning for three-dimensional analysis of multiapical angular deformities

in corrective procedures are those related to external fixation. With careful technique, the risk of external fixation problems can be reduced, but not eliminated.

There remain many unanswered biomechanical questions in distraction osteogenesis (Table 2.2). They range from the molecular mechanisms of distraction osteogenesis to computer-assisted surgery planning, and to better design of distraction devices capable of multiplanar correction of complex deformities.

CLASSIFICATION OF TREATMENT MODALITIES

There are four distraction treatment techniques: (1) pure lengthening procedures; (2) corrective distraction osteotomies; (3) bone segment transportation (transport distraction); and (4) stimulation of growth within a growth plate by distraction in corrective procedures of children. The latter treatment, so-called epiphyseolysis (72), involves the risk of fracture through the growth plate, leading to growth reduction.

In recent clinical reports (8–10), experimental distraction osteogenesis has been applied in the field of craniofacial reconstruction to lengthen the mandible (unifocal corticotomy) (11) and to advance the midface (12,13), to reconstruct a mandibular defect by using transport distraction (bifocal distraction treatment) (14,15), and to perform trifocal distraction treatment in the reconstruction of mandibular symphyseal defect (transportation of two separate bone fragments) (Figure 2.1) (16). Bone transportation involves moving a segment of living bone to fill an intercalary bone defect (3,4,17). The trailing end of the transport bone segment maintains continuity with the host bone surface by distraction of new bone. The leading end of the transport bone segment fuses to the target bone surface by nondistraction osteogenesis with or without the supplemental need of inductive bone graft.

PRIMARY TARGET OF DISTRACTION FORCES

The classic concept of bone formation mechanisms includes the concept that different types of tissue may form or remodel under a specific stress or loading condition (Figure 2.2) (18). Chondrogenic and fibroblastic expression of osteogenic cells is assumed to be the result of an unfavorable mechanical environment that leads to indirect bone formation through a cartilage intermediate (endochondral ossification) or even to fibrous union. Direct intramembranous new bone formation occurring during distraction is considered to be a

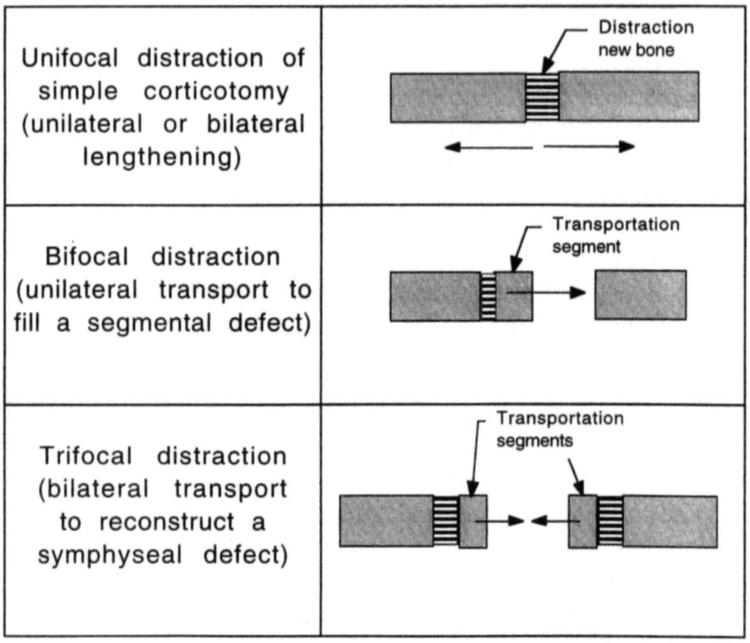

Figure 2.1. Schematic of the three types of distraction osteogenesis in mandibular reconstruction.

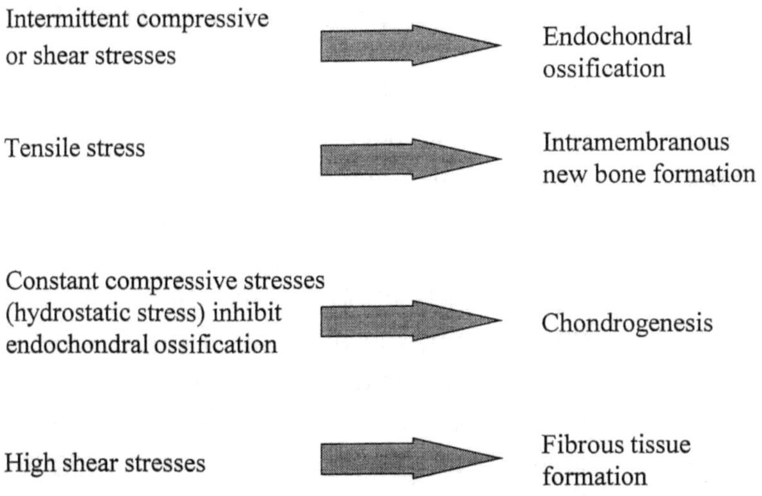

Figure 2.2. Hypothetical mechanisms involved between mechanical stresses and connective tissue formation.

response of osteogenic cells to the applied tensile stress.

The characteristics of distraction osteogenesis have been studied in detail both at the cellular (1,20) and ultrastructural levels (1,21), and at the biochemical level (1,22). The process is poorly understood at the molecular level, and the basic molecular phenomena existing between the applied mechanical environment (cyclic distraction stress) and the cellular response have not yet been defined.

The mechanical window for distraction osteogenesis is fairly wide, since a high variety of external skeletal fixators with different stiffness properties have been successfully applied in numerous experimental and clinical studies with the same result. In vitro studies designed to verify the sensitivity of human osteoblasts to cyclic mechanical stretching have suggested only a narrow range of optimal cyclic strain (approximately 1% strains) for activation of osteoblastic proliferation (23). In fact, the primary target of the applied tensile stress may not be the osteoblasts but the induction of angiogenesis, which is known to precede osteogenic activity.

Whether a primary or secondary effect, the angiogenic action of distraction explains why the method is applicable even in infected long-bone nonunions (3,4). Similarly, it explains why distraction osteogenesis is efficient even in irradiated mandibles, as observed in a recent experimental study (5). As reported by Ilizarov (1), distraction osteogensis is associated with intense angiogenic activity which is reflected in the growth of newly formed capillaries along the direction of the distraction vector. A recent experimental study (2) confirmed the presence of a prolonged hypervascular state at the site of distraction bone formation. Additional studies of distracted canine mandibles (biofocal distraction) have demonstrated the expression of constituents of the vascular basement membrane (laminin and type IV collagen) both at the site of distraction osteogenesis and at the interface area of the transported bone and the target bone (21).

The application of strain during distraction treatment may even induce systemic osteoblast stimulating factors that enhance osteoblast activity both locally and systematically. Holbein and associates (24) demonstrated that sera of patients with distraction osteogenesis have mitogenic effects on osteoblastic cells. Sera harvested from control patients with regular osteotomies did not exert such an effect. The authors could also show a difference in the serum concentration of transforming growth factor (TGF) between the patient groups. In contrast, the groups showed a similar increase in the concentration of platelet-derived growth factor (PDGF).

A case report described an osteogenic sarcoma arising from fibrous dysplasia tissue after the distraction of the affected bone (25). The case raises the question whether the biologic stimulus of distraction osteogenesis through abnormal metaplastic bone increases the risk of malignant neoplasia. As expected, skeletal deformities resulting from metabolic bone diseases do not represent contraindications to distraction treatment (26), although pathologic conditions appear to slow the process of distraction osteogenesis (6).

DISTRACTION MECHANICAL FORCES

The process of distraction involves an interaction of mechanical and biologic factors that influence each other. The factors that determine the local mechanical environment at the distraction site include the applied distraction forces, the rigidity of the fixation, the amount of physiological loading (muscle action), and the properties of the soft tissues, including the tissue formed at the distraction site (Figure 2.3).

In individual cases, it is impossible to define the existing mechanical conditions at the distraction tissue level. Measuring external distraction forces during limb lengthening involves dealing with combined forces. A percentage of the distraction forces can be attributed to muscle forces and to the soft-tissue resistance of the attached structures. If a significant percentage of the distraction load is generated by the tissue at the distraction site, the measurement of the distraction load could provide indirect information about the biologic status of the tissue under distraction (27).

Instrumented external fixators allow monitoring of bone healing—for example,

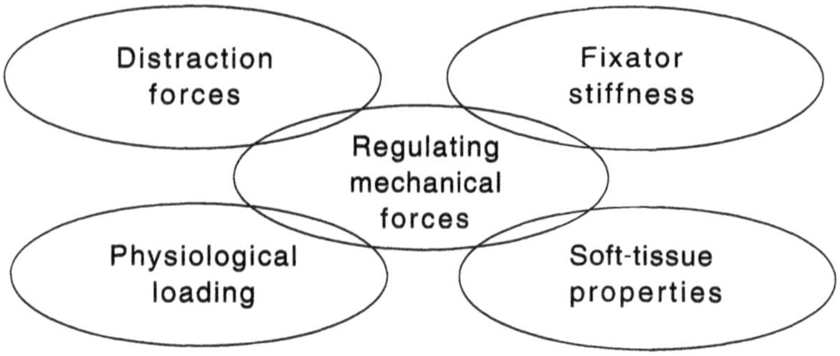

Figure 2.3. The mechanical milieu at the distraction site. The biologic process of osteogenesis is largely determined by four major interacting factors (modified from ref. 18).

the measurement of bending stiffness of a healing tibial fracture (28). The distraction devices can be instrumented in a similar way for recording the reactive forces during distraction. There are several published studies concerning the forces related to experimental distraction osteogenesis (27) and clinical limb lengthening procedures (29,30) as well as bone segment transportation procedures (31). The studies have demonstrated that distraction loads increase with time during the process of lengthening. Elastic tissue resistance of the distraction site is the most likely cause of the force increase. In human lengthening procedures, the maximum measured loads have ranged between 163 N and 236 N in tibias (29) and between 428 N and 673 N in femurs (30). A high early load is a sign of premature consolidation, whereas delayed unions are characterized by low resistance to distraction.

The model of bone segment transport by means of an intramedullary nail is relevant for measuring the forces within the regenerate since the percentage of muscle and soft-tissue forces of the total force measured is low. This type of distraction model of a sheep tibia was applied in the study of Brunner et al. (31). The study included daily measurements of the pretraction force, the peak force during the distraction cycle, and the posttraction force. The study was able to demonstrate the changes of stress relaxation (ie, the viscoelasticity of the distraction tissue during the bone transportation). Maximum stress relaxation was observed between the third and sixth week of distraction.

SIGNIFICANCE OF THE CORTICOTOMY TECHNIQUE, LATENCY PERIOD, RATE OF DISTRACTION, AND DIRECTION OF DISTRACTION FORCE

To minimize the risk of delayed consolidation, the corticotomy should involve minimal damage of the endosteum and periosteum. Translation of the osteotomy should also be avoided (6) since it may delay consolidation.

A comparison of different corticotomy techniques in distraction osteogenesis of canine tibia (32) showed no significant differences between a true corticotomy technique and an osteotomy performed by multiple drill holes and osteotome. The study, however, confirmed the detrimental effect of an oscillating saw on bone formation.

To optimize the response of osteogenic tissue to distraction, a latency period has been suggested for early callus formation (mesenchymal tissue reaction) (Figure 2.4). Different latency periods, ranging from 5 to 21 days, have been reported in clinical treatment and animal experiments. The biologic significance of the length of the latency delay is controversial based on the conflicting results of recent experimental studies (33,34).

The rate of distraction has been approximately 1 mm per day, regardless of species, bone segment distracted, and age of the subject. The rhythm of distraction has varied from one cycle per day to 0.25 mm four times per day.

Although longitudinal long-bone lengthening can be carried out almost routinely at a rate of 1 mm per day, angular

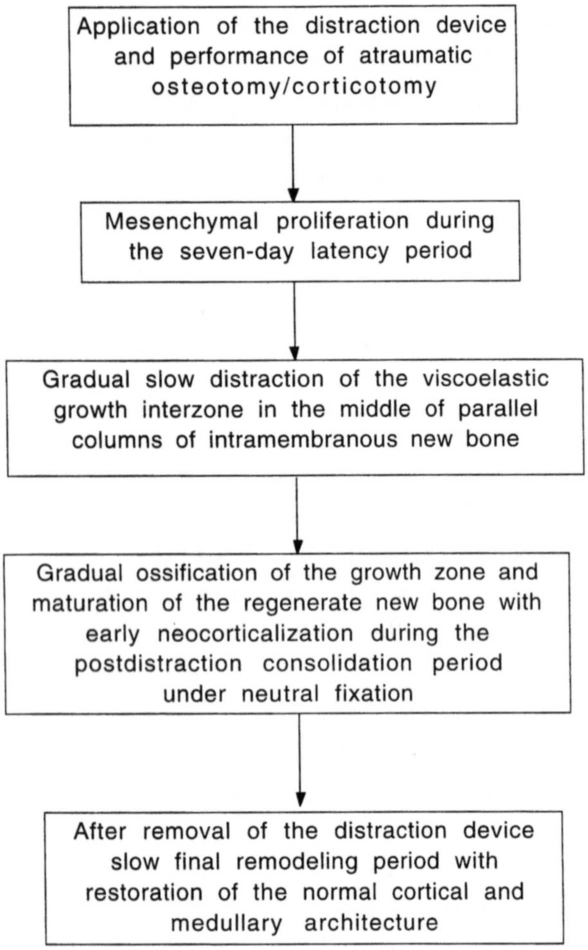

Figure 2.4. Distraction procedure divided into the major five chronological steps according to the morphologic process of new bone formation and remodeling.

corrections of deformed long bones require an adjustment of the rate of distraction according to the geometry of the external fixator relative to the lengthened bone. Modeling the deformity correction with simple geometric principles allows calculation of both the rate of correction and the expected duration of distraction (35). Corrective procedures of the craniofacial area might benefit from a similar approach although the modeling may become more complex.

Most of the distraction procedures are unidimensional and the corticotomized or osteotomized bone is distracted in the direction of its major axis. Does it make a biologic difference if the distraction is aligned away from the dominant axis of the bone? The answer is no. The regeneration process does not seem to sense the direction of the distraction vector. For example, Ilizarov (1) demonstrated in a cortical segment model that canine tibiae can be widened by means of distraction without any difficulties. In this experiment, distraction new bone grew perpendicular to the bone's mechanical axis. Similarly, the growth of new blood vessels followed the vector of distraction. The canine zygoma has also been experimentally distracted away from the dominant axis (36).

NONINVASIVE MONITORING

Noninvasive quantification of the mineralization of the regenerating tissue and the remodeling process of its neocorticalization is definitely needed. When such methods are applied, the biologic pathway proceeding to union can be monitored in order to regulate treatment. The methods may serve as a tool for optimizing early distraction rates in patients at risk for rate-related consolidation problems. In addition, the rigidity of the fixation could be optimized during the course of treatment. Precise measurement of mineral density and bone geometry might also allow prediction of late bowing of the regenerate segment or even a complete stress fracture after removal of the external fixator.

Potential methods of noninvasive quantitative imaging of bone healing and remodeling include: quantitative computerized axial tomography (QCT), ultrasound and magnetic resonance imaging (MRI), single-photon (SPA) and dual-photon (DEXA) absorptiometry, and acoustic ultrasound attenuation (37). Each of these methods has advantages and limitations. Each may prove helpful in examining a different aspect of the process of distraction osteogenesis. Quantitative measurement of mineral content (true density per volume unit) serves as a satisfactory predictor of the local material properties of the forming new bone (38) (Figure 2.5).

Previous studies have shown that QCT, SPA, and DEXA have the greatest promise in prediction of the ultimate torque of an osteotomized canine tibia healing under an external fixation (39,40). This parameter should have a close relationship with the risk of refracture after removal of the fixation device in patients with bone lengthening or transport distraction (37). A recent study by Harp and associates (41) confirmed that the stiffness properties of distracted tubular bones can also be predicted by noninvasive QCT.

Ultrasound attenuation measurements parallel computed tomography as a measure of bone formation within the distraction gap. However, future studies are needed to improve acoustic attenuation data acquisition techniques (42).

Plain radiographs have limitations in detecting the small amounts of new bone formation that occur at the distraction site in the early stages of distraction. In clinical conditions, ultrasound has proved to detect the early new bone at the distraction site (43). A recent comparative clinical study of Eyres and associates (44) confirmed that both ultrasound and DEXA can detect new bone within 1 or 2 weeks of distraction, compared with 4 to 8 weeks by plain radiographs. With ultrasound, the distraction interzone appeared as an echolucent window that narrowed progressively, producing a hyperflecting line during further consolidation. At this stage of healing, the mineral density of the new bone measured by DEXA was approximately 45 percent of control values. Eyres and coworkers (44) concluded that

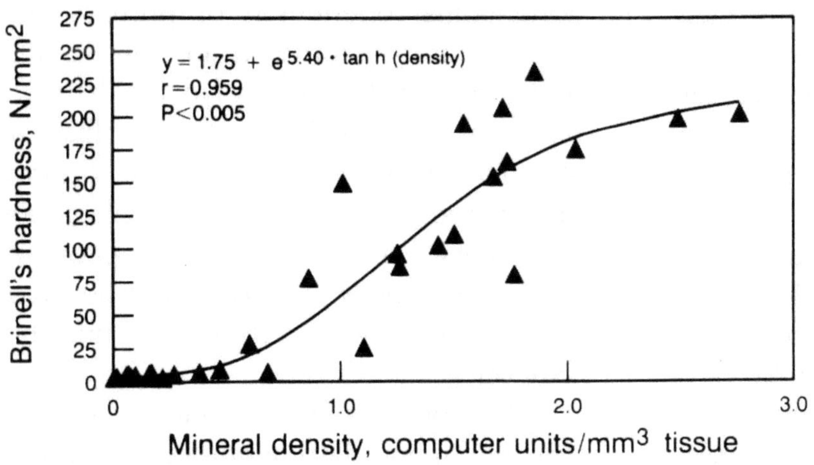

Figure 2.5. The hardness of the bone callus tissue (newton/mm^2) correlates significantly with the mineral density of the callus (computer units/mm^3) as measured by microbone densitometry (adapted from ref. 37).

ultrasound could be used to identify defects in mineralization (and also occasional cysts within the regenerate) and to determine the timing of the fixator dynamization, whereas DEXA could be used to measure the quantity and rate of formation of bone.

BIOMECHANICAL QUALITY OF THE REGENERATE

The structural strength and stiffness of the distraction site in a distracted bone is governed by the material properties of the new bone and the intervening tissue of the distraction growth zone (its strength and modulus) and the cross-sectional geometric factors (the area moments of inertia of the cross-section of the regenerate segment). The characterization of these properties is needed for an accurate determination of the biomechanical quality of the distraction regenerate. At present, little data are available on the biomechanical properties of the distraction regenerate and its incorporation within the host bone.

There are no indications that the structural properties of new bone formed during distraction is poorer than so-called normal new bone. Constantino and associates (14) showed in a canine mandibular model of bifocal distraction that after one year the ultimate strength of the regrown segment was up to 77 ± 6 percent of normal mandibular bone. Using a distraction model of canine tibia, Schickendantz and co-workers (45) demonstrated a mean difference of approximately 20 percent in torsional stiffness of distracted bone segments compared with controls. At present, no data are available on the material properties of early distraction new bone.

EFFECT OF INSTABILITY

One of the original basic concepts of Ilizarov was the need for stable external fixation for the successful outcome of distraction osteogenesis. He demonstrated the deleterious effect of fixation instability on new bone formation under distraction (1).

Using a canine tibial osteotomy model stabilized with a transfixation-wire circular external fixator, Ilizarov (1) compared three different fixator configurations that differed in stability (Table 2.3). The first group showed relatively marked mobility between fragments, the second group was more stable, and the third group was the most stable. Although the actual rigidity of the different configurations was not determined, the experiments clearly showed that increased fixation stability enhances bone formation during distraction treatment. In fact, the experiment demonstrated that the basic phenomenon of distraction osteogenesis (longitudinal orientation of primary collagen in association with fibroblastic cells and the spatial growth of osteoid tissue) does not occur without adequate fixation stability. It is noteworthy that Ilizarov considered the presence of cartilaginous connective tissue (ie, endochondral ossification) as a sign of a low level of osteogenic activity induced by unstable fixation.

Instability of an external fixation system has many detrimental consequences

Table 2.3. Role of fixation stability on distraction osteogenesis.

Osteotomy group	Histomorphometry of the distraction gap tissue
Unstable (two-ring configuration)	Poorly differentiated connective tissue with large islands of cartilage
Moderate stability (tensioned two-ring configuration)	Cone-shaped segments of regenerated osseous tissue separated by a fibrocartilage layer. No definite spatial orientation of the collagen structure and osteoid trabeculae.
Stable (four-ring configuration)	Highest osteogenic activity. The distraction space filled with longitudinally oriented new bone. The growth zone gradually ossifying after the elongation period.

From ref. 1.

during distraction treatment (Figure 2.6). In the clinical setting, many of the bone-healing complications (Table 2.4) have been associated with failure to reconstruct a stable fixation system (6).

What is a "stable" external fixation configuration as recommended by Ilizarov? The only way to define the stability of different fixation systems and to compare the results of different experimental and clinical studies is to use the well-established parameters of biome-

Table 2.4. Bone healing complications of distraction procedures.

- Acute translation of the corticotomy
- Gradual axial deviation at the distraction site
- Premature consolidation—incomplete corticotomy
- Delayed consolidation
- Late bowing of the regenerate
- Complete stress fracture of the regenerate after fixator removal
- Incomplete lengthening
- Incomplete deformity correction
- Recurrent shortening deformity

From ref. 6.

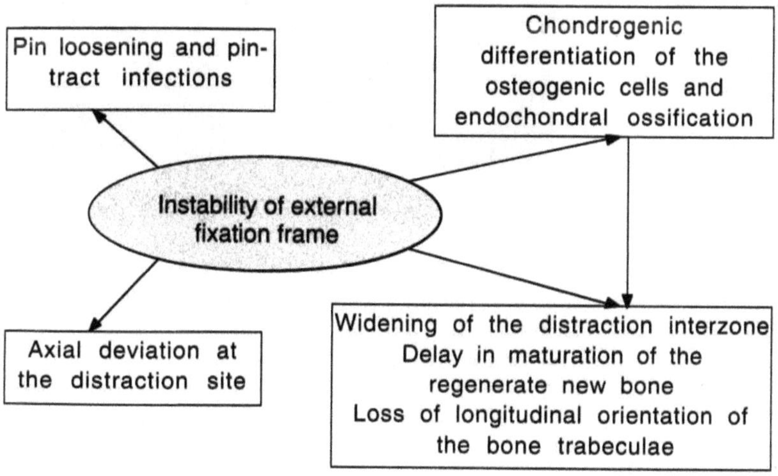

Figure 2.6. Failure to create a stable external fixation configuration increases the risk of delayed consolidation, axial deviation, and pin loosening.

chanical testing. Most of the experimental studies on distraction osteogenesis have neither defined the rigidity of the fixation systems nor quantitatively monitored pin loosening. As a result, the reason for the prominence of endochondral ossification in certain rabbit models of distraction remains unclear.

DEFINITIONS OF FIXATION RIGIDITY

Understanding the basic definitions of structural rigidity or stiffness of bone fragment fixation is essential in the evaluation of the factors that determine the biomechanical properties of a fixation method (46). Such knowledge is clinically important not only when one applies the fixation, but also when one considers and evaluates the biologic consequences of the selected fixation rigidity. This knowledge is especially critical in external fixation, for which many types of frames and fixation configurations are available.

External fixators must satisfy two fundamental requirements. First, the device should possess adequate fatigue resistance, as the apparatus will be required to remain on the patient under varying loading conditions for a long period of time. Second, the fixator must have the adjustability to realign bone fragments and to vary bone fixation rigidity and compression status during the course of treatment.

Theoretical models can be used to predict the stiffness of external fixators under any combination of pin and frame parameters (46,47). The structural rigidity (or stiffness) of a fixation device can be accurately determined in vitro using a universal material testing machine. The fixation device is constructed using the recommended application technique on an osteotomized cadaver or synthetic bone (Figures 2.7, 2.8). The bone ends are loaded under axial compression, bending in two planes, and torsion. During each mode of loading, the load versus deformation curve is recorded and subsequently analyzed to define the three basic stiffness parameters: axial, bending (flexural), and torsional. In each load-deformation curve, the slope of the linear portion of the curve is defined as the

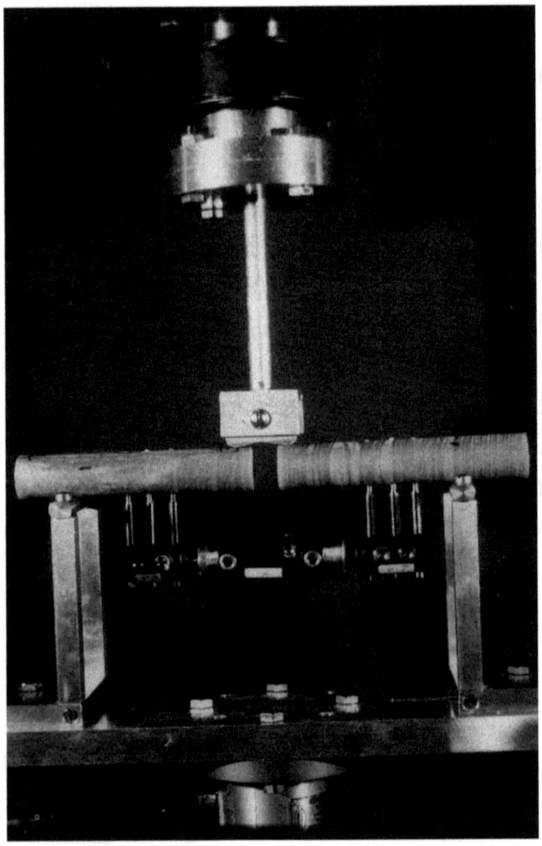

Figure 2.7. Experimental setup for the determination of structural rigidity of a unilateral external fixator (small Orthofix) using a universal mechanical testing machine. The fixator was applied to an osteotomized synthetic bone model and loaded under different loading modes, including four-point lateral bending (adapted from ref. 50).

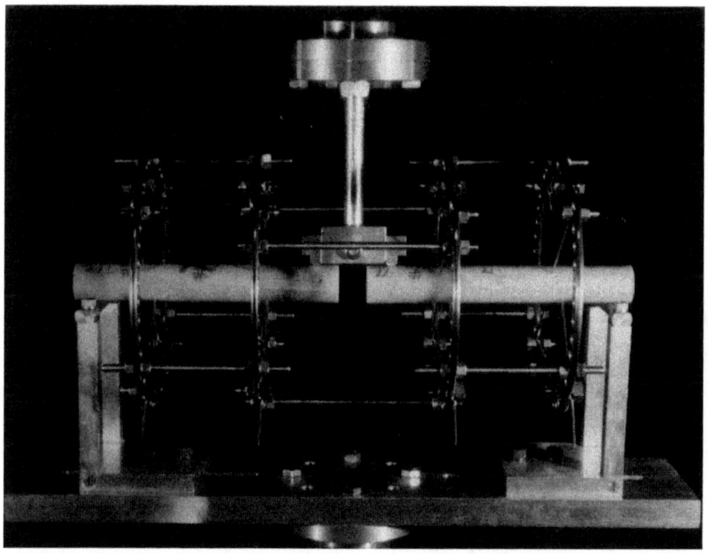

Figure 2.8. The experimental setup of the Ilizarov fixator applied to a synthetic bone model with an osteotomy gap under four-point-bending test (adapted from ref. 50).

fixation rigidity or stiffness (Figure 2.9). Using this testing procedure, it is possible to compare the fixation stiffness of different types of fixation (46).

The rigidity of a unilateral external fixation system (Figure 2.10) can be increased by a number of factors, including increased pin diameter, increased number of pins, decreased side-bar separation, decreased pin separation, increased pin group separation, and the application of pins in different planes. These variables have different effects on the axial, bending, and torsional stiffness, and, by varying these key parameters, it is possible to achieve a desired fracture stability. Pin diameter is the most important parameter to influence fixator rigidity (47,48). At best, the stiffness of an external fixation system can duplicate that of a bone-plate system. As shown in a following experiment, the pattern of primary bone union

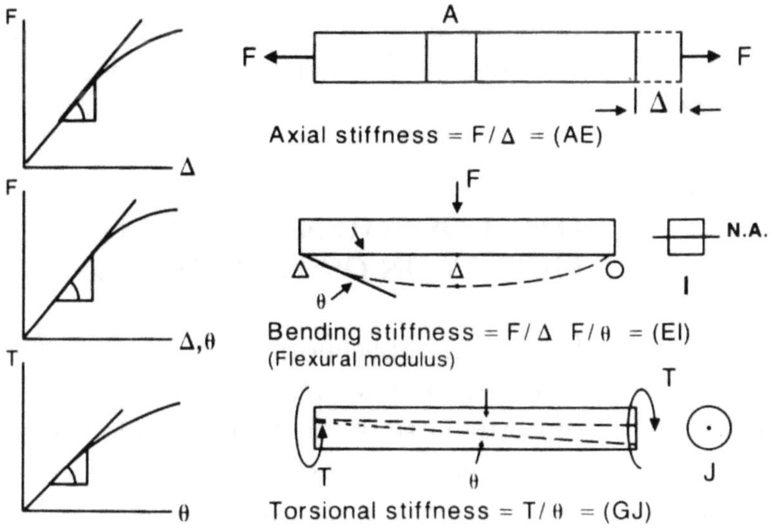

Figure 2.9. Determination of structural rigidity (or stiffness) of a bone-fixation device. Using the load deformation curve for each loading mode, the slope of the linear portion of the curve is used to define the fixation rigidity of an intact control bone or the bone fragments fixed with the fixation device.

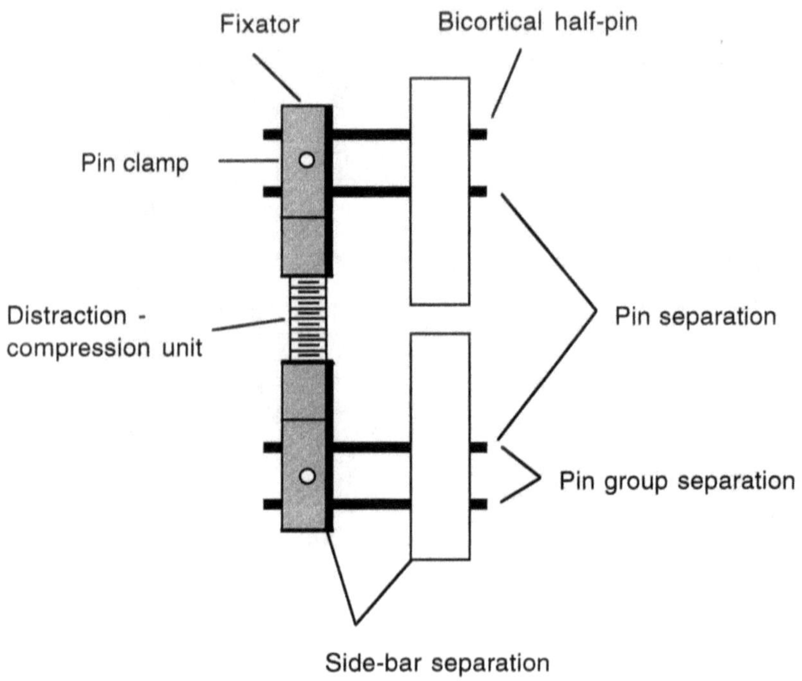

Figure 2.10. Schematic of the important parameters affecting the rigidity of a unilateral external fixator.

typical of compression-plated osteotomies does occur in osteotomies stabilized under rigid external fixation. These findings mean that the rigidity of the fixation and not the type of fixation (plating versus external fixation) determines the pattern of union.

External fixators with different structural designs—such as unilateral fixators with cortical screws (Orthofix®, Figure 2.7) and circular external fixators with tensioned wires (Figure 2.8; (1))—have different mechanical properties. Both of these fixators have been popular in limb lengthening procedures (7). Several recent studies (49,50) have shown that the overall stiffness of the Ilizarov device in proper configurations is close to that of unilateral external fixators, especially in bending and torsion. Under axial compression, the circular fixator has, however, a nonlinear stiffness behavior that varies with wire pretension (49,50). The nonlinear stiffness behavior, reflecting mostly the large deflection of the thin wire, is less pronounced under torsion and bending loads.

In the clinical situation, the overall rigidity of a fixation system (ie, clinical stability of the bone-fixator system) is not dependent only on the frame stiffness and the pins. Other important factors include the type of fracture, the accuracy of reduction, the amount of physiologic loading, and the performance of the pin–bone interface.

EFFECT OF EXTERNAL FIXATION RIGIDITY ON OSTEOTOMY HEALING

In clinical applications of distraction it is essential to understand the characteristics of normal osteotomy healing under external fixation. A series of experiments has been carried out for this purpose (51–54).

The experiments were designed to demonstrate the model of healing expected by each type of fixation rigidity under standardized healing conditions. The experiments used the same experimental model (canine tibial shaft osteotomy stabilized under a custom-designed Orthofix external fixator) (Figure 2.11) to eliminate other variables such as the extent of soft-tissue injury and the accuracy of reduction, variables that are known to influence bone healing under clinical conditions. The use of intra-animal comparison in analysis also minimized the many inter-animal variables, such as individual differences in age, biological responses, temperament, functional activity, and loading magnitude. The animals were divided into groups according to the osteotomy pattern (transverse or 60-degree oblique), the mode of fixation (osteotomy ends reduced in contact, with 0.8-mm osteotomy gap or with 2-mm gap) and the change of fixation rigidity during the treatment (early or delayed dynamization). In vitro experiments (Figure 2.12) showed that the torsional and lateral bending stiffness provided by the fixation system resembled that of intact bone (canine tibia) values, whereas anteroposterior bending stiffness was 32 percent of intact bone. Axial dynamization (the release of the telescoping mechanism of the fixator body) was aimed to allow full axial loading of the healing bone under external fixation.

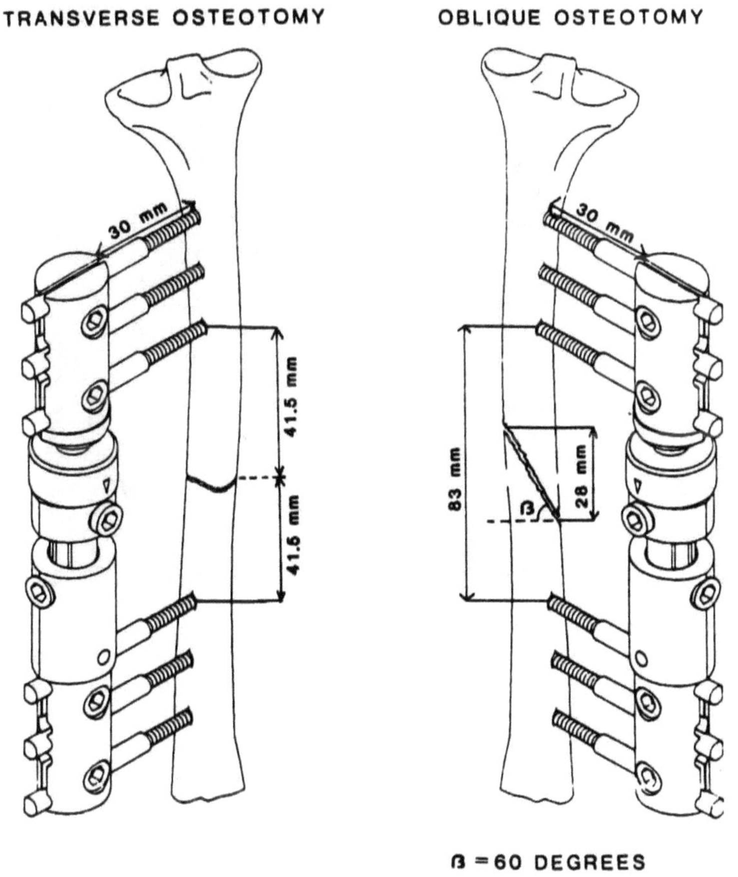

Figure 2.11. The experimental canine tibial model of external fixation used to study bone-healing biology and biomechanics associated with different osteotomy types, gap conditions, and dynamization effects (adapted from ref. 52).

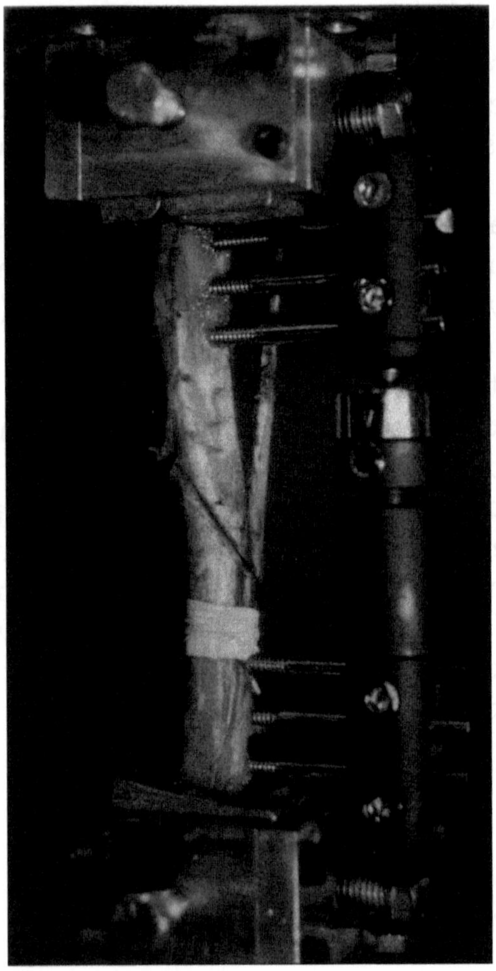

Figure 2.12. Experimental setup to define the axial and rotational rigidity of a unilateral external fixator (custom-modified Orthofix) applied to a canine tibia with a 60-degree oblique osteotomy.

The paired comparison of transverse and oblique osteotomies (52) showed that the osteotomy morphology per se does not dictate the bone union pattern. The transverse osteotomies, and occasionally even the oblique osteotomies, showed the growth of secondary osteons across the fracture site (Figures 2.13, 2.14). Despite evidence of early cortical healing (fulfilling the classic criteria of primary cortical bone union), the osteotomies also formed periosteal callus. The oblique osteotomy pattern had a retarding effect on the return of bone structural stiffness and on the rate of cortical bone repair. However, it had less effects on the return of bone torsional strength. The paired comparison of constant rigid fixation and early axial dynamization of transverse osteotomies (55) demonstrated that rigid external fixation prevents periosteal callus formation under low loading conditions. At 12

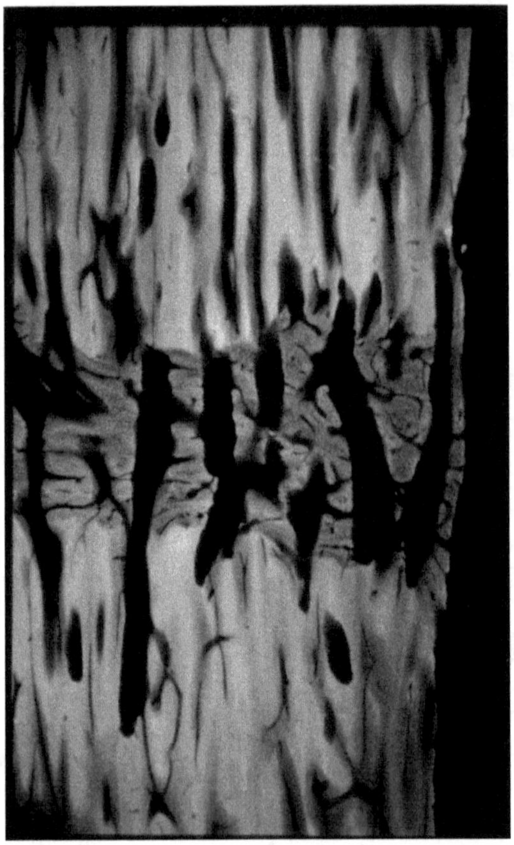

Figure 2.13. Primary bone union (gap type) of a transverse canine tibial osteotomy under rigid external fixation (90 days after osteotomy). There is lamellar new bone (dark zone in the center) between the osteotomy surfaces associated with growth of secondary osteons (resorption canals) across the osteotomy site (microradiograph from a longitudinal undecalcified section).

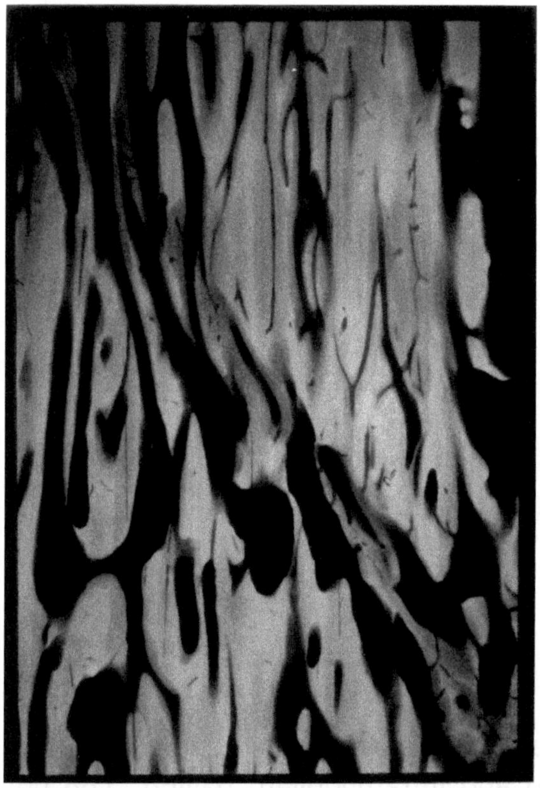

Figure 2.14. Sixty-degree oblique osteotomy of the canine tibia after 90 days of healing under rigid external fixation demonstrating primary contact union. The microradiograph shows the intimate contact of the oblique osteotomy ends and the growth of secondary osteons (dark resorption canals) across the osteotomy line.

weeks, the torsional strength and stiffness of both dynamized and nondynamized tibiae were already reaching the level of intact tibiae and no significant differences were found between the two sides. The study of Egger and associates (53) investigated the effects of early axial dynamization (7 days) in the osteotomy model with a significant 2-mm fracture gap. In torsional testing at 6 weeks, the dynamized osteotomies were significantly stiffer than controls, but the difference in torsional strength was not significant. The study suggested that very early dynamization may improve fracture healing by reducing fracture gap size. In the study of Aro and Chao (54), an unstable fracture model of the canine tibia (60-degree oblique osteotomy with a 2-mm gap) was used to study the effects of delayed dynamization (four weeks). This study showed that even a delayed dynamization may close an unintentional fracture gap, with a positive effect of enhanced axial loading on fracture callus remodeling. A fracture gap caused by unintentional distraction of bone fragments, and augmented by fracture end resorption, is one of the obvious reasons for bone healing problems under external fixation. Unintentional osteotomy diastasis is also one of the reasons for delayed consolidation under distraction treatment (6). The study of Markel (56) used a fracture union model with a large 2-mm osteotomy gap under bilateral external fixation, and the results demonstrated the detrimental effect of fracture gap on osteotomy healing under the external fixation. The osteotomies gained only approximately 44% of intact bone strength by 12 weeks. The experiments demonstrated that osteotomized bones heal without delay under external fixation if the osteotomy ends are reduced in contact. In contrast, diastasis of an osteotomy definitely inhibits bone healing under external fixation.

The externally fixed bones demonstrated three major union patterns under different healing conditions. The results obtained gave a compelling reason to modify the commonly used classification of bone-healing patterns (primary versus secondary bone union). In the modified classification (54), three major types were proposed: nonosteonal bone healing,

Figure 2.15. Schematic illustrating the three major union patterns observed in osteotomized canine tibias healed under external fixation. Non-osteonal healing is characterized by callus formation without early healing of the cortical bone by secondary osteons. Primary (no callus formation) and secondary (callus formation) osteonal healing shows early direct healing of the cortical bone.

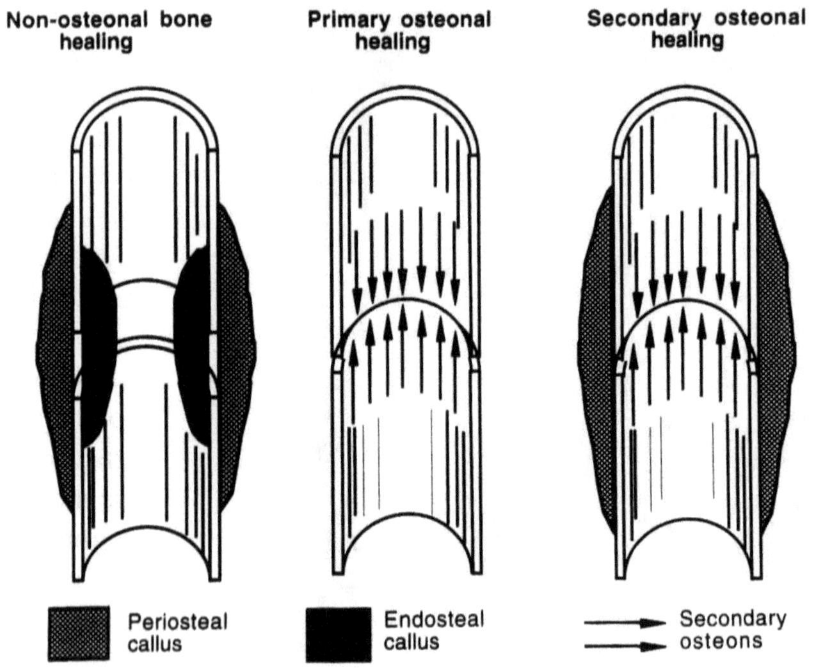

primary osteonal healing, and secondary osteonal healing (Figure 2.15). One of the most interesting findings was related to the biomechanical efficiency of the union patterns in restoring the structural properties of the healing bone. Neither the cortical healing alone (the characteristic of primary osteonal healing) nor the predominance of periosteal callus formation (the characteristic of nonosteonal bone healing) seemed to be more desirable over the other in the restoration of bone mechanical properties. In contrast, the combination of these two bone union mechanisms, characterized by early cortical healing and concomitant periosteal callus formation (secondary osteonal healing), appeared to be optimal to meet the time-related mechanical requirements of a healing diaphyseal bone.

These experiments confirmed the results of the previous studies of the same model (57), which had compared osteotomy healing under different external fixation systems and also under plate fixation and intramedullary nailing. The uniform result of all studies was that the stability of the fixation, and not the mode of fixation, is the most important single factor in bone healing. The results were in agreement with the results of Ilizarov on osteotomized canine tibias under distraction treatment. The failure to create a stable external fixation causes significant problems during distraction osteogenesis (see Figure 2.6), including delayed consolidation and the risk of axial deviation and deformity as well as the risk of pin loosening.

Biomechanical studies have shown that shear and axial osteotomy site motion differed significantly under simulated weight-bearing conditions when unilateral half-pin fixators (such as the Orthofix and Wagner devices) were compared with the Ilizarov circular wire fixator (58). Therefore, it is reasonable to assume that the quality of distracted new bone also depends on the type of external fixation. Indeed, Aronson and associates (17) could demonstrate qualitative histologic differences in the comparison of Ilizarov and Wagner external fixators in the lengthening of canine tibiae. As expected, the multiplanar, full-pin circular Ilizarov system induced perfectly parallel columns of distraction new bone, a finding suggesting concentric loading of the distraction tissue. The uniplanar, half-pin Wagner system induced angulation of the collagen and subsequent bone columns on the basis of eccentric loads to the distraction tissue. There were no major differences between the fixators in the volume of osteogenesis. It seems that the circular ring fixators do not provide any miracles in promotion of distraction osteogenesis, although they certainly have unique features under axial loading.

Is it possible that the rigidity of external fixation is too high? Indeed, Goodship and colleagues have demonstrated that excessively high rigidity of external fixation inhibits healing in an osteotomy model of the ovine tibia with a significant gap (59). This finding is in agreement with other studies. High rigidity of an external fixation with diastasis of the osteotomy, as seen in the study of Markel and associates (56), represented the worst combination for bone healing. As observed in other experiments, high fixation rigidity with close apposition of the osteotomy ends ensures rapid bone healing (54). Goodship and Kenwright (60) have also confirmed that induced axial micromotion is beneficial for new bone formation in healing human tibial fractures (61). The same response was also seen in sheep osteotomy models with a gap (60). Micromotion appears to compensate for any factor which delays healing.

Bone is sensitive to mechanical influences and the presence of any fixation device will impose constraints on the physiological mechanical loading that may influence subsequent remodeling. O'Doherty and colleagues (62) recently demonstrated that rigid external fixation causes significant stress protection with subsequent bone loss both on the endosteal and the periosteal surfaces. Thus, dynamization (decrease of stiffness) of rigid external fixators may help to promote remodeling and decrease the risk of a stress fracture after fixator removal.

MECHANICAL PERFORMANCE OF EXTERNAL FIXATION PINS

The pin-bone interface is the most critical factor for the performance of external fixators. The immediate holding power of external fixation pins is usually satisfactory; early pull-out of an external fixation pin is extremely rare. In contrast, loosening of an external fixation pin is not uncommon. A major effort must be focused to create and maintain the optimal conditions for the performance of the external fixation pins.

One common mistake is to assume that the use of external fixators does not require learning or mastering the surgical techniques. A majority of pin-tract complications is related to technical errors of surgery, such as unicortical pin placement. Optimal bicortical placement and insertion of fixation pins may be especially difficult in the craniofacial area, including

Table 2.5. Biomechanical factors in the prevention of pin-tract problems.

- Selection of an appropriate pin design (cortical vs. cancellous bone) and the maximum pin diameter
- Selection of appropriate sites for pins through the maximum diameter of the bone (bicortical fixation)
- Low-speed predrilling (and tapping, if necessary) through a drill guide (avoidance of bone and soft-tissue necrosis)
- Creation of a rigid frame configuration
- Skin release around the pins and reduction of soft-tissue motion

deformed mandibles with abnormal bone structure.

Pin-tract problems can be controlled, but the established regimens must be followed during insertion and postoperative care (Table 2.5). The most important single factor causing pin loosening is unstable fixation (see Figure 2.6). In the craniofacial region the thin layer of subcutaneous tissue, minimal pin-skin motion, relatively satisfactory soft tissue vascularity, and high wound-healing capacity may decrease the number of pin-skin tract complications.

The time sequence of events in pin-tract sepsis is controversial (63). First, mechanical loosening of a pin, as a result of thermal bone necrosis or mechanical cortical bone failure, carries a risk of subsequent pin–tract infection. Second, bacterial colonization from the pin–skin interface to the pin–bone interface may lead to bone resorption and subsequent pin loosening.

Pin geometry and thread design (Figure 2.16), as well as bone thread preparation, are critical biomechanical factors in bone screw performance (64). Improved cutting technology, with effective chip elimination, is important to minimize maximum temperatures during pin insertion. The inability of a pin to remove cut chips results in increased frictional forces relating to both higher temperatures and increased insertion torques (65). Many

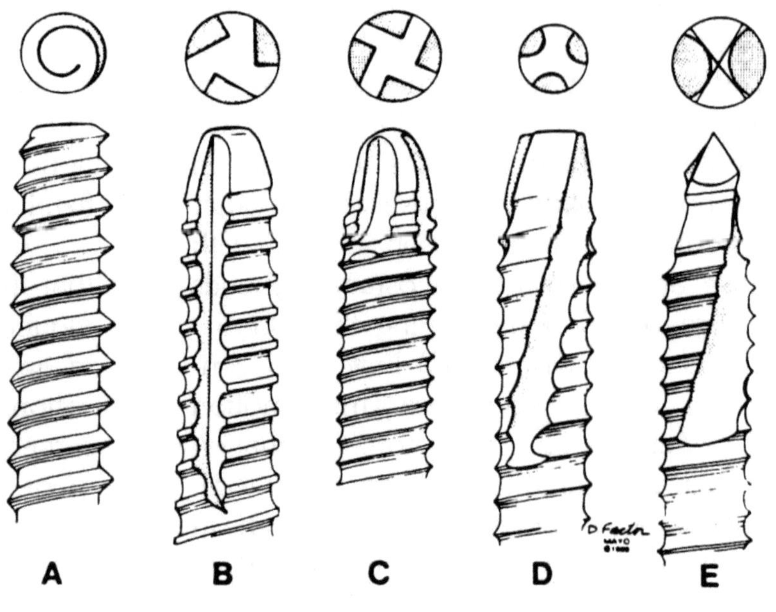

Figure 2.16. Cortical half-pin geometry with longitudinal and cross-sectional views of five different pins (A = Orthofix, B = Hoffmann, C = Ace, D = Apex Blunt, E = Apex Sharp) (adapted from ref. 68).

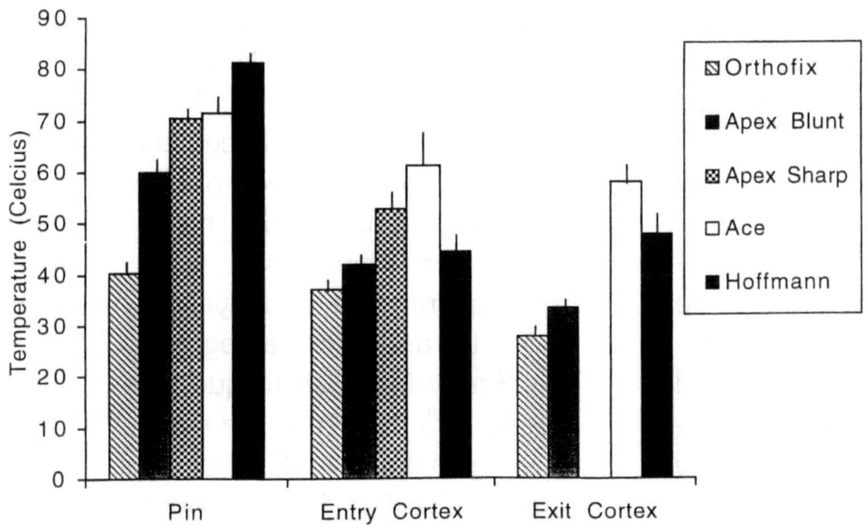

Figure 2.17. Measured pin and local bone temperatures during insertion of five different external pins in bone. The bars represent mean ± *SEM* (data adapted from ref. 67).

factors are involved in efficient bone chip removal during drilling. One of these is the presence or absence of flutes at the pin tips and the various orientation of the flutes. Predrilling is the most effective measure to prevent thermal necrosis during pin insertion (66). The technique of bone thread preparation is of particular importance when the bone quality is less than optimal for pin insertion.

A recent in vitro study (67) was carried out to compare the mechanical performance of five external fixation pins (Figure 2.16) with respect to insertion torque, pull-out strength, heat generation, and microdamage at the pin–bone interface. The results showed that pin-tip design plays a significant role in affecting insertion torque, heat generation (Figure 2.17), and pullout strength (Figure 2.18). High temperatures were measured both within pins and in bone tissue during insertion. The thermocouples placed within the pin tip often recorded temperatures well above known thermonecrotic ranges (ie, 50 °C). The insertion torque and

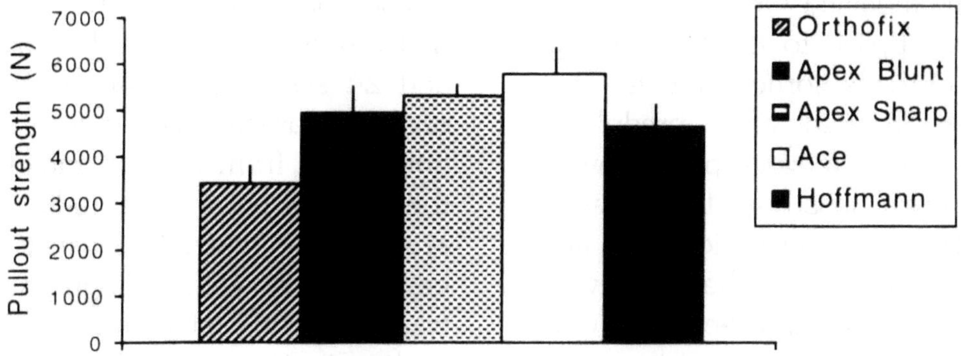

Figure 2.18. Pull-out strength (newtons) of five different external pins from artificial bone material. The bars represent mean ± *SEM* (data adapted from ref. 67).

temperature curves correlated closely. Pins with straight flute design had higher heat generation and insertion torques than helical fluted designs.

The biomechanical aspects of pin–bone interface performance have been studied in detail by using both three-dimensional and two-dimensional finite element analyses (47,48,68). Local pin-bone stresses may reach high levels, and there are chances for local bone yielding failure and pin loosening under heavy loading conditions.

CORTICAL BONE REACTIONS AROUND FIXATION PINS

The finite element analyses also suggested that the use of half-pins (ie, cortical screws in unilateral external fixators) involves a potential risk of local yielding failure at the entry cortex because of high local pin-bone stresses. Therefore, the canine model applied for osteotomy healing studies (see Figure 2.11) was also used to characterize the nature of cortical bone reactions at the pin-bone interface of the external fixation pins (cortical screws) (63). Custom modified Orthofix external fixators were applied to the tibiae using six tapered Orthofix cortical screws. The screws were inserted after predrilling both cortices with a slow-speed power drill, and screw insertion torque was measured. The screws were tightened until the threaded portion of the screw was through both cortices and the screw was clinically tight. The torque resistance of the screw during the final tightening was measured with an instrumented torque wrench. Free, unrestricted weight bearing was allowed immediately after surgery. At designated time periods, the screw-skin interfaces were examined, the external fixators were removed, and the screw-removal torques were measured. Pin tracts were processed and analyzed using quantitative tetracycline histomorphometry and microradiography.

Screw insertion torque was approximately 20% higher in the tibial shaft than in its proximal and distal metaphyseal regions. Taking into account only the screws with no radiographic changes, the screw removal torques decreased over time (Figure 2.19). The percentage reduction of insertion torque value by 12 weeks was uniform among screws of different locations.

The comparison of the osteotomy groups performed at 12 weeks showed highly significant differences in average screw-removal torque. The screw-removal torques were highest in stable transverse osteotomies fixed under cortical bone contact and lowest in unstable osteotomy models (transverse osteotomies with a large gap and oblique osteotomies).

Altogether, 243 screws (65% of the screws analyzed at 12 weeks) showed no radiographic changes; 105 screws (28%) had rarefaction only at the entry cortex; and 24 screws (7%) showed rarefaction on both cortices. The extent of rarefaction varied from a slight radiolucency of the cortical bone to a radiolucent halo around the screw. At 12 weeks, the number of screws with radiographic changes was lowest in stable fracture models. In each osteotomy model, rarefaction was most commonly observed only at the entry cortex.

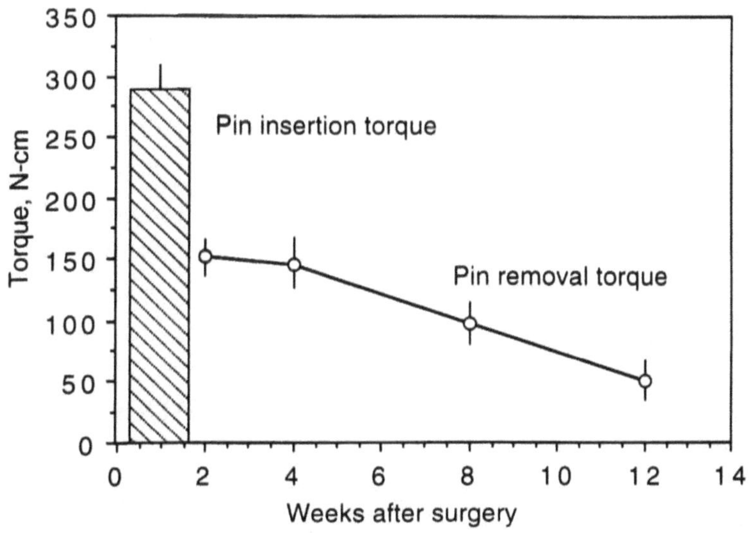

Figure 2.19. Insertion and removal torques (newton-cm) of stable external fixation pins, measured by using an instrumented torque wrench, at sequential experimental periods after canine tibial osteotomy. The values represent the averaged values of six pins for each animal (the means ± *SEM*, *n* = 7–8).

On microradiographic study the screws with no radiographic changes (so-called stable pins) showed well-preserved bone threads on both cortices (Figure 2.20). The endosteal and periosteal surfaces, as well as the medullary cavity, showed newly formed bone threads. Secondary osteons were seen invading into the well-preserved bone threads, a finding indicating the process of creeping substitution. The amount of new bone was approximately 43% of the total cortical bone space both at the entry and exit cortices of the stable screws (Figure 2.21). The corresponding cortical bone porosity (12%) was approximately four times higher than that of the intact canine cortical bone (3%), a sign of enhanced vascularization.

The screws with radiographic rarefaction at the entry cortices (unstable screws) showed marked porosity and complete or incomplete resorption of the bone threads at the entry cortex (Figure 2.22). The porosity of the entry cortex was increased approximately twofold compared with

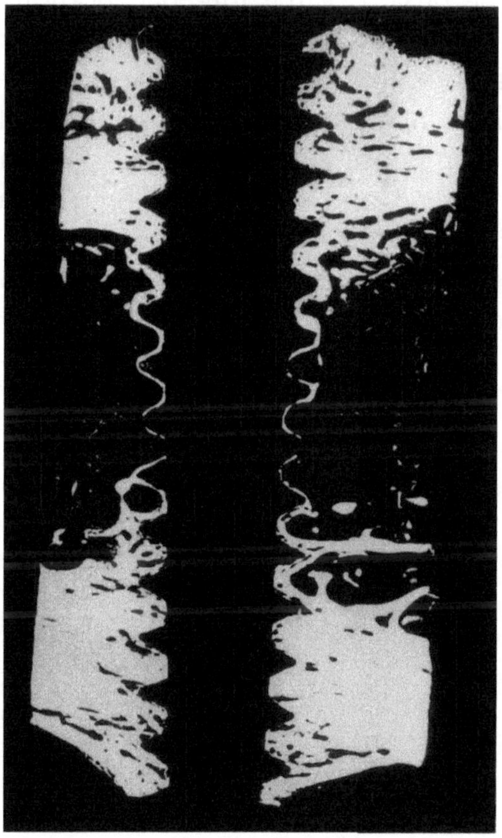

Figure 2.20. A microradiograph showing the pin tract of a stable external fixation pin (90 days after osteotomy of the canine tibia). The pin tract shows well-preserved bone threads of both cortices and newly formed bone threads on the periosteal surface and in the medullary cavity (adapted from ref. 63).

that of the stable screws (see Figure 2.21). The remodeling of the exit cortex showed no significant differences from that of the stable screws (see Figure 2.21).

Implantation of any bone screw results in cortical bone remodeling. A similar phenomenon of creeping substitution (Haversian remodeling) was evident around the external fixation screws. This beneficial biologic process replaces any damaged lamellar bone next to the screw while it obviously results in a time-related decrease of screw removal torque. The phenomenon does not seem to be related to the physiologic loading of the screw or to the design of the threaded portion of the screw. Coating of the external fixation screws with osteoconductive materials such as hydroxyapatite (69,70) may ideally compensate for the effects of bone remodeling and reverse the time-related decrease of screw anchorage.

The models of heavy loading conditions demonstrated bone thread resorption and adverse cortical bone remodeling at the entry cortex of the fixation screws. This type of uricortical screw loosening represents a consequence of micromotion and local bone yielding failure caused by excessively high dynamic stresses at the entry cortex of the pin–bone interface.

STRETCHING OF SOFT TISSUES

Reconstruction of skeletal defects by distraction requires the stretching of soft tissues such as muscle, fascia, and skin. In limb lengthening procedures, the most common complications are related to soft tissue contracture and joint stiffness. In the craniofacial area these complications obviously are rare. Distraction rates exceeding 1 mm per day cause damage and proliferation of fibrous tissue between the muscle fibers, and muscle responds more favorably at distraction rates slower

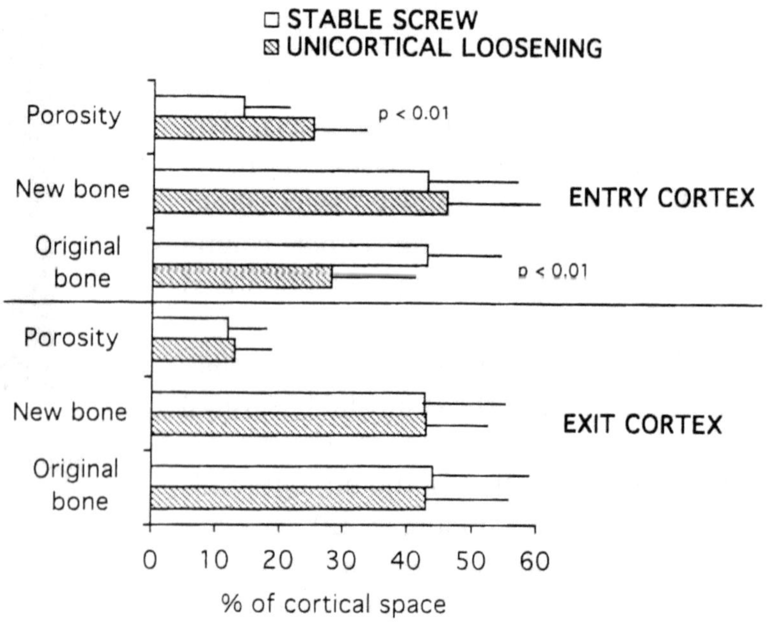

Figure 2.21. The histomorphometric features of cortical bone remodeling around external fixation pins. The bars represent the means ± *SD* ($n = 14$) for Orthofix pins 90 days after canine tibial osteotomy (data adapted from ref. 63).

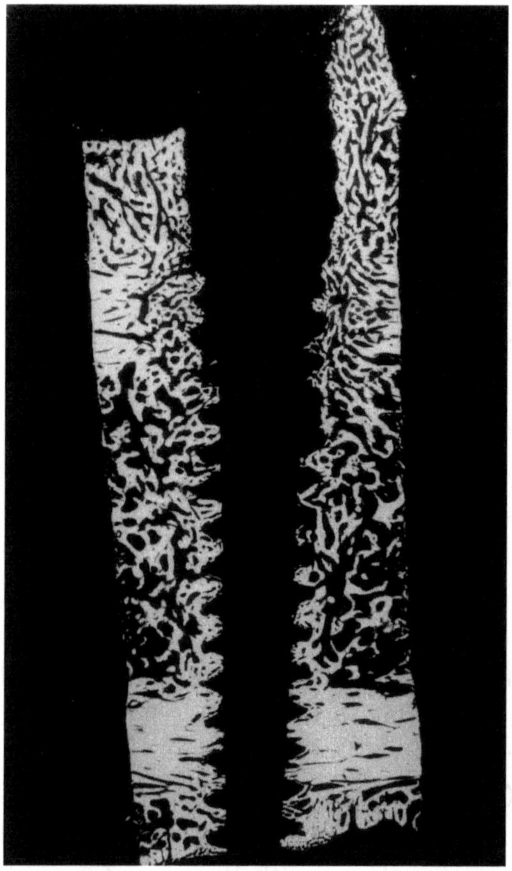

Figure 2.22. A corresponding microradiograph, compared with Fig. 2.20, demonstrating the pin tract characteristics of an unstable external pin. The entry cortex (the upper cortex) shows a partial loss of bone threads with marked osteoporotic transformation of the cortical bone. The exit cortex shows well-preserved bone threads (adapted from ref. 63).

than those that result in the most prolific bone formation (61). Therefore, it seems advisable to use a slower rate of distraction in patients with poor muscle compliance associated with the skeletal pathology. This principle may be applicable also in special cases of craniofacial distraction treatments. In the craniofacial area, most concern has been related to the possible stretching of the inferior alveolar nerve (12,71).

REACTION FORCES ACROSS JOINTS

During limb lengthening, the forces at the joints increase. In cases of large femoral lengthening, the reaction forces across the joints are so great that knee and hip subluxations have occurred. Hip dislocation is a particular concern in femoral lengthening of patients with acetabular dysplasia. Is an equal complication possible during mandibular distraction of a patient with temporomandibular joint (TMJ) instability (see Chapter 8)?

The reaction forces across the involved joints during bone lengthening theoretically depend on the strength and stiffness characteristics of the muscles and soft tissues that cross the joint. From a theoretical point, greater pressure across a particular joint occurs if the lengthening gap is between the origin and insertion of the major muscles that cross it. Based on a cadaver study (72,73), the level of osteotomy affects the forces across the proximal and distal joints. For example, if instability of the hip is a concern during femoral lengthening, a distal osteotomy should be used. The same cautious principle may be reasonable in lengthening procedures of the mandibular ramus with a dysplastic condyle.

DESIGN OF NEW DISTRACTION DEVICES

In a tubular bone, transport distraction is possible over a guiding intramedullary nail (31). A recent study even demonstrated the feasibility of bone transport and distraction osteogenesis in the presence of an internal distraction device with plate

Figure 2.23. Schematic of the consequence following malposition of the fixations pins in a unilateral external fixator. Rotational malposition of the pins in one of the fragments (A) causes translation at the osteotomy site after application of the distraction device (B). As a result, the distracted bone may show permanent axial deformity (C).

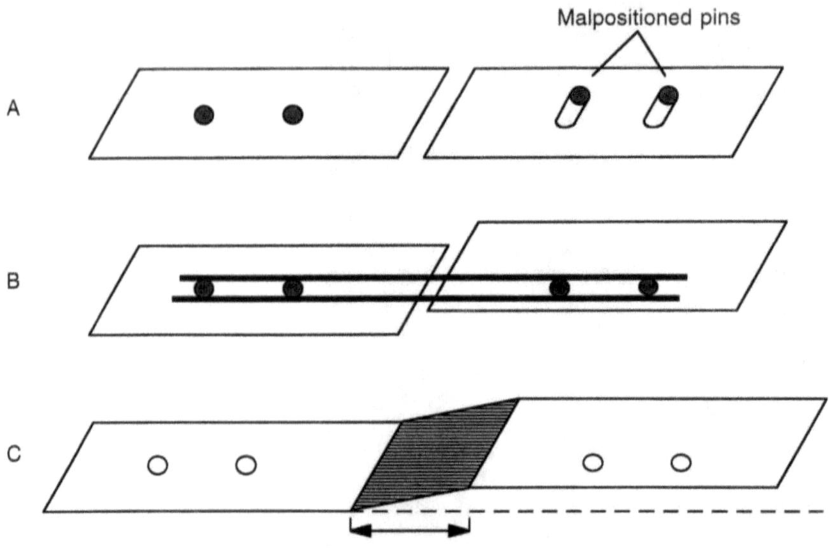

osteosynthesis in the sheep femur (74). Although desirable, there seem to be no solutions to avoid external skeletal fixation devices in most cases of more advanced distraction of craniofacial lamellar bones. External fixators are a relatively inconvenient form of treatment for the patient and labor intensive for the surgeon.

It should be understood that the method of distraction osteogenesis, either a monolateral external fixator or a circular wire fixator, is not exclusive to one device. In limb reconstruction procedures, many orthopedic surgeons use different devices to achieve the desired result (7). In each patient, the selection of a specific device depends only on the needs of the distraction procedure and on the patient-related factors. In the case of craniofacial reconstruction, the same scenario of the treatment strategy is inevitable. There are different procedures that may optimally need different types of distraction devices. A fairly simple design of lengthening devices is excellent in unifocal distraction of the mandible (75), but it may not fulfill all of the requirements for multidirectional or multiplanar corrections of complex deformities.

Optimal design of any distraction device allows free placement of individual fixation pins. Even with the use of a guiding instrument, the placement of fixation pins in one plane may be challenging. Malposition of the pins causes difficulties in maintenance of the osteotomy reduction during the application of the distraction device (Figure 2.23). As a result, the osteotomy develops acute translation, which would require a ball-joint structure for correction. The overall design of pin clamps is important for the optimal performance of the device (76). One of the common difficulties encountered during distraction is the maintenance of axial reduction. Distraction with a unilateral external fixator (and even with circular fixators) may cause gradual axial deviation of the corticotomy fragments, reflecting mostly pin bending (Figure 2.24).

For correction of complex limb deformities, Ilizarov fixators provide a mult-

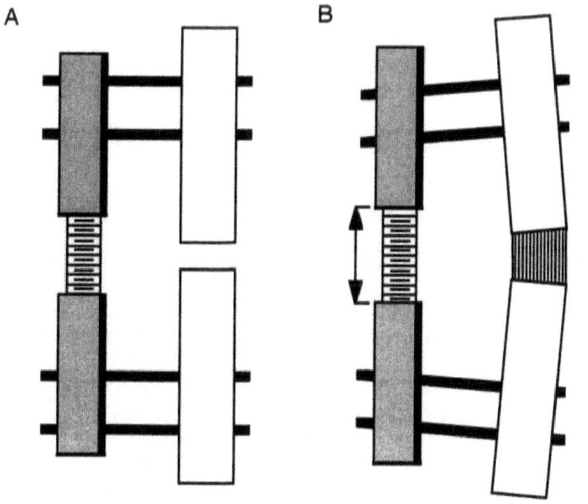

Figure 2.24. Schematic of a distraction osteotomy fixed with a unilateral external fixator (A) which develops gradual axial deviation during distraction osteogenesis (B), reflecting pin bending caused by large reactive forces.

iplanar system that uses circular external fixation with tensioned wires or a combination of half-pins (cortical screws). These fixators provide for multilevel, multiapical, and juxta-articular corrections, but the fixator design is not applicable in craniofacial areas. Therefore, there is a clear need for new designs of distraction devices for craniofacial distraction. Glat and colleagues (36) have indicated that miniaturization and internalization of the devices may allow for more precise changes in the amount and direction of craniofacial lengthening.

Certain goals can be established for the designs of new external distraction devices for craniofacial application (Table 2.6). The principle of a multiplanar distraction-compression device is already adapted to the structure of certain unilateral external fixators, principally aimed for accurate reduction of tibial fractures.

Table 2.6. Design considerations for new external distraction devices for craniofacial applications.

- There should be capabilities to allow a controlled multiplanar (three-dimensional) distraction and compression of the corticotomy site
- The device should allow distraction around a smooth arc, facilitating reconstruction of any bone curvature
- Pin clamps should allow placement of the fixation pins in any plane independently of each other
- Pin clamps should allow the use of pins with different diameters in order to allow the use of pins of the maximum thickness in each location
- Fixator body should involve a ball-joint type of structure to compensate for any pin malposition
- Thread designs of the pins should be matched with the specific anatomy of craniofacial lamellar bone
- Fixator should be of small size, MRI compatible, and radiolucent if possible
- For specific indications, a model of the device should include an option for instrumental monitoring of the distraction force

BIOMECHANICAL PREOPERATIVE PLANNING

Surgical methods of distraction osteogenesis represent a rather reliable biologic approach to correct difficult congenital, post-traumatic, or other acquired skeletal deformities. Correction of a skeletal deformity by distraction osteogenesis is similar to lengthening with respect to new bone formation but it necessitates complex three-dimensional planning and a specific distraction device. The success of such salvage procedures largely depends on the quality of preoperative planning.

As emphasized by Paley and Tetsworth (77), it is important to delineate the level, plane, direction, and magnitude of the deformity for each apex of multiapical deformities in the correction of lower extremity deformities. Without doubt, the same principle is equally important in the correction of craniofacial deformities. In both cases, the ultimate goal is to restore normal anatomy as much as possible and to improve function.

In the long bones, correction of multiapical angular deformities usually require more than one osteotomy (77). The same is evident in craniofacial structures. Glat and associates (36) have already demonstrated the biologic feasibility of multidimensional bone lengthening using a canine model of zygomatic arch osteotomies. Multiplanar distraction, as mandated by the patient's specific deformity, is possible, for example, in micrognathia (75).

Successful multiplanar correction of difficult skeletal deformities is dependent on the availability of advanced distraction devices (external fixators) that allow controlled multidirectional advancement of transportable bone fragments. The use of such devices requires careful preoperative analysis of the imaging results. In the future, computer software programs would allow simulation of the planned osteotomies in three-dimensional reconstructions of the preoperative CT scans. The results would predict the anatomical and biomechanical end result of the planned surgery before the procedure.

Such advanced systems of computer-aided surgery planning, albeit still based on the analysis of plain radiographs and two-dimensional graphic programs, are already in use in preoperative planning of knee osteotomies (78), a technique allowing prediction of the loading forces within the knee joint after osteotomy. The computer-assisted surgery planning has also been applied in the correction of lower extremity deformities by distraction osteogenesis (79). The latter software package also generates an ideal three-dimensional Ilizarov frame construction for each case.

FUTURE PERSPECTIVES

This chapter has briefly reviewed the basic biomechanics of distraction osteogenesis as a potential tool in reconstruction of difficult craniofacial deformities. The biological feasibility of distraction osteogenesis in guided regeneration of human bones is indisputable. Modern tools of molecular biology will provide additional insight into the basic molecular mechanisms of distraction osteogenesis in the near future. Experimental studies have emphasized the significance of fixation stability in the promotion of direct intramembranous new bone formation (without a cartilage intermediate) during distraction. Most of the current distraction devices were originally designed for fracture treatment and subsequently adapted directly or secondarily with small modifications for distraction treatment. Improved designs of the distraction devices and their fixation screws will improve their performance. Internal distraction devices with plate osteosynthesis are an attractive new option for selected cases. The new designs should allow controlled multiplanar distraction correction of complex deformities. These procedures would greatly benefit from the development of computer-assisted preoperative planning systems, which theoretically have the potential for improving the accuracy of the correction procedures and their clinical outcome. The application of modern quantitative noninvasive monitoring techniques in the evaluation of the healing wound may optimize the distraction protocols, shorten the length of treatment, and allow prediction of the risk of stress fracture through the regenerated bone.

References

1. Ilizarov GA. The tension-stress effect on the genesis and growth of tissues. Part I. The Influence of stability of fixation and soft-tissue preservation. *Clin Orthop* 238:249–281, 1989.
2. Ilizarov GA. Temporal and spatial increases in blood flow during distraction osteogenesis. *Clin Orthop* 301:124–131, 1994.
3. Marsh JL, Prokuski L, Biermann JS. Chronic infected tibial nonunions with bone loss. Conventional techniques versus bone transport. *Clin Orthop* 301:139–146, 1994.
4. Cierny G, Zorn K. Segemental tibial defects. Comparing conventional and Ilizarov methologies. *Clin Orthop* 301:118–123, 1994.
5. Gantous A, Phillips JH, Catton P, Holmberg D. Distraction osteogenisis in irradiated canine mandible. *Plast Reconstr Surg* 9:8, 1994.
6. Paley D. Problems, obstacles, and complications of limb lengthening by the Ilizarov Technique. *Clin Orthop* 250:81–105, 1990.
7. Dahl MT, Gulli B, Berg T. Complications of limb lengthening. A learning curve. *Clin Orthop* 301:10–18, 1994.
8. McCarthy JG, Schreiber J, Karp N, Thorne CH, Grayson BH. Lengthening the human mandible by gradual distraction. *Plast Reconstr Surg* 89:1–10, 1992.
9. Havlik RJ, Bartlett SP. Mandibular distraction lengthening in the severely hypoplastic mandible: a problematic case with tongue aplasia. *J Craniofac Surg* 5:305–310, 1994.
10. Pensler JM, Goldberg DP, Lindell B, Carroll NC. Skeletal distraction of the hypoplastic mandible. *Ann Plast Surg* 34:130–136, 1995.
11. Costantino PD, Shybut G, Friedman CD, Pelzer HJ, Masini M, Sisson GA. Segmental mandibular regeneration by distraction osteogenesis. *Arch Otolaryngol Head Neck Surg* 116:535, 1990.
12. Block MS, Cervini D, Chang A, Gottsegen GB. Anterior maxillary advancement using tooth-supported distraction osteogenesis. *J Oral Maxillofac Surg* 53:561–565, 1995.
13. Rachmiel A, Jackson IT, Potparic Z, Laufer D. Midface advancement in sheep by gradual distraction: a 1-year follow-up study. *J Oral Maxillofac Surg* 53:525–529, 1995
14. Costantino PD, Friedman CD, Shindo ML, Housten G, Sisson GA Sr. Experimental mandibular regrowth by distraction osteogenesis. *Arch Otolaryngol Head Neck Surg* 119: 511–516, 1993.
15. Ganey TM, Klotch DW, Slater-Haase AS, Sasse J. Evaluation of distraction osteogenesis by scanning electron microscopy. *Otolaryngol Head Neck Surg* 111:265–272, 1994.
16. Annino DJ Jr, Goguen LA, Karmody CS. Distraction osteogenesis for reconstruction of mandibular symphyseal defects. *Arch Otolaryngol Head Neck Surg* 120:911–916, 1994.
17. Aronson J, Harrison BH, Stewart CL, Harp JH Jr. The histology of distraction osteogenesis using different external fixators. *Clin Orthop* 241:106–116, 1989.
18. Chao EYS, Aro HT, Inoue N. Engineering principles for bone fracture fixation and repair. In: *Biomedical Applications of Synthetic Biodegradable Polymers*. Boca Raton, FL: CRC Press; 1995:145–172.
19. Delloye C, Delefortrie G, Coutelier L, Vincent A. Bone regenerate formation in cortical bone during distraction lengthening. An experimental study. *Clin Orthop* 250:34–42, 1990.
20. Karp NS, McCarthy JG, Schreiber JS, Sissons HA, Thorne CH. Membranous bone

lengthening: A serial histological study. *Ann Plast Surg* 29:2–7, 1992.

21. Ganey TM, Klotch DW, Sasse J, Odgen JA, Garcia T. Basement membrane of blood vessels during distraction osteogenesis. *Clin Orthop* 301:132–138, 1994.
22. Karaharju EO, Aalto K, Kahri A, Lindberg LA, Kallio T, Karaharju-Suvanto T, Vauhkonen M, Peltonen J. Distraction bone healing. *Clin Orthop* 297:38–42, 1993.
23. Neidlinger-Wilke C, Wilke HJ, Claes L. Cyclic stretching of human osteoblasts affects proliferation and metabolism: A new experimental method and its application. *J Orthop Res* 12:70–78, 1994.
24. Holbein O, Neidlinger-Wilke C, Suger G, Kinzl L, Claes L. Ilizarov callus distraction produces systemic bone cells mitogens. *J Orthop Res* 13:629–638, 1995.
25. Harris NL, Eilert RE, Davino N, Ruyle S, Edwardson M, Wilson V. Osteogenic sarcoma arising from bony regenerate following Ilizarov femoral lengthening through fibrous dysplasia. *J Pediatr Orthop* 14:123–129, 1994.
26. Stanitski D. Treatment of deformity secondary to metabolic bone disease with the Ilizarov Technique. *Clin Orthop* 301:38–41, 1994.
27. Aronson J, Harp JH. Mechanical forces as predictors of healing during tibial lengthening by distraction osteogenesis. *Clin Orthop* 301:73–79, 1994.
28. Richardson JB, Cunningham JL, Goodship AE, O'Conner BT, Kenwright J. Measuring stiffness can define healing of tibial fractures. *J Bone Joint Surg* 76:389–394, 1994.
29. Leong JC, Ma RY, Clark JA, Cornish LS, Yau AC. Viscoelastic behavior of tissue in leg lengthening by distraction. *Clin Orthop* 139:102–109, 1979.
30. Younger ASE, Mackenzie WG, Morrison JB. Femoral forces during limb lengthening in children. *Clin Orthop* 301:55–63, 1994.
31. Brunner UH, Cordey J, Schweiberer L, Perren SM. Force required for bone transport in the treatment of large bone defects using medullary nail fixation. *Clin Orthop* 301: 147–155, 1994.
32. Frieson M, Ibrahim K, Boles M, Bote H, Ganey T. Distraction osteogenesis. A comparison of corticotomy techniques. *Clin Orthop* 301:19–24, 1994.
33. White SH, Kenwright J. The importance of delay in distraction osteotomies. *Orthop Clin North Am* 22:659–579, 1991.
34. Aronson J, Shen X. Experimental healing of distraction osteogenesis comparing metaphyseal with diaphyseal sites. *Clin Orthop* 301: 25–30, 1994.
35. Hertzenberg JE, Waanders NA. Calculating rate and duration of distraction for deformity correction with the Ilizarov technique. *Orthop Clin North Am* 22:601–611, 1991.
36. Glat PM, Staffenberg DA, Karp NS, Holliday RA, Steiner G, McCarthy JG. Multidimensional distraction osteogenesis: the canine zygoma. *Plast Reconstr Surg* 94:753–758, 1994.
37. Chao EYS, Aro HT, Markel MD, Kuo RF. Application of non-invasive techniques in the determination of fracture callus property and bone strength. In: Campilho A, Barbosa MA, eds. *Imaging Techniques in Biomaterials.* Elsevier Science; 1994:307–323.
38. Aro HT, Wippermann BW, Hodgson SF, Wahner HW, Lewallen DG, Chao EYS. Prediction of fracture callus properties by measurement of mineral density using microbone densitometry. *J Bone Joint Surg* 71-A:1026–1036, 1989.
39. Markel MD, Wikenheiser MA, Chao EYS. A study of fracture callus material properties: relation to the torsional strength of bone. *J Orthop Res* 8:843–850, 1990.
40. Markel MD, Wikenheiser MA, Morin RL, Lewallen DG, Chao EYS. Quantification of bone healing—comparison of QCT, SPA, MRI and DEXA in dog osteotomies. *Acta Orthop Scand* 61:487–498, 1990.
41. Harp JH, Aronson J, Hollis M. Noninvasive determination of bone stiffness for distraction osteogenesis by quantitative computed tomography scans. *Clin Orthop* 301:42–48, 1994.
42. Daneil BL, Waanders NA, Zhang Y, Moskalik A, Fowlkes JB, Rubin JM, Goulet KA, Adler RS. The use of ultrasound mean acoustic

attenuation to quantify bone formation during distraction osteogenesis performed by the Ilizarov method. Preliminary results in five dogs. *Invest Radiol* 29:933–939, 1994.

43. Young JW, Kostrubiak IS, Resnik CS, Paley D. Sonographic evaluation of bone production at the distraction site in Ilizarov limb-lenghtening procedures. *Am J Roentgenol* 154:125–128, 1990.
44. Eyres KS, Bell MJ, Kanis JA. Methods of assessing new bone formation during limb lengthening. Ultrasonography, dual energy X-ray absorptiometry and radiography compared. *J Bone Joint Surg* 75-B:358–364, 1993.
45. Schickendantz MS, Watson JT, Sferra JJ, Kambic HE. A model for evaluating the strength of bones lengthened by distraction osteogenesis. *Clin Orthop* 275:248–252, 1992.
46. Chao EYS, Aro HT. Biomechanics of fracture fixation. In: Mow VC, Hayes WC, eds. *Basic Orthopaedic Biomechanics*. New York: Raven Press; 1991:293–336.
47. Chao EYS, Kasman RA, An KN. Rigidity and stress analysis of external fracture fixation devices—a theoretical approach. *J Biomech* 15:971–983, 1982.
48. Huiskes R, Chao EYS. Guidelines for external fixation frame rigidity and stresses. *J Orthop Res* 4:68–75, 1986.
49. Fleming B, Paley D, Kristiansen T, Pope M. A biomechanical analysis of the Ilizarov external fixator. *Clin Orthop* 241:95–105, 1989.
50. Podolsky A, Chao EYS. Mechanical performance of Ilizarov circular external fixators in comparison with other external fixators. *Clin Orthop* 293:61–70, 1993.
51. Aro HT, Hein TJ, Chao EYS. Mechanical characteristics of an upper extremity external fixator. *Clin Orthop* 253:240–250, 1990.
52. Aro HT, Wahner HT, Chao EYS. Healing patterns of transverse and oblique osteotomies in the canine tibia. *J Orthop Trauma* 5:351–364, 1991.
53. Egger EL, Gottsauner-Wolf F, Palmer J, Aro HT, Chao EYS. Effects of axial dynamization on bone healing. *J Trauma* 34:185–192, 1992.
54. Aro HT, Chao EYS. Bone healing patterns affected by loading, fracture fragment stability, fracture type, and fracture site compression. *Clin Orthop* 293:8–17, 1993.
55. Aro HT, Kelly PJ, Lewallen DG, Chao EYS. The effects of physiologic dynamic compression on bone healing under external fixation. *Clin Orthop* 256:260–273, 1990.
56. Markel MD, Wikenheiser MA, Chao ETS. Formation of bone in tibial defects in a canine model. *J Bone Joint Surg* 73-A:914–923, 1991.
57. Chao EYS, Aro HT, Lewallen DG, Kelly PJ. The effect of rigidity on fracture healing in external fixation. *Clin Orthop* 241:24–35, 1989.
58. Paley D, Fleming B, Catagni M, Kristiansen T, Pope M. Mechanical evaluation of external fixators used in limb lengthening. *Clin Orthop* 250:50–57, 1990.
59. Goodship AE, Watkins PE, Rigby HS, Kenwright J. The role of fixator frame stiffness in the control of fracture healing. An experimental study. *J Biomech* 26:1027–1035, 1993.
60. Goodship AE, Kenwright J. The influence of induced micromotion upon the healing of experimental tibial fractures. *J Bone Joint Surg* 67-B:650–655, 1985.
61. Simpson AH, Williams PE, Kyberd P, Goldspink G, Kenwright J. The response of muscle to leg lengthening. *J Bone Joint Surg* 77-B:630–636, 1995.
62. O'Doherty DM, Butler SP, Goodship AE. Stress protection due to external fixation. *J Biomech* 28:575–586, 1995.
63. Aro HT, Markel MD, Chao EYS. Cortical bone reactions at the interface of external fixation half-pins under different loading conditions. *J Trauma* 35:776–785, 1993.
64. Ansell RH, Scales JT. A study of some factors which affect the strength of screws and their insertion and holding power in bone. *J Biomech* 1:279–302, 1968.
65. Wiggins KL, Malkin S. Drilling of bone. *J Biomech* 9:553–559, 1976.
66. Matthews LS, Green CA, Goldstein SA. The thermal effects of skeletal fixation—pin

insertion in bone. *J Bone Joint Surg* 66A:1077–1083, 1984.

67. Wikenheiser MA, Markel MD, Lewallen DG, Chao EYS. Thermal response and torque resistance of five cortical half-pins under simulated insertion technique. *J Orthop Res* 13:615–619, 1995.

68. Huiskes R, Chao EYS, Crippen TE. Parametric analyses of pin-bone stresses in external fracture fixation devices. *J Orthop Res* 3: 341–349, 1985.

69. Augat P, Claes L, Hanselmann KF, Suger G, Fleischmann W. Increase of stability in external fracture fixation by hydroxyapatite-coated bone screws. *J Appl Biomater* 6:99–104, 1995.

70. Moroni A, Orienti L, Stea S, Visentin M. Improvement of the bone-pin interface with hydroyapatite coating: an in vivo long-term experimental study. *J Orthop Trauma* 10: 236–242, 1996.

71. McCarthy JG. The role of distraction osteogenesis in the reconstruction of the mandible in unilateral craniofacial microsomia. *Clin Plast Surg* 21:625–631, 1994.

72. Eyres KS, Bell MJ, Kanis JA. Methods of assessing new bone formation during limb lengthening. Ultrasonography, dual energy X-ray absorptiometry and radiography compared. *J Bone Joint Surg* 75:358–364, 1993.

73. Olney BW, Jayaraman G. Joint reaction forces during femoral lenthening. *Clin Orthop* 301:64–67, 1994.

74. Windhager R, Großschbmidt, Tsuboyama T, Siegl H, Heinzl H, Seidl G, Plenk H Jr. Recorticalization after bifocal internal bone transport in the double-plated sheep femur. *J Orthop Res* 14:94–101, 1996.

75. De Bastiani G, Aldegheri R, Renzi-Brivio L, Trivella G. Limb lengthening by distraction of the epiphyseal plate. *J Bone Joint Surg* 66B: 545–555, 1986.

76. Aro HT, Hein TJ, Chao EYS. Mechanical performance of pins clamps in external fixators. *Clin Orthop* 248:246–253, 1989.

77. Paley D, Tetsworth K. Mechanical axis deviation of the lower limbs. Preoprative planning of multiapical frontal plane angular and bowing deformities of the femur and tibia. *Clin Orthop* 280:65–71, 1992.

78. Chao EY, Sim FH. Computer-aided preoperative planning in knee osteotomy. *Iowa Orthop J* 15:4–18, 1995.

79. Lin H, Birch JG, Samchukov ML, Ashman RB. Computer-aided preoperative planning of lower extremity deformity correction. *Proc. of 14th Annual International Conference IEES/EMBS*, Vol 3, 1992: 1278.

CHAPTER 3

Principles of Distraction Osteogenesis

The Orthopedic Experience*

James Aronson

Distraction osteogenesis, also called callostasis, was introduced by Ilizarov in 1951 (1,2). Ilizarov initially treated patients in Siberia with fractures and nonunions following World War II. He utilized a primitive external ring fixator to compress the injured bone ends. By chance, a patient reversed the compression rods, thereby distracting the bone fragments. Ilizarov observed new bone formation radiographically and pursued this new method both experimentally and clinically (2). Initially his patients were treated for fractures and nonunions. Without the benefit of antibiotics, Ilizarov was also able to cure cases of chronic osteomyelitis using only this method. Later, he developed the techniques of bone transportation (3,4,6,7) and limb lengthening (8,9).

Sporadic recognition of his work has appeared in the English literature (10–13), but in the early 1980s a group of orthopaedic surgeons in Italy dedicated themselves to understanding and applying his method (14,15). The author was fortunate to observe this method while on a traveling fellowship in Italy and later to learn the techniques from Ilizarov himself in Kurgan, Siberia.

In 1984, the first experiments utilizing the Ilizarov model for canine tibial lengthening (16) were initiated. Since 1985, the author has applied his method clinically (17). In 1987, this research was presented at the first Ilizarov meeting in New York. Since that time, interest in this method, both experimentally and

*This chapter is reprinted in part and with permission from the *Cleft Palate-Craniofacial Journal*, 31:473, 1994.

clinically, has grown exponentially in the orthopedic community (9,18).

Based upon my experimental and clinical experience, this article provides biologic guidelines for applying this method to craniofacial surgery.

DEFINITIONS

- *Distraction osteogenesis* is the regeneration of bone between vascularized bone surfaces that are separated by gradual distraction. The bone is most commonly separated by a low-energy osteotomy or corticotomy stabilized by external fixation. Following a 5-day latency period, the daily rate of distraction (1 mm) is divided into a rhythm of 0.25 mm four times a day.
- *Corticotomy* is a low-energy osteotomy of the cortex preserving the local blood supply to both the periosteum and the medullary canal.
- *Latency* is the time following the osteotomy when initial fracture healing bridges the cut bone surfaces prior to initiating distraction.
- *Rate* is the number of millimeters per day at which the bone surfaces are stretched.
- *Rhythm* is the number of distractions per day, usually in equally divided increments to total the rate.
- *Transformation osteogenesis* is the conversion of nonosseous interpositions (eg, fibrocartilage in nonunion, synovial cavities in pseudarthrosis, or muscle in delayed unions) into normal bone by combined compression and distraction forces, sometimes augmented by a nearby corticotomy.
- *Bone transportation* is the regeneration of intercalary bone defects by combined distraction and transformation osteogenesis.
- *Healing index* is the number of days or months from the operation to full, unprotected loadbearing for each centimeter of new bone length.

EXPERIMENTAL EXPERIENCE

By varying the *stability of fixation*, the *displacement of the osteotomy*, and the *rate* and *rhythm* of distraction, Ilizarov postulated that all four factors were critical to osteogenesis. In over 60 experimental lengthenings using Ilizarov's original model of the adult canine tibia, the author attempted to reproduce his results. All experiments have followed the same model using four animals in each group and the contralateral tibia as a control (19). The results have been reported using the Wilcoxon nonparametric statistical analysis.

The hypothesis was tested that rate and rhythm are critical to distraction osteogenesis. The null hypothesis tested the potential for bone bridging across a distraction gap created on day 7 immediately following the osteotomy. All of the bones went on to atrophic nonunions. When the same distraction gap was created at irregular rate and rhythm, the bones went on to fibrous nonunions. The third group of animals, which were distracted at the recommended rate of 1 mm per day and rhythm of 0.25 mm four times a day, all went on to bridge the 28 mm distraction gap with new bone that quickly remodeled to normal by radiography (healing index 31 days/cm).

Subsequent experiments sought to characterize the nature of this bone formation histologically and biochemically. The dogs were sacrificed at various time points during distraction, and both decalcified and nondecalcified histology was carried out. Prior to distraction, the traditional reparative response of normal fracture healing was observed. Once distraction had begun, however, the local histology was transformed from mixed endochondral intramembranous ossification (a reparative response) to well-organized longitudinal intramembranous ossification (a regenerative response).

Throughout the distraction phase, a transverse, undulating central radiolucent band 4 to 6 mm in thickness persisted radiographically. On histological examination, the fibrous interzone (FIZ) corresponded to a longitudinal arrangement of spindle cells with dense collagen production arranged parallel to the distraction force. At both edges of the FIZ, primary mineralization occurred in the regions of newly formed capillaries and vascular sinuses, the *primary mineralization front* (PMF) (Figure 3.1).

More recently, unpublished data using in situ hybridization have demonstrated that a majority of cells in the adjacent zones of primary mineralization stained heavily for basic fibroblast growth factor. Numerous plump osteoblasts appeared at the osteoid surface of each new bone column. Along with the adjacent collagen bundles, the osteoblasts became incorporated into the longitudinal microcolumns of bone, which expanded to diameters of 150 to 200 μm. The bone columns did not contain Haversian systems, but instead were surrounded by large, thin-walled blood vessels. The microcolumns attached to the entire cross-section of cut bone on both ends of the distraction gap, including periosteum, cortex, and medullary spongiosa.

When distraction was discontinued, the PMF advanced from each end toward the center, bridging the FIZ. At the same time, the longitudinal microcolumns of bone began to form transverse bone

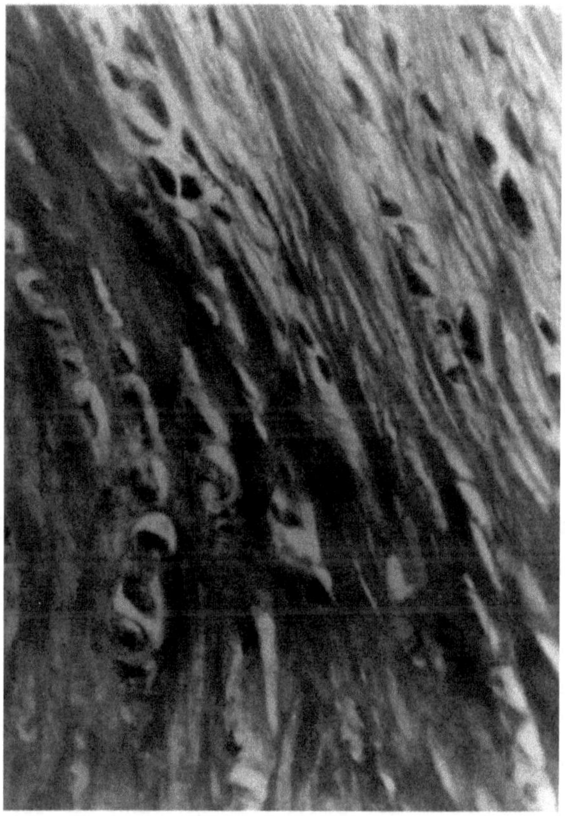

Figure 3.1. Histology of primary bone formation during distraction osteogenesis (canine tibial lengthening, ×20, H&E). Note the mesenchymal cells producing a collagen matrix (upper right) that consolidates into a microcolumn of bone with incorporated osteoblasts.

bridges, taking on the appearance of a honeycomb structure.

Six weeks after the completion of distraction, when the external fixators were removed, the 28-mm distraction gap was fully bridged with honeycomb bone in the adult canine tibial lengthening model. The dogs routinely bore weight on this leg for 6 more weeks until staged sacrifice. The distracted bones demonstrated remodeling to mature, lamellar bone with bone marrow present in the medullary region. By this time (day 119), the cortical structure was reconstituted both radiographically and histologically.

The addition of new bone to the existing tibia was demonstrated by gravimetric studies where increased mass and volume were measured commensurate with the amount of lengthening. Both decalcified and nondecalcified histology confirmed the presence of well-organized collagen bundles and normal bone formation. Back-scattered scanning electron microscopy detailed the three-dimensional honeycomb microstructure. Quantitative biochemistry measured increasing calcium and phosphate in relation to collagen until mature ratios were achieved, a finding consistent with hydroxyapatite.

The overall histologic picture correlated directly with the periosteum surrounding a growth plate at the zone of Ranvier (Figure 3.2). Just as the cartilage physis is believed to push the epiphysis away from the bony metaphysis, stretching the peripheral periosteum, the external fixator stretched the FIZ in distraction osteogenesis.

The overall blood supply to the distraction zone, as measured by quantitative technetium scintigraphy, reached maximum levels of seven times that of the normal contralateral side during distraction and remained at approximately three times normal for the next 3 months of remodeling. The relative increase in blood flow seemed to exceed the amount measured for simple fracture healing (20).

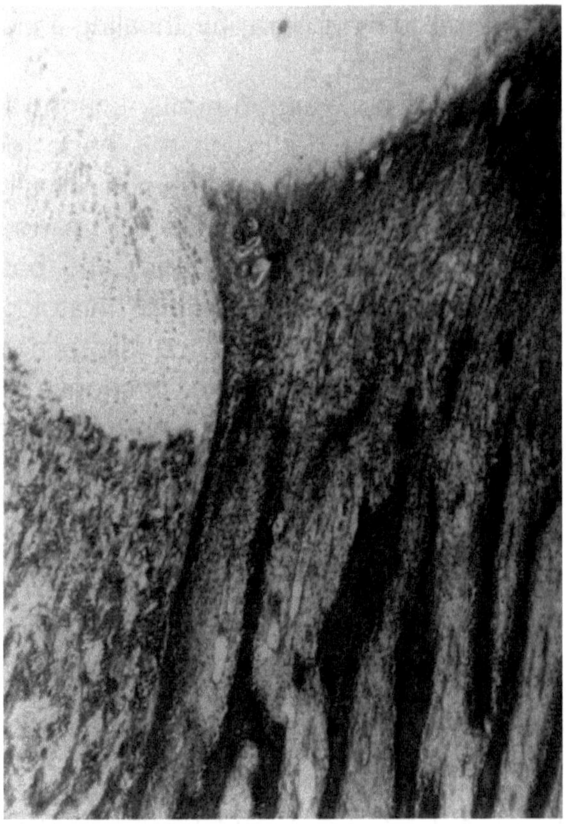

Figure 3.2. The proximal tibial growth plate in young canine demonstrates the two major pathways of bone formation: indirect via enchondral sequence from the cartilaginous physis (upper left) and direct via periosteal stretching (along the right) with intramembranous ossification into primary bone columns identical to distraction osteogenesis (×4, H&E).

Delloye et al. (21) and Yasui et al. (22) have examined the importance of preservation of blood supply in performing the osteotomy. By locally inhibiting either the medullary blood supply, the cortical blood supply, or the periosteal blood supply, these investigators have demonstrated that the periosteum is probably the most important structure for successful regeneration of bone.

In both experimental and clinical cases where distraction osteogensis failed, histologic preparations demonstrated that lack of local blood supply inhibited the process. Each bone surface that is being distracted must contain viable osteocytes in the bony lacunae with an intact blood supply in order to initiate and perpetuate the distraction osteogenesis process. Although it is not mandatory to perform the classical corticotomy, certain techniques such as the use of the oscillating saw, which can create thermal necrosis of bone, should be avoided in order to maximize the available blood supply to both surfaces.

In another series of experiments, the importance of the latency period for distraction osteogensis was tested. It was hypothesized that different latency periods would be optimal, depending on where the bone was broken, comparing metaphyseal to diaphyseal sites in the adult canine tibia. It was found that premature consolidation of the cut metaphyseal bone surfaces was predictable whether following a 14-day or a 21-day latency period. Even at the diaphyseal site, a 21-day latency was too long in 50% of the animals. Of the four latency periods tested (0, 7, 14, and 21 days), contrary to other findings (23), the most reliable bone production occurred after a 0-day latency in both metaphyseal and diaphyseal groups, a finding indicating that a latency may not be necessary (24).

Different rates of distraction have been tested to find the optimal range for the rate of distraction. In patients undergoing angular lengthening for deformity, the distraction osteogenesis zone follows a radial pattern (Figure 3.3), in order that bone formation must necessarily occur at different rates (4). Based upon the experimental evidence, distraction osteogenesis can occur at rates from 0.5 to 2 mm per day; however, 1 mm per day is optimal. At 2 mm a day, a 15% metaphyseal lengthening eventually bridged after some delay. This accelerated rate is not recommended, however, for less metabolically active regions, such as the diaphysis. A

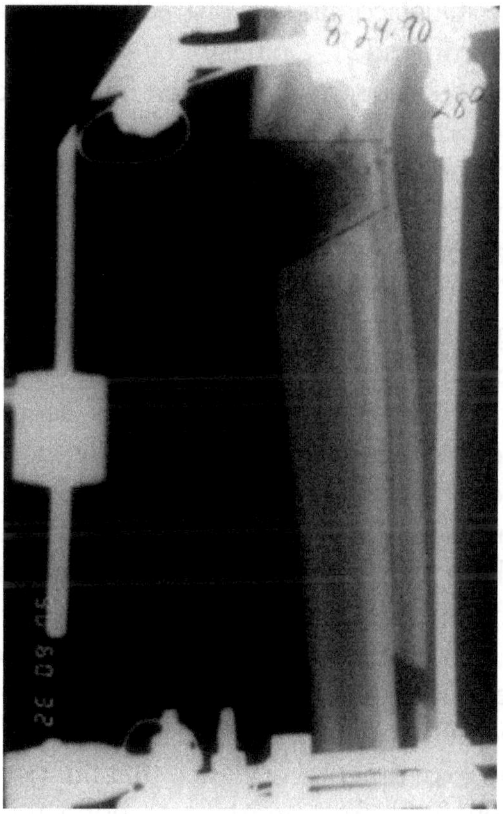

Figure 3.3. Lateral radiograph of a proximal tibia in an adolescent male undergoing angular distraction osteogenesis to correct shortening and a recurvatum deformity. The triangular zone of new bone (28°) had to form at different rates of distraction.

rate of 0.5 mm a day may be acceptable in diaphyseal bone, but may be too slow for metaphyseal bone, risking premature consolidation.

The rhythm of distraction, as recommended by Ilizarov, is 0.25 mm four times a day (1,2,25). The experimental work demonstrated that sporadic rhythms seemed to inhibit bone formation. However, it was possible to create successful distraction osteogenesis at a rhythm of two increments a day in animal models, including the dog, rabbit, and rat. For shorter distraction gaps, other investigators have produced adequate distraction osteogenesis at a rhythm of once a day.

Quasicontinuous distraction has been recommended, initially by Ilizarov (2) and subsequently by other investigators. Motorized distraction devices have been produced, but the experimental proof of improved osteogenesis remains limited to Ilizarov's own experiments (1,25).

Stable fixation is important for adequate formation of microcolumns of bone during distraction osteogenesis (Figure 3.4). Bending or shear forces seem to induce fractures of the microcolumns with local hemorrhage and resultant histologic cartilage interposition. Stable fixation, which allows controlled axial compression or distraction, is optimal (26).

Successful distraction osteogenesis has been demonstrated over an intramedullary nail (27,28). This is based on the experimental evidence that the periosteum is more important to bone formation, especially in the diaphyseal region. The intramedullary nail seems to increase the stability of the distracted segments and has real potential for providing an internal distraction method, which would obviate the need for external fixation pins or wires.

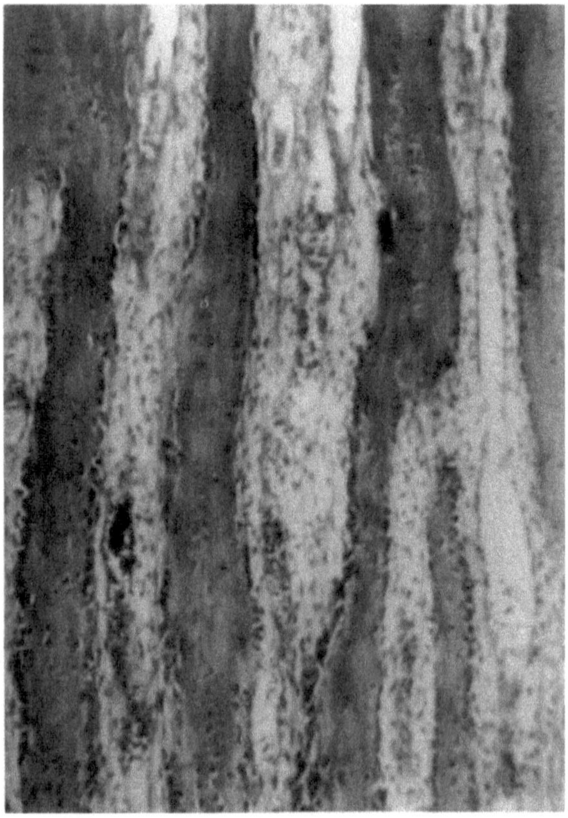

Figure 3.4. Uniform microcolumns of new bone bridge the distraction gap from each cut bone surface, each separated and surrounded by fibrovascular tissue. (Canine tibial lengthening, ×10, H&E).

Different external fixation frames have been used to create distraction osteogenesis (29). The Ilizarov device is a ring external fixator that utilizes tensioned transosseous wires in multiple planes for fixation (30,31). This type of modular system is constructed based on the biomechanical requirements for each case. It allows for multiplanar mechanical correction, including axial distraction, angular distraction, translation, and rotation. It also permits the frame to be built across joints to adjacent limb segments for both multifocal treatment and protection of the joint cartilage from joint compression forces (arthrodiastasis) (29). As long as the wire tension is maintained by adequate friction fit of the fixation bolts to the rings and an appropriate distribution of wires is achieved for each bone segment, this system is quite stable and well suited for distraction osteogenesis (30,31). Several biomechanical studies have demonstrated that tensioned wires have a self-stiffening effect such that deflection of the wire increases its stiffness (17,30,31).

Half-pin, uniplanar, monolateral, external fixation devices are commercially available. These devices are user-friendly but rely on cantilever loading of the bone with asymmetrical stiffness in different planes (18,29). Internal fixation devices, such as special unicortical plates or intramedullary nails, have also been devised and used, creating successful distraction osteogenesis.

CAUSES OF DISTRACTION FAILURE

Distraction osteogenesis can fail in at least four ways: (1) ischemic fibrogenesis (with failure of mineralization); (2) cystic degeneration; (3) fibrocartilage nonunion; and (4) late buckling, bending, or fracture of the regenerate bone.

Ischemic fibrogenesis occurs from inadequate local blood supply during distraction. Although fibrous tissue forms in the distraction gap, it appears loose and bone columns do not form from the avascular host bone surfaces (Figure 3.5).

Cystic degeneration seems to occur when there is blockage of venous outflow from the system. The large vascular channels contain a fluid more like lymph than blood, and the distraction gap is filled either completely, or in part, with a cystic cavity and cyst-like fluid (Figure 3.6).

Fibrocartilage nonunion occurs usually with unstable external fixation where microfractures, hemorrhage, and cartilage interposition occurs (Figure 3.7).

Buckling or bending of the regenerate bone occurs when the fixation device is destabilized or removed prematurely. Plain radiography is helpful to determine the maturity of the regenerate bone. If the

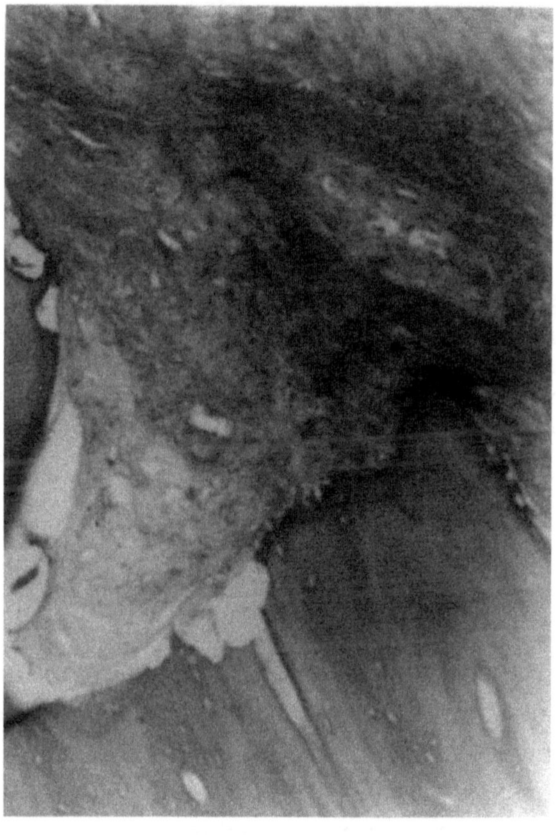

Figure 3.5. A zone of ischemic fibrosis in a failed distraction osteogenesis between avascular bone ends. The empty lacunae are from an attempted bone transportation in a sclerotic proximal tibia. The patient had cavitary osteomyelitis that healed by transporting a different, well-vascularized segment in a subsequent procedure (×10, H&E).

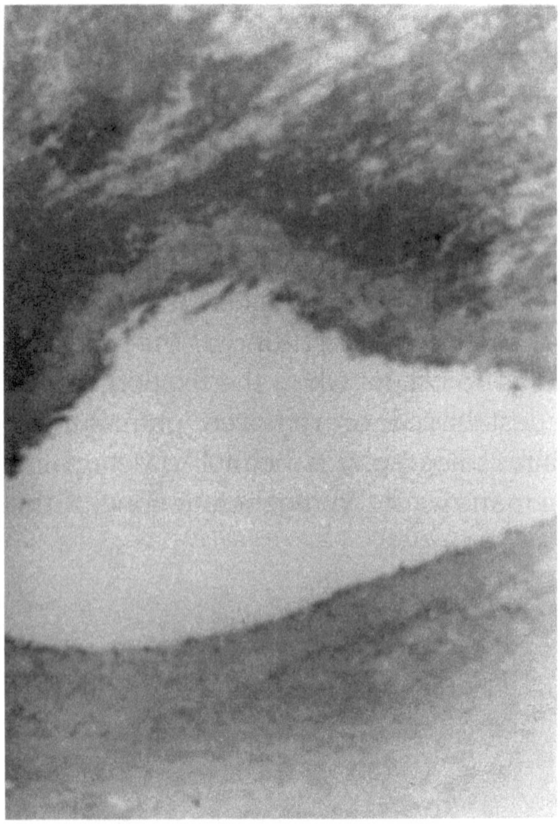

Figure 3.6. Cystic degeneration in an adult male during proximal tibial lengthening to correct a post-traumatic, infected nonunion. He developed swelling with reduced venous outflow associated with a preexisting dysvascular limb (multiple scars, free flap, and skin grafts). The cyst was removed and bone grafted. (×4, H&E).

new bone has a radiodensity equivalent to the host bone surfaces and a macrostructure resembling that of host bone with an equivalent cross-sectional area and the formation of cortex and a medullary canal, the fixator can be removed.

Certain types of external fixators allow for "dynamization," where the fixator itself can be selectively destabilized to allow for axial compression of the distraction gap while resisting bending or shear forces. Trials of weightbearing with the dynamized fixator can then be carried out, with radiographic follow-up to measure the distraction gap. By this trial method, relative gap stiffness can be determined prior to device removal. Experiments are in progress to utilize in-line strain gauges to measure the actual stiffness of the distracted segment (32,33).

Quantitative computed tomography (CT) scans measure the relative bone density and the cross-sectional geometry of the new bone. Quantitative CT scans have

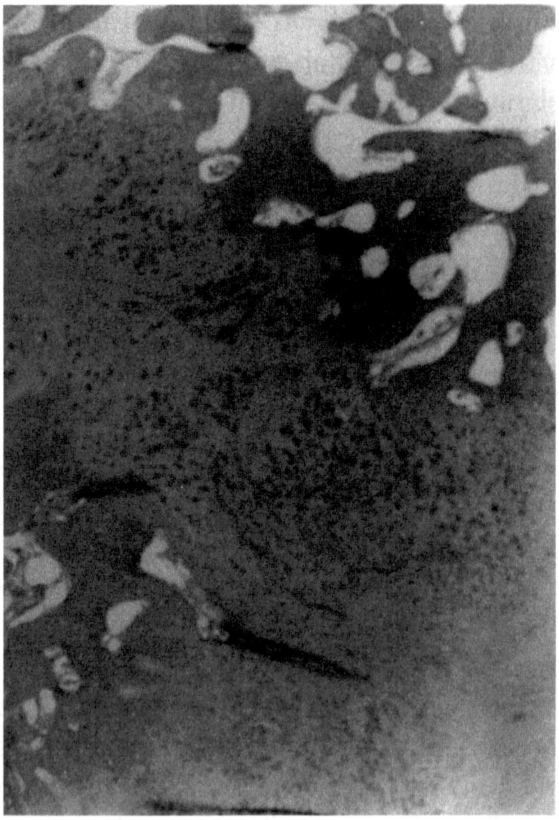

Figure 3.7. Unstable external fixation in a canine tibial lengthening led to disruption of the new bony microcolumns with fibrocartilage replacement leading to nonunion (×4, H&E).

been moderately successful in predicting the strength of the new bone both experimentally and clinically (34,35).

CLINICAL APPLICATIONS

In the first one hundred cases, 70 patients were children and 30 were adults (over 17 years of age). The age of the patients ranged from 18 months to 49 years.

In order of descending frequency, the anatomic segments that have been treated include: 62 tibiae, 30 femora, 24 feet, 6 humeri, 6 ulnae, 5 radii, 4 hands, and 2 iliac crests. Initially, monolateral frames with half-pins were used in ten cases. However, the majority of patients have undergone ring fixation for more complex treatment and three-dimensional mechanical control.

In the 100 cases, more than 1000 pins were used with none resulting in osteomyelitis, although 10% demonstrated evidence of pin tract inflammation. Some of the patients required antibiotics for soft tissue infection.

The cases included the following applications: 87 lengthenings, 76 deformity corrections (66 bony, 10 soft tissue), 40 arthrodiastasis (36), 17 nonunion treatment, 9 bone transportations, and 4 acute fracture care. The lengthenings were mainly carried out in the tibia, followed by the femur, forearm, and foot.

Bifocal lengthenings, where the bone is lengthened at two sites simultaneously, were most successful in the tibia. In this manner, 1 mm of distraction was carried out at each of two sites for 2 mm of lengthening a day. The healing index overall, for bifocal tibial lengthenings, was approximately 25% faster than for monofocal lengthening.

The healing index in the 70 children was measured at 0.87 months (26 days) per cm of new bone treatment time. Adults took longer, healing at 1.5 months (47 days) per cm. The healing index can be translated into a rate of bone growth measured at 385 μm a day in children and at 213 μm a day in adults. These growth rates fell between the growth rates of the adolescent distal femur at 50 μm a day and the fetal femur at 400 μm a day.

The longest lengthenings measured in centimeters and in percentage of the original bone length were performed in the forearm of patients with the radial deficiency syndrome. The congenitally short, one-bone (the ulna) forearm has been lengthened in two patients by more than 100% of the original bone length, totaling 10 to 11 cm of new bone formation, without adverse sequelae (Figure 3.8).

The longest bone regeneration by distraction osteogenesis for a given limb was 18 cm of new bone produced during bone transportation. The patient was a 30-year-old mother of two who had undergone replacement of her distal femur with an allograft for a recurrent giant cell tumor. Bone transportation was carried out after resection of the failed allograft. The 18-cm gap between her remaining femur and proximal tibia was bridged with the ring external fixation frame from the hip to the ankle utilizing an intermedullary rod for further stability.

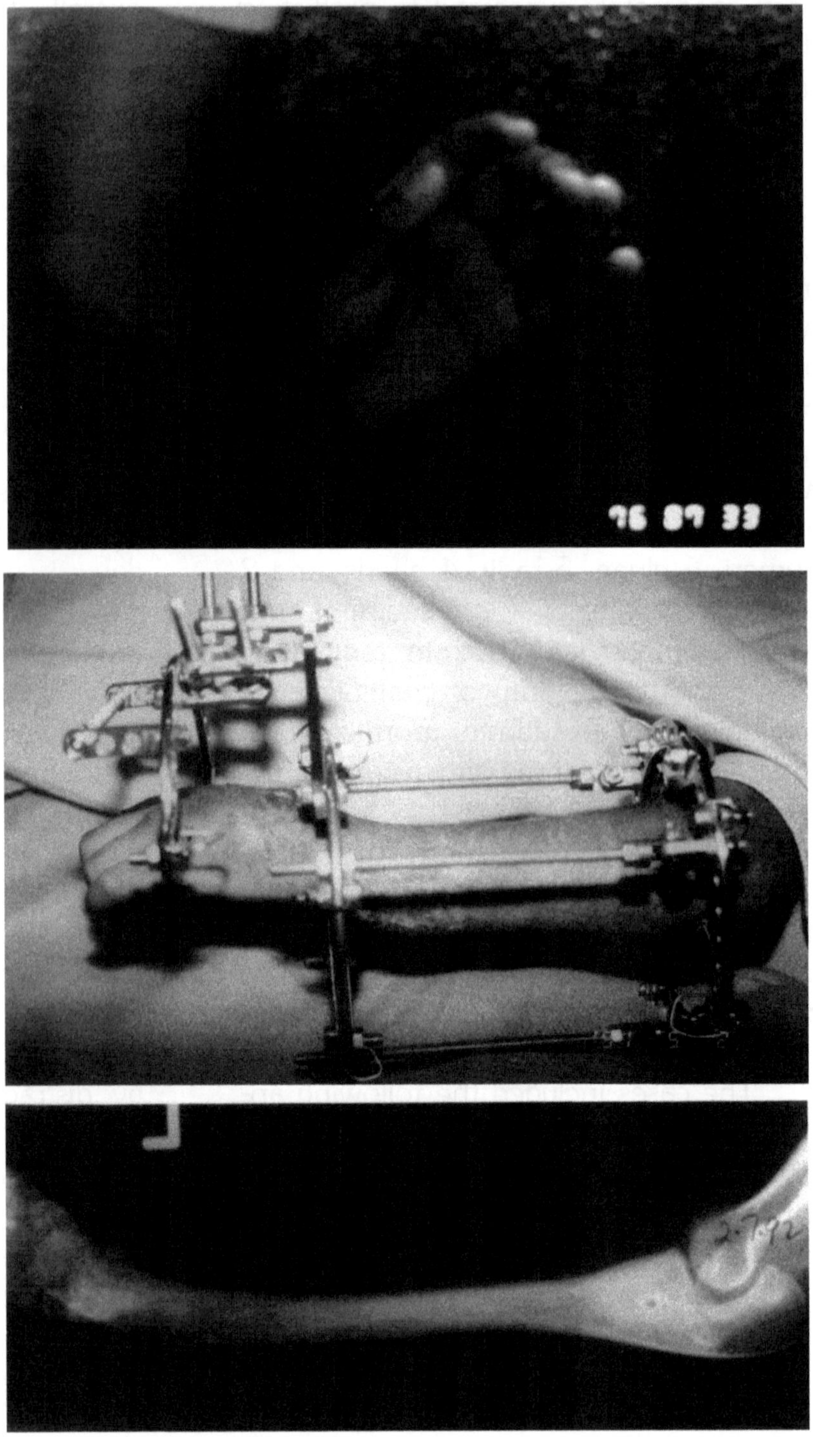

A

B

C

Figure 3.8. Clinical example of lengthening of the forearm by 10 cm (100%). (A). Preoperative radial clubhand with a shortened ulna and radially deviated hand. (B). After distraction is complete, the bone must consolidate. The hand is held by a separate half-ring; the forearm, now 100% longer, is held by two full rings and four threaded rods. (C). The newly lengthened ulna appears solid with normal bone size, shape, and density following device removal.

Bone transportation was carried out at two sites; the distal end of the residual femur was distracted toward the knee while the proximal end of the remaining tibia was also distracted toward the knee. The two transport segments of bone met at the new knee joint where they fused by transformation osteogenesis supplemented by local bone grafting. The treatment time for this patient's massive bone regeneration was 1 year. She is continuing to do well at 2-year follow-up.

The greatest number of osteogenic foci in one limb was five, as achieved in several patients. For example, one patient underwent simultaneous correction of a deformity in the proximal femur, lengthening of the distal femur, lengthening at the proximal tibia, lengthening at the distal tibia, and lengthening of the foot. At the same time, the knee and ankle joints were protected by hinge connections of the frame so that, in essence, seven foci of treatment were carried out simultaneously (Figure 3.9).

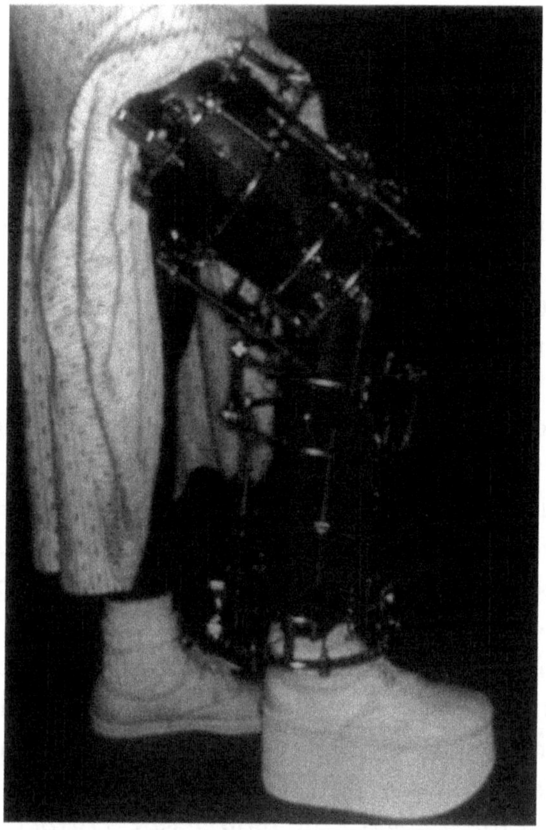

Figure 3.9. Congenitally short femur and tibia undergoing simultaneous lengthening after acute correction of the deformity. The knee is protected from excessive forces by a distraction hinge, allowing movement and weightbearing. The built-up shoe has layers that are removable as the limb is progressively lengthened.

Hypertrophic nonunions of bone have been successfully treated by primary distraction to restimulate active bone formation, followed by compression at the same site in order to bridge a long-standing nonunion with new bone. More commonly, however, nonunions were atrophic with a dysvascular soft tissue interposition. Like chronic osteomyelitis, the focus of hypovascular soft tissue was surgically removed prior to treatment with the Ilizarov device. The freshened bone surfaces were then acutely opposed with compression by the device while the bone was lengthened at a distant site to accommodate the overall bone loss. This form of bifocal treatment is similar to that used in bone transportation. Cases of cavitary osteomyelitis have been successfully treated by transporting a vascularized piece of cortex across the cortical defect to reestablish a true medullary canal (7).

Overall, 105 sites of distraction osteogenesis were evaluated in this series of patients (excluding the fibula, which in some cases was purposefully resected to prevent premature consolidation). Ninety-seven healed primarily by spontaneous bone formation, while eight required bone grafts. Four of the eight underwent cystic degeneration, which required excision of the cyst and insertion of a bone graft, while the other four failed to mineralize the fibrous matrix. Three additional sites of transformation osteogenesis also required bone grafting. All of the 11 failures of spontaneous bone formation were successfully bridged by secondary bone autografts.

Complications included pain, to some degree, in all 100 patients during distraction (37). Ninety-five patients experienced at least one site of pin inflammation. Eleven patients had problems with bone formation requiring bone grafting. Nine patients experienced late deformity of the new bone; six were residual or incomplete corrections of deformity, while three patients experienced bending of the regenerate bone from premature removal of the device. All nine cases corrected with repeat application of the device. Joint contracture occurred in seven patients, most commonly at the knee and ankle. Neuropraxia occurred in three patients, all of whom recovered. All patients regained baseline muscle strength.

Pain was most severe during foot lengthenings or extended bony lengthenings beyond five centimeters. The pain was generally controlled with low-grade analgesics and mild narcotics. All cases of pin inflammation resolved with local pin care, oral antibiotics and, in three patients, parenteral antibiotics.

CONCLUSION

Distraction osteogenesis is a reliable method for regeneration of bone deficiencies; the technique depends upon the local blood supply, stable fixation, and gradual stretching. Different devices that provide stable fixation (eg, external fixators, plates, intramedullary nails) can propagate distraction osteogenesis and, therefore, allow for creative applications to areas such as the facial bones. The principles of preservation of blood supply, close apposition of cut bone surfaces to allow early bridge formation, and gradual distraction at regular rhythm allow successful application of this method to most skeletal structures. The surrounding soft tissues remain as the primary obstacles to this method, although a small percentage of these cases require bone grafting for failure of osteogenesis.

References

1. Ilizarov GA. The tension-stress effect on the genesis and growth of tissues. Part I. The influence of stability of fixation and soft-tissue preservation. *Clin Orthop* 238:249–281, 1989a.
2. Ilizarov GA. *Transosseous Osteosynthesis—Theoretical and Clinical Aspects of the Regeneration and Growth of Tissue*. New York: Springer-Verlag, 1992.
3. Martini Z, Castaman E. Tissue regeneration of lost bone and soft tissue in lower limbs: a preliminary report. *Br J Plast Surg* 40:142–148, 1987.
4. Aronson J, Harrison B, Stewart C. The histology of distraction osteogenesis using different external fixators. *Clin Orthop* 241:106–116, 1989.
5. Aronson J, Johnson E, Harp J. Local bone transportation for intercalary defects by the Ilizarov technique. *Clin Orthop* 243:71–79, 1989.
6. Catagni M. Classification and treatment of nonunion. In: Bianchi Maiocchi A, Aronson J, eds. *Operative principles of Ilizarov—Fracture Treatment, Nonunion, Osteomyelitis, Lengthening, Deformity Correction*. Baltimore: Williams & Wilkins, 1991.

7. Aronson J, Harp J. Cavitary osteomyelitis treated by partial cortical transport. *Clin Orthop* 280:153–159, 1992a.
8. Dal Monte A, Donzelli O. Tibial lengthening according to Ilizarov in congenital hypoplasia of the leg. *J Pediatr Orthop* 7:135–138, 1987.
9. Paley D. Current techniques of limb lengthening. *J Pediatr Orthop* 8:73–92, 1988.
10. Styazhkin N. Surgeon Ilizarov and his method. *Australas Nurses J* 2:8, 1973.
11. Liberman SB, Semenova VD. Investigation of the strength and rigidity of Kirschner spokes in the apparatus of G.A. Ilizarov. *Biomed Mater Eng* (NY) 7:226–227, 1974.
12. Fishbane BM, Riley LH. Continuous transphyseal traction: a simple method of bone lengthening. *Johns Hopkins Med J* 138:79–81, 1976.
13. Alho A, Bang G, Karaharju E, Armond I. Filling of a bone defect during experimental osteotaxis distraction. *Acta Orthop Scand* 53:29–34, 1982.
14. Aronson J. The biology of mechanical distraction osteogenesis. In: Bianchi Maiocchi A, Aronson J, eds. *Operative Principles of Ilizarov—Fracture Treatment, Nonunion, Osteomyelitis, Lengthening, Deformity Correction.* Baltimore: Williams & Wilkins, 1991.
15. Bianchi Maiocchi A, Aronson J. Indications. In: Bianchi Maiocchi A, Aronson J, eds. *Operative principles of Ilizarov—Fracture Treatment, Nonunion, Osteomyelitis, Lengthening, Deformity Correction.* Baltimore: Williams & Wilkins, 1991.
16. Aronson J, Harrison B. Mechanical induction of osteogenesis: preliminary studies. *Ann Clin Lab Sci* 18:195–203, 1988.
17. Aronson J, Harrison B, Cannon DJ, Lubansky HJ. Mechanical induction of osteogenesis: the importance of pin rigidity. *J Pediatr Orthop* 8:396–401, 1988.
18. Price CT, Cole JD. Limb lengthening by callotasis for children and adolescents: early experience. *Clin Orthop* 250:105–111, 1990.
19. Aronson J. The biology of distraction osteogenesis. In: Chapman MW, ed. *Operative Orthopaedics.* Philadelphia: JB Lippincott, 1993.
20. Aronson J. Temporal and spatial increases in blood flow during distraction osteogenesis. *Clin Orthop* 301:124–131, 1993b.
21. Delloye C, Delefortrie G, Coutelier L, Vincent A. Bone regenerate formation in cortical bone during distraction lengthening: an experimental study. *Clin Orthop* 250:34–42, 1990.
22. Yasui N, Kojimoto H, Shimizu H, Shimomura Y. The effects of distraction upon bone, muscle and periosteum. *Orthop Clin North Am* 22:563–567, 1991.
23. White SH, Kenwright J. The importance of delay in distraction osteotomies. *Orthop Clin North Am* 22:569–579, 1991.
24. Aronson J, Shen X. Experimental healing of distraction osteogenesis comparing metaphyseal to diaphyseal sites. *Clin Orthop* 301:25–30, 1993.
25. Ilizarov GA. The tension-stress effect on the genesis and growth of tissues. Part II. The influence of the rate and frequency of distraction. *Clin Orthop* 239:263–285, 1989b.
26. Paley D, Fleming B, Catagni M, Kristiansen T, Pope M. Mechanical evaluation of external fixators used in limb lengthening. *Clin Orthop* 250:50–57, 1990.
27. Cole JD, Morandi M, Price CT. Extremity lengthening and bone transport over an intramedullary nail. American Academy of Orthopaedic Surgeons Final Program, 1993 (Abstract).
28. Paley D, Goulet JA, Herzenberg JE, Maab DC, Tetsworth K. Femoral lengthening over intramedullary rods. American Academy of Orthopaedic Surgeons Final Program, 1993 (Abstract).
29. Aronson J. Factors influencing the choice of external fixation for distraction osteogensis. In: Barr JJ Jr., ed. *Instructional Course Lectures.* Vol. 38. Park Ridge, IL: American Academy of Orthopaedic Surgeons, 1989.
30. Aronson J. Proper wire tensioning for Ilizarov external fixation. *Tech Orthop* 5:27–32, 1990.
31. Aronson J, Harp J. Mechanical considerations in using tensioned wires in a

transosseous external fixation system. *Clin Orthop* 280:23–29, 1992b.

32. Wolfson N, Hearn TC, Thomason JJ, Armstrong PF. Force and stiffness changes during Iliazov leg lengthening. *Clin Orthop* 250:58–60, 1990.
33. Aronson J, Harp J. Mechanical forces as predictors of healing during tibial lengthening by distraction osteogenesis. *Clin Orthop* 301: 73–79, 1993.
34. Aronson J, Good B, Stewart C, Harrison B. Preliminary studies of mineralization during distraction osteogenesis. *Clin Orthop* 250:43–49, 1990.
35. Aronson J, Harp J. Noninvasive determination of bone stiffness for distraction osteogenesis by quantitative computed tomography scan. *Clin Orthop* 301:42–48, 1993.
36. Grill F, Franke J. The Ilizarov distractor for the correction of relapsed or neglected clubfoot. *J Bone Joint Surg Br* 69B:593–597, 1987.
37. Paley D. Problems, obstacles and complications of limb lengthening by the Ilizarov technique. *Clin Orthop* 250:81–104, 1990.

Part 2

The Mandible

CHAPTER 4

Distraction of the Mandible

Experimental Studies

Paul M. Glat and Joseph G. McCarthy

The surgical technique of distraction osteogenesis has long been used in the reconstruction of defects of the long bones of the extremities. The technique has only recently become popular in surgical reconstruction of the craniofacial skeleton. In the plastic surgery literature, the mandible is the anatomic site that has received the most attention, both in experimental and human models.

The majority of the early experimental work in membranous bone lengthening was performed in the mandible. The first report of experimental distraction of the craniofacial skeleton was reported by Snyder and associates in 1973 (1). After creating a crossbite by removing a 1.5-cm segment of the canine mandible, they distracted the mandible back to its original length by using a modified external fixator device. Following a one-week delay after the osteotomy, the bone was distracted at the rate of 1 mm/day for 14 days. Fixation was maintained for an additional 6 weeks.

This concept was next applied in 1977 by Michieli and Miotti in Italy (2). The investigators performed a unilateral osteotomy in the canine mandible in order to create an anterior crossbite. The mandible was lengthened 15 mm at a rate of 0.5 mm/day followed by 40 days of fixation. Microscopic evaluation showed active formation of new cortical bone at the site of lengthening. Of note, this study utilized an intraoral distraction device (as compared to the extraoral device of Snyder and his group).

The next application of this technique did not appear in the literature until 1990. Karp and his associates at New York University performed a unilateral angular osteotomy in the canine mandible (Figure 4.1) (3). After 10 days of external fixation, the mandible was distracted at the rate of 1 mm/day for 20 days and then held in fixation for 56 days. Fluorochrome labels of oxytetracycline (30 mg/kg), xylenol orange (80 mg/kg), and alizarin complexone (20 mg/kg) were administered. All dogs demonstrated evidence of a crossbite after distraction as well as an increase in the height of the mandibular ramus on the operated side (Figure 4.2). On histologic evaluation, the zone of distraction showed new cortical bone, which was less organized and had larger vascular channels than the control bone.

In order to understand better what was occurring microscopically, a follow-up study by the same group at New York University serially examined the histology of the distraction zone (4). The same canine mandible model was employed. The bone was harvested after 10 and 20 days of distraction, as well as at 14, 28, and 56 days after the completion of distraction. The histologic study demonstrated early new bone formation at the periphery of the radiolucent distraction zone. The new bone spicules were oriented in the direction of distraction (Figure 4.3). By 8 weeks of fixation, the entire distraction zone was bridged with new bone (Figure 4.4). In the early stages of distraction, the gap was occupied by fibrous tissue. After 10 days of distraction, the new tissue (collagen fibers) in the distraction gap was oriented in the direction of the distraction forces (Figure 4.5). By 14 days after distraction, osteoclastic resorption of bone was evident, indicating remodeling of the new trabeculae (Figure 4.6). The new trabeculae eventually coalesced to reestablish bony continuity, usually by 28 days. Continued remodeling led to an increased amount of more mature lamellar bone, approaching that of normal cortical bone. The authors did not find evidence of cartilage present as a precursor stage to bone formation, in contrast to the findings in long-bone distraction.

In summary, there were four stages in

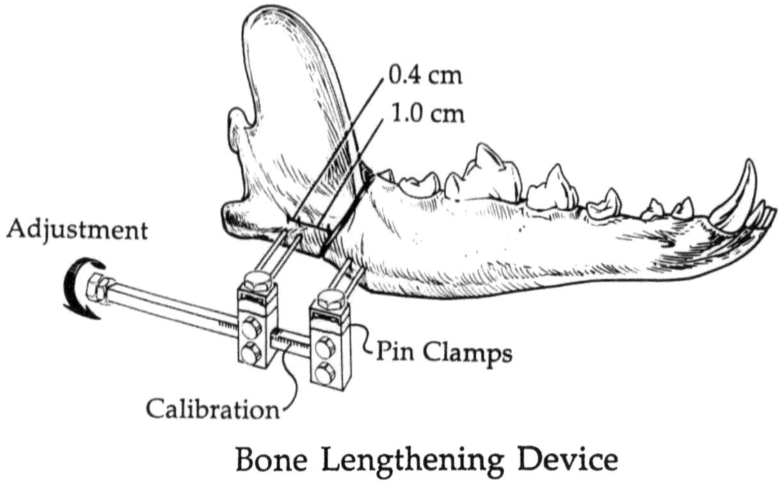

Figure 4.1. Drawing demonstrating the canine model and the site of osteotomy with the bone distraction device in place. Reprinted with permission from *Ann Plast Surg* 24: 232, 1990.

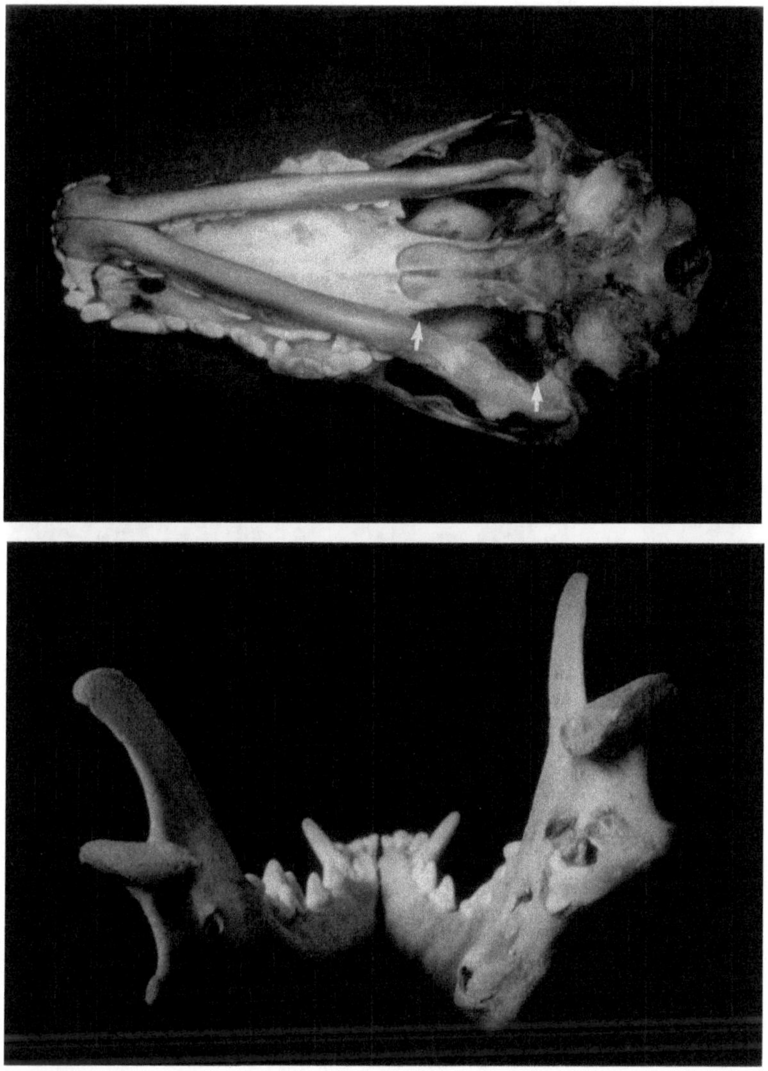

A

B

Figure 4.2. Gross pathological canine specimen. The site of distraction is located between the arrows. (A) Ventral view of articulated specimen demonstrating the increase in the length of the body of the mandible on the operated side. Note the associated crossbite. Reprinted with permission from *Ann Plast Surg* 24:233, 1990. (B) Posterior view of disarticulated specimen showing an increase in the length of the body and the height of the ramus of the operated side of the mandible compared with the unoperated side. Reprinted with permission from *Ann Plast Surg* 24:233, 1990.

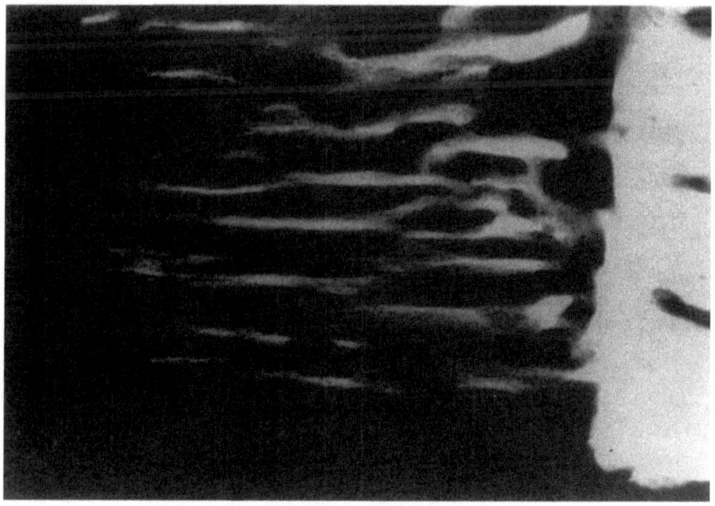

Figure 4.3. Microradiograph (original magnification, undecalcified specimen) demonstrating slender bone trabeculae extending from the divided surface of the cortical bone (seen on the right). After 10 days of distraction, note that the new bone spicules are oriented in the direction of the vector of distraction. Reprinted with permission from *Ann Plast Surg* 29:4, 1992.

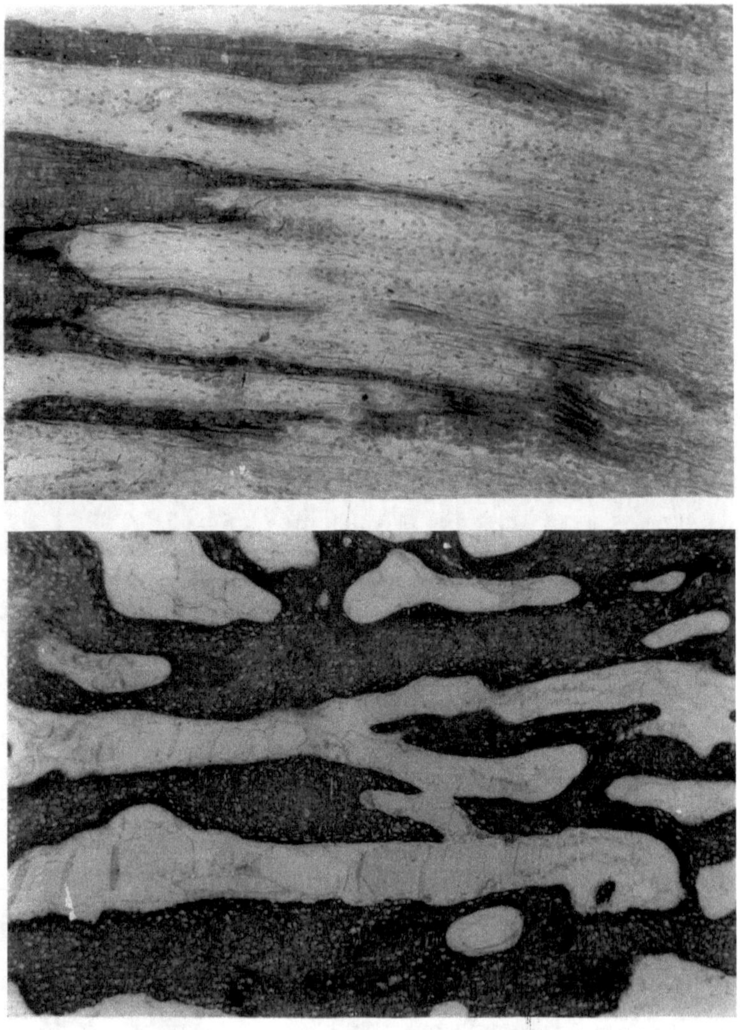

A

B

Figure 4.4. (A) Fifty-six days after the completion of distraction. Dense cortical bone has bridged the gap between the distracted bone ends. (Microradiograph, original magnification ×92). Reprinted with permission from *Ann Plast Surg* 29:6, 1992. (B) Fifty-six days after distraction, the histologic appearance of the specimen demonstrates dense cortical bone. Undecalcified specimen. (Masson stain, original magnification ×92). Reprinted with permission from *Ann Plast Surg* 29:6, 1992.

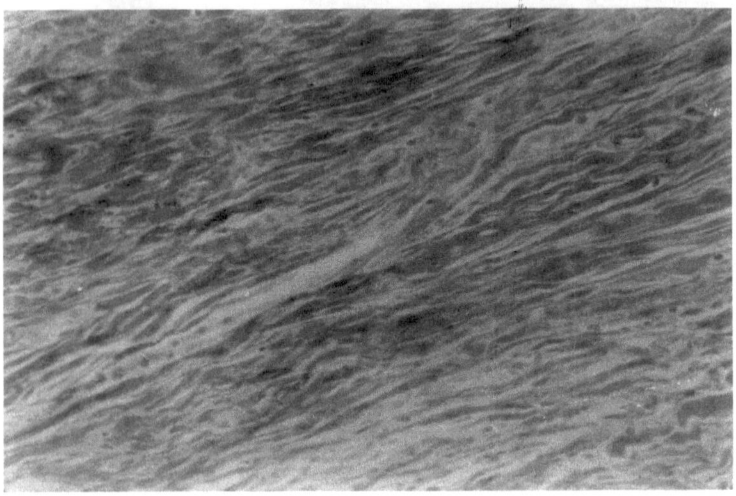

Figure 4.5. Ten days after distraction. The collagen fibers are preferentially oriented in the direction of distraction. Undecalcified section. (Original magnification ×183). Reprinted with permission from *Ann Plast Surg* 29:6, 1992.

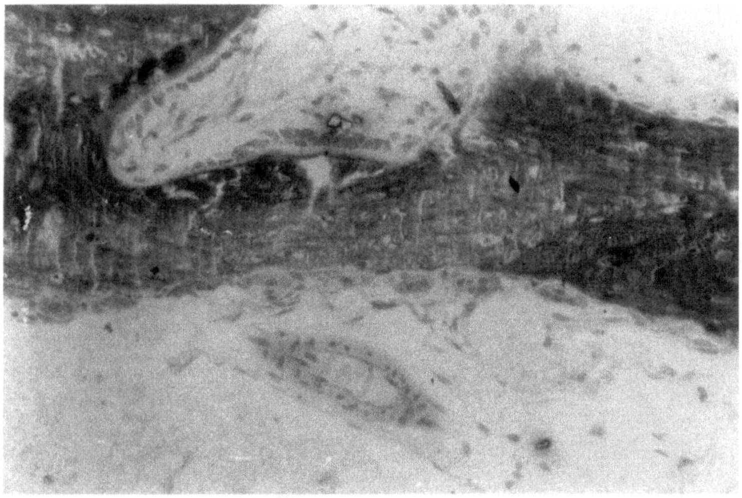

Figure 4.6. Fourteen days after distraction. Osteoclastic resorption can be seen on the surfaces of the bone trabeculae. Note the multinucleated osteoclasts. Undecalcified section. (Masson stain; original magnification ×235). Reprinted with permission from *Ann Plast Surg* 29:6, 1992.

the development of the bony regenerate (Figure 4.7):

1. The "stage of fibrous tissue" consisting of highly organized, longitudinally oriented parallel strands of collagen with spindle-shaped fibroblasts and undifferentiated mesenchymal precursor cells throughout the matrix.

2. The "stage of extending bone formation" in which fibroblasts and undifferentiated precursor cells of the matrix were in continuity with osteoblasts. The osteoblasts had a longitudinal orientation. The osteoblasts arose from transformed spindle-shaped fibroblastic cells located between the collagen bundles.

3. The "stage of bone remodeling" consisting of advancing fields of bone resorption and apposition. There were increased numbers of osteoclasts.

4. The "stage of mature bone" in which compact cortical bone was located adjacent to the mature bone in the nondistracted areas. The bone spicules were thicker and less longitudinal than in the remodeling stage.

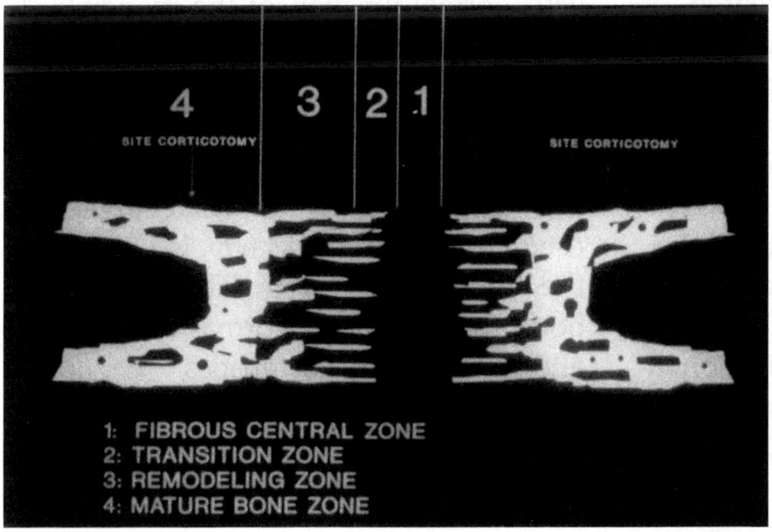

Figure 4.7. Schematic of the stages of formation of the bone regenerate in distraction. (1) Central Zone of Fibrous Tissue. (2) Transition Zone of Extending Bone Formation. (3) Bone Remodeling Zone. (4) Mature Bone Zone. Reprinted with permission from *Ann Plast Surg* 29:6, 1992.

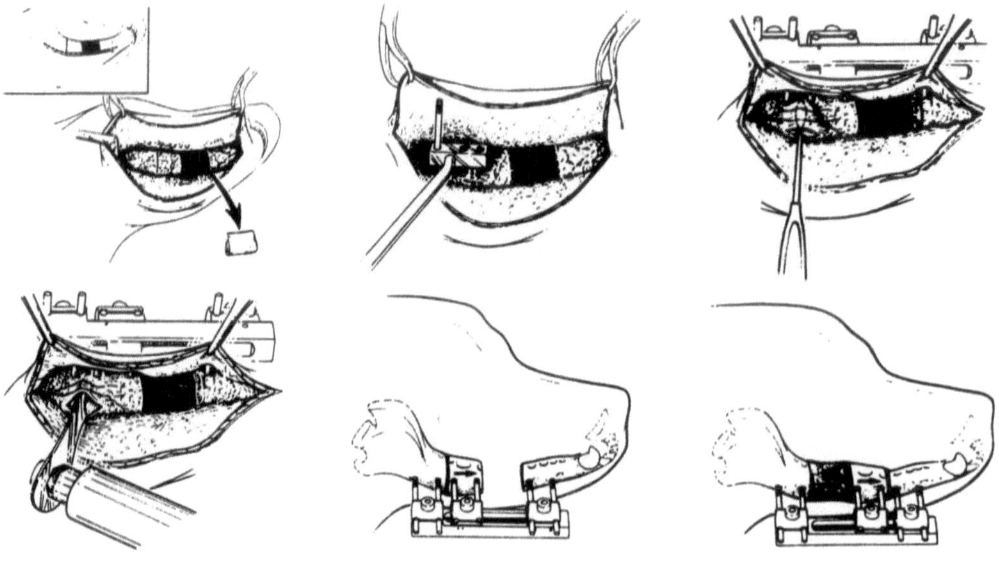

Figure 4.8. Technique demonstrating bifocal (transport) osteogenesis. Top left, Exposure of the mandibular body with preservation of the surrounding soft tissue and periosteum. Shaded region shows where the segmental defect will be created. Top center, Placement of the drill template and bicortical pins. Top right, Circumferential elevation of the periosteum off the mandible where the transport disk osteotomy will be made. With the distraction appliance in place, the segmental defect was created. Bottom left, Placement of the osteotomy with an oscillating saw. Bottom center, Device in place. Bottom right, Early bone regenerate formation between the transport disk and the proximal stump. Arrow indicates direction of movement of the transport disk during distraction. At the completion of distraction, the transport disk is in contact with the distal mandibular stump and the segmental defect is filed with regenerate. Reprinted with permission from *Arch Otolaryngol Head Neck Surg* 116:538, 1990. Copyright 1990–94, American Medical Association.

Costantino and associates reported an experimental model of segmental mandibular regeneration by distraction osteogenesis (5). In a canine model, a 2.5-cm segmental mandibular defect was created. The defect was filled with regenerate bone in 25 days at the rate of 1.0 mm/day by using bifocal distraction ("transport") osteogenesis. This technique involves the use of a transport disk of bone, in this case 1.5 cm in width, which was distracted across the mandibular defect (Figure 4.8). The authors began distraction 10 days after the creation of the defect. Fixation was maintained for 4 weeks. The new bone was evaluated histologically by H&E and trichrome stains. It was found to consist of partially calcified woven bone in all specimens. Various stages of maturity were found within the same specimen. All animals developed stable regenerate bone with normal function of the mandible. In 1993 Costantino and his associates reported a follow-up of their original study, reporting the one-year results after bifocal distraction (transport) osteogenesis (6). The same methods of distraction were used as in the original study. In all animals, the bone defects were filled with stable bone that exhibited normal macroscopic and histologic characteristics.

Karaharju-Suvanto and Karaharju, in 1990, applied the technique of distraction osteogenesis to the mandible of sheep

(7). A unilateral osteotomy was made in the ramus, fixation applied for 5 days and distraction performed from 0.5 to 1.5 mm/day for 16 days. New bone was demonstrated 25 days after cessation of distraction.

In 1993 Block and his colleagues described the changes that occur in the inferior alveolar nerve after unilateral distraction of the canine mandible (8). After osteotomy, one week of fixation (latency) was maintained, followed by distraction at the rate of 1.0 mm/day. Inferior alveolar nerve function was assessed by measuring jaw-jerk reflex testing. There was no difference in these measurements when compared to control. On histologic examination, the distracted nerves showed a 9.1% incidence of Wallerian degeneration of the large nerve fibers and a 15.9% incidence of degeneration of the small fibers, a significant increase over controls. There were small areas of demyelination, axonal swelling, and axoplasmic darkening, findings indicative of mild nerve injury.

In 1994 Annino and colleagues used trifocal distraction (using two transport disks) around an arc in order to reconstruct mandibular symphyseal defects in a canine model (Figure 4.9) (9). Distraction was initiated on postoperative day 11 and it proceeded at the rate of 1 mm/day. It was discontinued when the two transport disks met in the midline (Figure 4.10). Fixation was maintained for 35 to 47 days. On histologic examination, there was evidence of membranous bone formation oriented in columns directly parallel to the force of distraction. This study demonstrated the ability to perform distraction osteogenesis around an arc, with an incremental gain of 4.5 to 5.5 cm of bone, thereby allowing recreation of the symphyseal region of the mandible in all anatomic dimensions.

In 1994, Gantous and colleagues performed distraction osteogenesis in the irradiated canine mandible (10). This study was undertaken to simulate the clinical situation occurring with reconstruction of the human mandible following resection

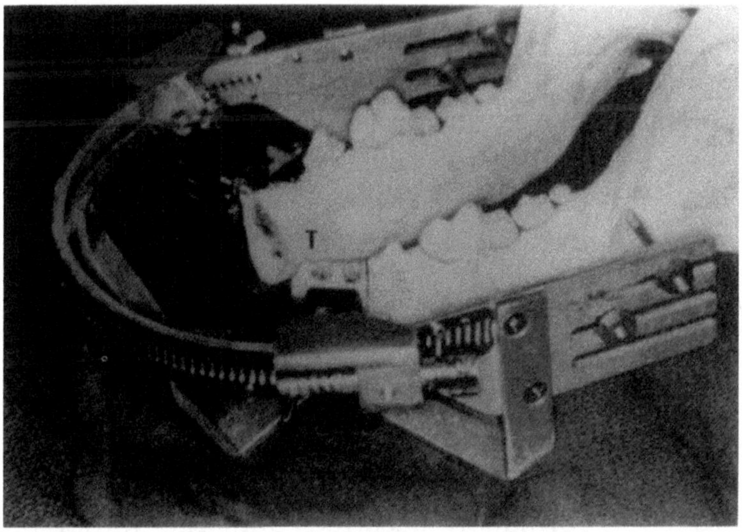

Figure 4.9. Demonstration of trifocal distraction in which bilateral transport disks (T) have been created. A preserved canine mandible is mounted on the distraction apparatus. An anterior symphyseal mandibulectomy defect has been created between the third premolar extraction sockets. Reprinted with permission by *Arch Otolaryngol Head Neck Surg*, 120:913, 1994. Copyright 1990–94, American Medical Association.

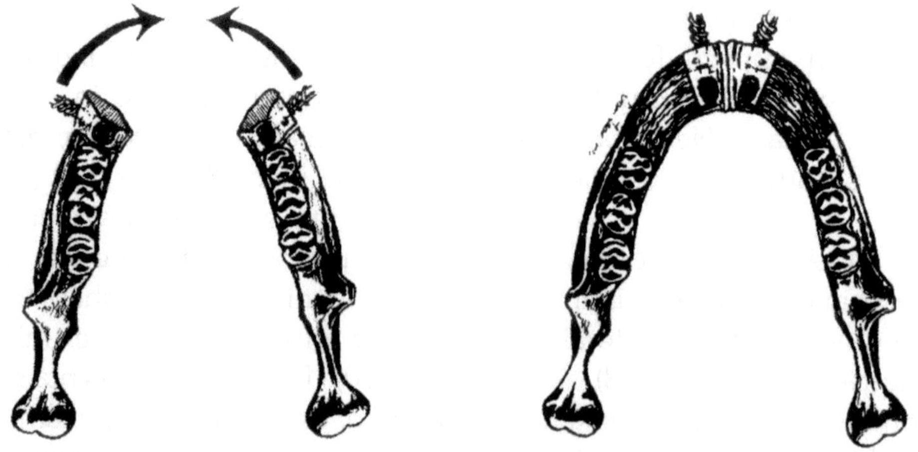

Figure 4.10. A segmental mandibular symphyseal defect before and after reconstruction with trifocal distraction osteogenesis. The transport disks are distracted towards the midline (arrows). The disks meet in the midline in compression. Reprinted with permission by *Arch Otolaryngol Head Neck Surg* 120:913, 1994. Copyright 1990–94, American Medical Association.

for head and neck cancer. The dogs were subjected to 50 Gy of external beam radiation. Six months later, a 2-cm gap was created in the mandible. Bifocal distraction osteogenesis was performed at the rate of 0.75 mm/day for 30 days, resulting in filling of the defect in 4 of the 5 operated dogs. The only failure was attributed to the formation of a large hematoma. Histology confirmed the formation of new cortical bone 7 weeks after the completion of distraction.

Two studies, also reported in 1994, confirmed that the technique of distraction osteogenesis was also applicable to the rabbit mandible. The first study was undertaken by Guerrissi and colleagues and demonstrated bilateral distraction of the rami as well as unilateral distraction of the mandible (11). This was successfully performed at the rate of 1.0 mm/day. The second study by Komuro and associates demonstrated unilateral distraction after corticotomy, 2 weeks of fixation, and distraction at the rate of 0.36 mm/day for 24 days (12). They documented early evidence of a central radiolucent zone within the distraction gap that was indistinguishable from the control by 10 weeks after distraction. Unlike other histologic studies, however, the authors found that both membranous and endochondral ossification had occurred (4). These findings suggest that the fixation may not have been rigid.

In 1995 Klotch and associates attempted to elucidate further the process that occurs during formation of new bone (regenerate) during distraction osteogenesis in a canine model (13). Using bifocal distraction, a transport disk was employed to close a 2-cm defect at the rate of 0.75 mm/day. Fixation was maintained for one week after distraction; after this interval the animals were sacrificed. The distraction zone was assessed histologically. No cartilage was documented. Bone formation occurred primarily within an angiogenic matrix, which was rich in basement membrane laminin and type IV collagen.

In 1995, McCarthy and his colleagues at New York University developed an intraoral device that was used to lengthen or distract the canine mandible (Figures 4.11, 4.12) (14). The application to human subjects is important because this technique would avoid external scarring. This same device was used to evaluate the effects of distraction osteogenesis on the temporomandibular joint (TMJ) and on the muscles of mastication (15,16).

The effects on the TMJ were assessed after unilateral distraction of the mandible in the previously described canine model (15). On gross examination, there was flattening of the posterior aspect of the ipsilateral condylar head with thinning of the condylar cartilage (Figure 4.13). New bone deposition was noted. There were no obvious changes in the joint on three-dimensional CT scan evaluation. On microscopic examination, there was no evidence of avascular necrosis, microfracture, or cystic degeneration (Figure 4.14). These data confirmed that morphologic changes can occur in the TMJ after distraction but that these effects are minimal and reversible (see Chapter 8).

The muscles of mastication are also altered by mandibular distraction (16). After unilateral distraction of the mandible in canines, biopsies of the masseter and digastric muscles were obtained from both the contralateral and ipsilateral sides. The biopsies were analyzed for both nucleic acid and protein content. The muscles lying parallel to the direction of distraction (eg, digastric) showed adaptation to the distraction by regeneration and hypertrophy. In contrast, the masseter, lying in a different plane from the direction of the distraction vector, showed persistent evidence of atrophy with decreased protein synthesis.

In an effort to develop multidimensional distraction of the mandible, a multiplanar device was developed that permits linear, angular, and transverse distraction (17). In this way, the surgeon can

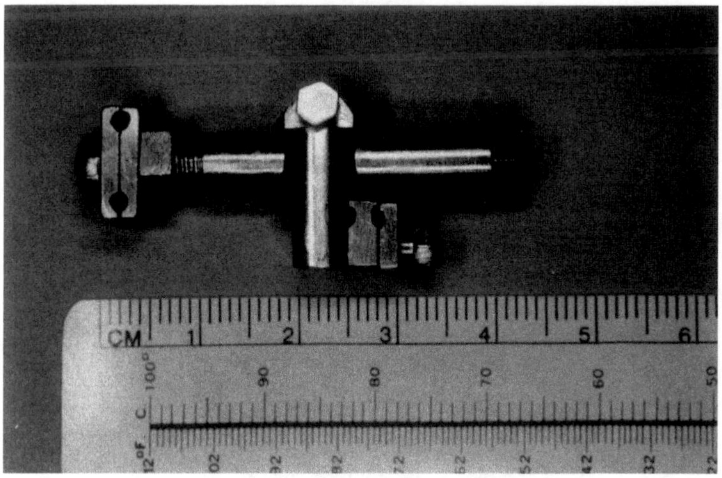

Figure 4.11. The intraoral distraction device in the fully collapsed position. The lengthening nut is at the extreme distal (right) end. Reprinted with permission by *Plast Reconstr Surg* 96:978, 1995.

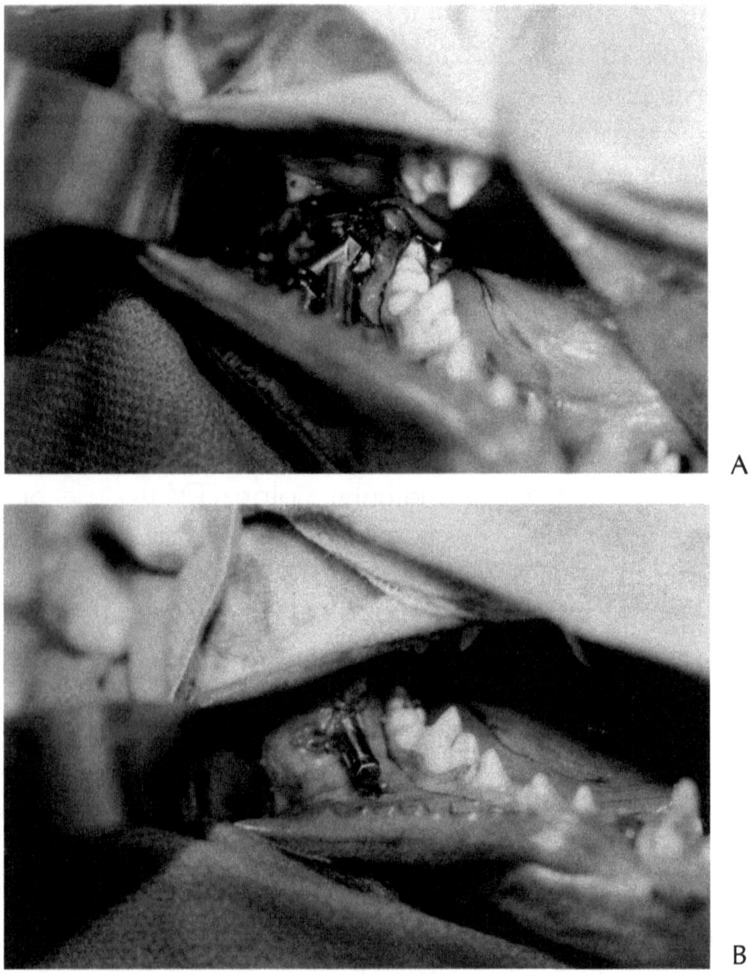

Figure 4.12. (A) Intraoral view showing the distraction device lying in the labiobuccal sulcus and mounted on half pins on the right side of the mandible. Immediately prior to completion of the osteotomy and closure of the mucosa. (B) The device is in place on the right side of the mandible. The osteotomy is complete and the mucosa is closed. Reprinted with permission from *Plast Reconstr Surg* 96:978, 1995.

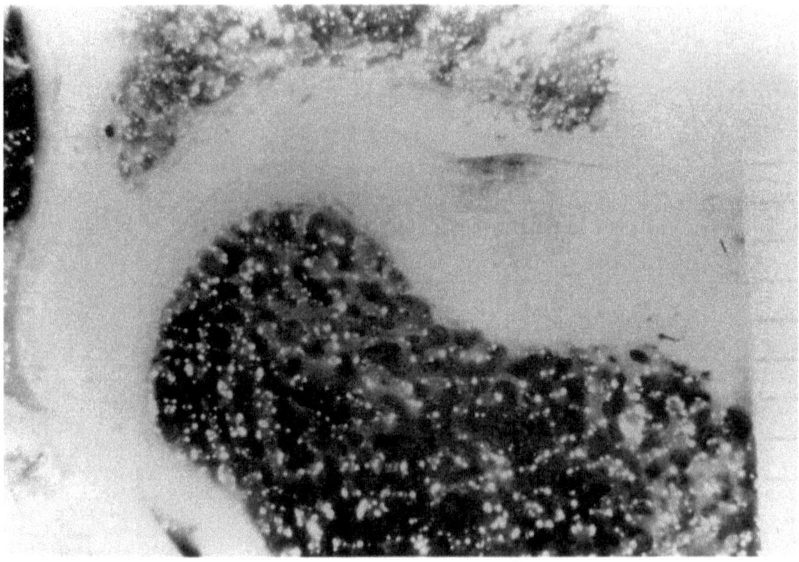

Figure 4.13. Canine temporomandibular joint (ipsilateral) after 20 mm of unilateral mandibular distraction. Gross examination shows posterior condylar flattening. Courtesy of Dr. Susan McCormick.

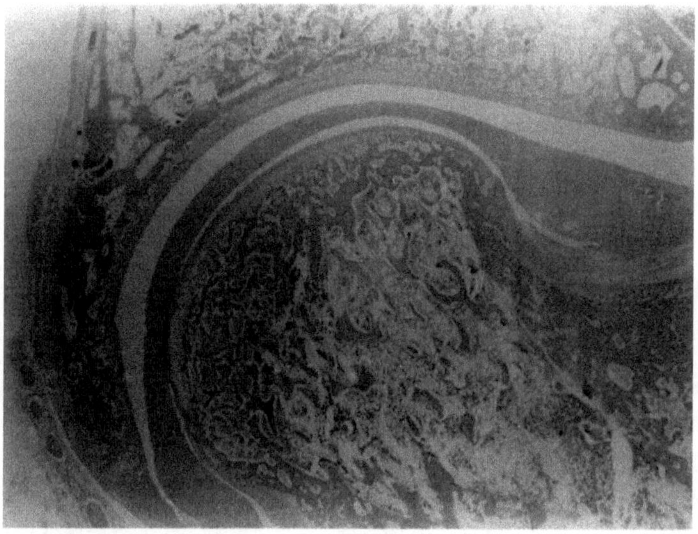

Figure 4.14. Microscopic specimen of canine temporomandibular joint (see Figure 4.13) after distraction (ipsilateral). Note posterior bony changes (×15 magnification). (Courtesy of Dr. Susan McCormick.)

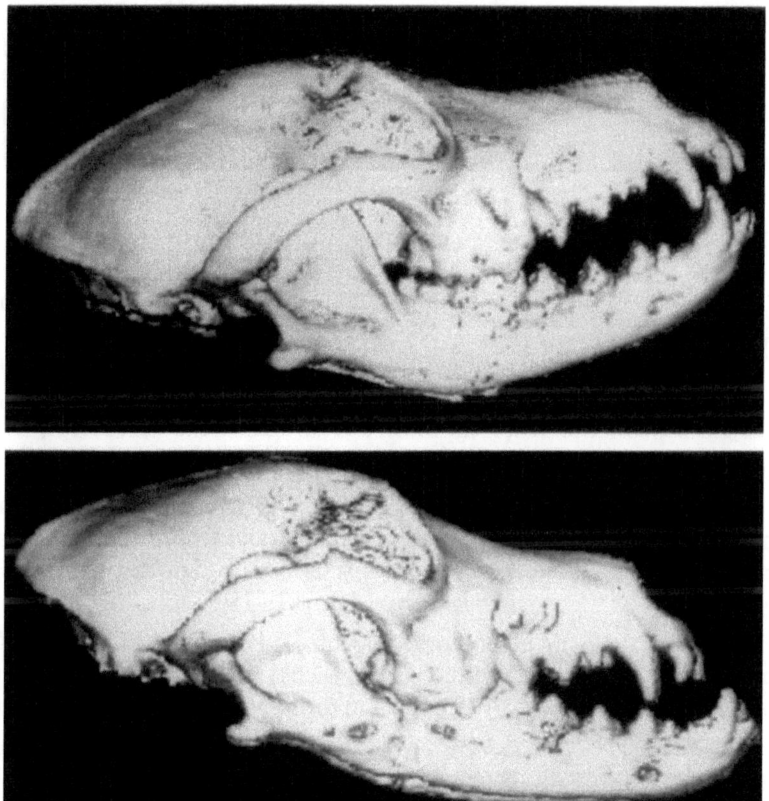

A

B

Figure 4.15. Canine mandibular distraction (bilateral) demonstrating linear and angular distraction. (A) Lateral view before distraction. (B) Lateral view after linear and angular distraction. Note the anterior open bite (the latter secondary to angular distraction).

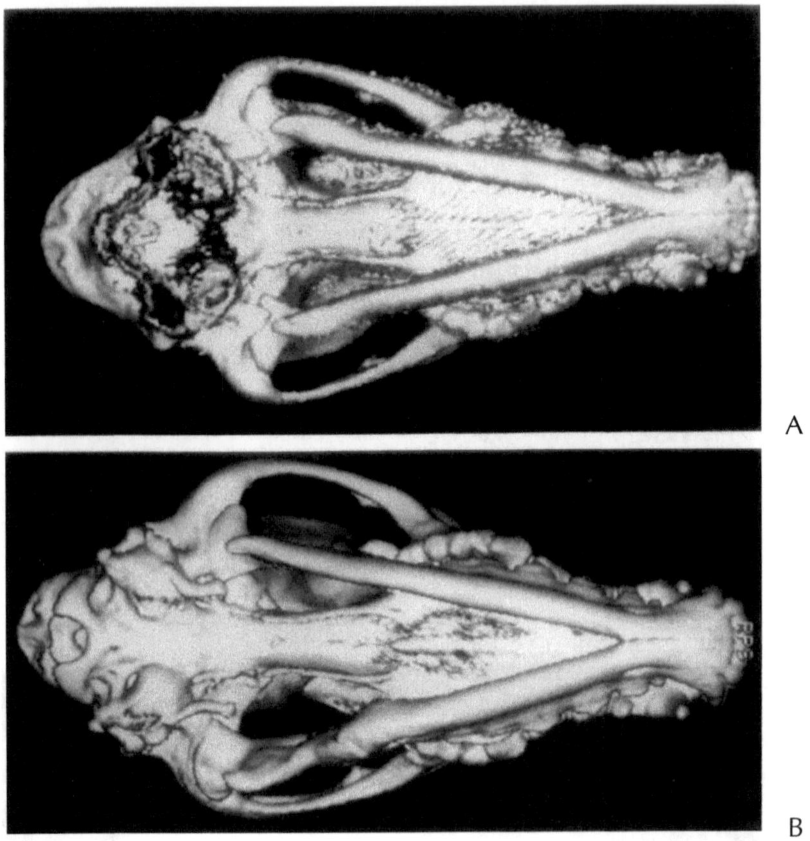

Figure 4.16. Canine mandibular distraction (unilateral) demonstrating linear and transverse distraction. (A) Basilar view before distraction. (B) Basilar view after linear and transverse distraction. Note the lateral deviation of the gonial angle and the increase in the bigonial distance.

manipulate the regenerate to reconstruct a three-dimensional mandible (Figures 4.15 and 4.16).

References

1. Snyder CC, Levine GA, Swanson HM, Browne EZ. Mandibular lengthening by gradual distraction: a preliminary report. *Plast Reconstr Surg* 51:506, 1973.
2. Michieli S, Miotti B. Lengthening of mandibular body by gradual surgical-orthodontic distraction. *J Oral Surg* 35:187, 1977.
3. Karp NS, Thorne CHM, McCarthy JG, Sissons HA. Bone lengthening in the craniofacial skeleton. *Ann Plast Surg* 24:231, 1990.
4. Karp NS, McCarthy JG, Schreiber JS, Sissons HA, Thorne CHM. Membranous bone lengthening: a serial histological study. *Ann Plast Surg* 29:2, 1992.
5. Costantino PD, Shybut G, Friedman CD, Pelzer HJ et al. Segmental mandibular regeneration by distraction osteogenesis. *Arch Otolaryngol Head Neck Surg* 116:535, 1990.
6. Costantino PD, Friedman CD, Shindo ML, Houston G, Sisson GA. Experimental mandibular regrowth by distraction osteogenesis: long term results. *Arch Otolarygol Head Neck Surg* 119:511, 1993.
7. Karaharju-Suvanto T, Karaharju EO, Ranta R. Mandibular distraction: an experimental study on sheep. *J Cranio-Max-Fac Surg* 18:280, 1990.
8. Block MS, Daire J, Stover J, Matthews M. Changes in the inferior alveolar nerve following mandibular lengthening in the dog using distraction osteogenesis. *J Oral Maxillofac Surg* 51:652, 1993.
9. Annino DJ, Goguen LA, Karmody CS. Distraction osteogenesis for reconstruction of mandibular symphyseal defects. *Arch*

Otolarygol Head Neck Surg 120:911, 1994.

10. Gantous A, Phillips JH, Catton P, Holmberg D. Distraction osteogenesis in the irradiated canine mandible. *Plast Reconstr Surg* 93: 164, 1994.
11. Guerrissi J, Ferrentino G, Margulies D, Fiz D. Lengthening of the mandible by distraction osteogenesis: Experimental work in rabbits. *J Craniofac Surg* 5:314, 1994.
12. Komuro Y, Takato T, Harii K, Yonemara Y. The histologic analysis of distraction osteogenesis of the mandible in rabbits. *Plast Reconstr Surg* 94:152, 1994.
13. Klotch D, Ganey TM, Slater-Haase A, Sasse J. Assessment of bone formation during osteoneogenesis: A canine model. *Head Neck Surg* 112:291, 1995.
14. McCarthy JG, Staffenberg DA, Wood RJ et al. Introduction of an intraoral bone-lengthening device. *Plast Reconstr Surg* 96:978, 1995.
15. McCormick SU, McCarthy JG, Grayson BH et al. Effect of mandibular distraction on the temporomandibular joint: Part 1. Canine Study. *J Craniofac Surg* 6:358, 1995.
16. Fischer E, Staffenberg DA, McCarthy JG et al. Histopathologic and biochemical changes in the muscles affected by distraction osteogenesis of the mandible. *Plast Reconstr Surg* 99:366, 1997.
17. McCarthy JG. Personal communication, 1998.

CHAPTER 5

Distraction of the Mandible
The New York University Experience

Joseph G. McCarthy, Barry Grayson,
Joseph K. Williams, and Andrew Turk

Ilizarov (1,2) demonstrated the scientific basis and clinical efficacy of distraction or lengthening of the long bones of the extremities. After preliminary studies in our laboratories (3,4), as well as those in others (5,6), which documented the feasibility of distraction of the membranous bones of the craniofacial skeleton (see chapter 4), we undertook a clinical program of mandibular distraction in May, 1989, the preliminary communication appearing in 1992 (7–10). This chapter documents the clinical experience with patients who underwent mandibular distraction at the New York University Medical Center (NYU).

CLINICAL PROTOCOL

Preoperative Evaluation

The patient (Figure 5.1) should first be examined with the head in a "neutral" position, a goal often rendered difficult because of craniofacial asymmetry and head tilt. One should note forehead, orbital, zygomatic, and external ear position and relationships by viewing the patient from the bird's eye and submental vertex positions. In patients with unilateral craniofacial microsomia, the position of the oral commissure should be documented and the distance between it and the external auditory canal (or ear remnant) recorded; the quality and thickness of the cheek soft tissue should also be observed. The position and contour of the chin (pogonion), as well as the inferior border and angle of the mandible (gonion) are likewise recorded. The external ear is graded according to the classification of Meurman (11).

The intraoral examination documents the status of the occlusion and presence or absence of crossbites. It is important

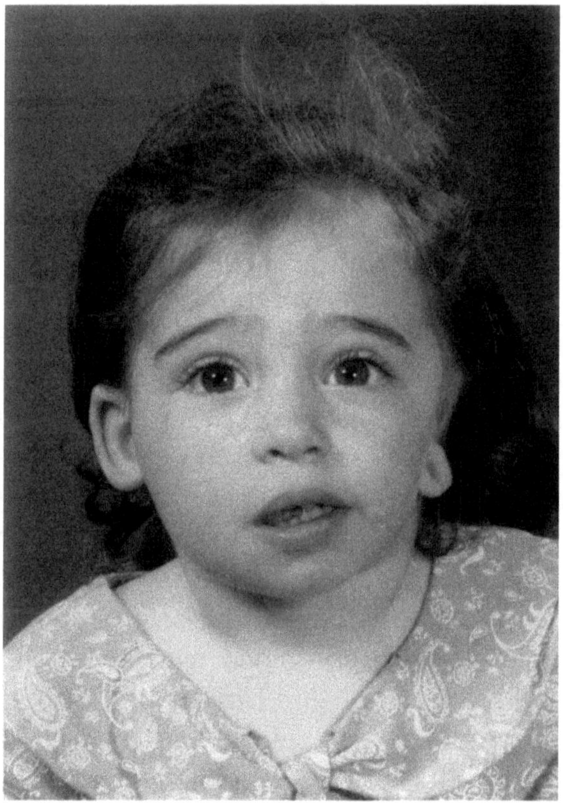

Figure 5.1. A patient with unilateral craniofacial microsomia. Note the deficiency of the cheek on the affected side with elevation of the oral commissure and a decrease in the distance between the latter and the ear remnant. The chin point is deviated to the affected side. Note the canting of the occlusal and pyriform aperture planes.

to relate the intraoral pathology to the extraoral skeletal and soft-tissue abnormalities. The occlusal plane/cant should be related to the transorbital plane, a determination later facilitated by examination of the posteroanterior cephalogram, which also allows analysis of the transmeatal and midsagittal (vertical) planes (Figure 5.2).

The functional clinical exam should include documentation of mandibular excursions, including maximum interincisal opening, since a transient limitation of opening can be observed at the end of distraction. It is, therefore, important to know what the original interincisal opening was, as an objective goal for posttreatment physical therapy. The role of the temporomandibular joint and its actual function prior to distraction are also documented, and the motor (muscles of mastication and facial expression) and sensory (infraorbital, inferior alveolar) nerve functions of the patient are likewise recorded.

Craniofacial pathology and asymmetry should be documented by facial

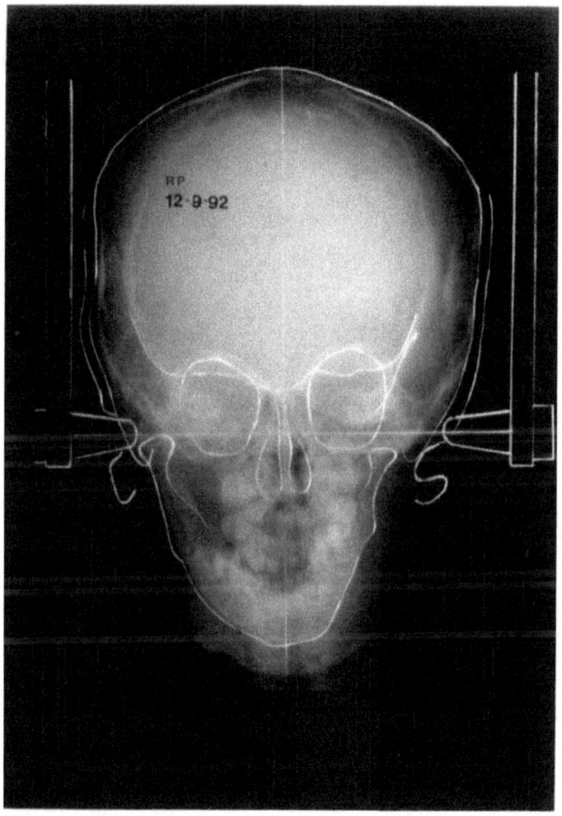

Figure 5.2. Posteroanterior cephalogram of a patient with unilateral craniofacial microsomia. Note that the ear rod is positioned in the ear canal on the unaffected side but is placed on the calvaria on the affected side. However, the midsagittal plane is perpendicular and the lateral borders of the orbital rims are likewise parallel to the lateral vertical plane.

photographs, (frontal, laterals, obliques, submental), a three-dimensional computed tomography (CT) scan (serial axial cuts from menton to cranial vertex), lateral and posteroanterior cephalograms, and a panoramic roentgenogram (panorex); sedation is usually required in the younger patient. In patients with unilateral craniofacial microsomia and microtia, particular attention must be paid to placing the head in the correct vertical or midsaggital plane when obtaining the cephalograms (12).

As illustrated in Figure 5.3, the ear rod is positioned in the ear canal on the unaffected side but is placed on the calvaria on the affected side. Note that the midsaggital plane is perpendicular and the

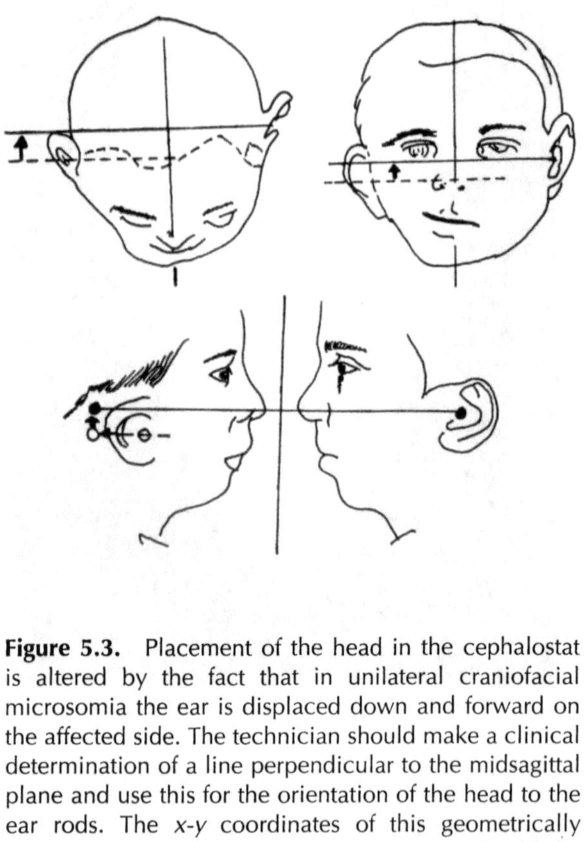

Figure 5.3. Placement of the head in the cephalostat is altered by the fact that in unilateral craniofacial microsomia the ear is displaced down and forward on the affected side. The technician should make a clinical determination of a line perpendicular to the midsagittal plane and use this for the orientation of the head to the ear rods. The *x-y* coordinates of this geometrically determined porion for the affected side should be recorded directly on the cephalometric film for future reference. Reprinted with permission from McCarthy, JG. Plastic Surgery, W.B. Saunders, Philadelphia, 1990.

lateral borders of the orbital rims are symmetrically positioned in relation to the lateral borders of the calvarium. This type of precise documentation must be done routinely in the preoperative period. The record of this discrepancy should be applied postoperatively. The lateral cephalogram is taken with the same protocol. The cephalograms still provide a significant advantage over CT scans in that the clinician can obtain serial records and evaluate long-term growth and developmental changes. In addition, a child cannot be exposed to high levels of radiation for CT scan documentation of long-term growth. The lateral and posteroanterior cephalograms, combined with a panoramic radiograph, are invaluable if they are produced accurately, and they allow classification of the mandible according to the system proposed by Pruzansky (13) and modified by Kaban, Moses, and Mulliken (14) (Figure 5.4).

The three-dimensional (3D) cephalogram is also used for documentation of craniofacial deformity. The lateral film is traced and digitized into a computer, the posteroanterior film is also traced and digitized. The computer integrates the X, Y, and Z coordinates of each landmark to create or establish the actual 3D location in space for those landmarks. In Figure 5.5 the 3D cephalometric image is represented by the landmarks along the mandible, the occlusal plane, the pyriform aperture, and the orbital rims. The 3D cephalogram can also be rotated into an atypical view (Figure 5.6A). The basilar view highlights the left and right asymmetry of the mandible. The posterior asymmetry in the orbital rims and rotation of the maxillary occlusal plane along the Y

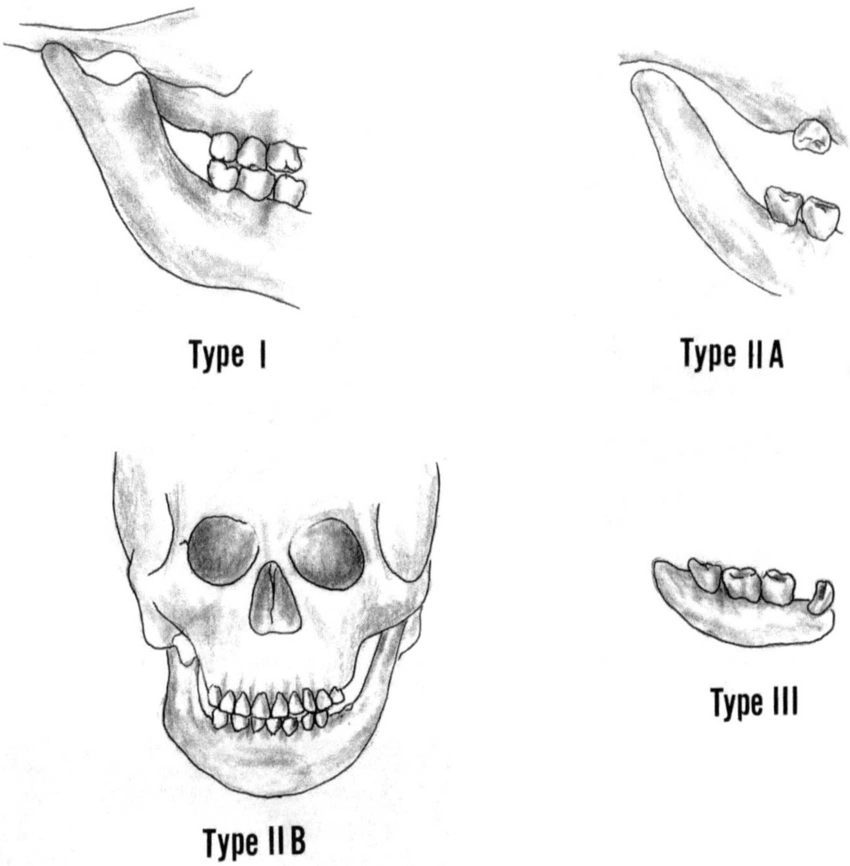

Figure 5.4. Classification of mandibular pathology in craniofacial microsomia. Type I—hypoplastic ramus and body but normal spatial relationship of the temporomandibular joint (TMJ). Type IIA-reduced volume of body and ramus and absence of coronoid process but normal spatial relationship of TMJ. Type IIB—Similar to IIA, but the TMJ or pseudoarticulation is medially displaced. Type III—absence of the ramus and TMJ. From Kaban LB et al. *Plast Reconstr Surg* 82:9, 1988. Reproduced with permission from Grabb & Smith's *Plastic Surgery*, 5th Ed. Little Brown, Boston, 1997.

axis are noted in this view (Figure 5.6B). Any number of views can be selected to assess the skeletal pathology.

The panorex is extremely valuable in documenting the size and shape of the condyle, ramus, and body, as well as the position of partially erupted teeth and tooth follicles (Figure 5.7).

The 3D CT scan reproduces the skeletal pathology in detail and also gives a baseline study for postdistraction documentation of the increase in bone volume and change in mandibular morphology (Figure 5.8).

The diagnostic records also include study models, which are three-dimensional representations of the occlusion (Figure 5.9). Study models can be mounted by a facebow to an articulator, while respecting the anatomical deformity in the external auditory canal. In this way one obtains preoperatively a fairly accurate set of three-dimensional records of the preexisting occlusion. Another impor-

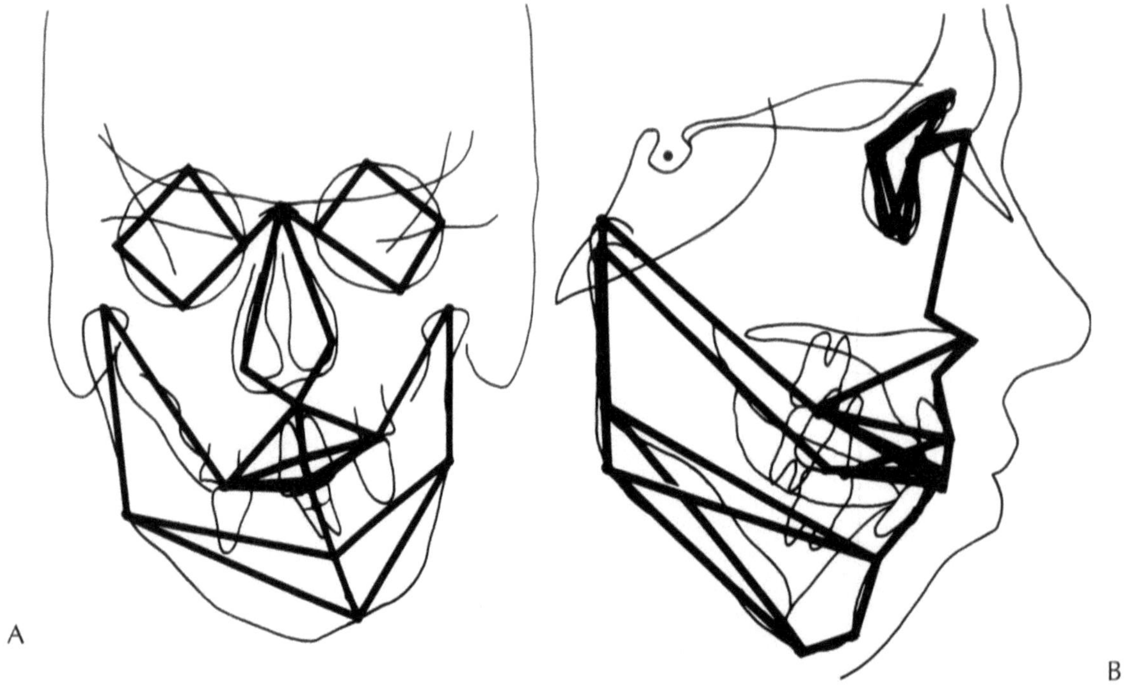

Figure 5.5. Three-dimensional cephalogram. (A) frontal view (B) lateral view. Reprinted from Grayson BH et al. Basilar multiplane cephalometric analysis. *Am J Orthod* 88:503, 1985.

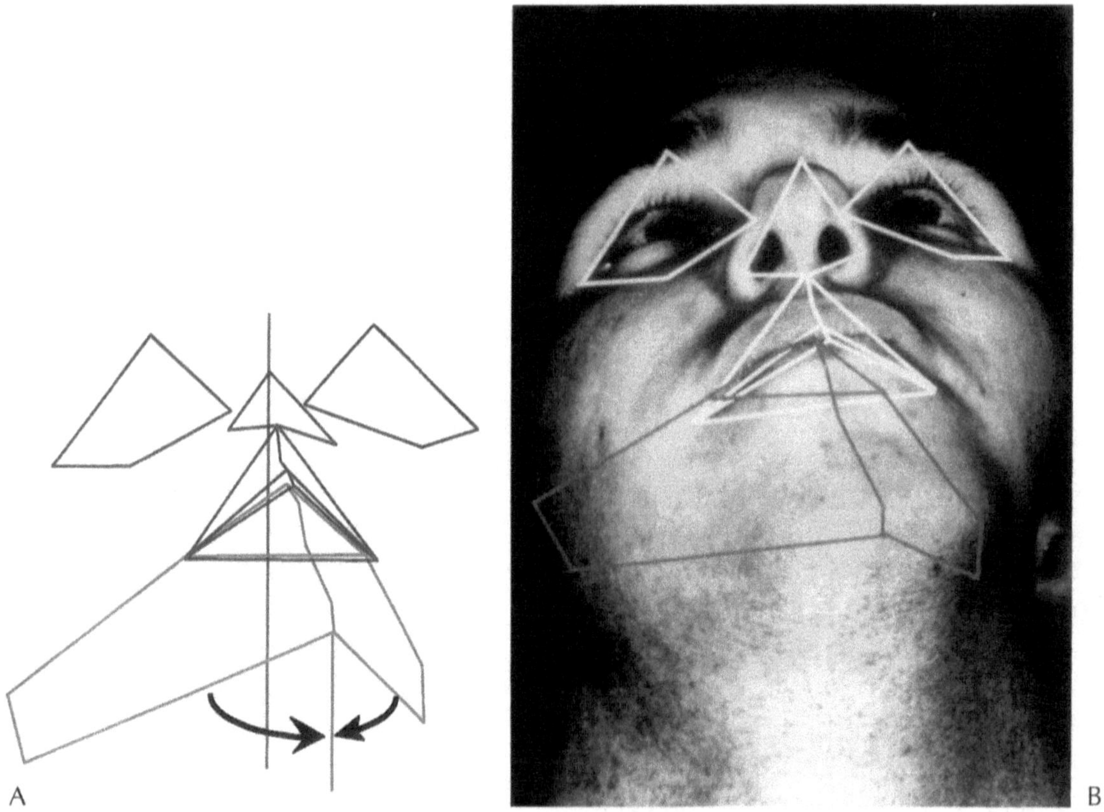

Figure 5.6. Three-dimensional cephalogram. (A) Basilar right oblique view. (B) Basilar right oblique view superimposed on photograph of patient with left-sided craniofacial microsomia. Reprinted from Grayson BH et al. Basilar multiplane cephalometric analysis. *Am J Orthod* 88:503, 1985.

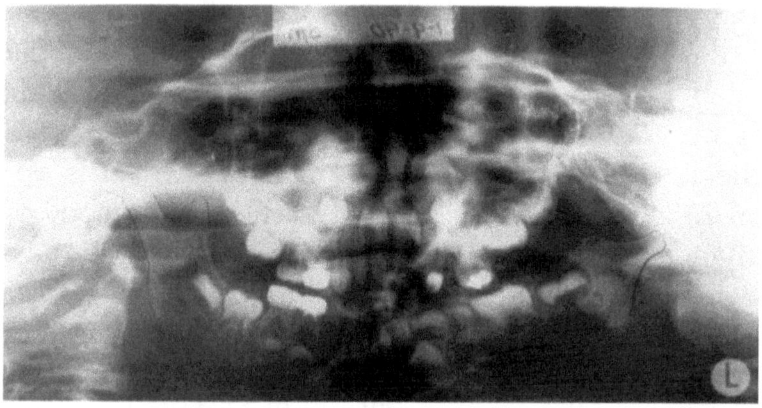

Figure 5.7. Panoramic roentgenogram (panorex) of a patient with left-sided craniofacial microsomia. Note the deficiency of the ramus and condyle. The coronoid process is absent.

tant role of pretreatment study models is the construction of postdistraction orthodontic treatment appliances. These orthodontic appliances need to be made on the preoperative study models, because, following distraction, a limited range of motion may prevent the orthodontist from obtaining impressions and study models for a variable period of time. The preoperative study model can be mounted on an occlusal bite registration from the postoperative period and used in the laboratory to construct the orthodontic appliance.

It was recognized early in the clinical study that in treatment planning there are

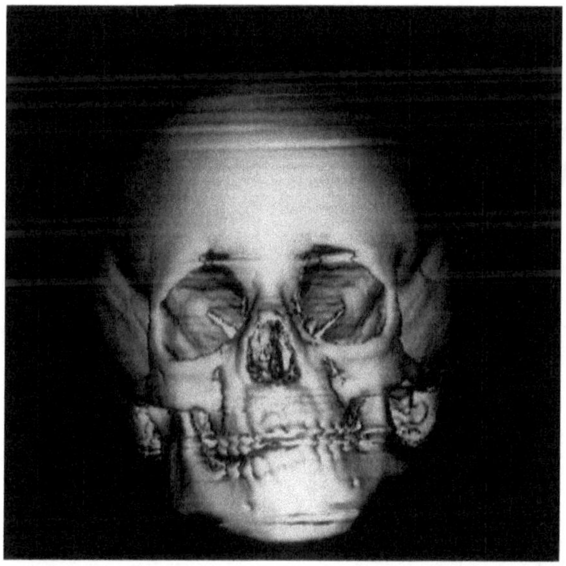

Figure 5.8. Three-dimensional CT scan of a patient with unilateral craniofacial microsomia. Note the occlusal cant, chin deviation, and left-sided mandibular hypoplasia.

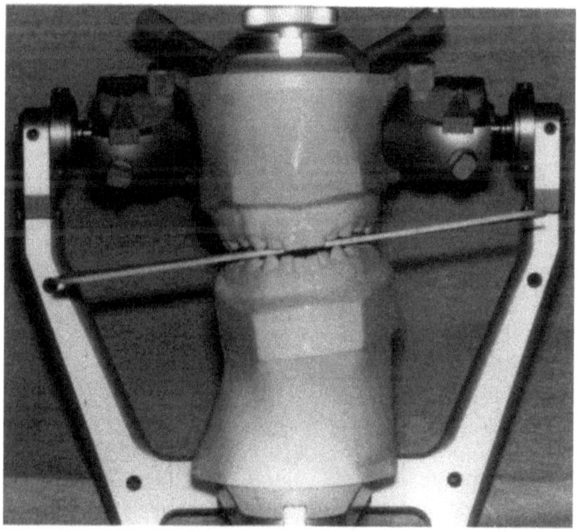

Figure 5.9. Dental models of a patient with craniofacial microsomia showing the occlusal cant and deviation of the mandibular midline.

several structural or architectural goals: (1) increasing the vertical dimension of the hypoplastic mandibular ramus; (2) reestablishing the transverse position of the ramus (bigonial distance) to improve cheek contour; (3) increasing the projection or anteroposterior dimension of the mandibular body and symphysis; (4) improving the dentoalveolar relations; (5) "leveling" the occlusal plane in the unilateral distraction case; (6) correcting any asymmetry of the oral commissure (in the unilateral case); and (7) increasing ("overcorrecting" in the growing patient) chin projection in bilateral cases and "overcorrecting" chin point (movement to the contralateral side) in unilateral cases.

A retrospective review of the clinical records has demonstrated that the shape of the neomandible (a term used to describe mandibular morphology postdistraction) is dependent on the *trajectory* or movement in space of the distraction device, which, in turn, reflects the positioning of the distraction device on the mandible at the time of surgery (the *vector of distraction*) (Figure 5.10). There are three vectors: the *vertical*, which is approximately perpendicular to the body of the mandible; the *horizontal* which is best described as parallel to the inferior border of the body or parallel to the occlusal plane; and the *oblique*, which bisects these two positions. This study has demonstrated that the vertical vector is most effective in lengthening the hypoplastic ramus in the vertical plane. It results in the greatest amount of posterior open bite and corrects a severe occlusal cant in the patient with deficient vertical ramus height. Vertically placed distraction devices will also drive the pogonion toward the midsagittal plane. The *horizontal* vector is parallel to the inferior border of the mandible and the occlusal plane. The devices are placed in this relationship when

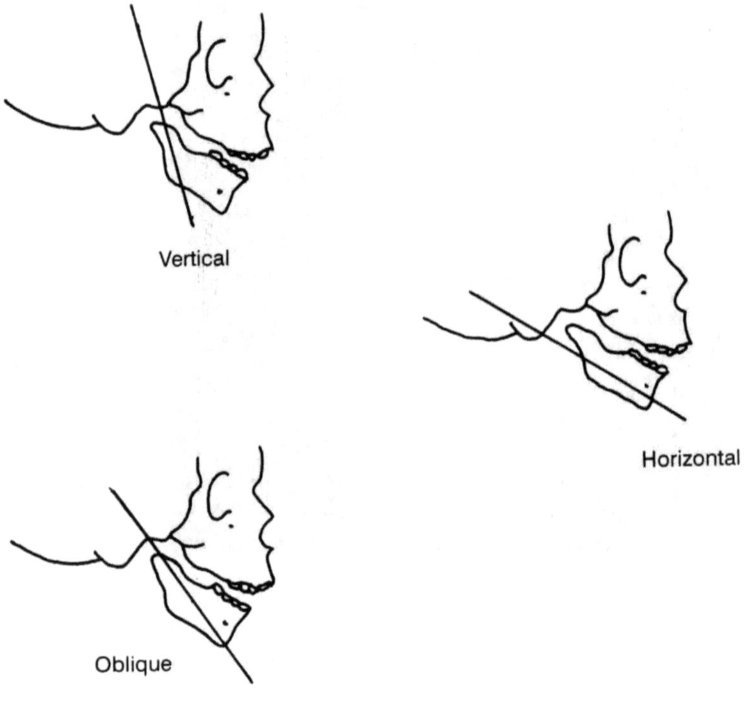

Figure 5.10. The vectors of distraction. The *vertical* vector is approximately perpendicular to the axis of the body of the mandible; the *horizontal* vector is parallel to the inferior border of the body or parallel to the occlusal plane, and the *oblique* vector is intermediary between the previous vectors. The vectors represent the position of the long axis of the distraction device, which, in turn, is determined by the positions of the pins in the mandible.

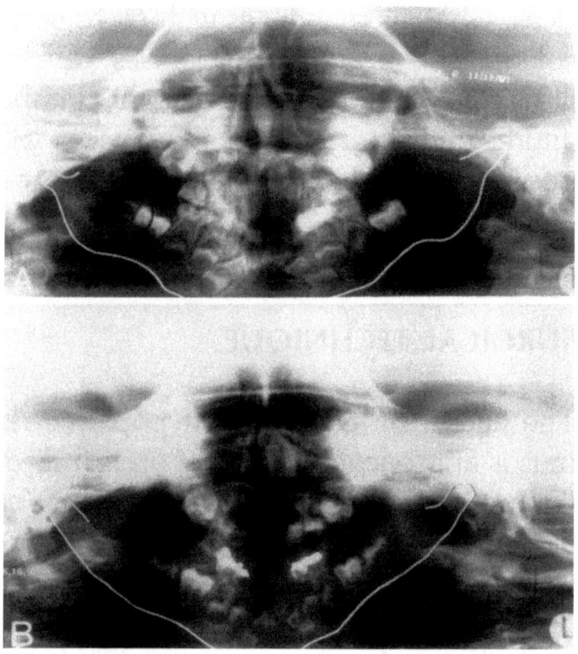

Figure 5.11. Change in gonial angle after distraction with horizontal vector. (A) Preoperative panorex demonstrating well defined gonial angle. (B) Postdistraction panorex demonstrating increase (or flattening) in gonial angle.

there is a marked overjet or micrognathia with mandibular retrusion as usually seen in bilateral mandibular deficiencies. The horizontal placement is most effective at thrusting the mandible in an anterior direction to correct the horizontal deficiency. Horizontal placement (vector) can occasionally change the gonial angle. In a preoperative tracing of the panorex (Figure 5.11A), a well-defined angle between the ramus and body is documented, and in the postdistraction tracing (Figure 5.11B), a straightening of the gonial angle or an alignment of the ramus and body is observed along the same axis. The *oblique* vector represents a bisector of the vertical and horizontal vectors and is best used when one wants to maintain the general morphology of the mandible but increase the vertical dimension of the ramus and the anteroposterior dimension of the body.

DISTRACTION DEVICES

The NYU group began their clinical mandibular distraction studies with the mini-Hoffman uniplanar device (extraoral), which was modified by the Howmedica Corp. (Figure 5.12). It is a four-pin device that allows calibrated lengthening for a total distance of 25 mm; however, additional noncalibrated lengthening is possible.

To obviate the need for an incision (and resulting scar) an intraoral device was designed (15) (Figure 5.13). It is also a four-pin device and can be used only for horizontal vector placement on the mandible. It has US Food and Drug Administration (FDA) approval for only extraoral placement.

In an effort to obtain multiplanar distraction (*X*, *Y*, *Z* planes) and to modify the trajectory during the activation phase a tridirectional device[R] (extraoral) was designed (Figure 5.14). A four-pin device, it has four operational sites: individual wheel adjustments (one quarter turn = 0.5 mm) at each of two limbs, an angle adjustor, and a varus-valgus (transverse) adjustor. It is used with a single mandibular osteotomy. The device was approved for extraoral use by the FDA in 1996.

The Normed Corporation in Germany, in conjunction with the Johann-Wolfgang Goethe University in Frankfurt, developed a bidirectional distraction device[R] (16). It is a six-pin device requiring one or two osteotomies to perform linear

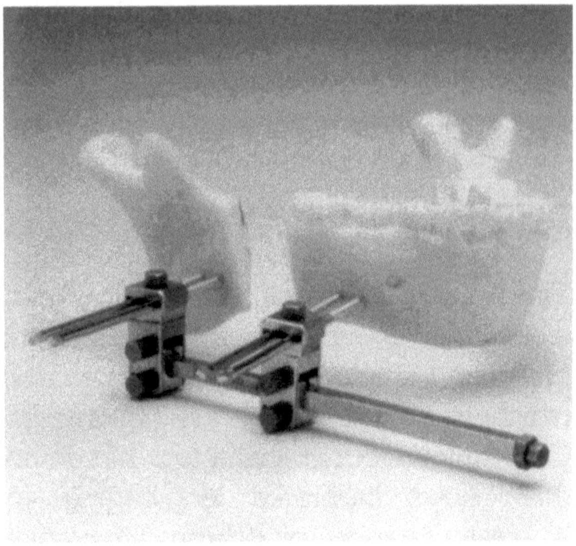

Figure 5.12. The mini-Hoffman uniplanar distraction device (Howmedica). It is a four-pin device that allows up to 25 mm of lengthening along one axis.

and angular mandibular distraction; it does not have the capability for varus-valgus (transverse) movements. Vazquez, Diner, Kollar, and associates developed an intraoral distraction device[R], but it is relatively large for application on the hypoplastic mandibular ramus in congenital anomalies (17). It can also be used for distraction of the mandibular body in bilateral deficiencies. An extension rod allows intraoral adjustments. Wangerin and Gropp (18) have also developed an intraoral device. The Mexico City group (19) has used a single-pin device[R] used with one or two osteotomies (see chapter 6). The central rod is malleable, a property that the authors contend gives improved projection of the gonial angle.

At the current time it appears that extremely hypoplastic rami are amenable only to the application of extraoral devices, whereas mandibles with more bone volume and bilateral deficiencies can be distracted with intraoral devices. In the future, miniaturization of the devices will possibly lead to an era of only intraoral distraction.

SURGICAL TECHNIQUE

The buccal surface of the hypoplastic ramus is approached via either an *intraoral* (Figure 5.15) or a *transcutaneous or extraoral* incision (modified Risdon) (Figure 5.16). The initial cases were done through an extraoral incision but, as clinical experience was accumulated, the intraoral approach, occasionally supplemented with a small 1.5-cm transcutaneous incision to improve visualization, has been used almost exclusively. In either incision a dilute solution of xylocaine and

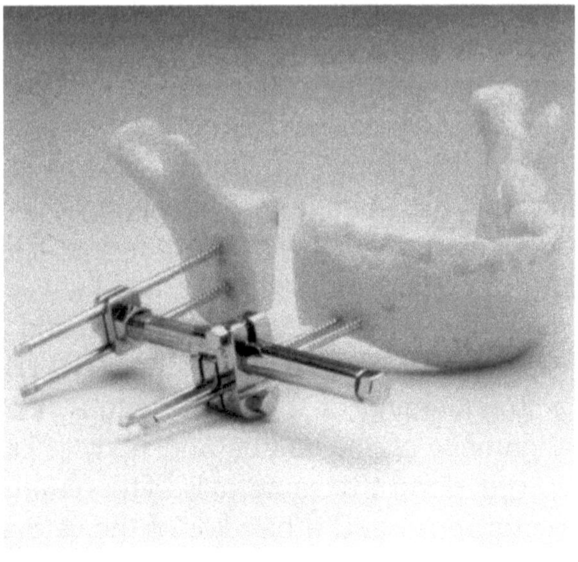

Figure 5.13. The intraoral device (Howmedica). It is a four-pin device to be used along a horizontal vector.

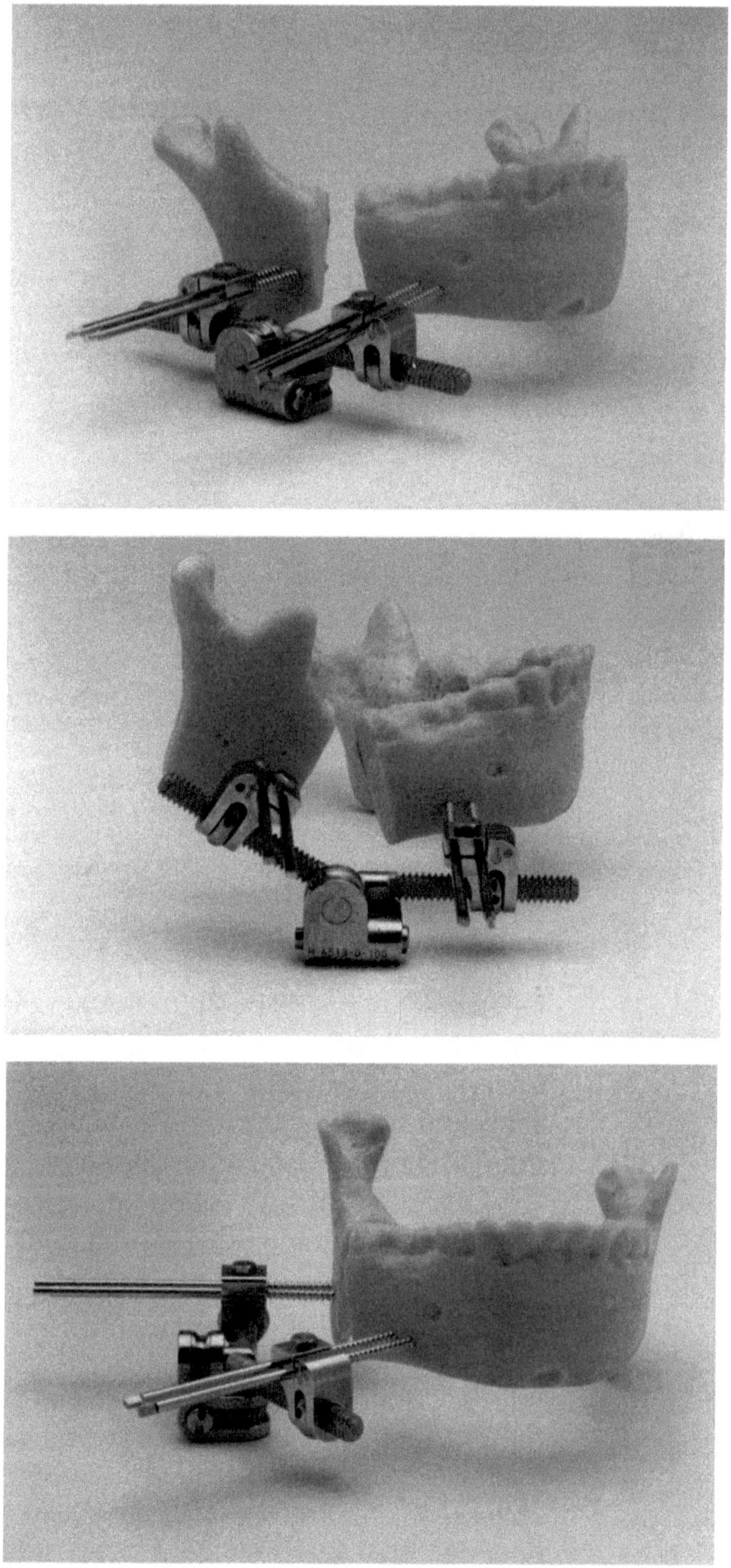

A

B

C

Figure 5.14. The multiplanar device (Howmedica). It is a four-pin device requiring a single osteotomy. It is capable of movement in the following dimensions: linear (A), angular (B), and transverse (C).

adrenalin is injected over the oblique line and buccal surface of the ramus.

In the intraoral approach (see Figure 5.15) an incision is made over the oblique line and the buccal surface is widely exposed in a subperiosteal plane. It should be noted that in the first ten patients the dissection was performed in a supraperiosteal plane, but this practice has been discontinued. Subperiosteal dissection is technically simpler and provides better exposure of the hypoplastic mandible.

In the transcutaneous approach (see Figure 5.16), a 3-cm incision is made in the skin lines of the submandibular fold at a position along the angle and inferior border of the mandible (at a somewhat higher position than the Risdon incision). Care is taken to identify and preserve the marginal mandibular nerve after the platysma muscle is incised. The masseter muscle is sharply dissected off the buccal aspect of the mandible in a subperiosteal plane.

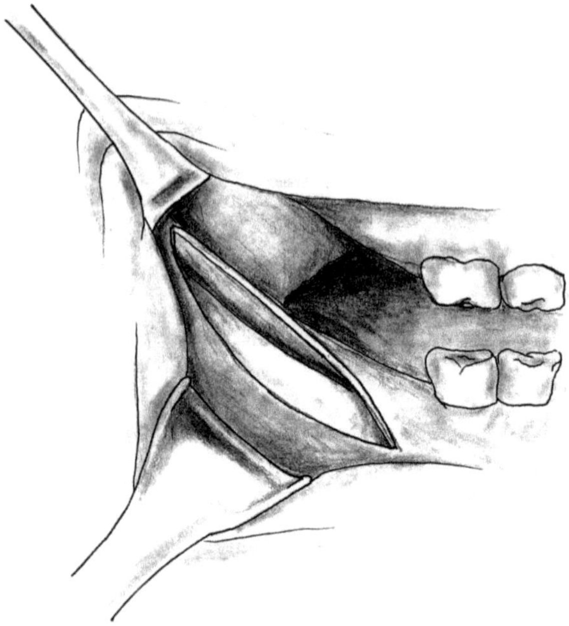

Figure 5.15. The intraoral incision along the oblique line of the affected mandible. The bony surface is exposed in the subperiosteal plane. Reprinted with permission from McCarthy JG. Craniofacial Microsomia: Grabb & Smith's *Plastic Surgery*, 5th Ed. Little Brown, Boston, 1997.

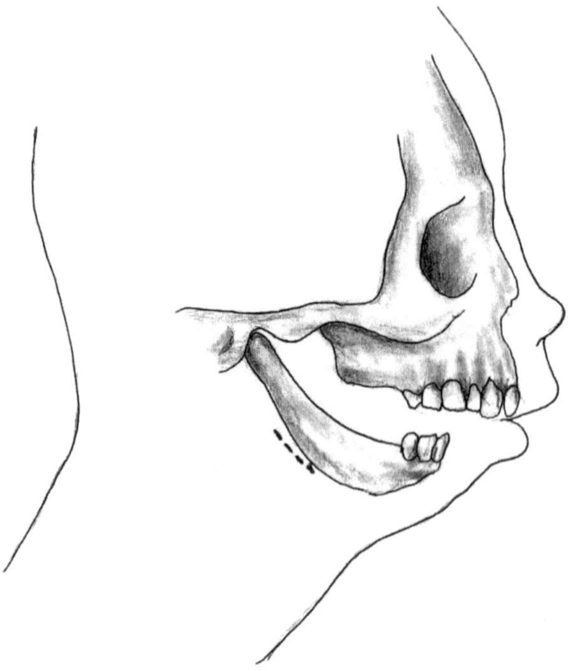

Figure 5.16. The transcutaneous (extraoral) incision. A 2- to 3-cm incision is made at the angle of the mandible in the skin lines. Access is provided to the buccal surface of the mandible in a subperiosteal plane. Reprinted with permission from McCarthy JG. Craniofacial Microsomia: Grabb & Smith's *Plastic Surgery*, 5th Ed. Little Brown, Boston, 1997.

Selection of the pin-hole sites requires careful attention to planning since they dictate positioning of the device (ie, the vector of distraction) (Figure 5.17). One must avoid drilling unerupted tooth follicles, and one must also be sure that the pins project sufficiently above the skin so that the distraction device clears the cheek skin or any auricular remnant. In general, the most cephalic drill holes should be placed first as they are usually the technically most difficult ones because

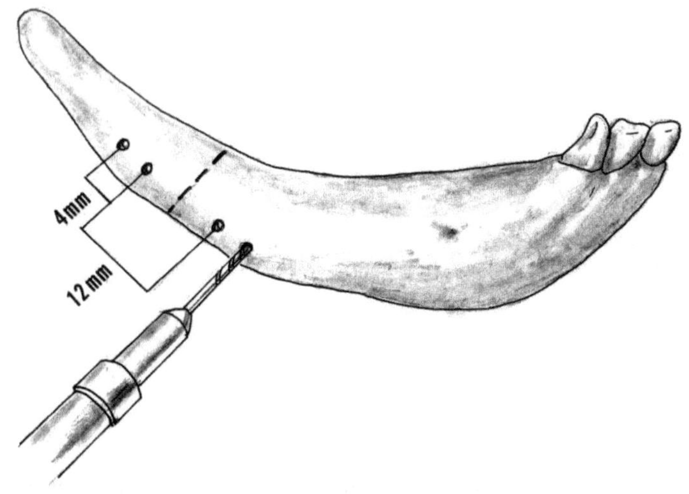

Figure 5.17. Selection of the drill holes determines the position of the distraction device and the vector. The distance between the drill holes is illustrated. Reprinted with permission from McCarthy JG. Craniofacial Microsomia: Grabb & Smith's *Plastic Surgery,* 5th Ed. Little Brown, Boston, 1997.

of the limited size of that portion of the affected mandible. The positions of the four drill holes dictate the orientation of the device and, thus, the vector of distraction. In the four-pin device, the skin and soft tissue are pinched between the two pairs of pins to reduce the length of the resulting scar, and the skin is also retracted in a superior direction so that the pins penetrate the skin in the submandibular fold and the resulting scar will fall in the latter, relatively camouflaged, site.

After the drill holes have been completed under saline irrigation, 50-mm half pins are inserted (Figure 5.18). In the intraoral approach a trocar is used to permit percutaneous drilling of the holes as well as insertion of the half pins. The recent development of self-drilling pins obviates the need for separate drill holes. The distraction device is then attached.

It is technically best to perform or complete the osteotomy after the distraction device has been applied and tightened. Alternatively, it can be removed and reapplied in its previously set position after completion of the osteotomy. The osteotomy can be performed in a variety of ways. A mechanical saw (Figure 5.19), supplemented by saline irrigation, can be used to interrupt the buccal surface (cortex) as well as the superior and inferior cortical borders of the affected mandible; the area of the lingula and path of the inferior alvealor nerve are thus spared. The osteotomy is completed by inserting

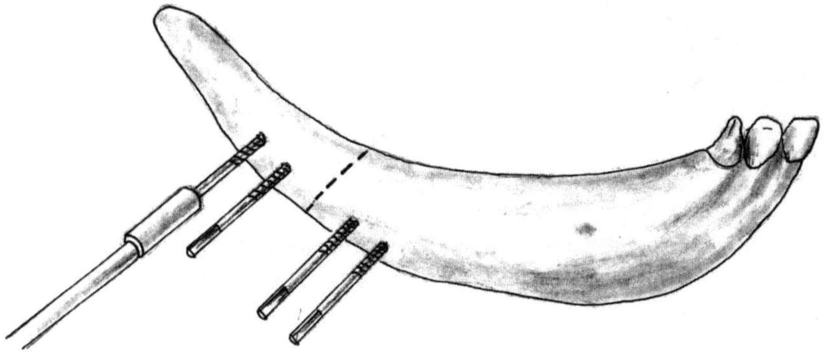

Figure 5.18. Insertion of 50-mm half pins into the drill holes. The interrupted line indicates the site of the projected osteotomy. Reprinted with permission from McCarthy JG. Craniofacial Microsomia: Grabb & Smith's *Plastic Surgery,* 5th Ed. Little Brown, Boston, 1997.

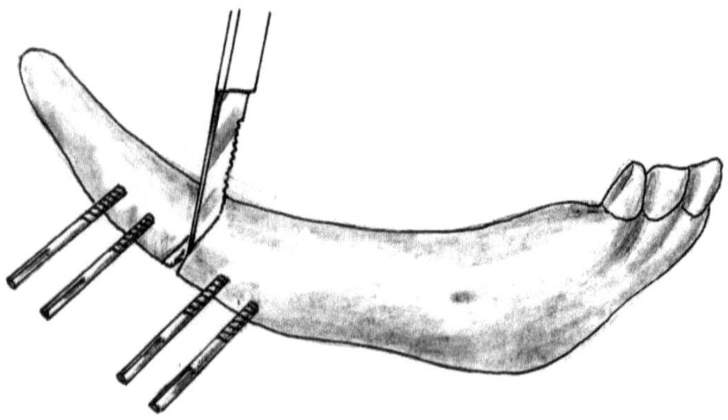

Figure 5.19. The osteotomy is performed with a small reciprocating saw under saline irrigation. The osteotomy is 90% completed before the distraction device is applied. The osteotomy is then completed. Reprinted with permission from McCarthy JG. Craniofacial Microsomia: Grabb & Smith's *Plastic Surgery,* 5th Ed. Little Brown, Boston, 1997.

and rotating an osteotome to demonstrate separation of the bony segments ("greenstick"). There is obvious disruption, albeit limited, of the periosteum and endosteum with the act of the osteotomy; the term corticotomy has, therefore, been abandoned (Figure 5.20).

The wound is irrigated with saline, and, if the transcutaneous approach is employed, the platysma muscle is approximated with interrupted 4-0 chromic catgut sutures and the skin margins are approximated with interrupted 6-0 nylon or vicryl sutures. In the intraoral approach, the wound is closed with a single layer of interrupted 3-0 chromic catgut sutures.

POSTOPERATIVE PERIOD

Photographs and cephalograms are also obtained on the day following insertion of the pins and expansion device. The man-

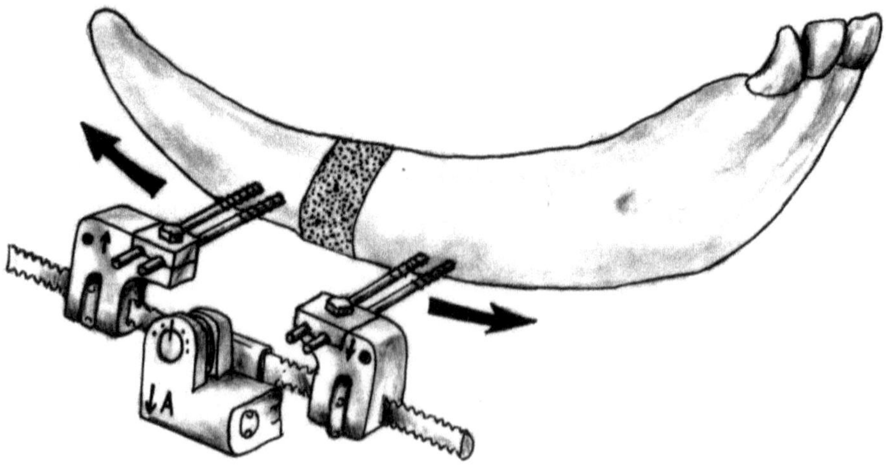

Figure 5.20. Application of the multiplanar distraction device. The distraction has begun in the direction of the arrows with the formation of bone regenerate at the distraction site. Reprinted with permission from McCarthy JG. Craniofacial Microsomia: Grabb & Smith's *Plastic Surgery,* 5th Ed. Little Brown, Boston, 1997.

dible is maintained in fixation for five to seven days (lag phase) before activation of the device is commenced (activation phase) at the rate of 1 mm per day (0.5 mm twice a day). In the child under six years of age a rate of 1.5 to 2.0 mm per day (0.5 mm thrice a day or 1.0 mm twice a day) can be considered to avoid premature consolidation at the distraction site.

The progress of distraction is monitored by documenting changes in the relationships of the anterior maxillary and mandibular occlusion and the position or level of the occlusal plane, oral commissure, and chin point. In general, and especially in the growing child, the deformity is overcorrected, or activation is continued until the above parameters are exceeded beyond the "normal" range.

After the completion of activation, the device is maintained in position for approximately 8 weeks (fixation phase). The device is not removed until there is radiographic evidence of a cortical outline or mineralization of the regenerate portion of the mandible (neomandible). Upon removal of the pins and distraction device (an office procedure), photographs, lateral and posteroanterior cephalograms, panorex, and 3D CT scan of the mandible are obtained.

In the unilateral series, if at the time of device removal there is a resulting leveling of the mandibular occlusal plane with a resulting posterior open bite, a bite plate (worn on the mandibular dentition) is constructed by the orthodontist to maintain the space in order to allow eventual but gradual eruption of the maxillary teeth into the open bite. Over the subsequent months the posterior portion of the prosthesis is serially reduced in size under the most terminal and distal maxillary molar to allow the latter to erupt down to the postdistraction occlusal plane, bringing with it the dentoalveolar process (Figure 5.21). Upon completion of hypereruption of the tooth, the occlusal plate is reduced under the more anterior pairs of teeth until the entire maxillary occlusal plane is leveled. In the younger patient (under 3 years of age) the maxillary teeth quickly fill the space, and the above orthodontic maneuver is often not necessary.

Following vertical distraction of the mandibular ramus, the mandible is deviated toward the midsaggital plane and a posterior crossbite can exist on the contralateral side. The maxilla may be expanded to correct the crossbite with a classical palatal expansion device (Figure 5.22). The maxillary expansion is typically a bilateral phenomenon, as the molar is corrected on the contralateral side and the maxillary molar on the distracted side may come out toward the buccal aspect. To correct the latter, intermaxillary elastics may be worn to bring the maxilla (the dentition and alveolus) down into occlusion (Figure 5.23A). In order to avoid tipping of the lower molar toward the buccal aspect, the lower molar can be joined to the contralateral side with a lingual arch (Figure 5.23B). The lingual arch is a heavy arch wire that runs along the lingual surface of the lower anterior teeth, connecting each molar and thus preventing the lower molar from responding to the intermaxillary elastics. The maxillary posterior dentition is gradually brought down into contact with the lower dentition, resulting in the leveling of the occlusal plane (Figure 5.23C). There are many different

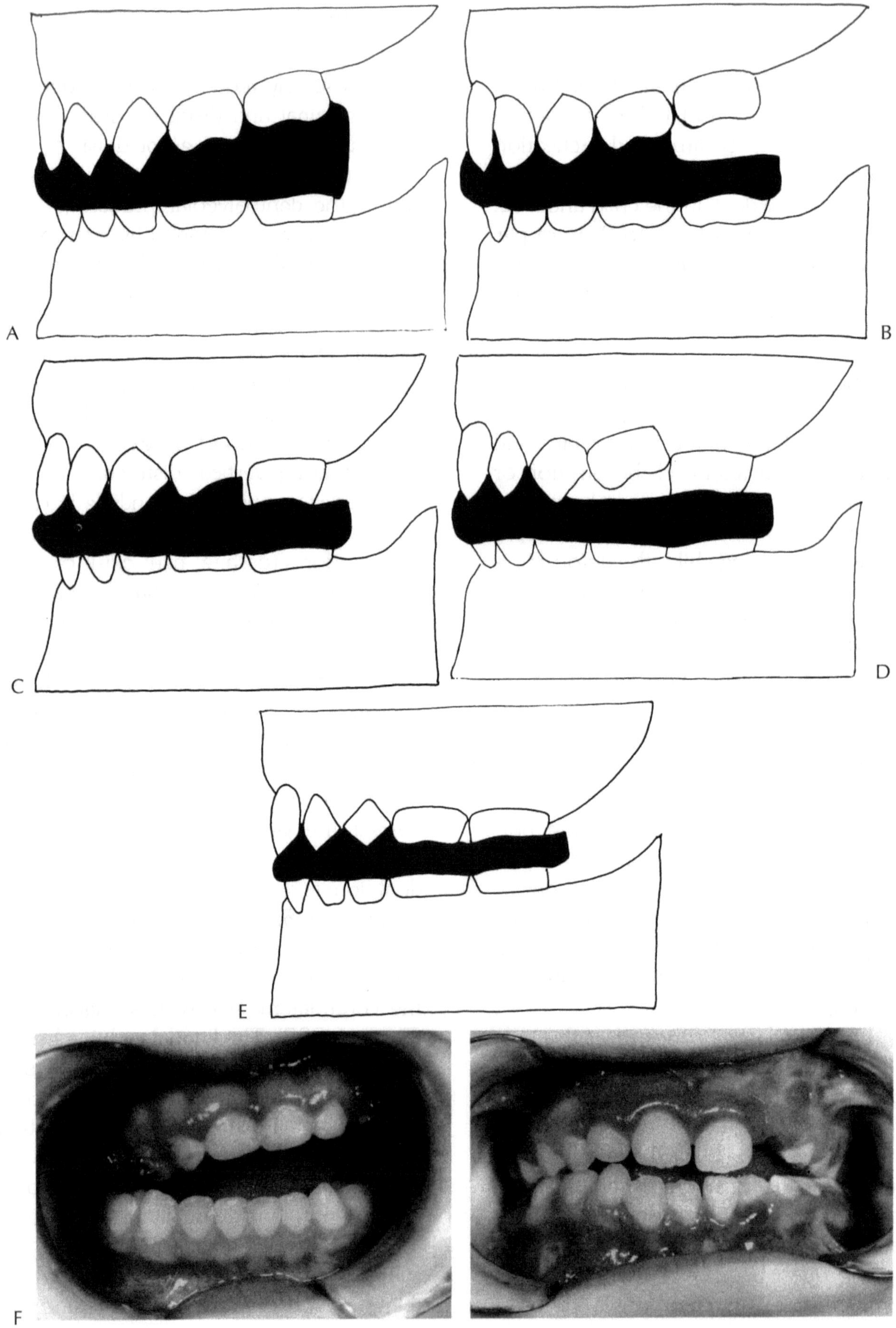
A
B
C
D
E
F
G

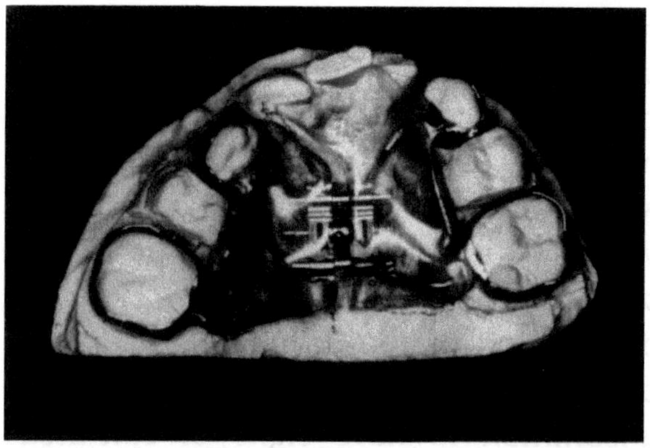

Figure 5.22. Maxillary arch constriction after distraction can be corrected by the application of a classical palatal expansion device (demonstrated on dental model).

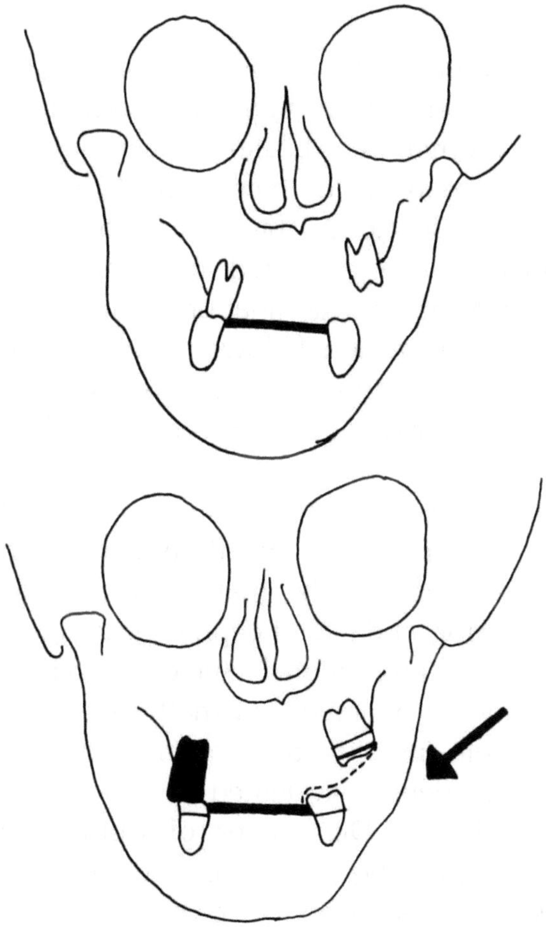

A

B

ways of orthodontically treating the post-distraction patient.

CLINICAL SERIES

The technique has been applied on patients with unilateral craniofacial microsomia (unilateral distraction) and micrognathia (bilateral distraction), ie, bilateral craniofacial microsomia, developmental micrognathia, Treacher Collins syndrome, and Nager syndrome.

Since the series began in May 1989, forty-eight patients (25 male and 23 female) have undergone mandibular distraction: thirty-five patients with unilateral

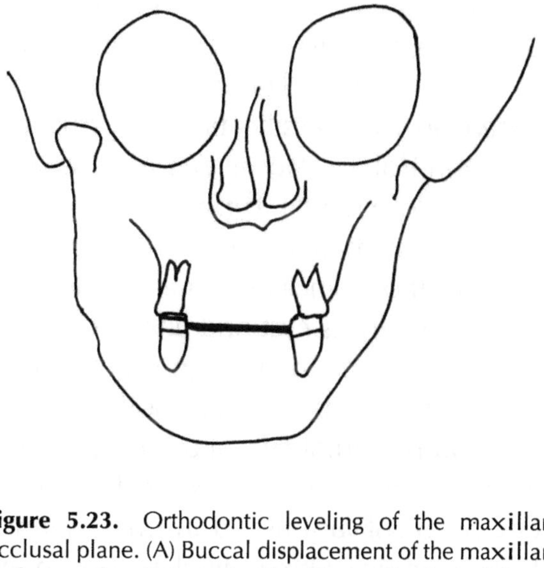

C

Figure 5.23. Orthodontic leveling of the maxillary occlusal plane. (A) Buccal displacement of the maxillary molar on the distracted side. (B) Application of intermaxillary elastics between the maxillary and mandibular molar with stabilization of the mandibular molar by a lingual arch joined to the contralateral side. (C) Final leveling of the occlusal plane.

Figure 5.21. Orthodontic correction of a posterior open bite after distraction. (A–E) A bite plate is inserted and gradually reduced to allow the descent and eruption of the maxillary molars and the associated dentoalveolar complex. (F) Occlusion at the completion of distraction. Note the open bite. (G) Occlusion at the completion of orthodontic treatment.

craniofacial microsomia (eight patients with Goldenhaar variant) and thirteen patients with bilateral deformity (two patients with bilateral craniofacial microsomia, four patients with developmental micrognathia, five patients with Treacher Collins syndrome, and two patients with Nager syndrome). In other words, there was unilateral distraction in thirty-five patients, bilateral distraction in thirteen patients, and transverse distraction in one patient (the latter also underwent bilateral distraction). Secondary distraction was performed in three patients and distraction was accomplished across a previously bone-grafted site in three patients.

The average patient age at the time of osteotomy and application of the distraction device was aged 5.9 years, and the age range of the patient population was 1.5 to 21 years. The average amount of lengthening was 23.3 mm with a range of 16 to 32 mm. The skeletal pathology, based on the classifications of Pruzansky (13) and Kaban, Moses and Mulliken (14), was predominantly Types I, IIA, and IIB.

In this patient series the observed complications included the development of a dentigerous cyst and unsuccessful distraction in one patient (presumably due to injury of an unerupted tooth follicle), a temporary partial buccal branch (VII) palsy in two patients with a vertically oriented device, a salivary fistula in one patient, a hypertrophic submandibular scar in two patients, and an ankylosis requiring bilateral coronoidectomy in another patient who had undergone bilateral distraction (and the osteotomy had been made posterior to the coronoid process). In one patient undergoing bilateral distraction after rib graft reconstruction of the ramus on each side, there was less lengthening on one side for an unknown reason. One patient accidentally dislodged his device, but this was successfully reapplied. Toward the end of the activation phase, two young patients demonstrated premature bony consolidation. There were no cases of infection or the development of temporomandibular joint problems. It was not uncommon to have signs of soft-tissue inflammation around the pins, but no patient required institution of intravenous antibiotic therapy.

LONG-TERM STUDIES

In a preliminary longitudinal study (20), ten patients with unilateral craniofacial microsomia and bilateral micrognathia, who underwent correction of their mandibular deficiency by distraction techniques, were evaluated by clinical and cephalometric examination. The period of postdistraction follow-up ranged from 12 to 70 months. Five patients underwent unilateral mandibular distraction and five patients underwent bilateral distraction with an extraoral device.

Preoperative, posttreatment, and annual radiographs (panoramic, posteroanterior, and lateral cephalograms) were obtained and studied. All cephalometric tracings were made on matte acetate by a single investigator. The tracings were independently evaluated by a second investigator. Differences of opinion regarding tracing or landmark identification were discussed and resolved among the investigators.

In the period of observation following distraction, the ten mandibles showed cephalometric and clinical evidence of

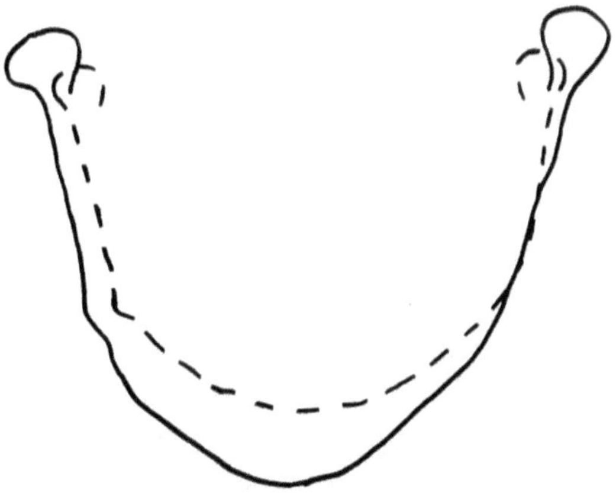

Figure 5.24. Serial tracings from a posteroanterior cephalogram. The interrupted line indicates the contour of the mandible approximately one year after rightsided distraction. The solid line represents the contour five years later. Note that there was growth on the distracted side at the site of the bone regenerate as well as in the adjacent body, ramus, and condylar head of the mandible. The chin point has remained in the midsagittal plane (see Case 1).

growth. In the five *unilateral* cases, the unoperated side grew in a pattern as would be expected for the unaffected side of a mandible with unilateral craniofacial microsomia. The distracted side, however, grew with a variable response (Figure 5.24). Growth occurred at the site of the bone regenerate as well as in the adjacent body, ramus, and the condylar head. *No evidence of relapse was noted in any patient*. The growth response of the operated side was variable and appeared to be dependent on the genetic program of the native bone and the surrounding soft-tissue matrix. Morphologic and volumetric improvements previously reported (21) for the condyle were maintained long term, with continued growth of the condyle without evidence of deformational changes (see Chapter 8).

In the five patients who underwent *bilateral* distraction, the neomandible grew without evidence of relapse during the period of observation. Both sides of the mandible grew at comparable rates. The unoperated sites, including the body and condyle, also showed evidence of growth throughout the study period.

Comparison of lateral cephalograms revealed that a clockwise rotation of the mandible occurred with the passage of time (Figure 5.25). Clockwise mandibular rotation occurred secondary to the expected vertical growth of the maxillary dentoalveolus as the children passed from the primary to the mixed and finally to the permanent stages of dentition. Tooth development and eruption occurred with no evidence of developmental delay.

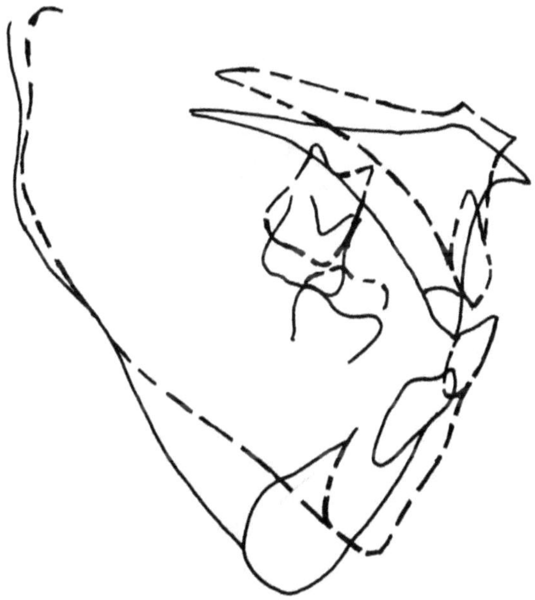

Figure 5.25. Serial lateral cephalograms of a patient who underwent bilateral distraction for the correction of a developmental micrognathia. The interrupted lines illustrate the position of the mandible immediately following distraction, and the solid lines are the contour almost two years later. Note that there has been clockwise mandibular rotation secondary to the expected vertical growth of the maxillary dentoalveolus.

The shape of the postdistraction mandible could be defined by the angular relationship formed by the long axis of the distractor device and the mandibular body (see Figure 5.10). As mentioned previously, the relationship of the distraction device to the mandible could be described as vertical, horizontal, or oblique. When the distraction device was placed vertically (ie, perpendicular to the mandibular body), ramal elongation and bone regeneration occurred in a superoinferior direction across the osteotomy site (Figure 5.26). As a consequence of vertical ramal lengthening, the patients developed a posterior open bite. In the unilateral cases, a shift of the mandible occurred with a rotation and displacement of the mandibular ramus and body toward the contralateral side. In those patients in whom the distraction device was placed horizontally (ie, parallel to the inferior border or body of the mandible), elongation occurred along the long axis of the body of the mandible with opening or obliteration of the gonial angle (Figure 5.27). In these cases, the distractor was placed at an angle (long axis of the device relative to sella nasion line)

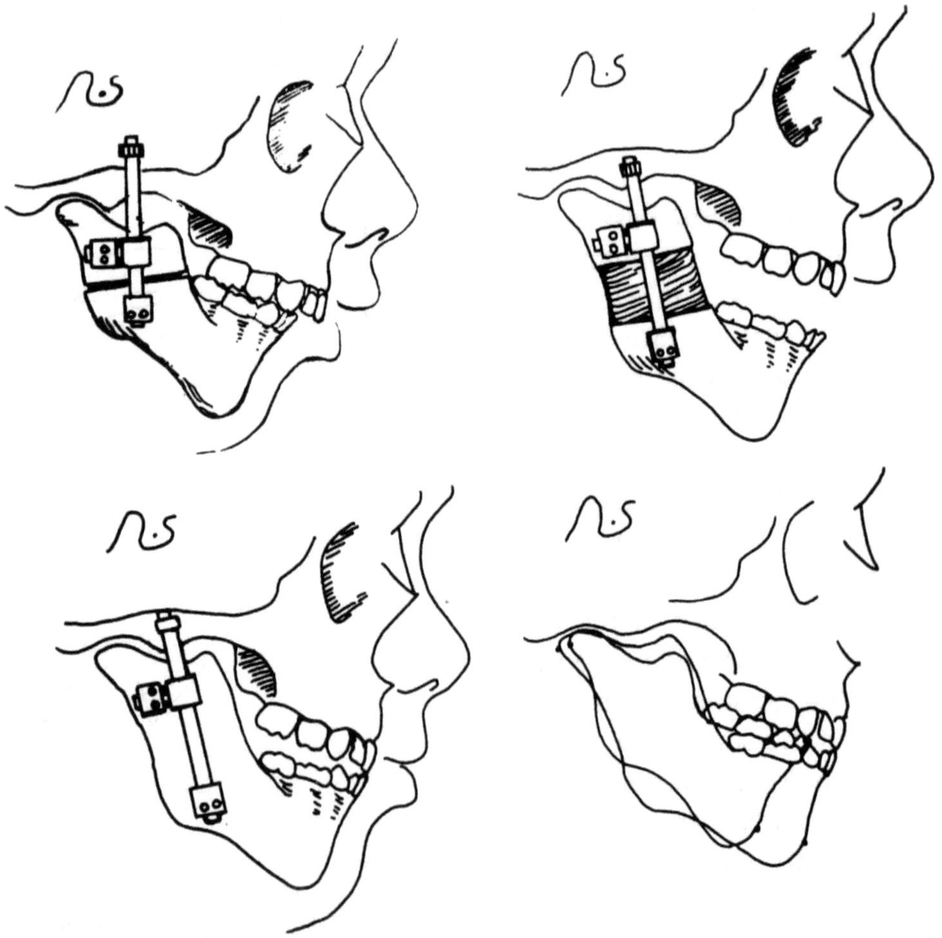

Figure 5.26. Vertical vector. *Upper Panel.* The diagram depicts the relationship of the device approximately perpendicular to the body of the mandible and the development of the bony regenerate. *Lower Panel.* After distraction there has been the development of a posterior open bite and a counter clockwise rotation of the mandible.

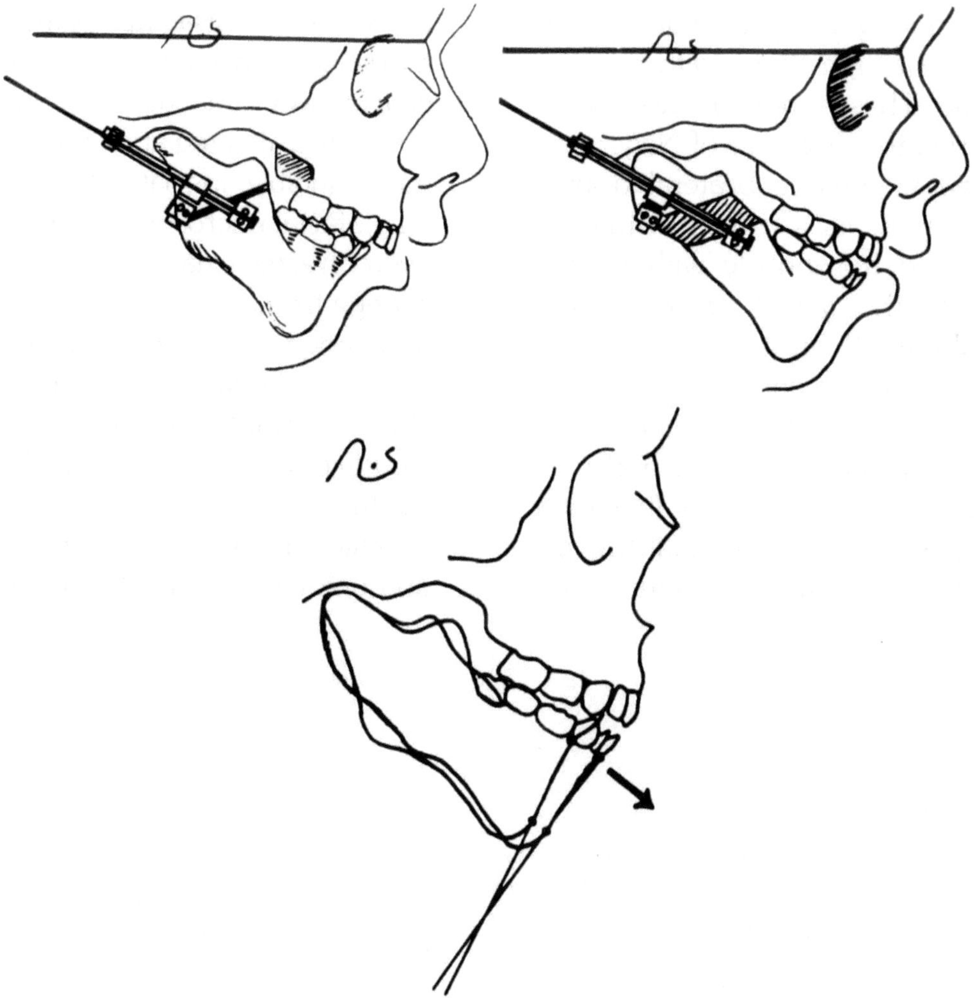

Figure 5.27. Horizontal Vector. *Upper Panel.* The diagram depicts the relationship of the device parallel to the long axis of the body or the inferior border of the mandible with subsequent development of the bony regenerate. *Lower Panel.* The mandible has been advanced. Note the correction of the overjet and the flattening of the gonial angle.

that was greater than 65°, in part due to the high mandibular plane angle. The distractor was actually positioned parallel to the inferior border of the mandibular body. If the distractor was placed oblique to both the posterior and inferior borders, the resultant neomandible maintained the original mandibular form, with preservation of the gonial angle. In the oblique pattern the bone regenerate occurred in two directions: vertically and horizontally, maintaining the original relationship of the mandibular ramus, gonial angle, and body. It should be emphasized, however, that the development of multiplanar distraction devices will give more control over the trajectory of distraction, and the precision of placement of the device will become less critical.

In 7 of 10 patients, the mandibles maintained their postdistraction morphology while demonstrating growth during the study period. Conversely, in three of the ten patients, mandibular morphology was altered during distraction but returned to the predistraction shape with the passage of time. These three patients, two of whom carried the diagnosis of Nager syndrome, had undergone bilateral distraction. These patients had their distraction devices placed horizontally with temporary loss of the gonial angle postdistraction. Within 2 years, the mandibles demonstrated growth but remodeled to assume the preexpansion shape with restitution of the gonial angle (Figure 5.28).

All asymmetric mandibles (unilateral distraction) were expanded until the pogonion, or chin point, was translocated beyond the midsagittal plane. The overcorrected chin position was noted to decrease over time as the relative growth rate of the affected and unaffected sides of the mandible in patients with unilateral craniofacial microsomia was unequal. The overcorrected mandibles were noted to change from a class III incisor relationship to an edge-to-edge relationship over time. This was thought to be secondary to the clockwise rotation of the mandible, as previously discussed (see Figure 5.25), as well as the reexpression of the syndrome-specific growth pattern of the affected and unaffected mandibular rami.

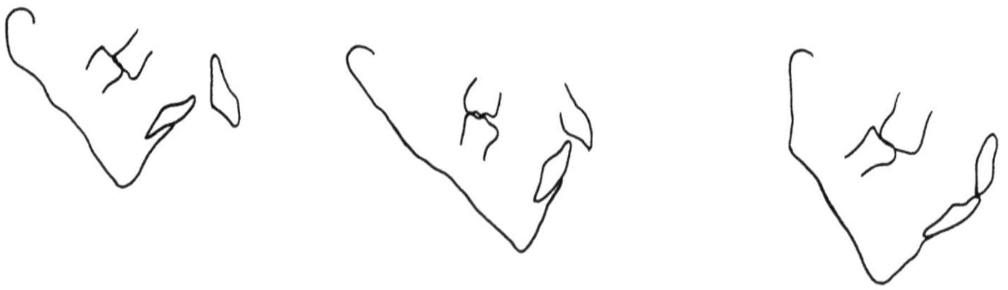

A B C

Figure 5.28. Serial lateral cephalograms of a patient who underwent bilateral distraction. (A) Predistraction tracing. (B) Lateral tracing following distraction. Note that the overjet has been reduced, but the overall mandibular morphology has been changed. (C) A lateral cephalogram 5 years later shows that the gonial angle has returned, and there is a more anatomic mandibular morphology.

Case Studies

CASE STUDIES: UNILATERAL DISTRACTION

Case 1. C.R. was an 18-month-old boy with right craniofacial microsomia involving the ipsilateral auricle, orbit, soft-tissue cheek, maxilla, and mandible (Pruzansky Class I) (Figure 5.29). His previous surgery has included an ipsilateral fronto-orbital advancement. In May 1989 he underwent unilateral, mandibular distraction (18 mm) with movement of his dental midline to the contralateral side. This was followed by 8 weeks of fixation. At the completion of distraction, a bite plate was placed in the resulting posterior open bite. Over the ensuing 12 months the prosthesis was reduced in size to allow the eruption of the maxillary dentoalveolus. He has now been followed for over 8 years. Note the multidimensional expansion of the craniofacial skeleton and the improvement in his right cheek contour. His bigonial distance has been significantly increased and he has a level occlusal plane. His chin point and mandibular dental midline remains slightly to the contralateral side. It has been recommended that he undergo transcranial correction of his residual orbital dystopia. Auricular reconstruction is currently underway (Dr. Bert Brent).

His serial cephalometric studies are also illustrated in Figure 5.29.

Figure 5.29. Case 1.

(A) Preoperative frontal view. Note the microtia, deviation of the chin to the right, hypoplasia of the affected cheek, and occlusal cant.

(B) Postoperative frontal view 7 years after completion of distraction. Note the position of the chin point in the midline and the relative symmetry of the oral commissures and the cheek contour. The affected auricle is in staged reconsruction.

(C) Preoperative submental view.

(D) Postoperative submental view showing improvement in chin position and symmetry as well as contour of the right cheek.

(E) Preoperative right profile with microtia.

(F) Postoperative right profile. Note the position of the scar and the increase in the oral commissure-tragal distance.

(G) Preoperative left profile.

(H) Postoperative left profile.

(I) Predistraction posteroanterior cephalogram.

(J) Postdistraction posteroanterior cephalogram.

(K) Predistraction lateral cephalogram.

(L) Postdistraction lateral cephalogram.

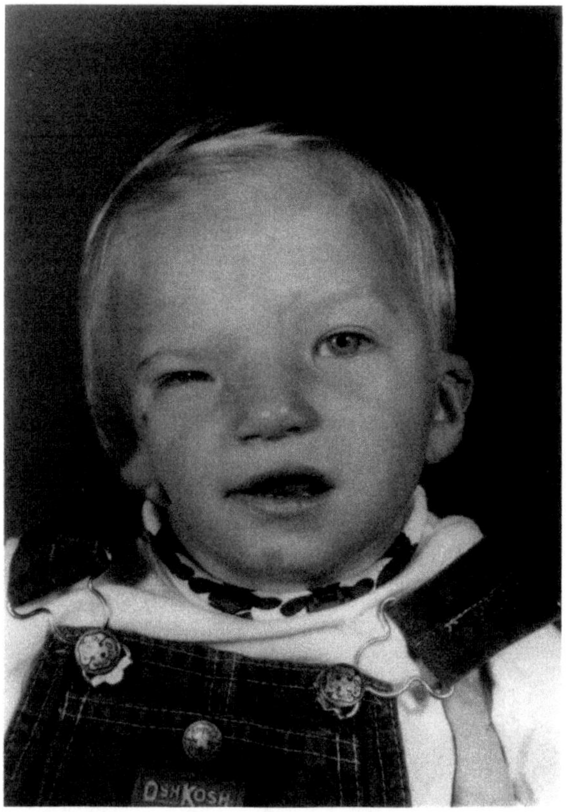

A

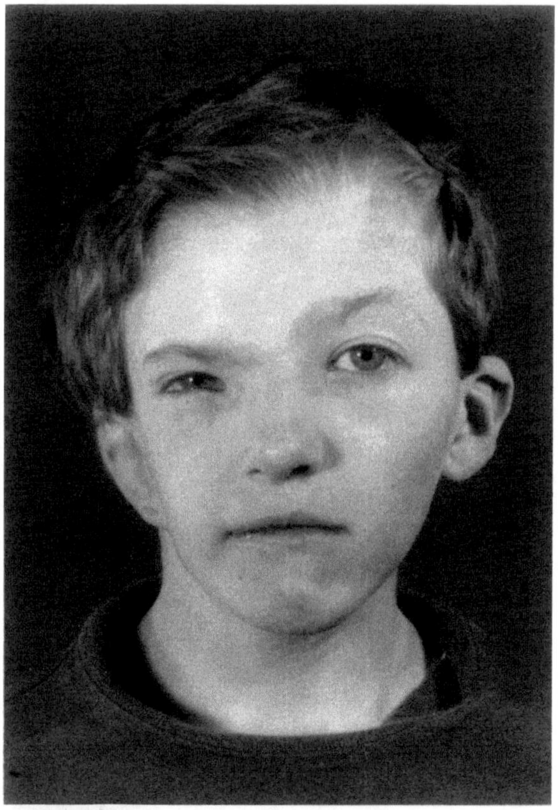

B

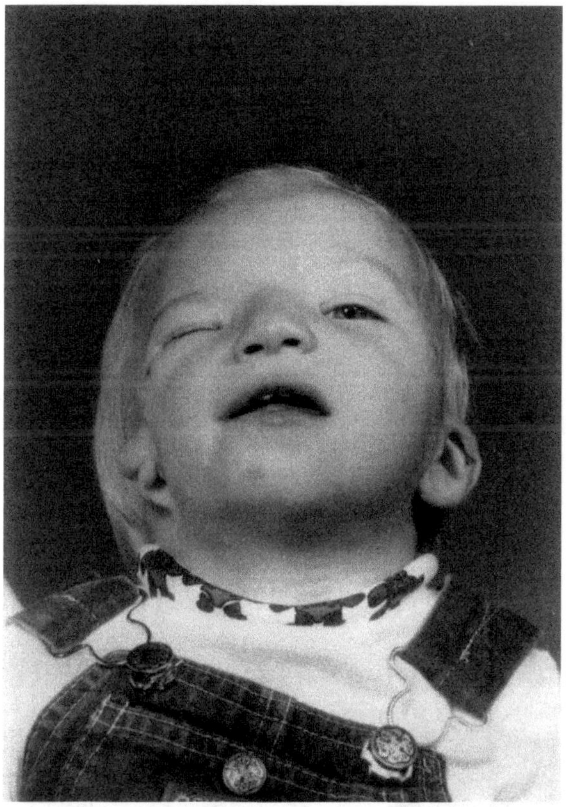

C

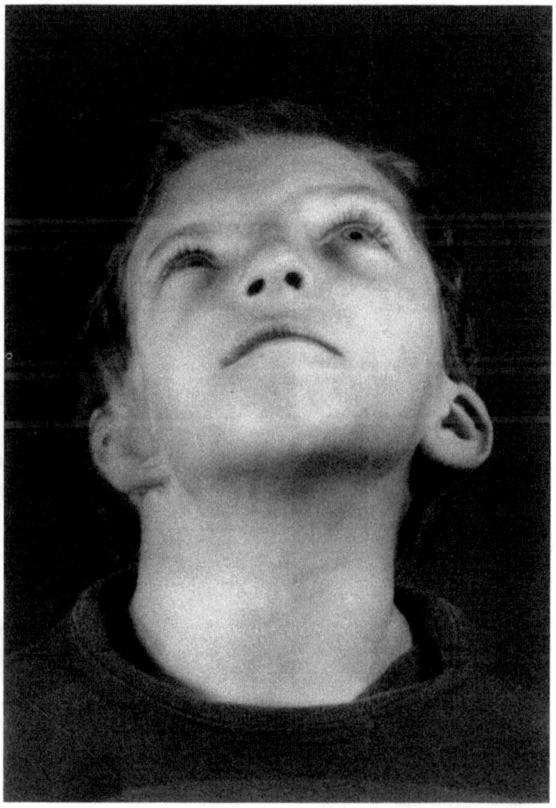

D

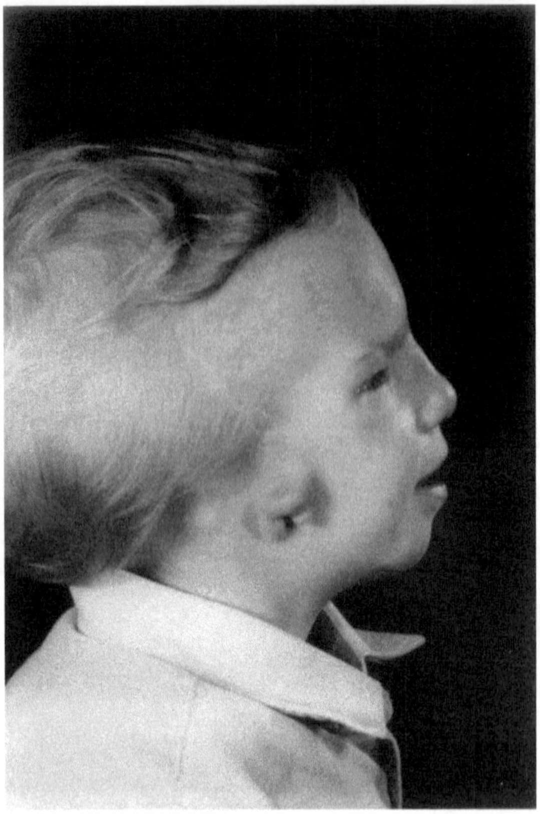

E

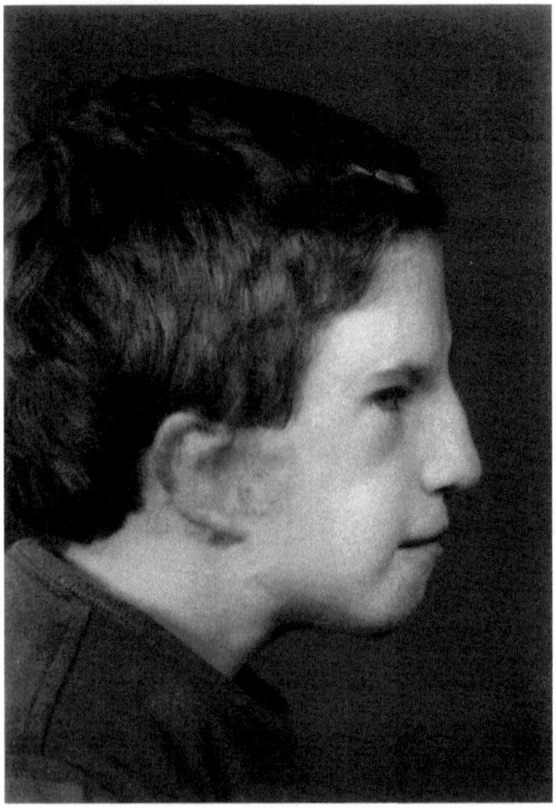

F

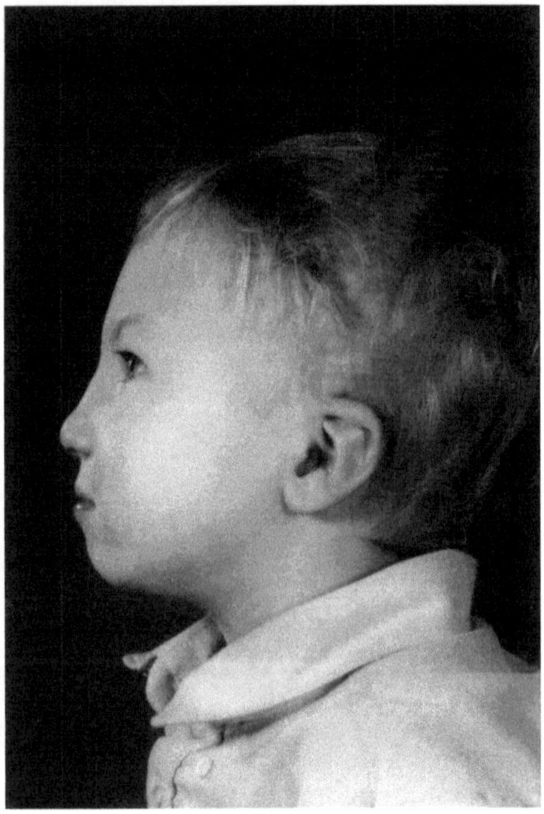

G

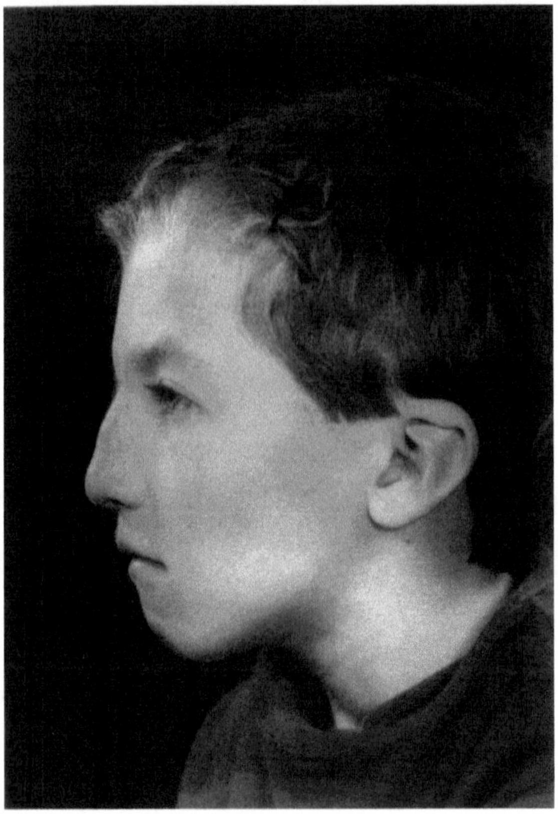

H

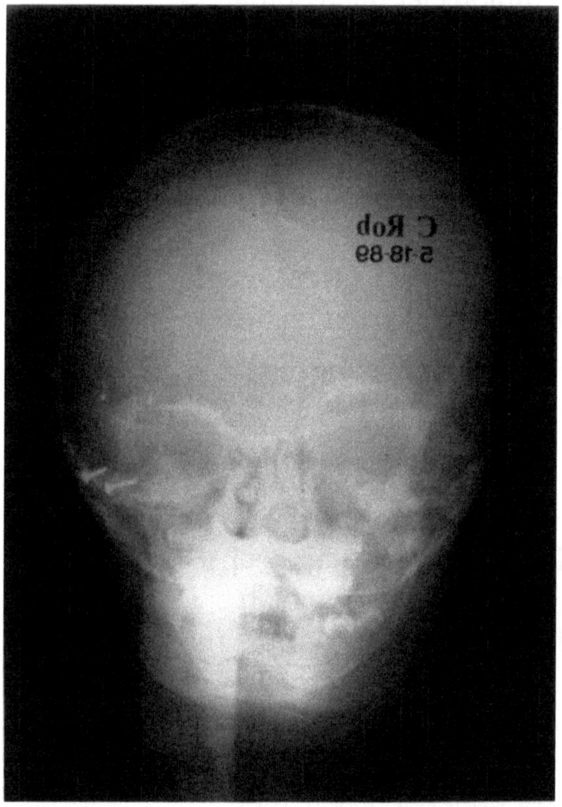

I

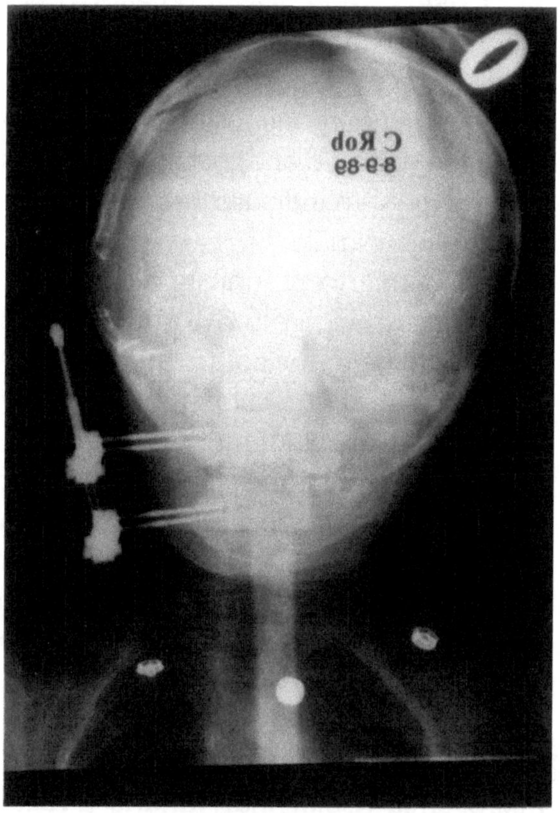

J

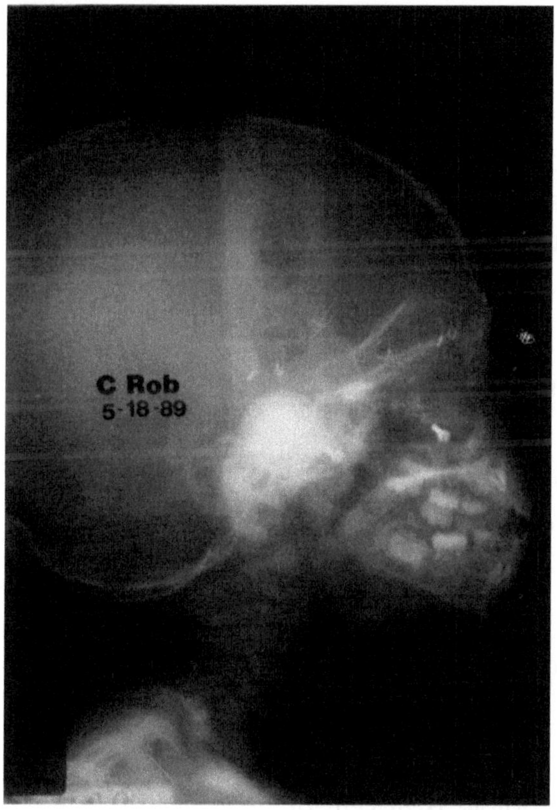

K

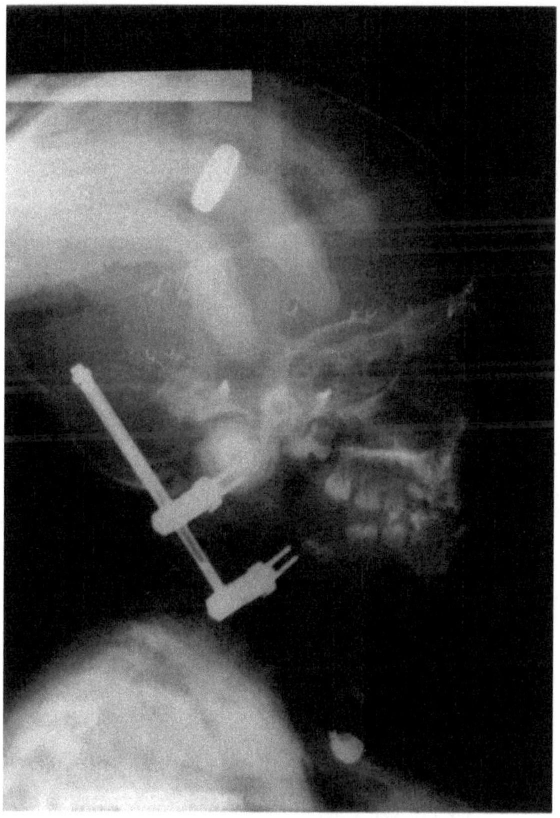

L

Case 2. J.D. was a 6-year-old boy with left craniofacial microsomia (Goldenhar variant) characterized by involvement of the frontal bone, orbit, maxilla, mandible (Pruzansky Class IIa), and auricle (Figure 5.30). He had previously undergone ipsilateral fronto-orbital advancement and excision of a midline dermoid and, because of a postoperative infection, an unsuccessful attempt at mandibular reconstruction with rib graft reconstruction of the hypoplastic ramus.

He underwent unilateral distraction (26 mm) with leveling of the occlusal cant (Figure 5.30) and relocation of his pogonion and mandibular dental midline to the contralateral side. After 8 weeks of fixation a bite plate was placed in the resulting intermaxillary void and was serially reduced in size in the ensuing months to allow eruption of the maxillary teeth. Following distraction he had significant increase in his bigonial distance. His soft-tissue contour was reestablished with the insertion of a microvascular parascapular free flap 9 months after distraction. He has been followed for 6 years. Note the satisfactory position of the oral commissure, chin point, and cheek contour. His serial cephalometric studies are also illustrated in Figure 5.30.

Figure 5.30. Case 2. A 6-year-old male with left craniofacial microsomia (Goldenhar variant) (Pruzansky IIa) who underwent left mandibular distraction (26 mm). An earlier surgical reconstruction with costochondral rib grafts was complicated by infection.

(A) Preoperative frontal view. Note the chin deviation to the affected side, elevation of the affected oral commissure and occlusal cant (mandibular).

(B) Postoperative frontal view 48 months after completion of distraction. He had also undergone insertion of a microvascular free flap in the left cheek. Note the position of the chin and the improved relationship of the oral commissures.

(C) Preoperative submental view.

(D) Postoperative submental view. The ill-positioned ear remnant was resected.

(E) Preoperative right profile.

(F) Postoperative right profile. Note the increased projection of the chin profile.

(G) Preoperative left profile.

(H) Postoperative left profile. The scar is satisfactory.

(I) Predistraction posteroanterior cephalogram (device in place).

(J) Postdistraction posteroanterior cephalogram. The inferior displacement of the inferior border of the affected mandible is apparent.

(K) Predistraction lateral cephalogram (before activation).

(L) Postdistraction lateral cephalogram. Note the horizontal vector and the increased sagittal thrust of the mandible.

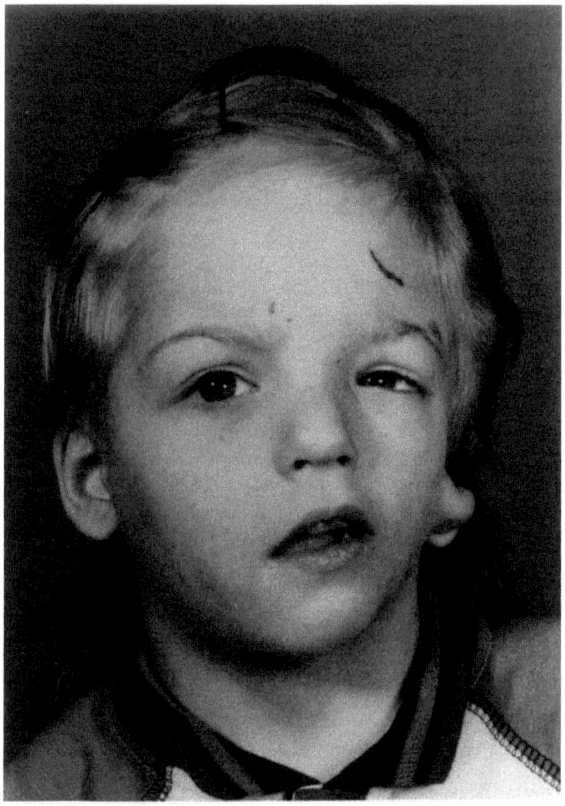

A

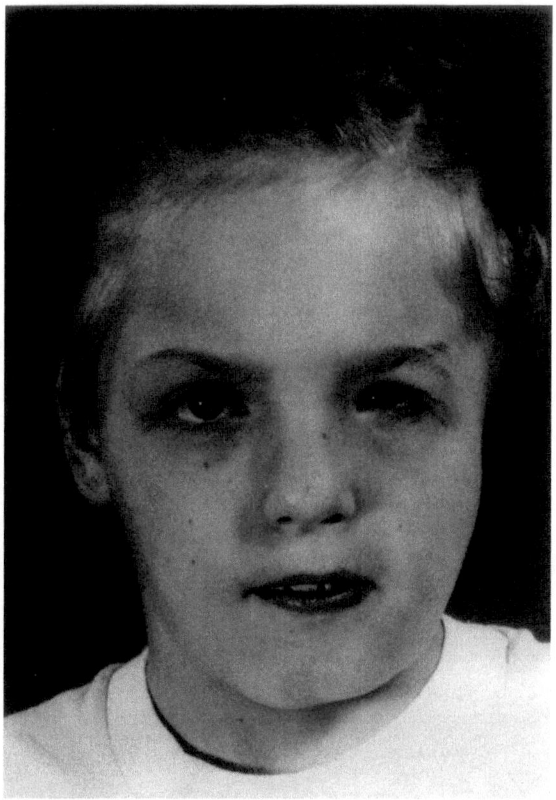

B

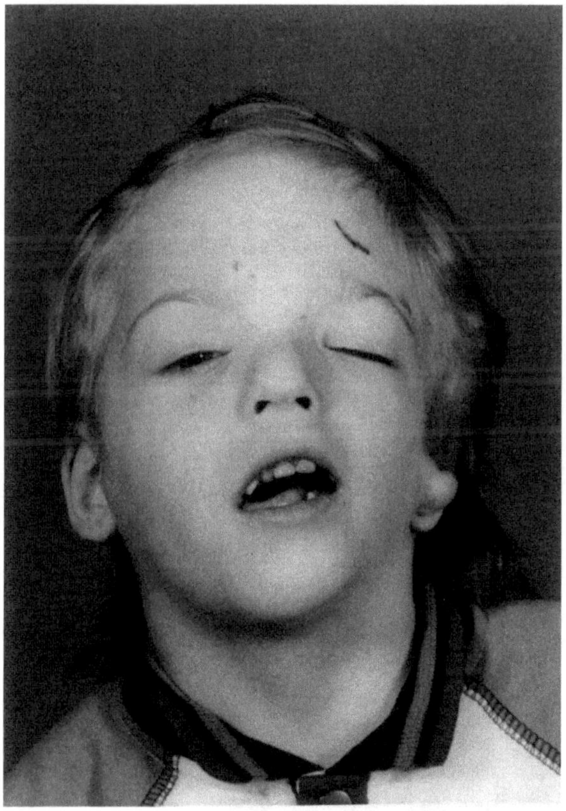

C

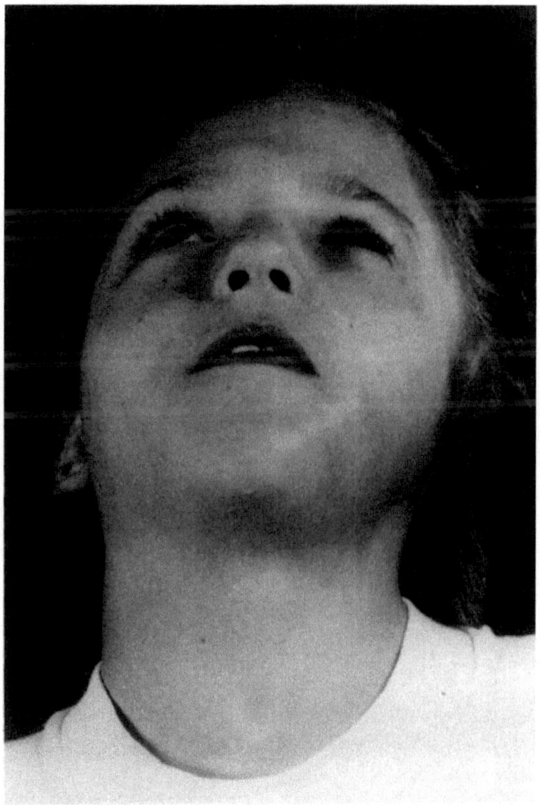

D

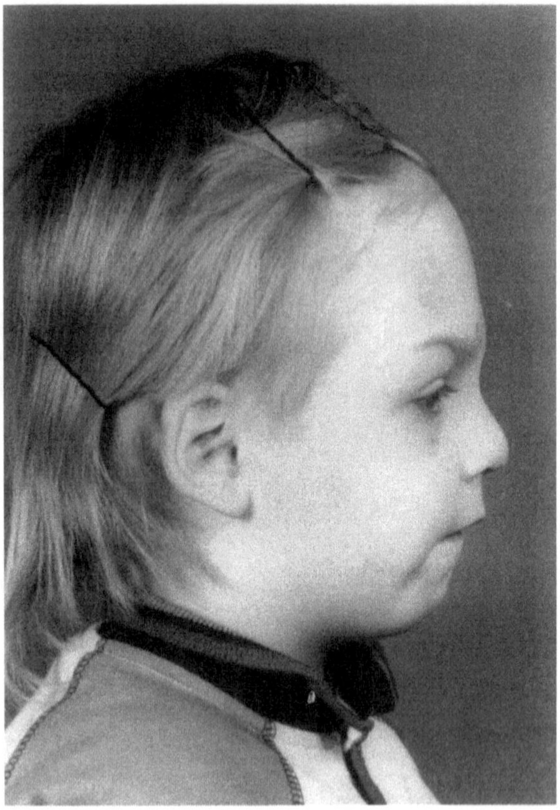

E

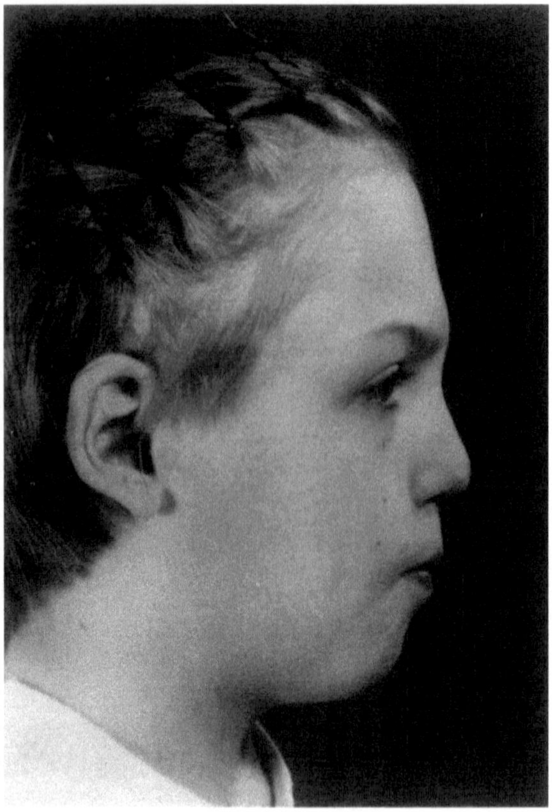

F

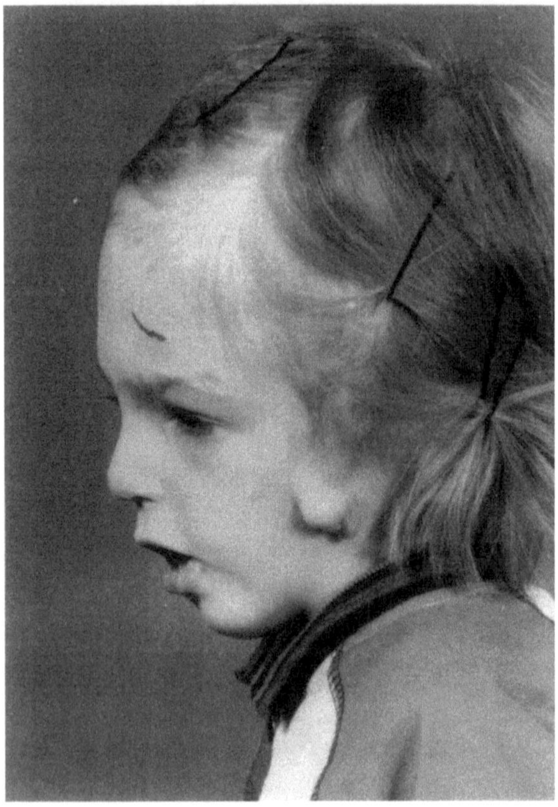

G

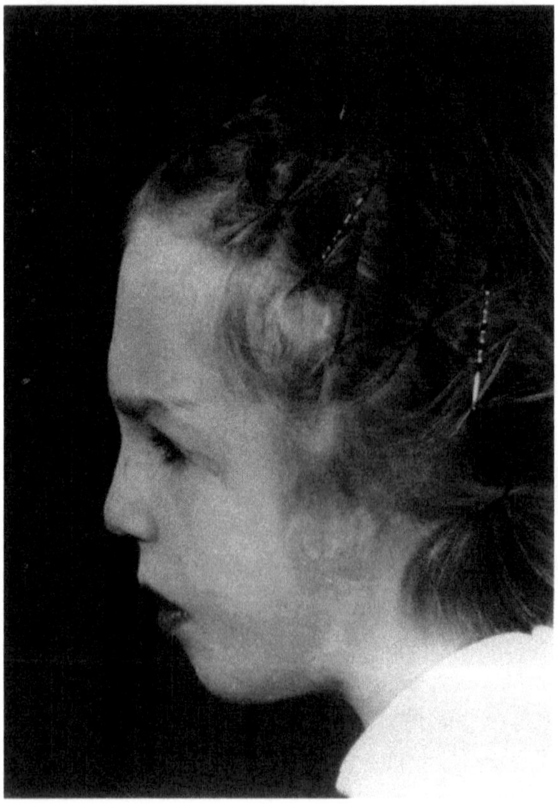

H

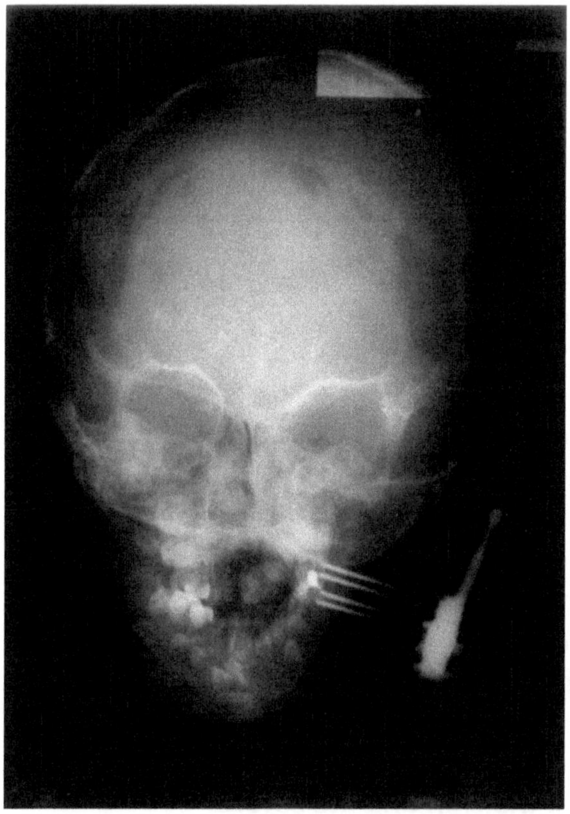

I

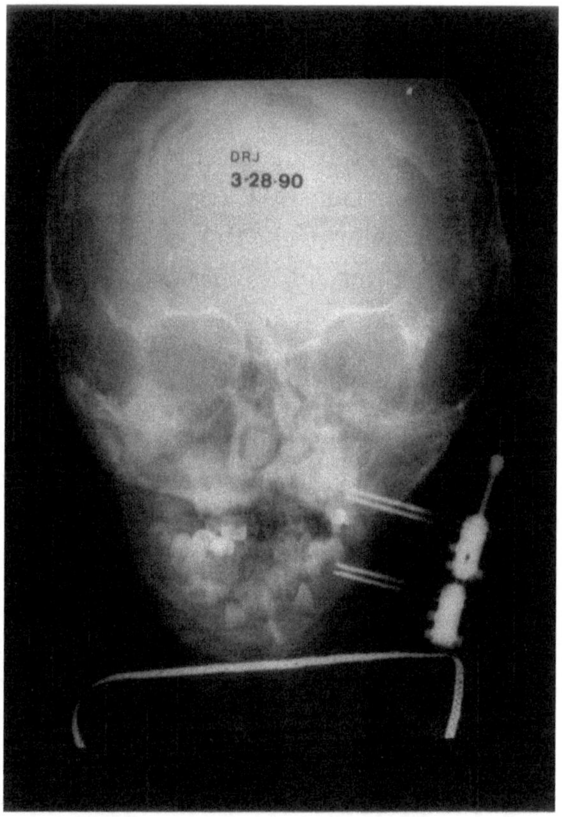

J

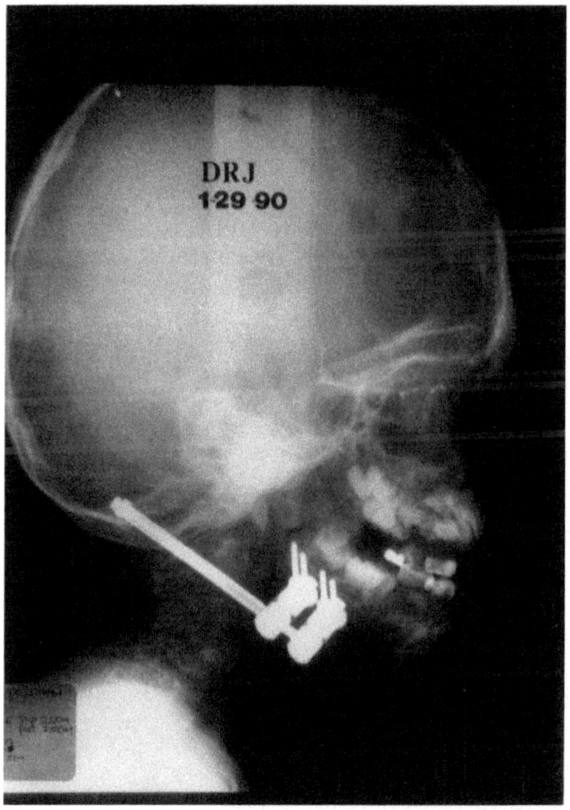

K

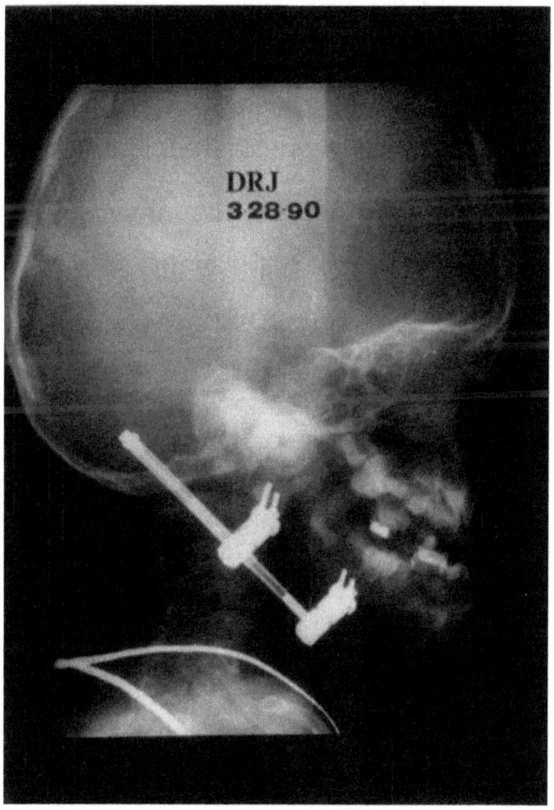

L

Case 3. R.P. was a three-year-old boy with left craniofacial microsomia characterized by a mini ear and involvement of the maxilla and mandible (Pruzansky Class IIa) with an occlusal cant upward on the affected side and deviation of the pogonion to the affected side (Figure 5.31).

He underwent unilateral mandibular distraction (25 mm). After 8 weeks of fixation, a bite plate was placed in the resulting intermaxillary void. The latter was gradually reduced by the orthodontist in the subsequent months. He has been followed for over 5 years.

Serial preoperative and postoperative cephalograms and 3D CT scans demonstrated elongation of the ascending ramus with forward projection of the body and chin (Figure 5.31I–P).

Figure 5.31. **Case 3.** A 3-year-old male with left craniofacial microsomia (Pruzansky IIa) who underwent left mandibular distraction (25 mm).

(A) Preoperative fronal view. Note the deviation of the chin and the severe occlusal cant.

(B) Postoperative frontal view 19 months after completion of distraction. Note the improvement in the position of the chin, oral commissure, and left alar base. The occlusal plane has been leveled. The cheek contours are more symmetrical.

(C) Preoperative submental view.

(D) Postoperative submental view.

(E) Preoperative right profile.

(F) Postoperative right profile. Note the increased thrust of the mandible.

(G) Preoperative left profile.

(H) Postoperative left profile.

(I) Predistraction posteroanterior cephalogram (before activation with device in place). Note the osteotomy.

(J) Postdistraction posteroanterior cephalogram.

(K) Predistraction lateral cephalogram (oblique vector).

(L) Postdistraction later cephalogram. Note the sagittal thrust of the mandible in an "overcorrected" position and the counterclock rotation of the mandible.

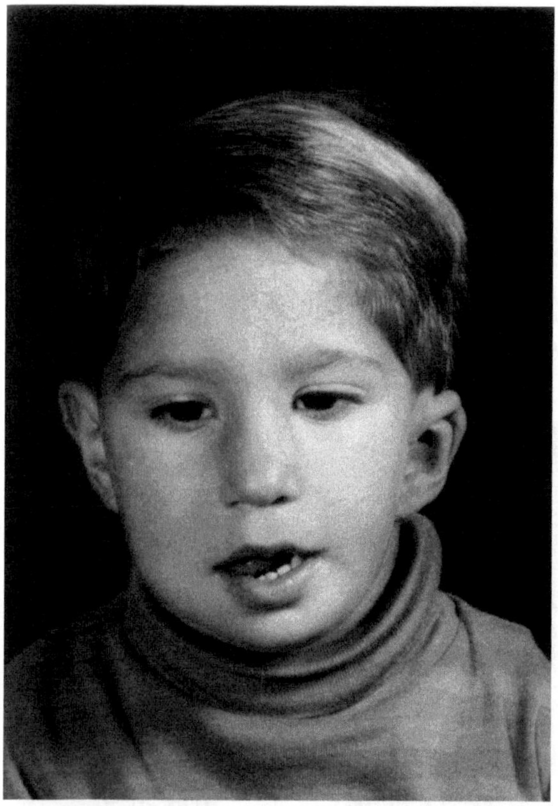

A

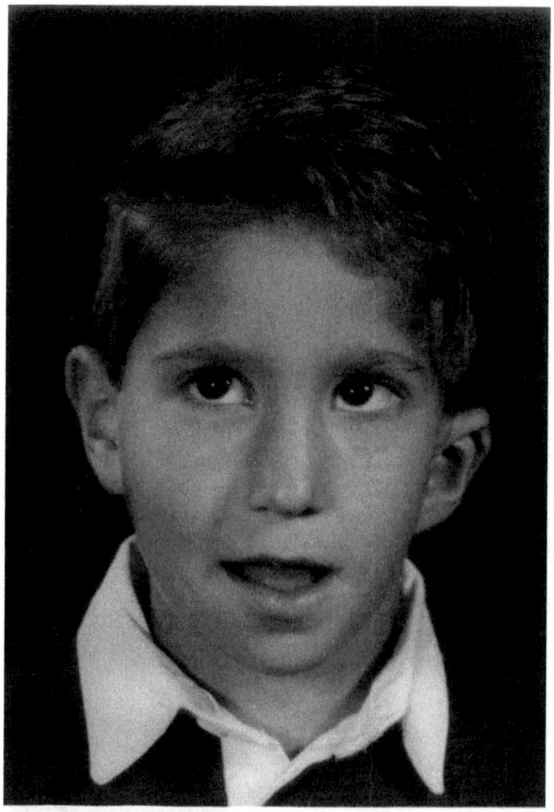

B

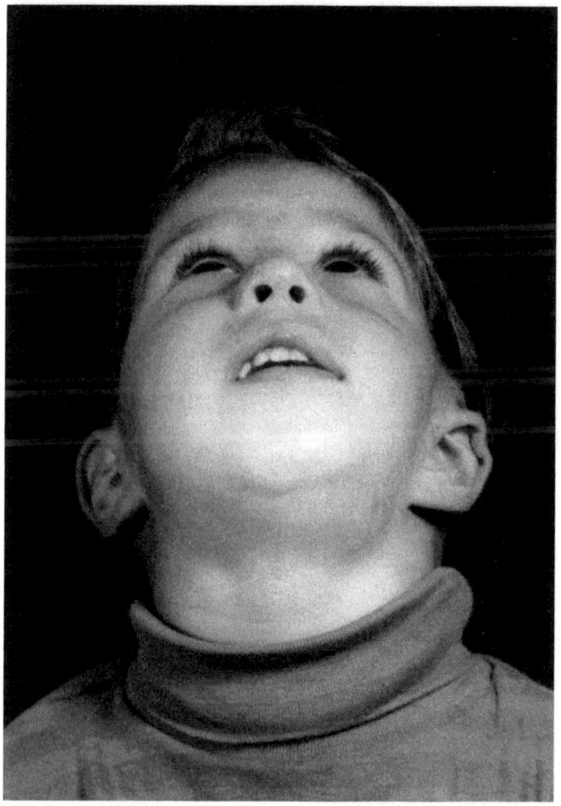

C

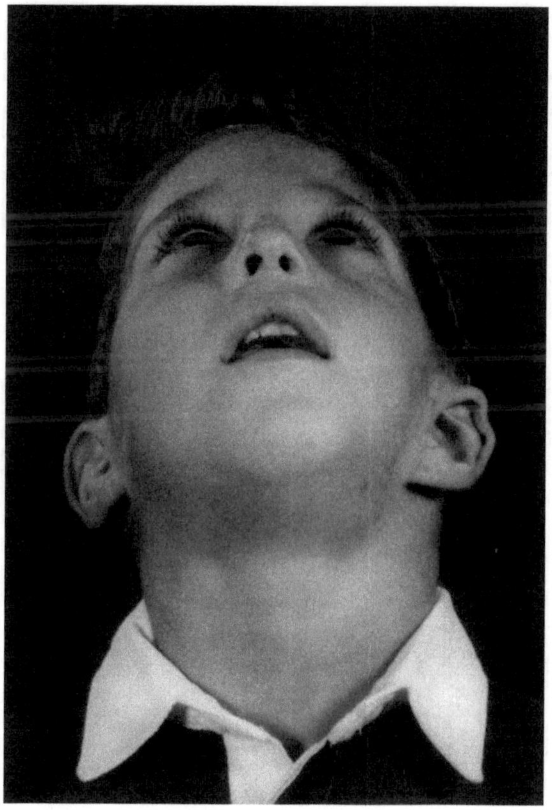

D

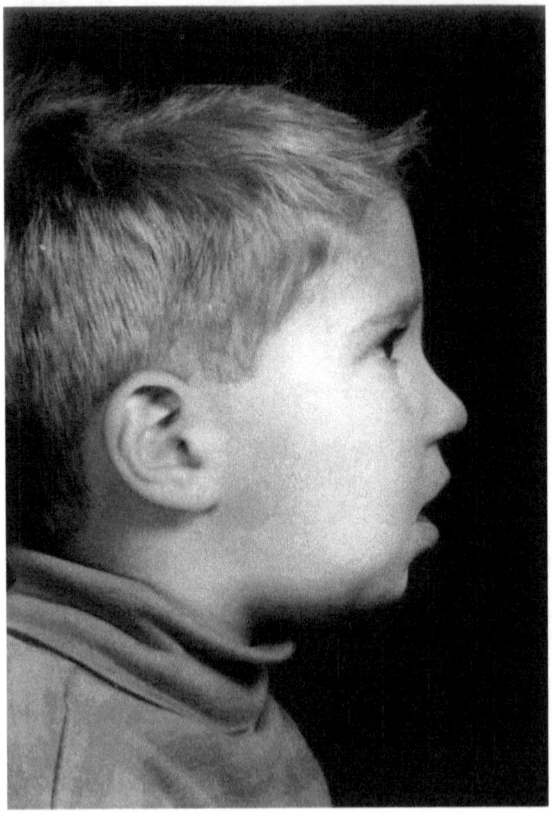

E

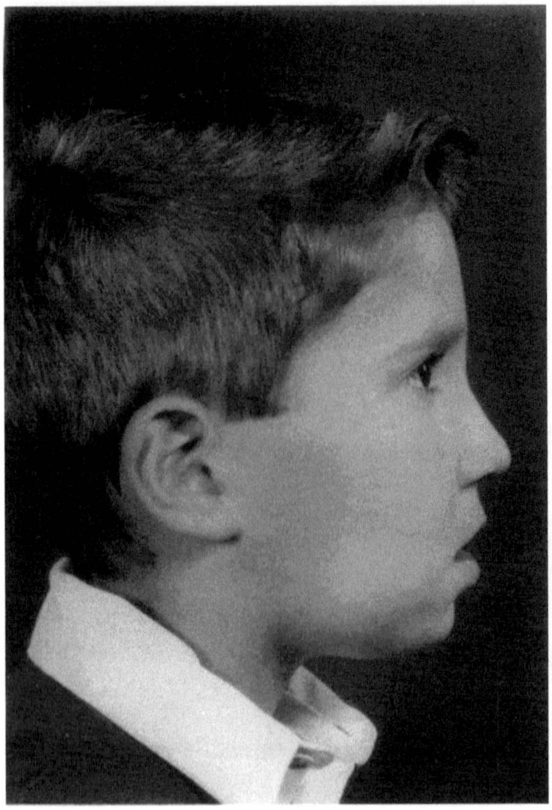

F

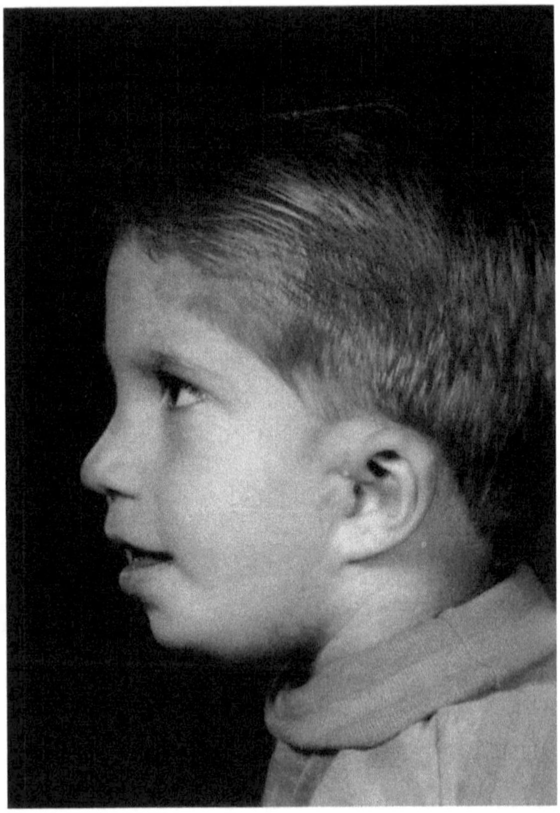

G

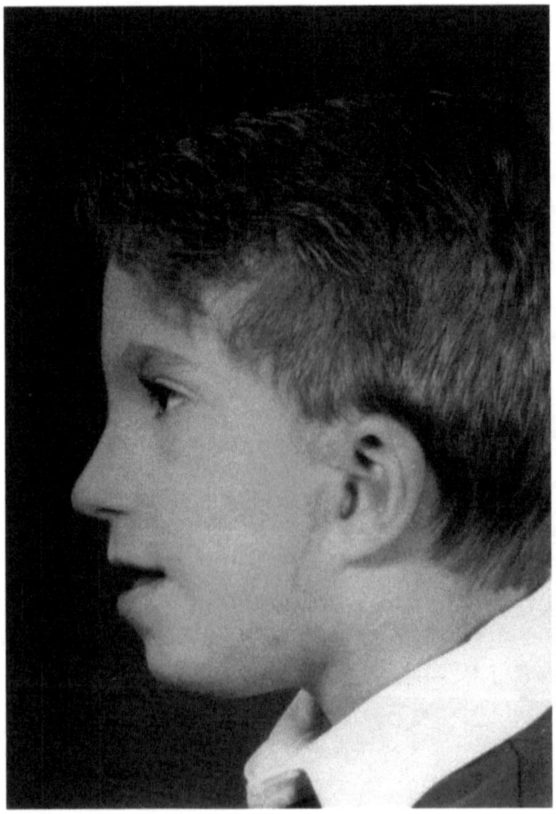

H

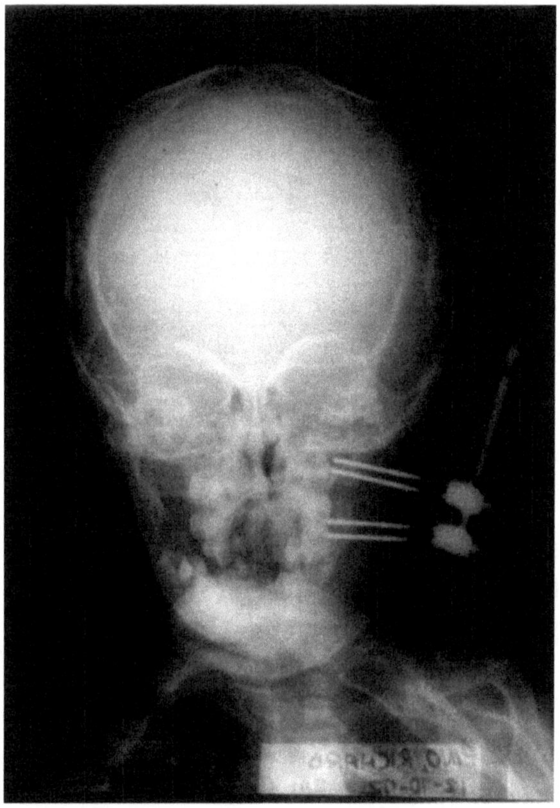

I

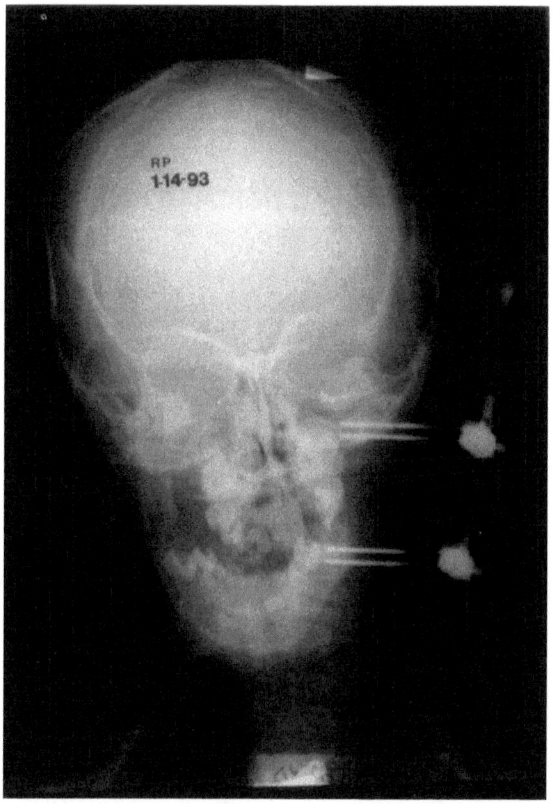

J

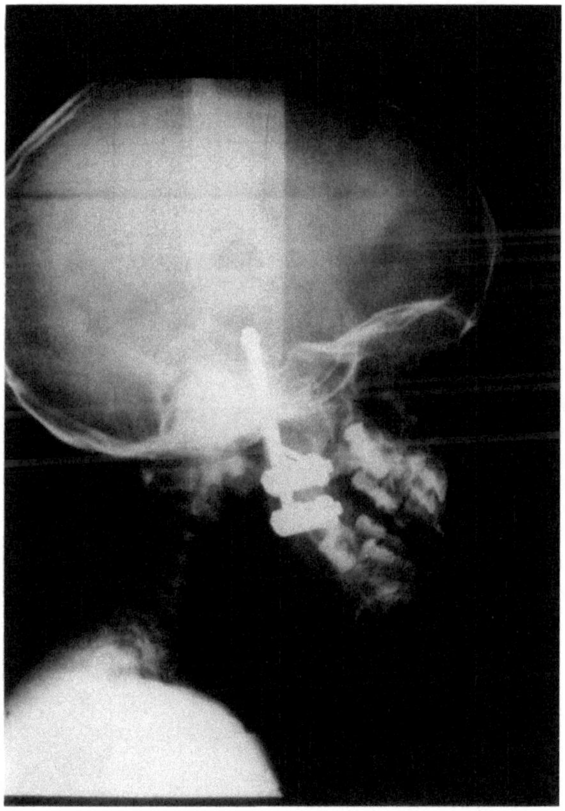

K

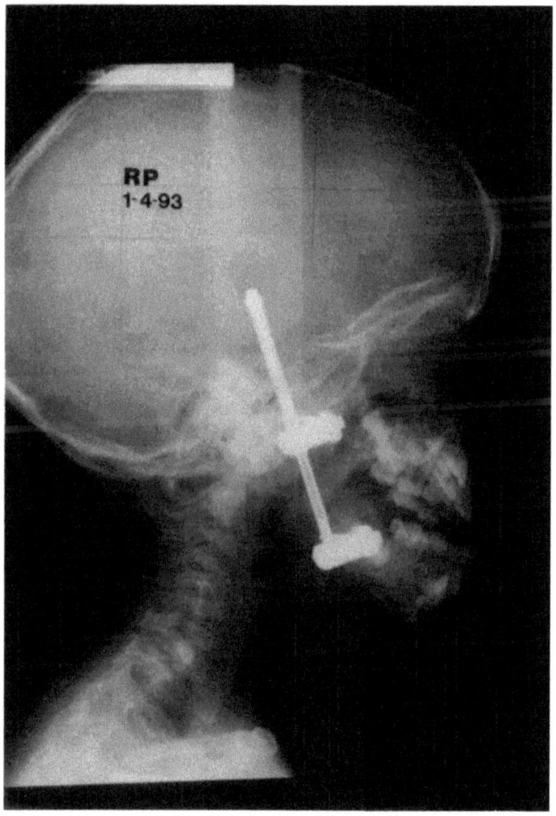

L

Figure 5.31. *Case 3. Continued*

(M) Predistraction frontal 3D CT scan. Note the occlusal cant and the chin position.

(N) Postdistraction frontal 3D CT scan 21 months after completion of distraction. Note the improvement in the occlusal plane and overall chin/mandible morphology.

(O) Predistraction lateral 3D CT scan showing hypoplasia of the affected ramus.

(P) Postdistraction lateral 3D CT scan. Note the increase in the vertical dimension of the ramus, the improvement in the gonial angle, and the clockwise rotation of the mandible.

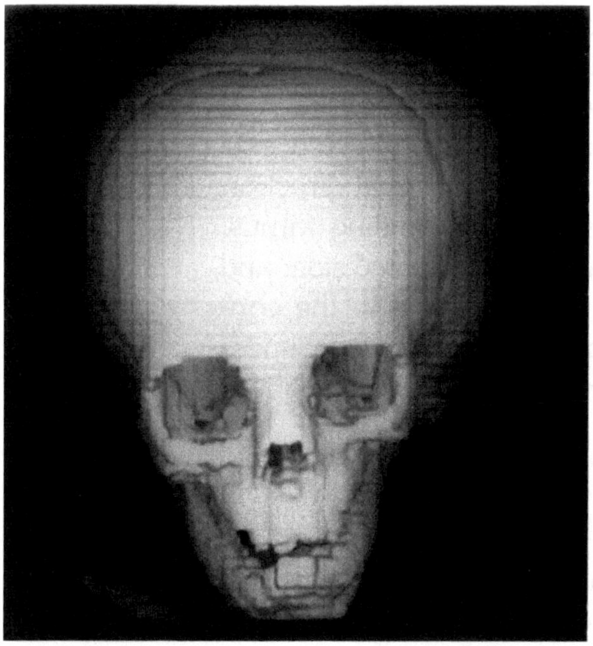

M

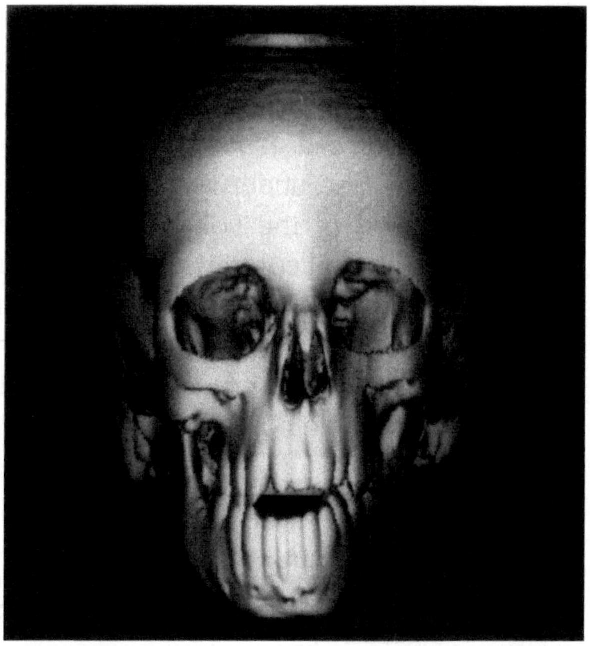

N

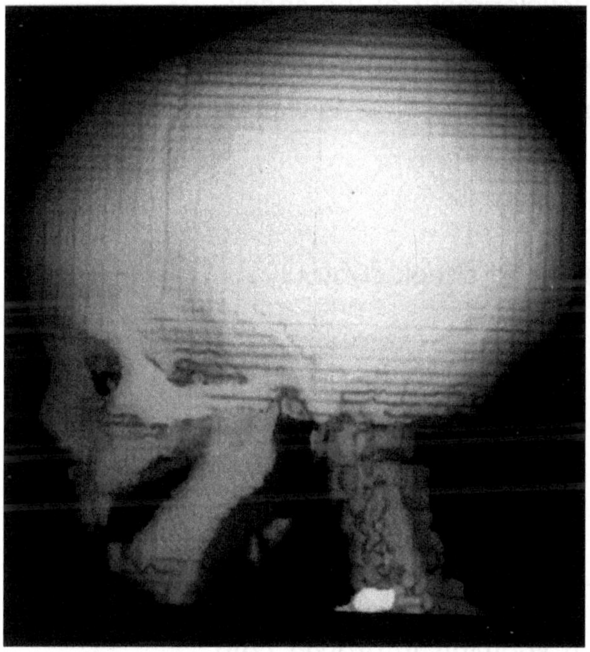

O

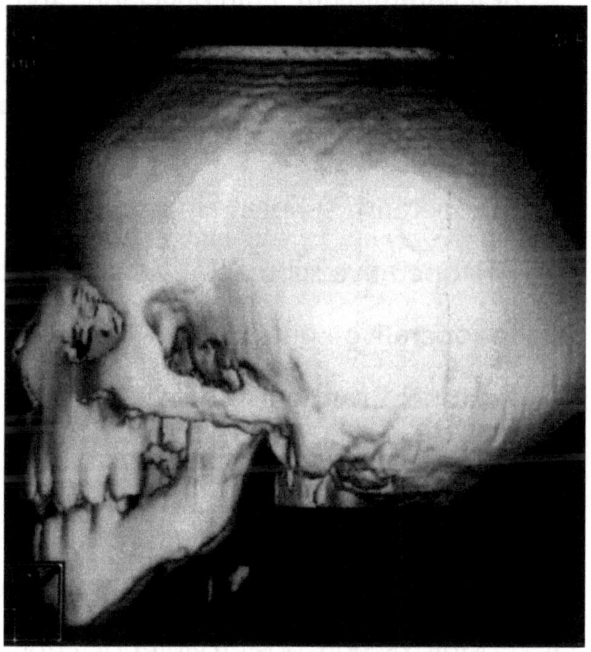

P

Case 4. S.R. was a 10-year-old girl (Figure 5.32) with right craniofacial microsomia (Goldenhaar variant) characterized by involvement of the maxilla and mandible (Pruzansky Class I). The occlusal plane and oral commissure were displaced in a cephalic direction on the affected side (Figure 5.32). She underwent 20 mm of distraction in a vertical direction with restoration of the volume and dimensions of her ascending ramus, lowering of the oral commissure and occlusal cant on the affected side, and repositioning of the pogonion and mandibular dental midline to the contralateral side. On the distracted side she showed temporary weakness (partial) of the buccal branch of the facial nerve over a 4-week period, followed by complete resolution.

Figure 5.32. Case 4. A 10-year-old female with right craniofacial microsomia (Goldenhar variant) (Pruzansky I) who underwent right mandibular distraction (20 mm).

(A) Preoperative frontal view showing canting of the occlusal plane and oral commissure, chin deviation, and underdevelopment of the cheek.

(B) Postoperative frontal view 26 months after completion of distraction showing improvement in chin and oral commissure position as well as the occlusal plane.

(C) Preoperative submental view.

(D) Postoperative submental view. Note the improved cheek contour.

(E) Preoperative right profile.

(F) Postoperative right profile.

(G) Preoperative left profile.

(H) Postoperative left profile.

(I) Predistraction posteroanterior cephalogram.

(J) Postdistraction posteroanterior cephalogram showing improved chin position and mandibular morphology with an increased bigonial distance.

(K) Predistraction lateral cephalogram.

(L) Postdistraction lateral cephalogram showing a vertical vector.

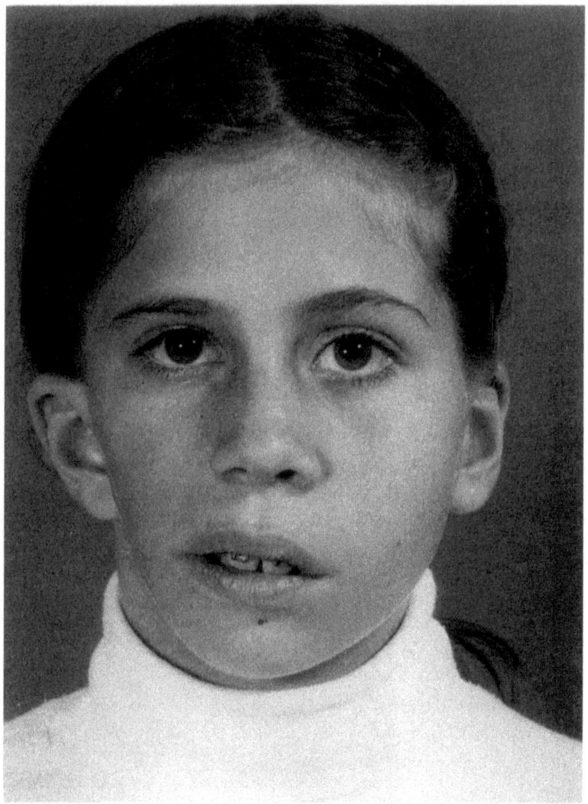

A

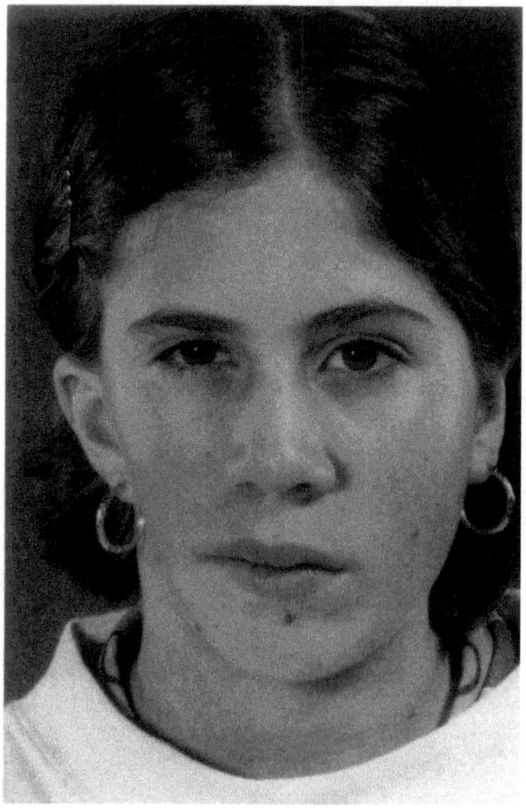

B

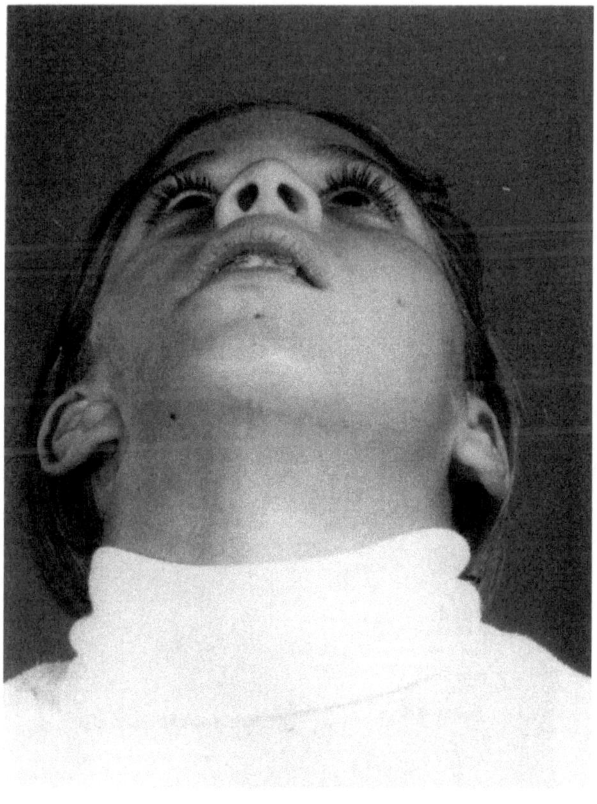

C

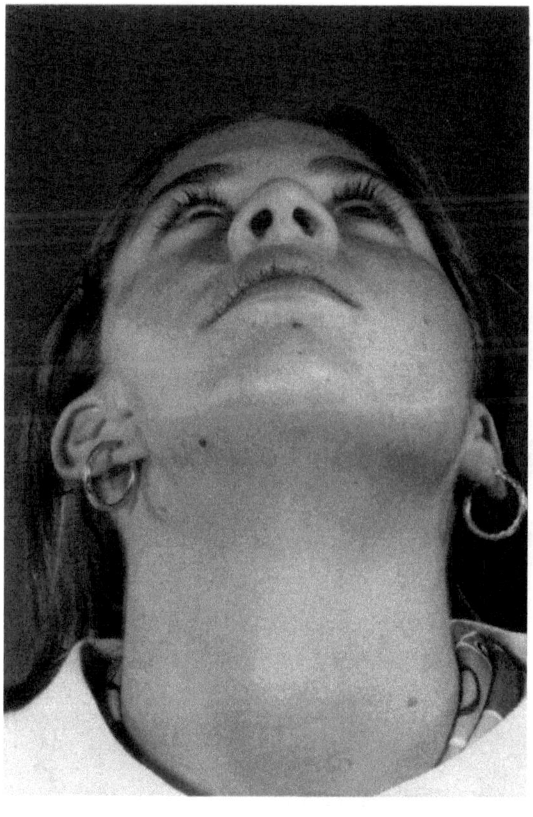

D

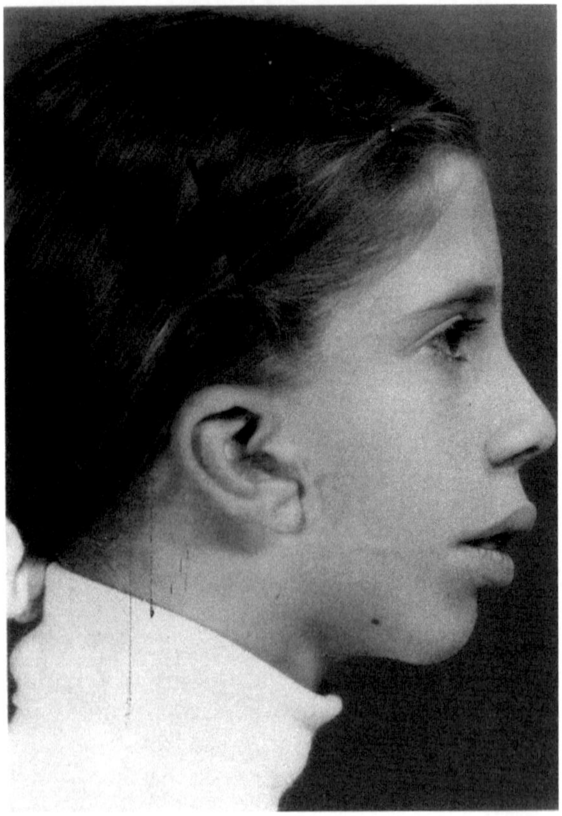

E

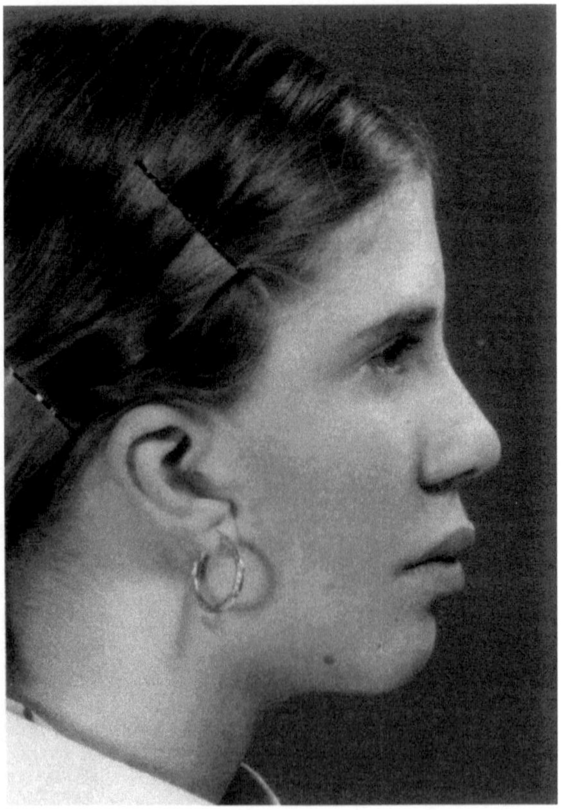

F

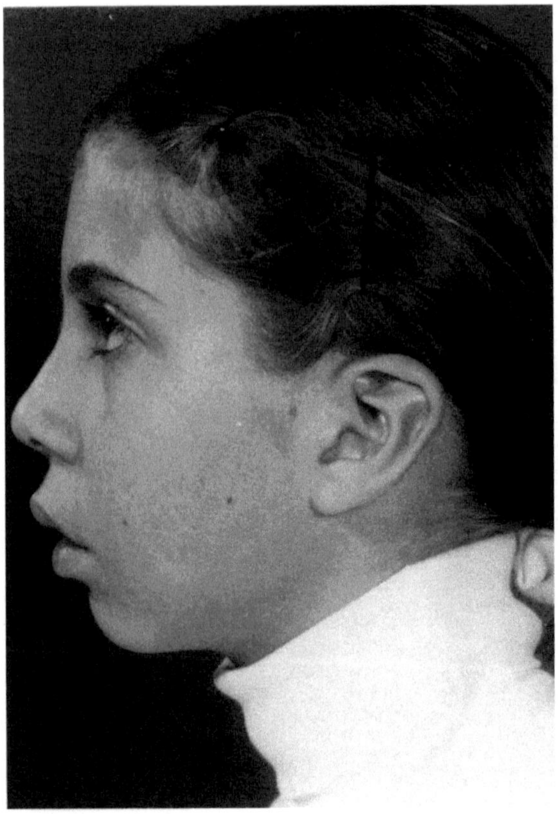

G

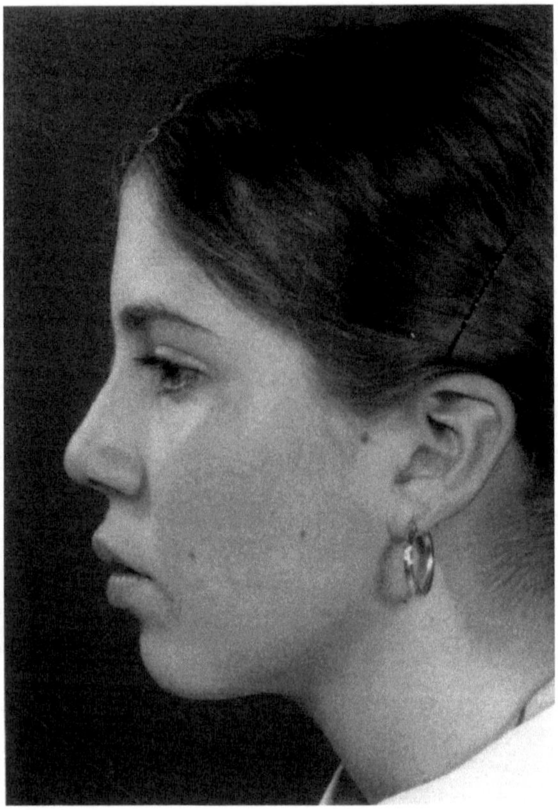

H

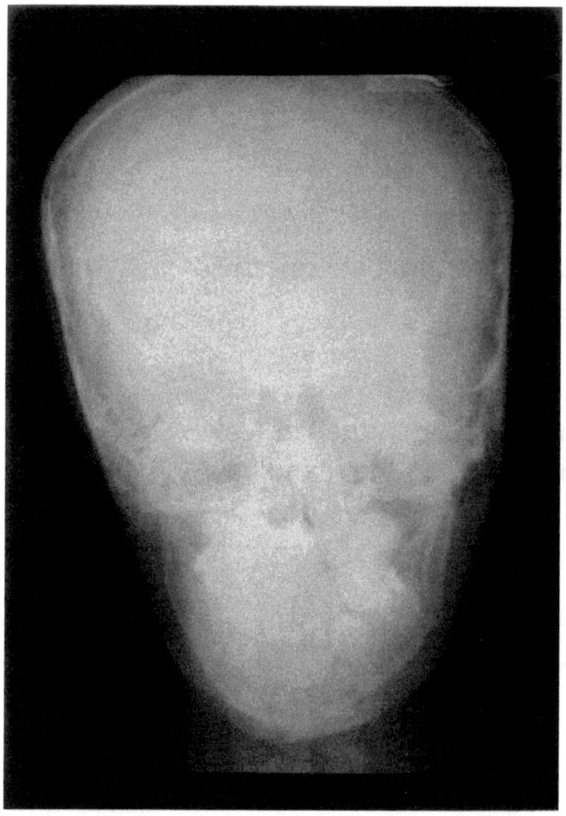

I

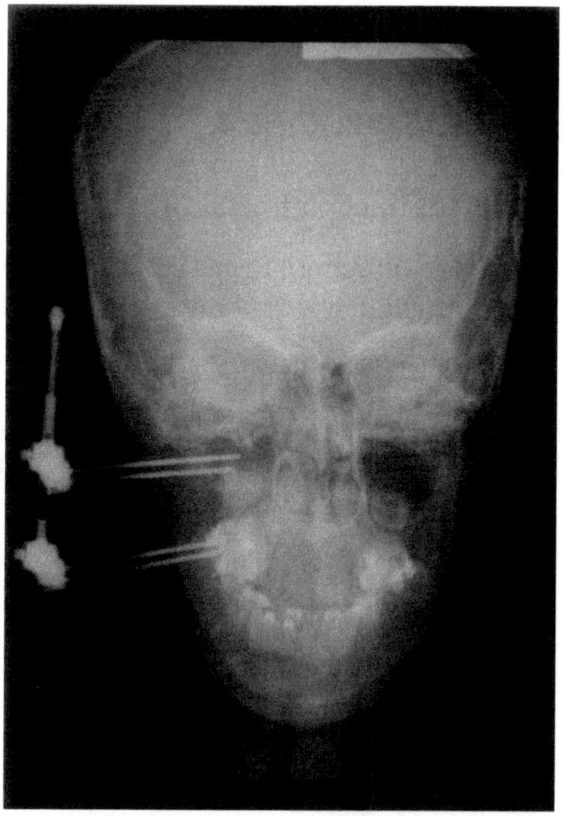

J

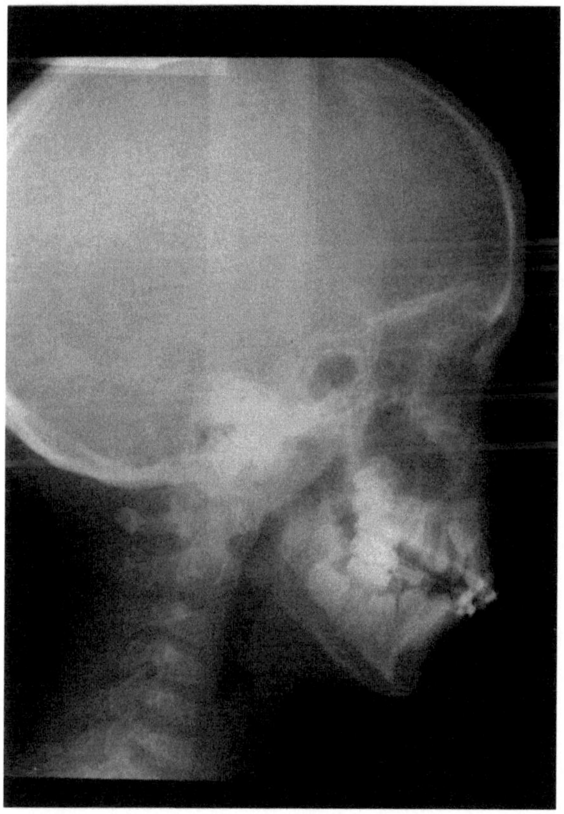

K

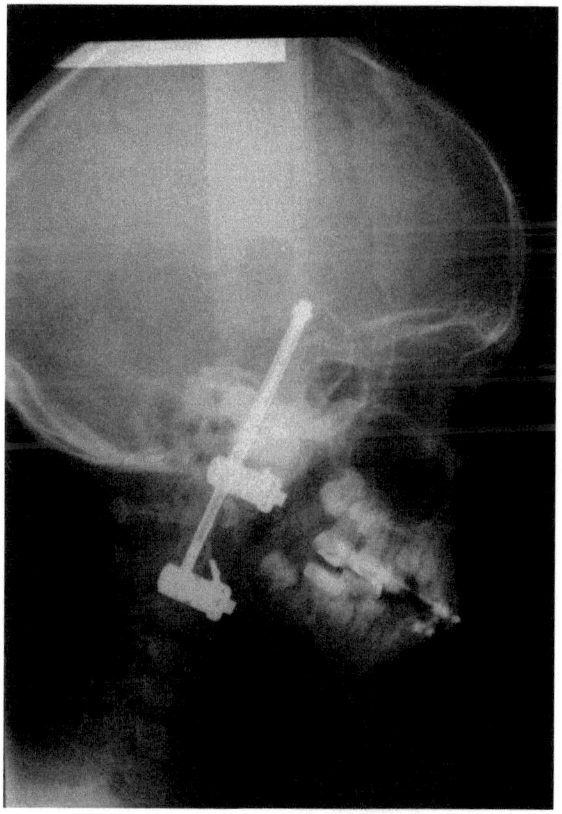

L

Figure 5.32. *Case 4. Continued*

(M) Predistraction frontal 3D CT scan.

(N) Postdistraction frontal 3D CT scan showing an open bite on the distracted side and an increase in the bigonial distance.

(O) Predistraction lateral 3D CT scan.

(P) Postdistraction lateral 3D CT scan showing an increase in the vertical dimension of the ramus. Note that the inferior borders of the mandibular bodies are on the same plane.

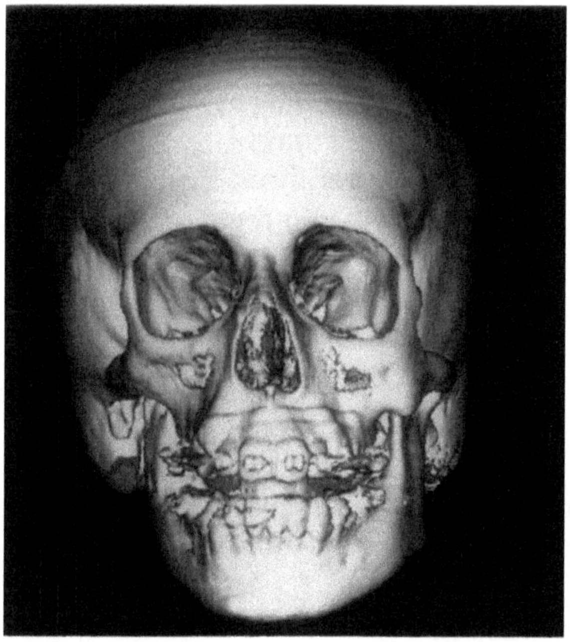

M

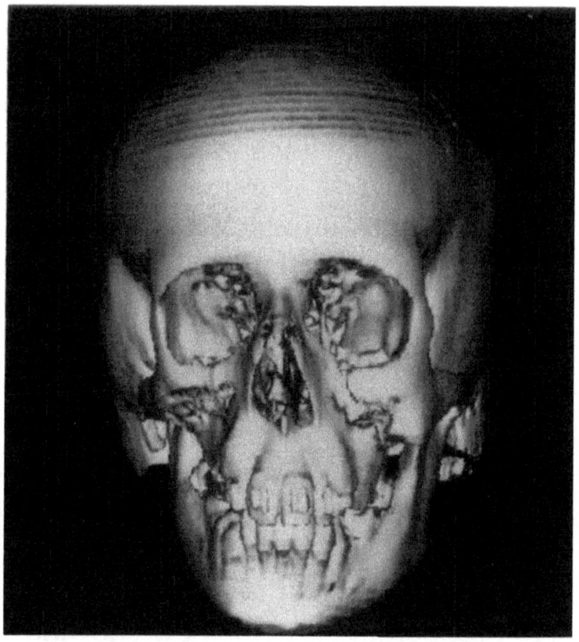

N

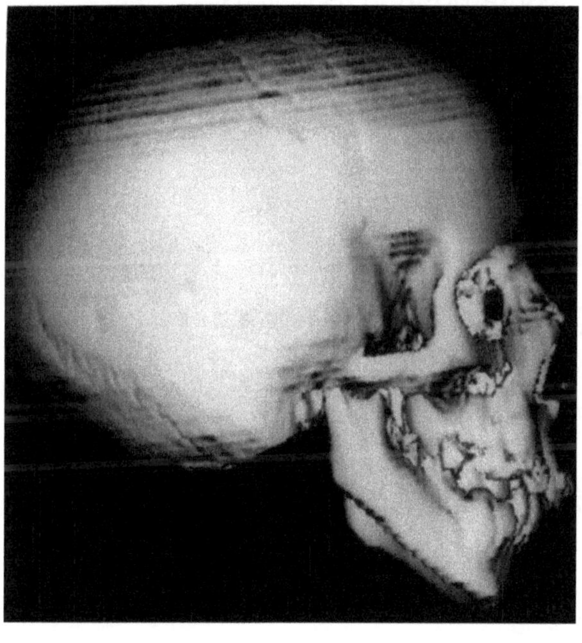

O

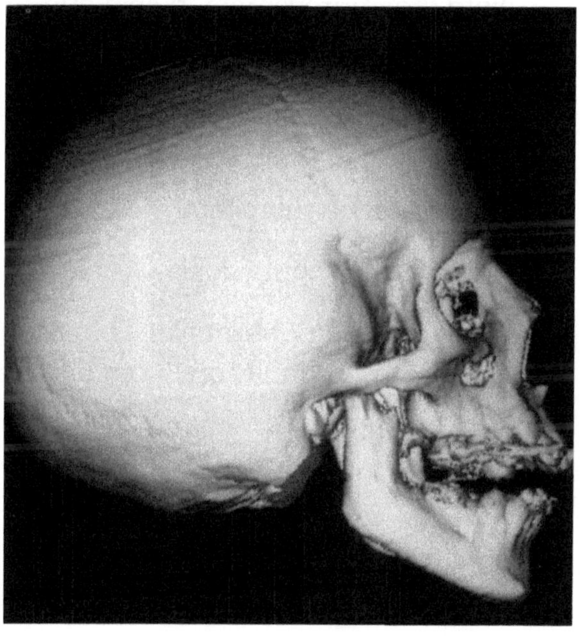

P

Case 5. M.P. was a 7-year-old girl with right craniofacial microsomia characterized by an upward occlusal cant, chin deviation to the affected side, and a severely constricted right ear (previously operated on with a resulting keloid) (Figure 5.33). She demonstrated approximately 11 mm of vertical deficiency of the ramus and 6 mm of deficiency in sagittal thrust (Pruzansky I). A unilateral distraction was completed predominantly in the vertical direction (17 mm). A marked increase was noted in the bigonial distance (cheek contour) and the chin was slightly overcorrected to the left of the craniofacial midline.

Figure 5.33. Case 5. A 7-year-old girl with right craniofacial microsomia (Pruzansky I) who underwent right mandibular distraction (17 mm).

(A) Preoperative frontal view showing the chin deviation, asymmetry of the oral commissure, and hypoplasia of the right cheek. There is a keloid of the affected auricle.

(B) Postoperative frontal view 16 months after completion of distraction. Note the improvement in chin and oral commissure position as well as cheek contour. There is less alar base asymmetry.

(C) Preoperative submental view showing hypoplasia of the affected cheek.

(D) Postoperative submental view showing increased cheek contour.

(E) Preoperative right profile.

(F) Postoperative right profile. The distraction scar has not matured. Note the increased tragal–oral commissure distance.

(G) Preoperative left profile.

(H) Postoperative left profile. Note the increased sagittal thrust of the mandible.

(I) Predistraction posteroanterior cephalogram (device in place).

(J) Postdistraction posteroanterior cephalogram. Note the improved chin and mandibular morphology and leveling of the occlusal plane.

(K) Predistraction lateral cephalogram (oblique vector).

(L) Postdistraction lateral cephalogram. The bite has been closed and there has been counterclockwise rotation of the long arm of the device.

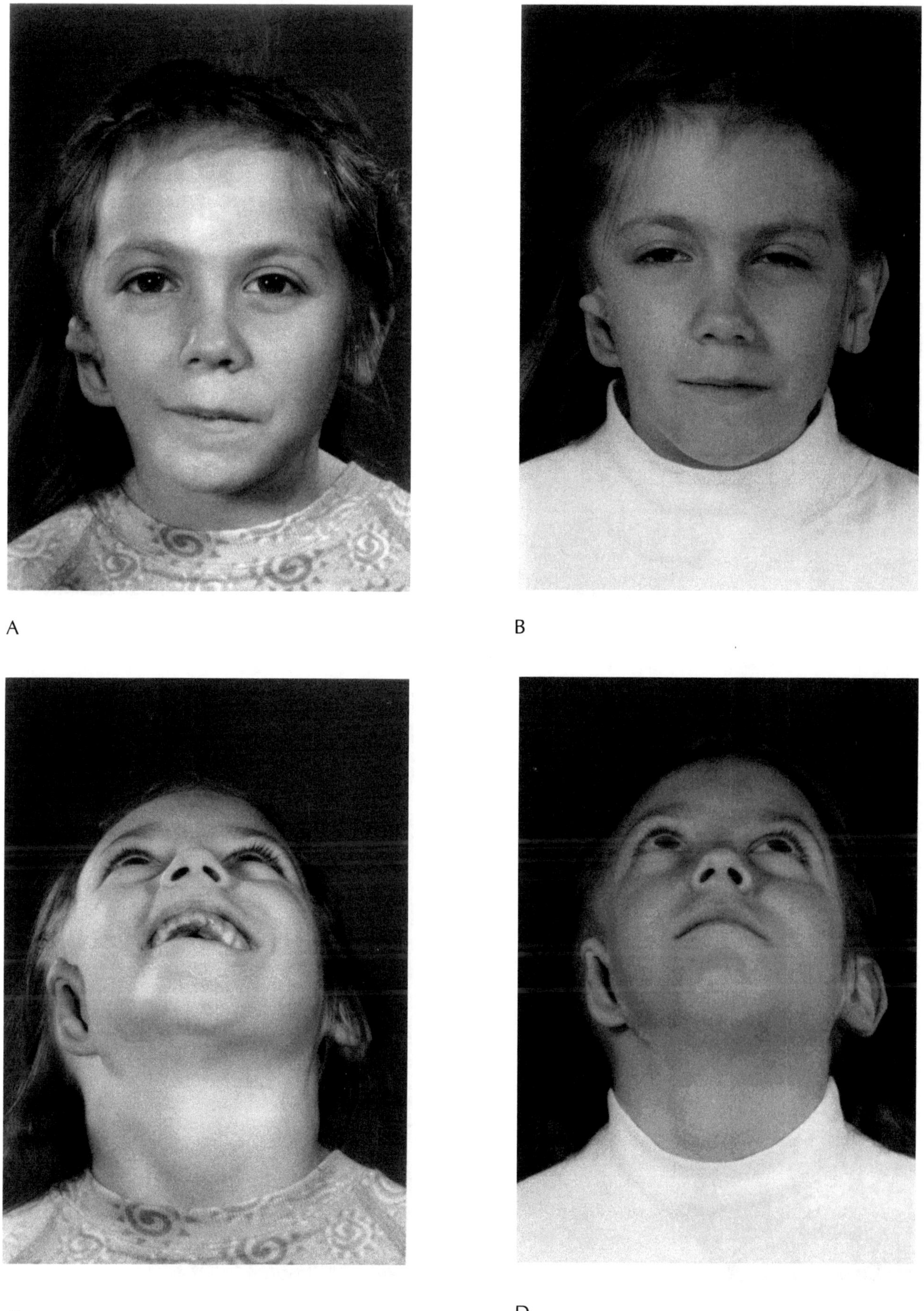

A B C D

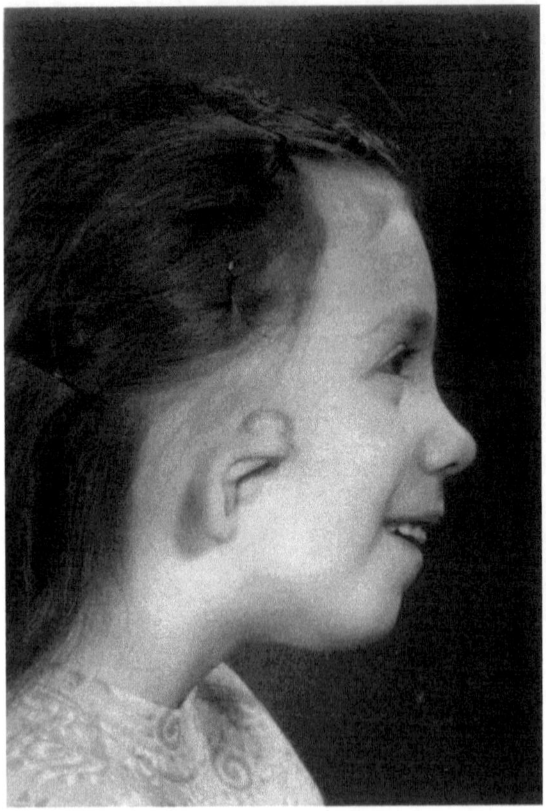

E

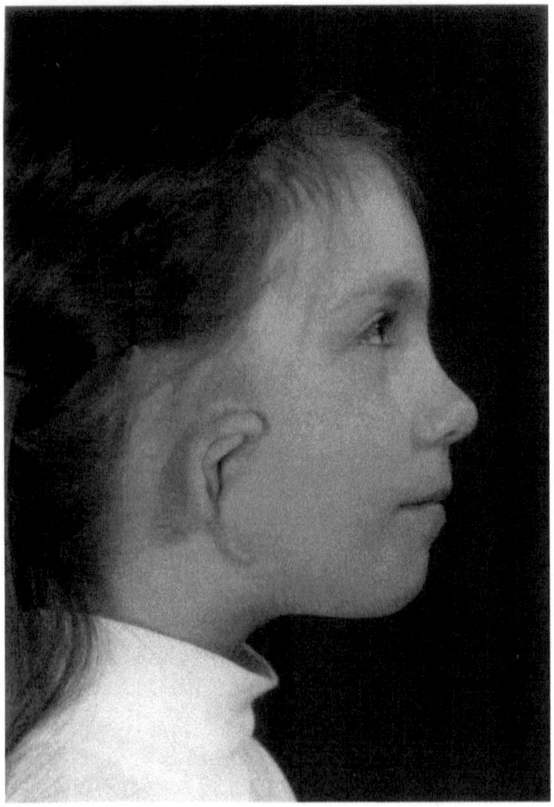

F

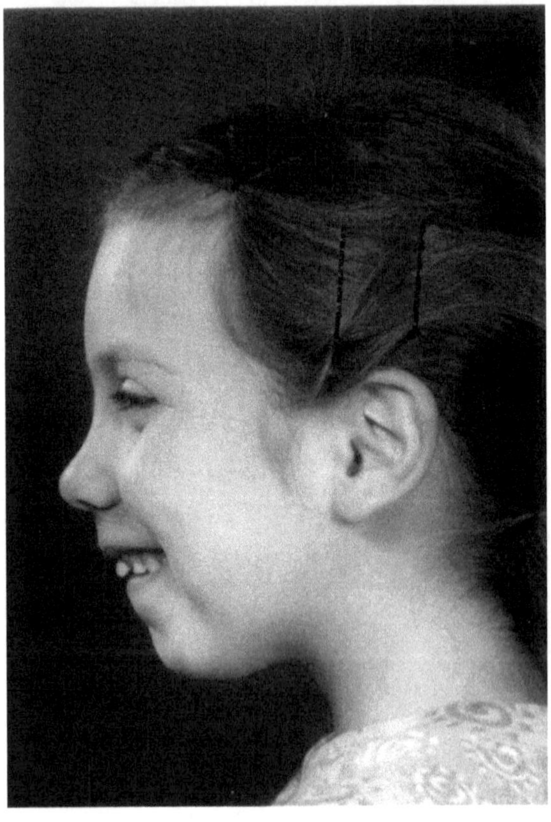

G

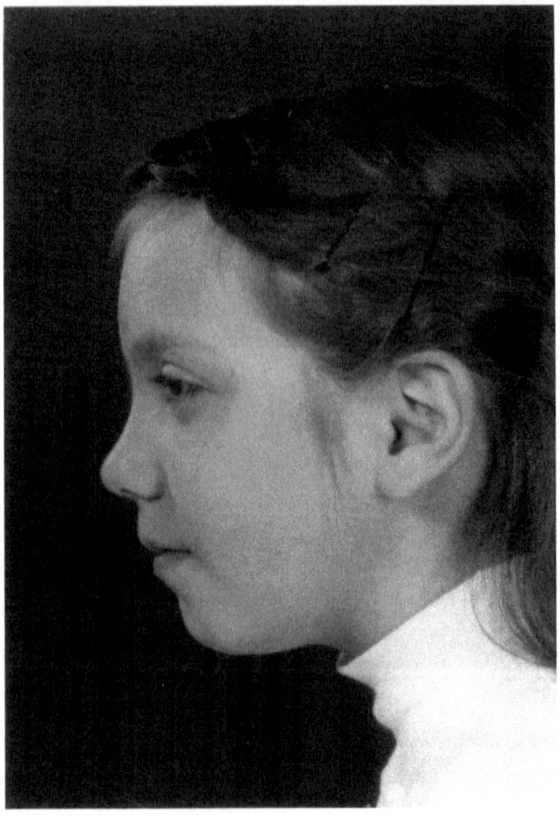

H

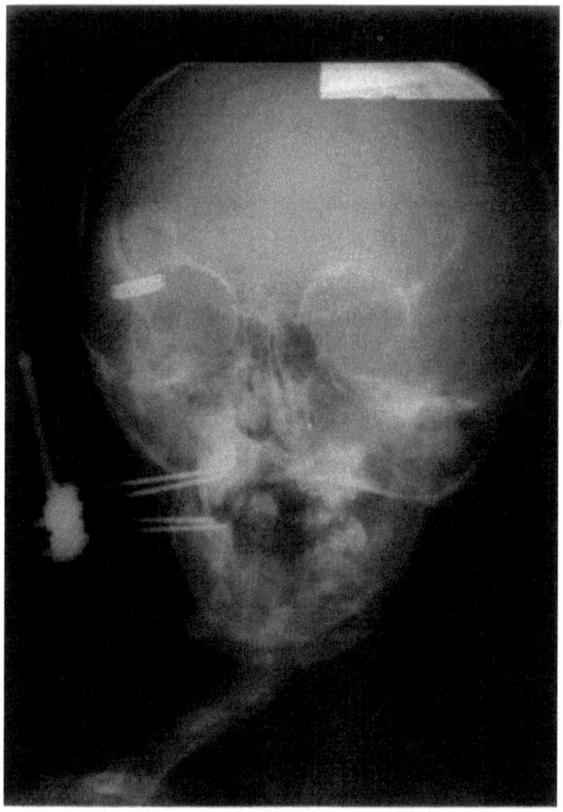

I

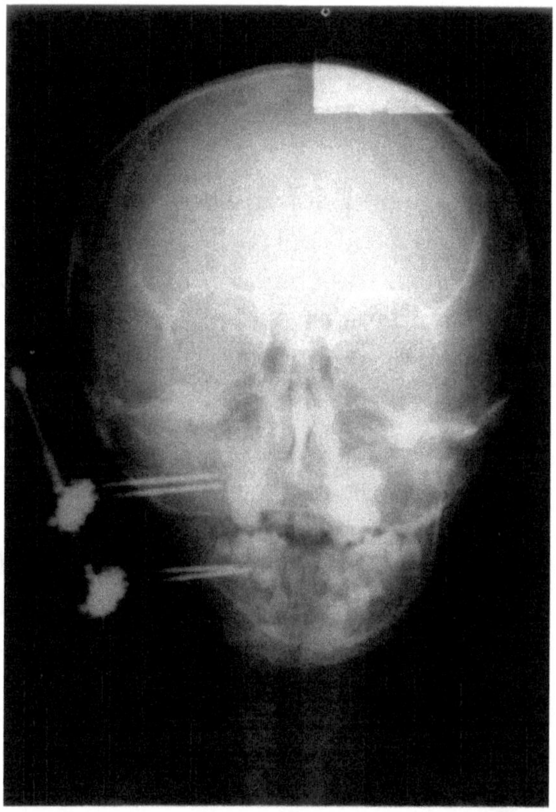

J

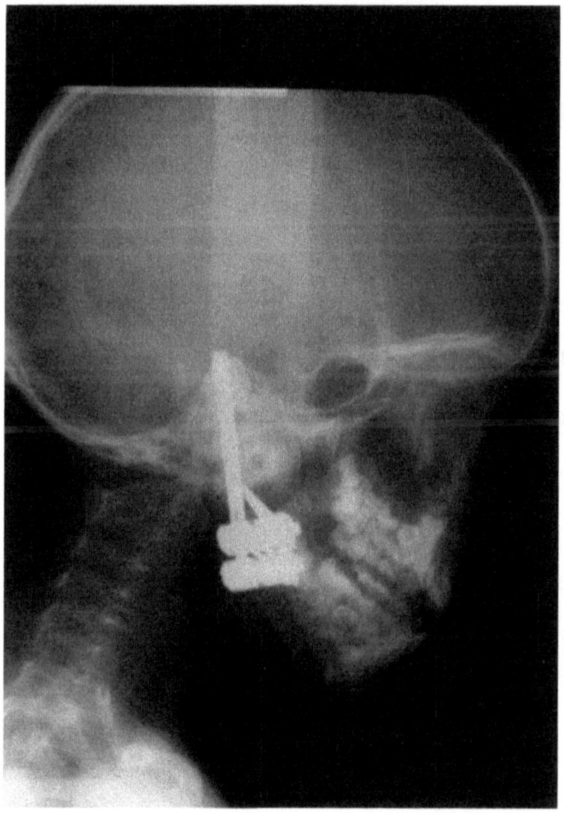

K

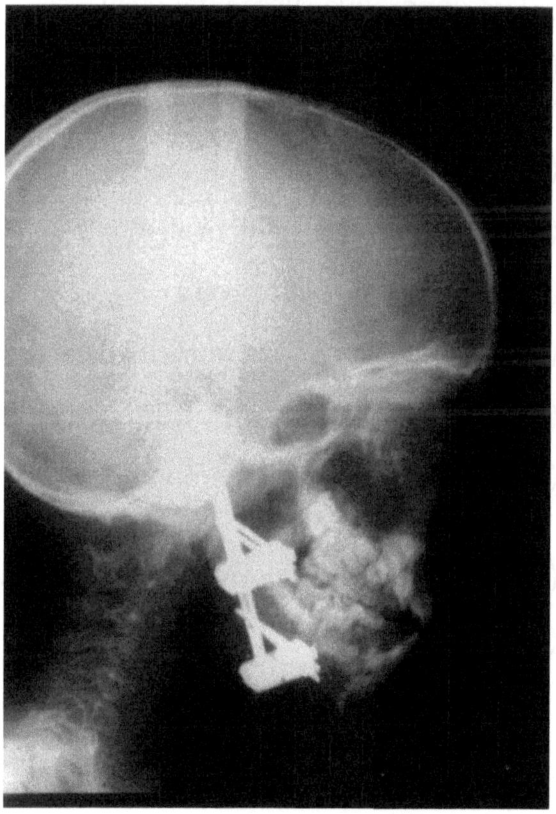

L

Case 6. R.M. was a five-and-a-half-year-old boy with the diagnosis of left craniofacial microsomia characterized by a deficiency of the maxilla, mandible, and soft tissues of the left face (Figure 5.34). He also had elevation of the oral commisure and occlusal plane on the affected side with deviation of the chin point to the left. Distraction of the left hemimandible was completed to 21 mm. Follow-up at 12 months demonstrated an increased bigonial distance and overcorrection of the chin point to the right of midline.

Figure 5.34. Case 6. A five-and-a-half-year-old boy with left craniofacial microsomia (Pruzansky I) who underwent left mandibular distraction (21 mm).

(A) Preoperative frontal view. Note the deviation of the chin and the severe occlusal cant.

(B) Postoperative frontal view 12 months after completion of distraction. Note the improvement in chin position and cheek contour.

(C) Preoperative submental view.

(D) Postoperative submental view showing improvement in chin position and symmetry of the inferior borders of the mandibular bodies.

(E) Preoperative right profile.

(F) Postoperative right profile.

(G) Preoperative left profile.

(H) Postoperative left profile. The scar is immature.

(I) Predistraction posteroanterior cephalogram (device in place).

(J) Postdistraction posteroanterior cephalogram. Note the leveling of the occlusal plane.

(K) Predistraction lateral cephalogram (vertical vector).

(L) Postdistraction lateral cephalogram. The long arm of the device has a more oblique orientation (counterclockwise rotation of the mandible).

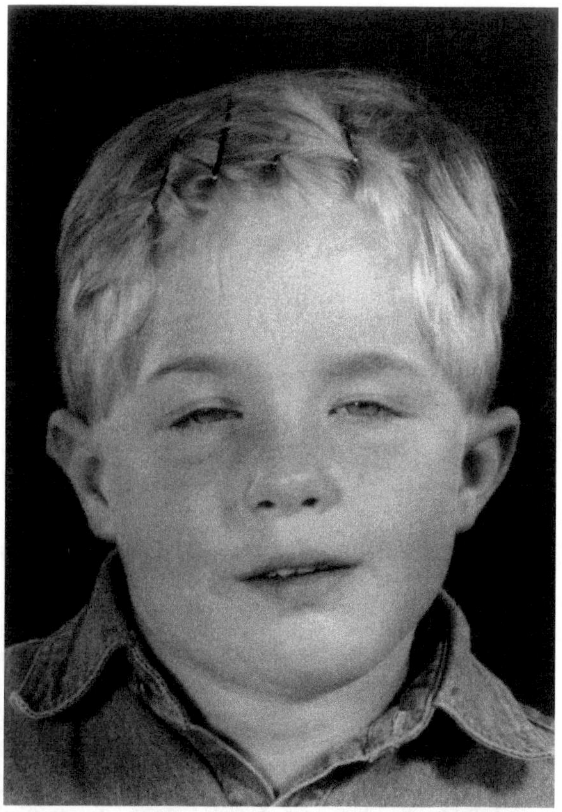

A

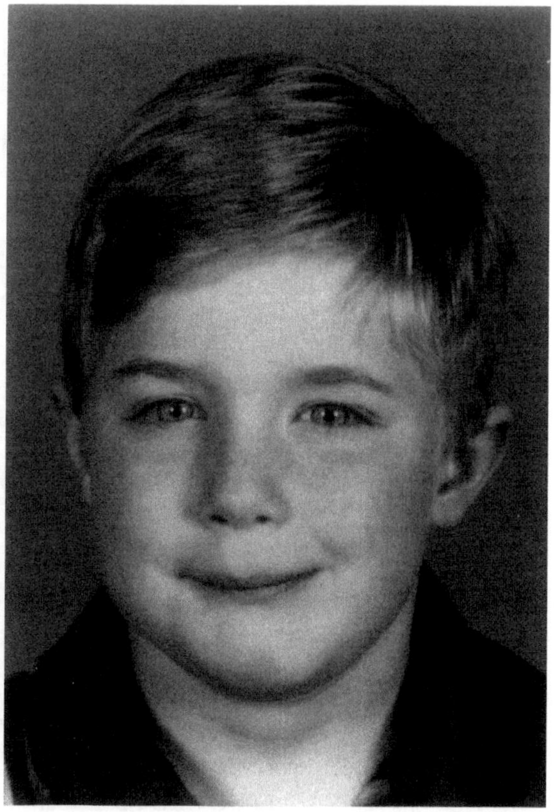

B

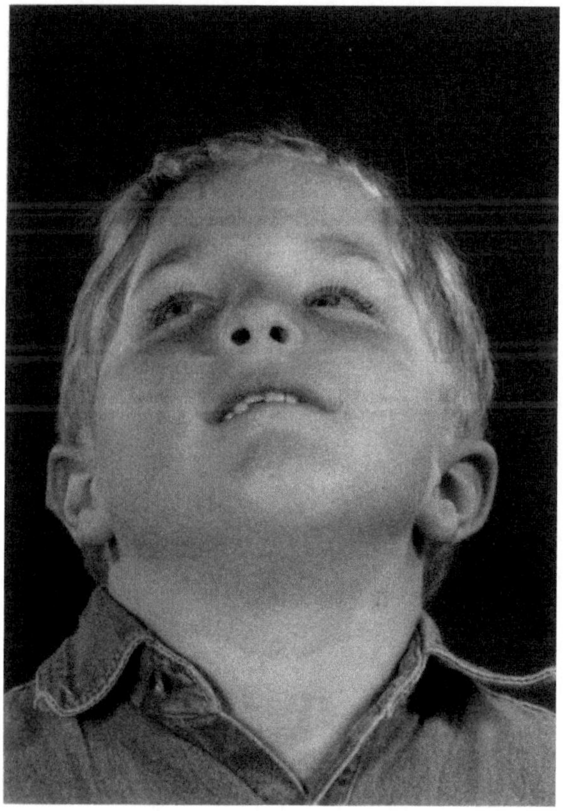

C

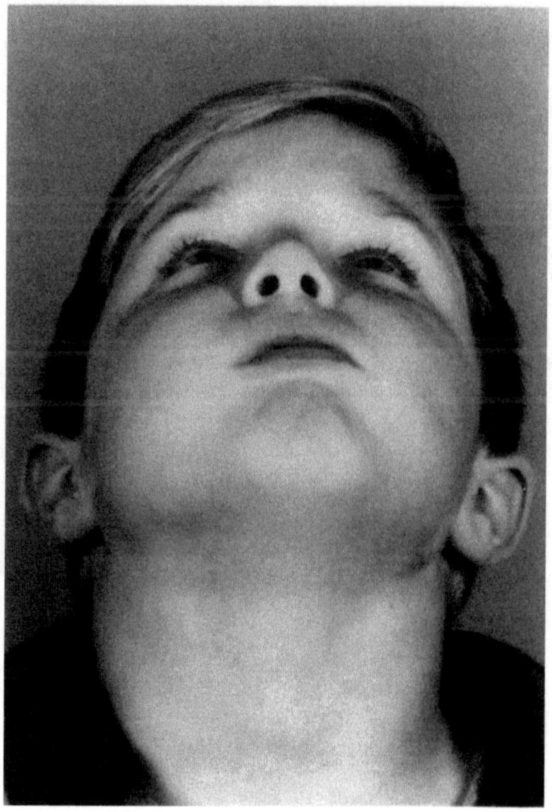

D

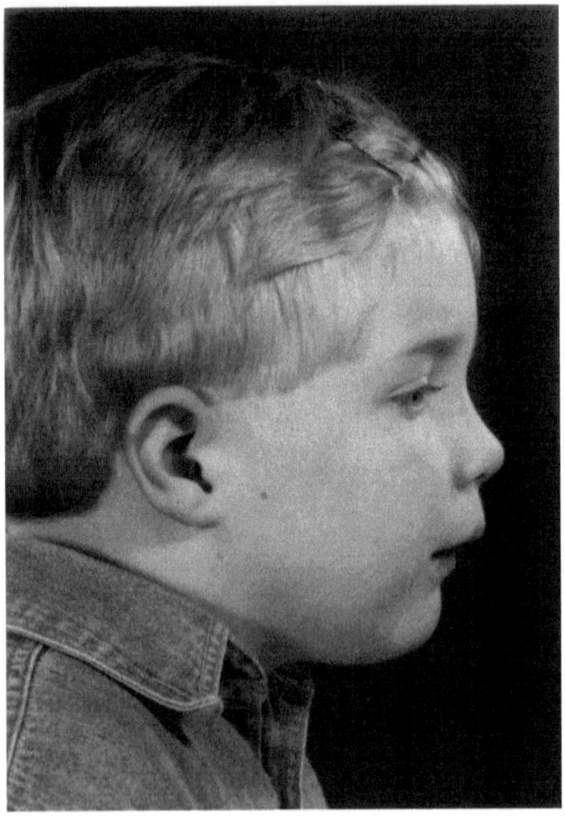

E

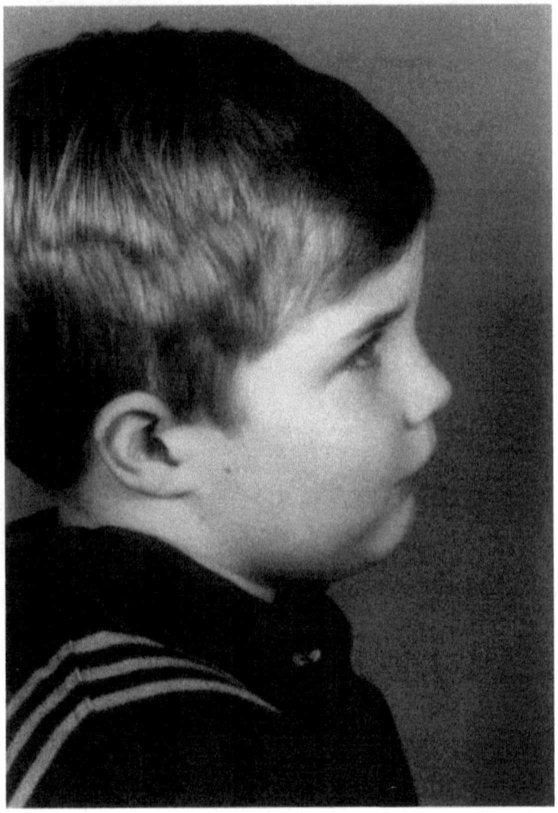

F

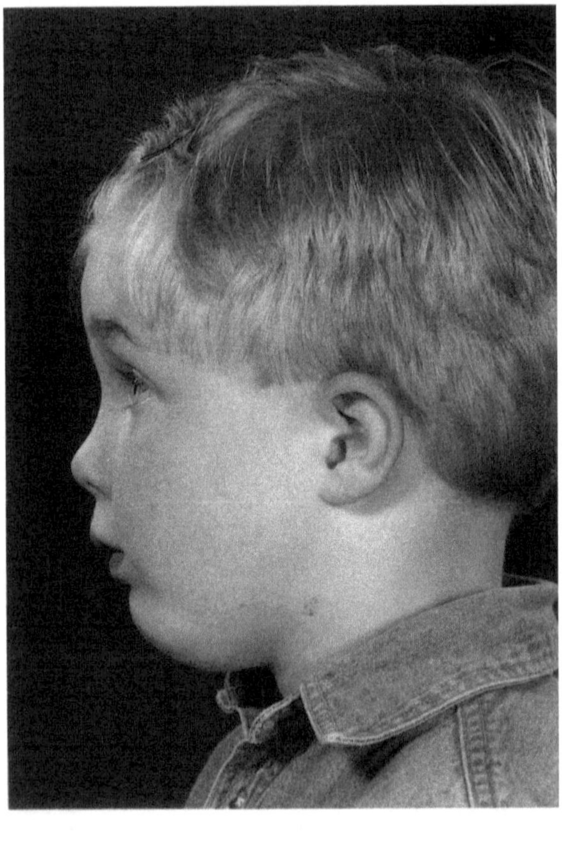

G

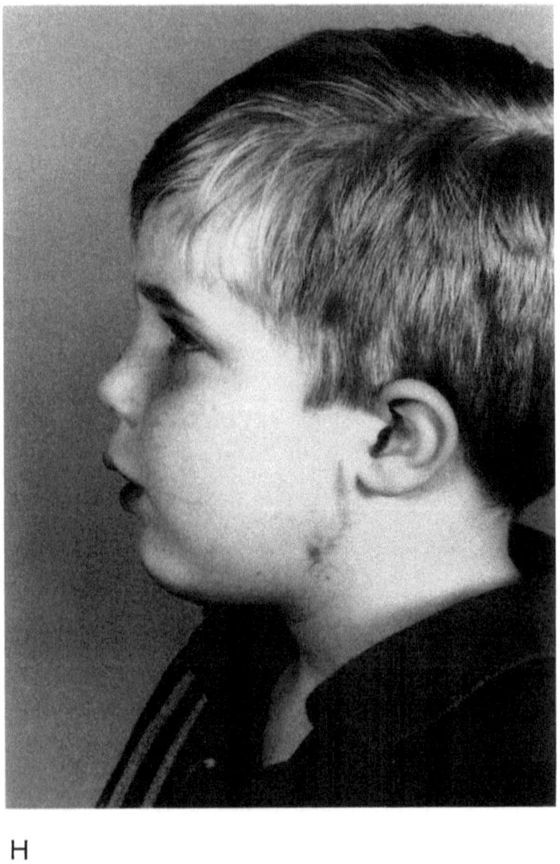

H

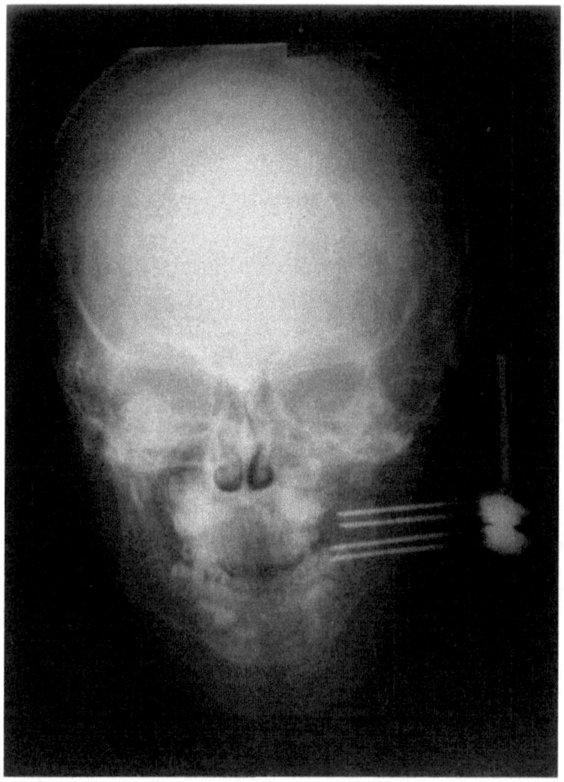

I

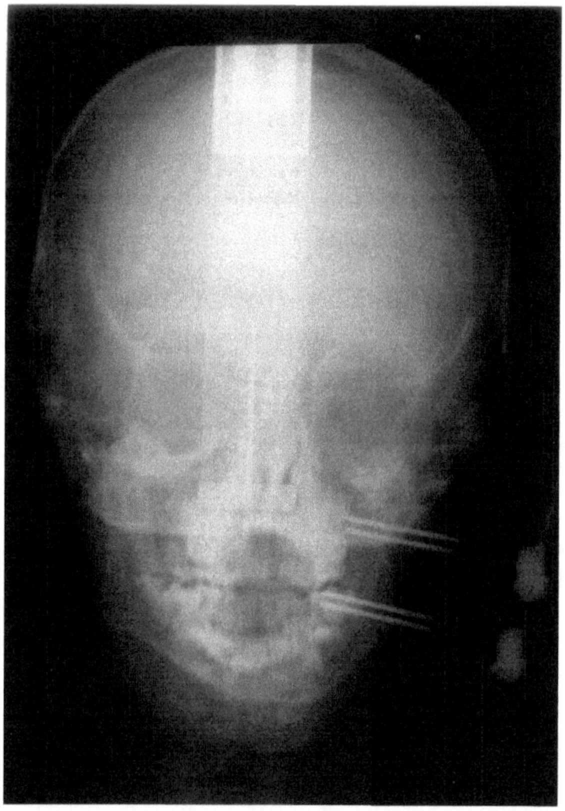

J

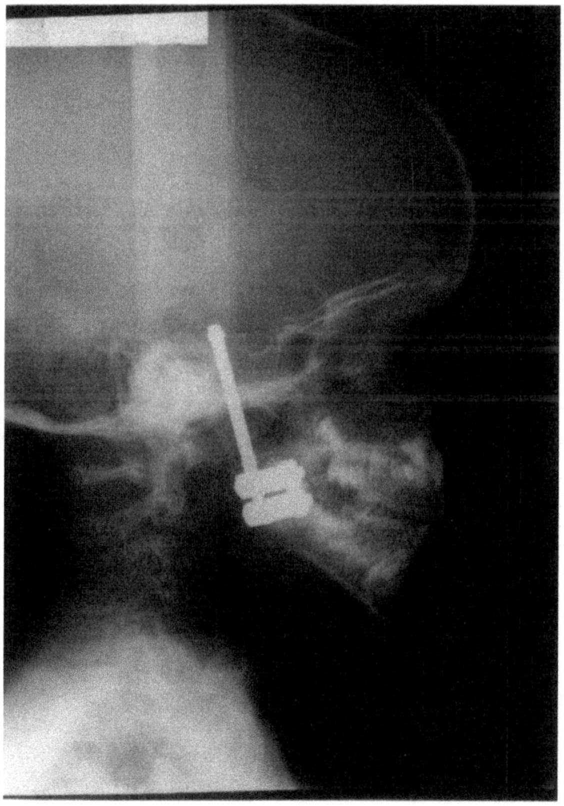

K

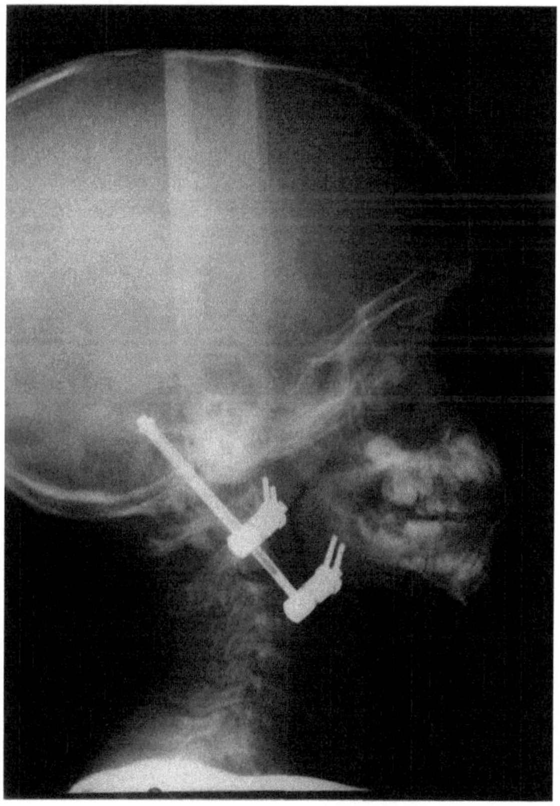

L

Figure 5.34. ***Case 6.*** *Continued*

(M) Predistraction frontal 3D CT scan showing the mandibular asymmetry and hypoplasia.

(N) Postdistraction frontal 3D CT scan showing leveling of the occlusal plane, improved mandibular morphology, and midline chin position. The gonions are on the same plane.

(O) Predistraction lateral 3D CT scan.

(P) Postdistraction lateral 3D CT scan showing augmentation of the affected mandibular body and ramus. The gonions, rami, and bodies of the mandible are symmetrical.

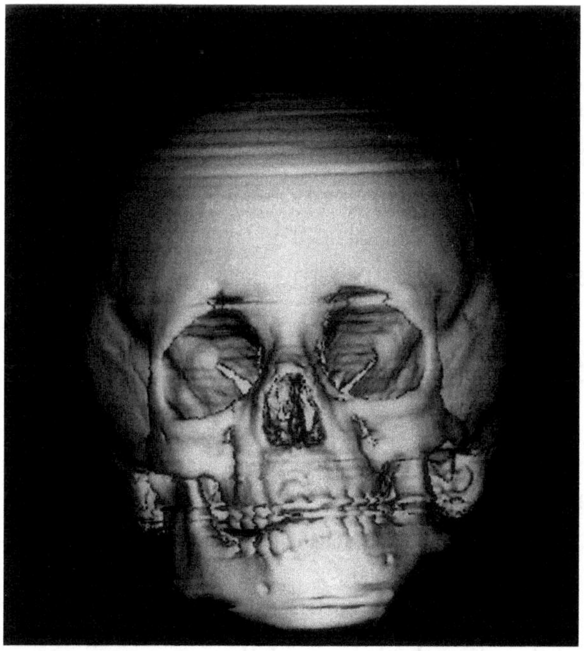

M

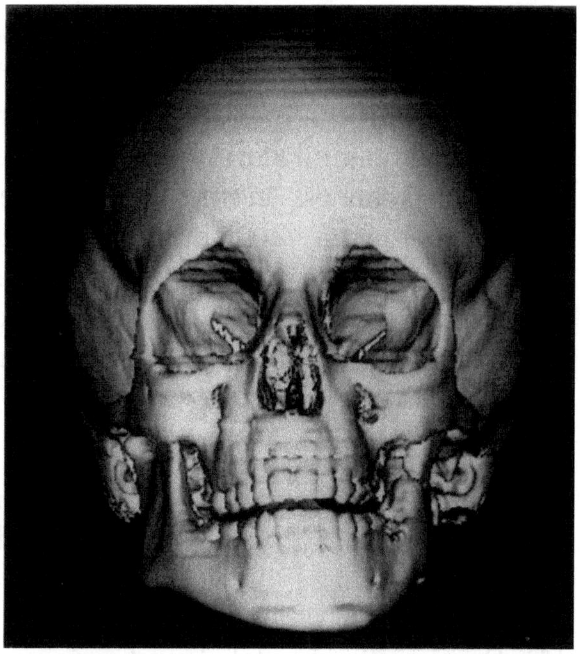

N

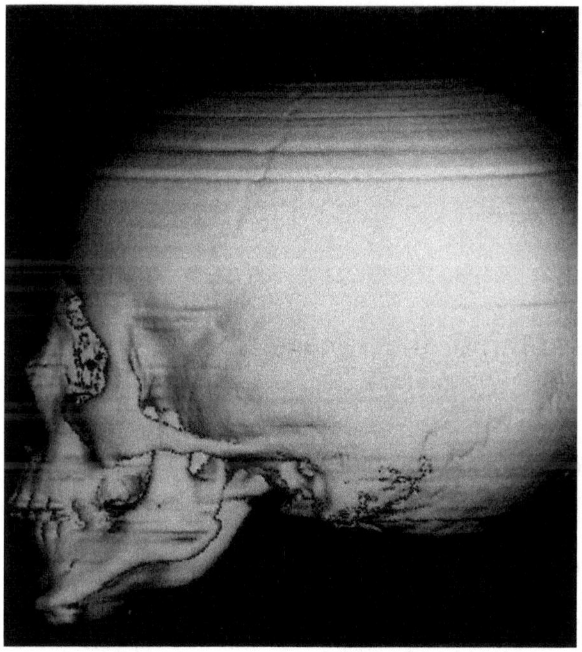

O

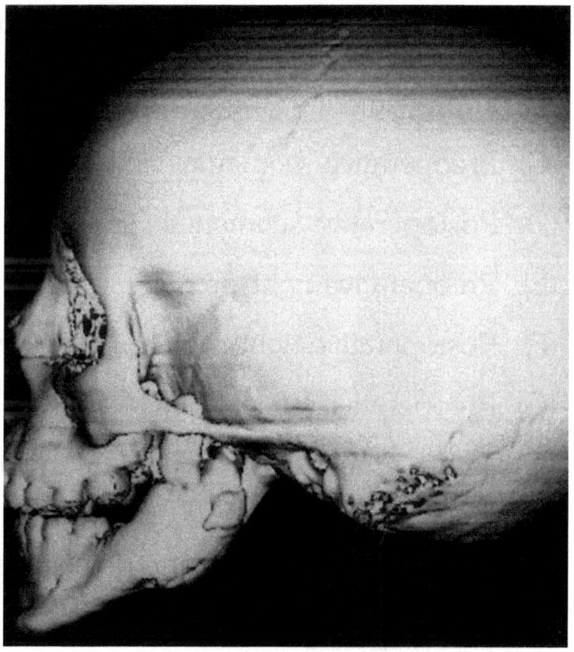

P

Case 7. C.R. is a two-and-a-half-year-old boy with left craniofacial microsomia characterized by generalized hypoplasia of the left face and involvement of the maxilla and mandible (Pruzansky I) with an ipsilateral auricular remnant (Figure 5.35). Examination of the left facial nerve demonstrated weakness in the area of the upper and lower lips and the zygomatic region. A slight macrostomia and upward occlusal cant on the affected side were also noted. After distraction to 25 mm, the left commisure was lowered to the level of the unaffected side. A slight overcorrection of the mandibular midline to the right of the maxillary midline was also noted.

Figure 5.35. Case 7. A two-and-a-half-year-old male with left craniofacial microsomia (Pruzansky I) who underwent unilateral mandibular distraction (25 mm).

(A) Preoperative frontal view showing unilateral microtia, deviation of the chin, and hypoplasia of the affected cheek.

(B) Postoperative frontal view 2 months after completion of distraction. Note the improvement in the position of the chin, oral commisure, and left alar base. The occusal plane has been leveled. There is a marked improvement in the symmetry of the cheek contour.

(C) Preoperative submental view.

(D) Postoperative submental view.

(E) Preoperative right profile.

(F) Postoperative right profile. Note the increased thrust of the mandible.

(G) Preoperative left profile.

(H) Postoperative left profile. Note the increased distance between the ear remnant and oral commissure. The scar is immature.

(I) Predistraction posteroanterior cephalogram.

(J) Postdistraction posteroanterior cephalogram. Note the restoration of the left gonial angle and the improved position of the chin. There is a lateral open bite.

(K) Predistraction lateral cephalogram (oblique vector).

(L) Postdistraction lateral cephalogram. Note the forward thrust of the mandible and slight anterior crossbite. The inferior borders of the mandible are almost parallel. There has been counterclockwise rotation of the long arm of the distraction device.

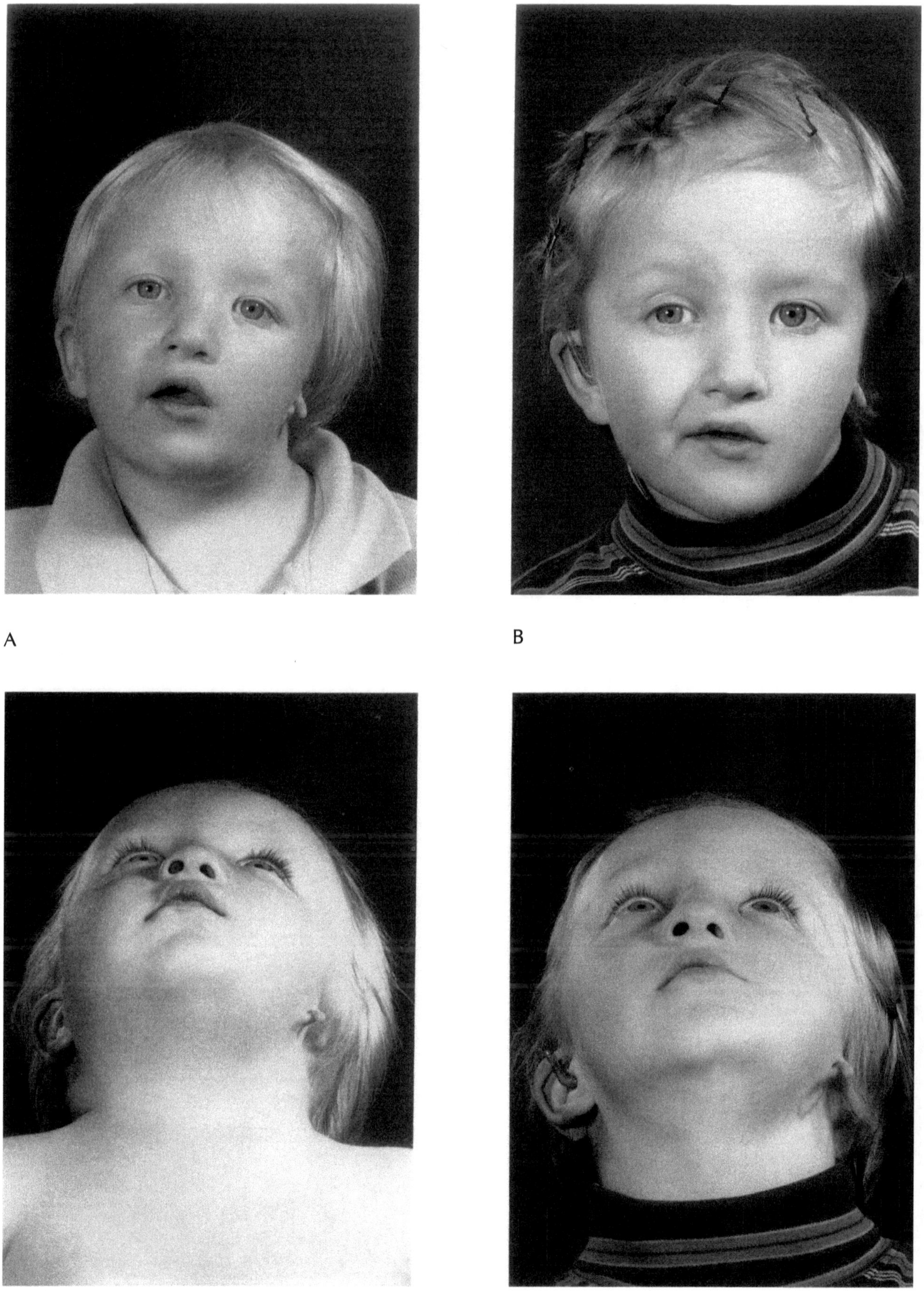

A

B

C

D

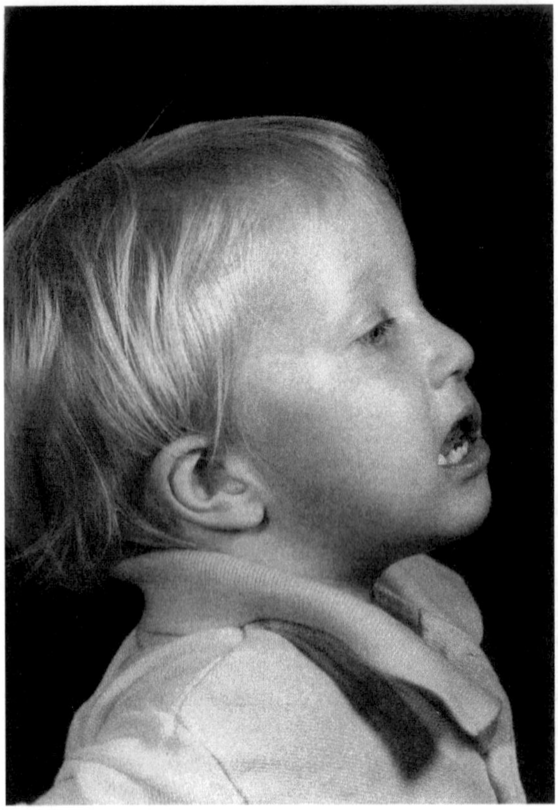

E

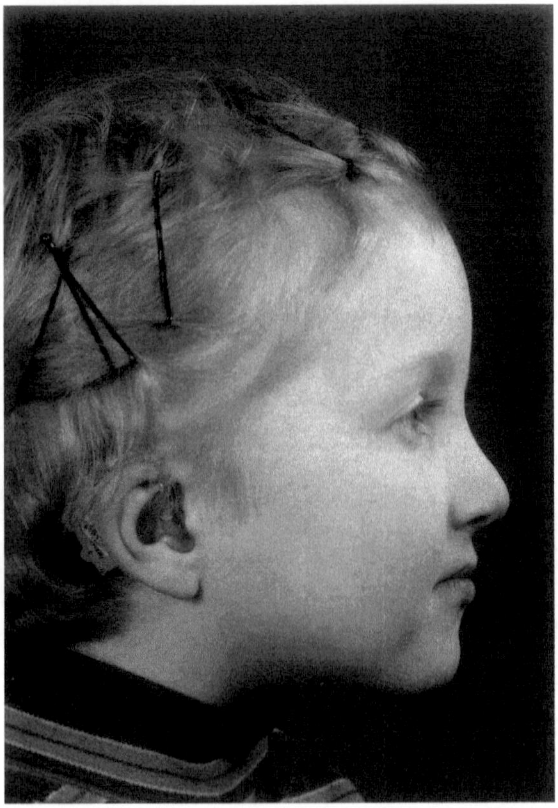

F

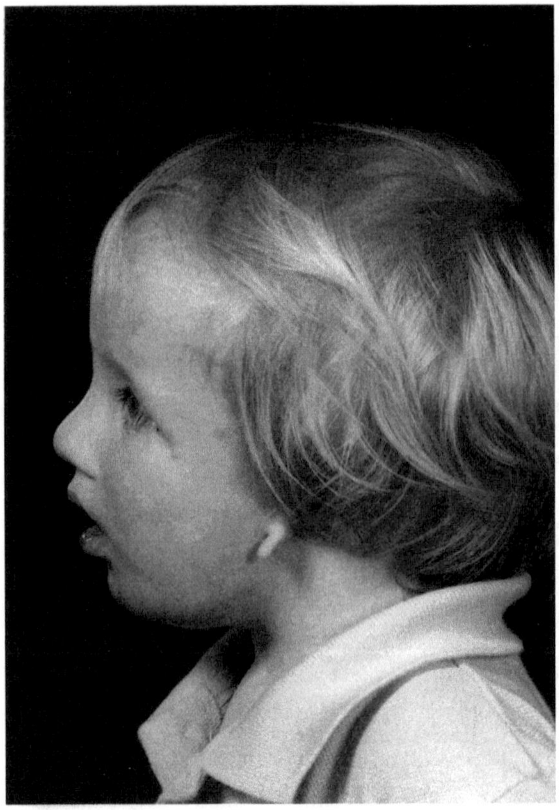

G

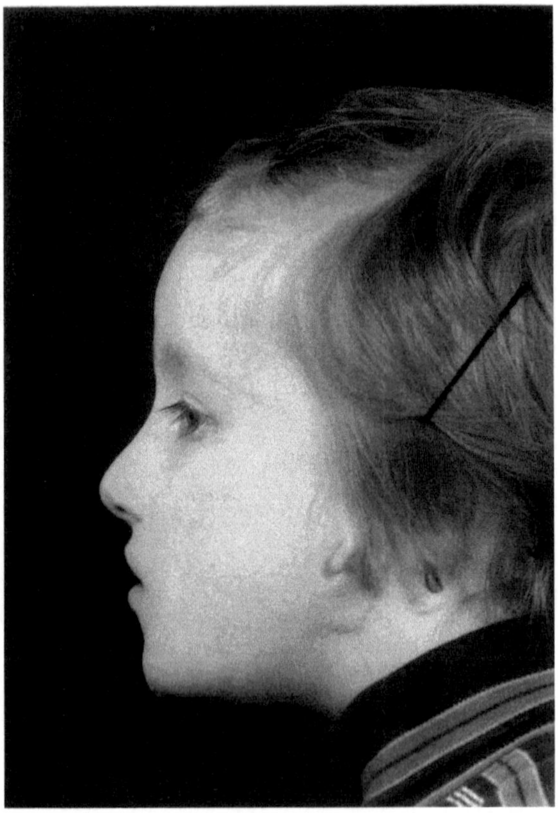

H

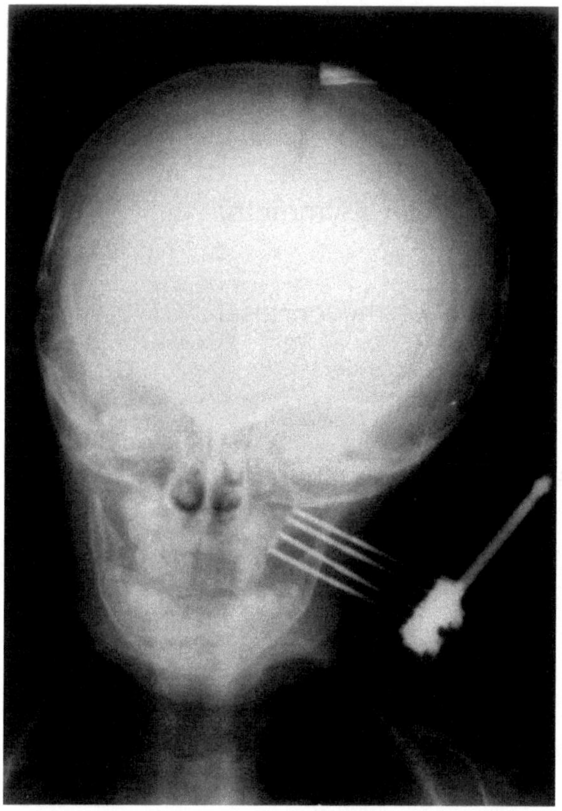

I

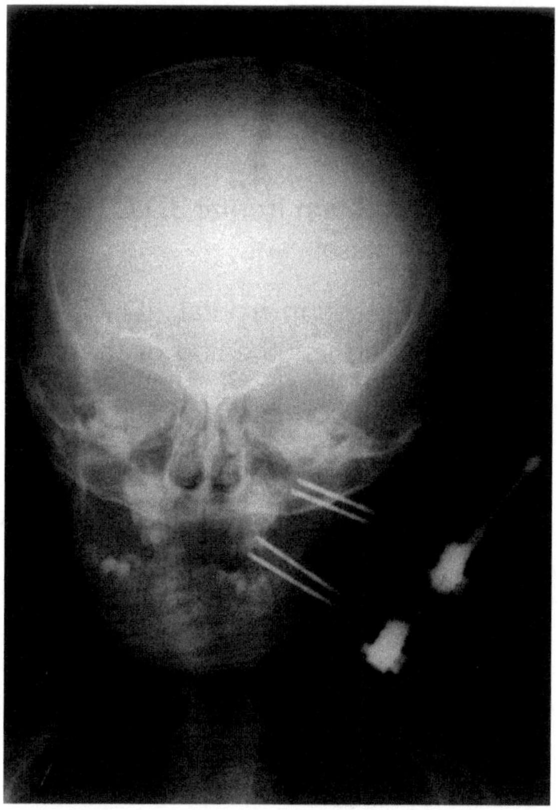

J

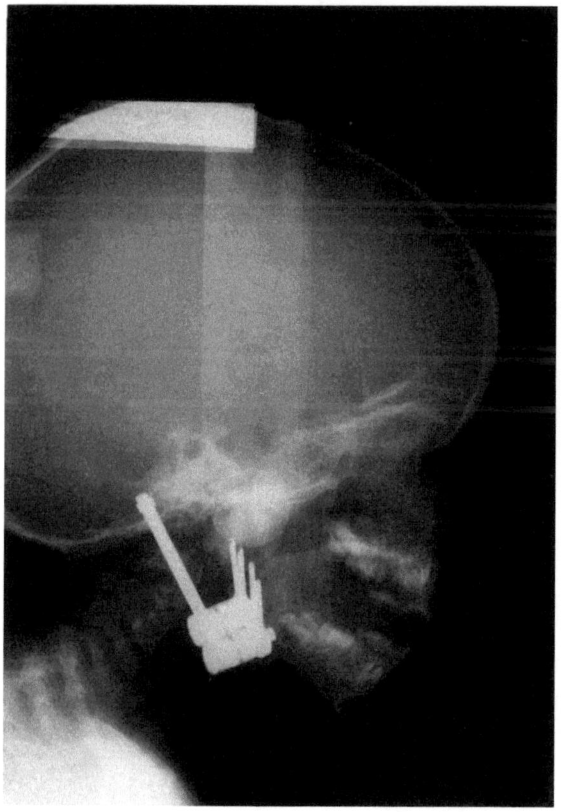

K

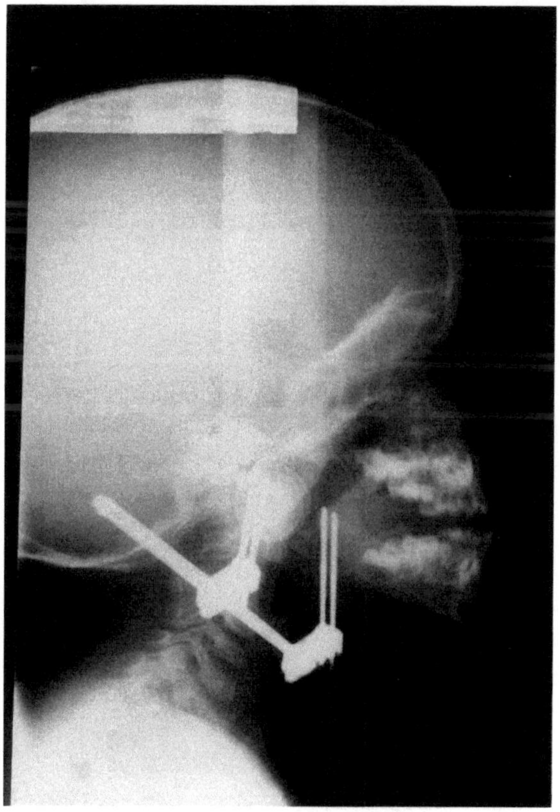

L

Figure 5.35. ***Case 7.*** *Continued*

(M) Predistraction frontal 3D CT scan showing the mandibular asymmetry and occlusal cant.

(N) Postdistraction frontal 3D CT scan showing leveling of the occlusal plane and lengthening of the affected ramus.

(O) Predistraction lateral 3D CT scan.

(P) Postdistraction lateral 3D CT scan showing lengthening and augmentation of the affected ramus and body.

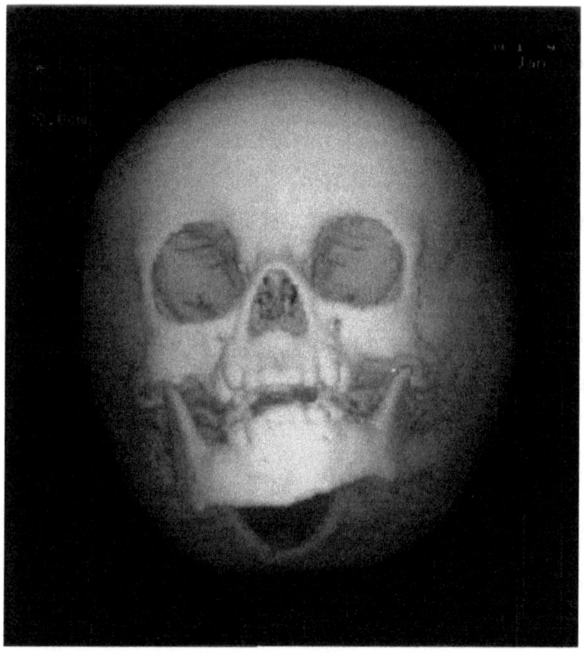

M

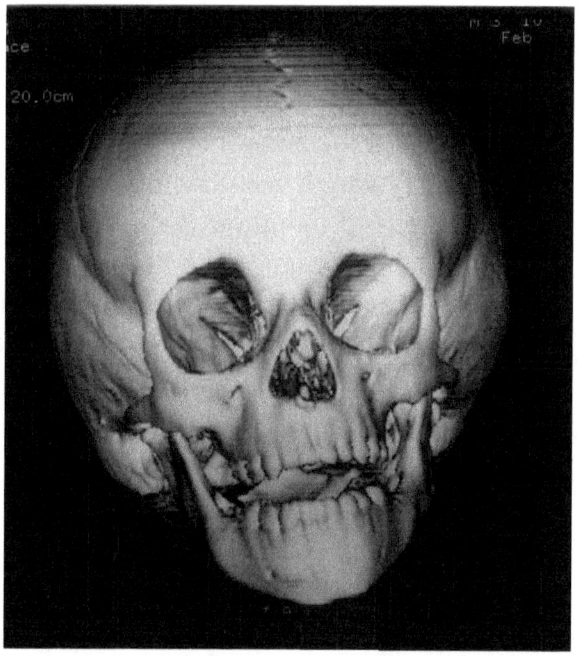

N

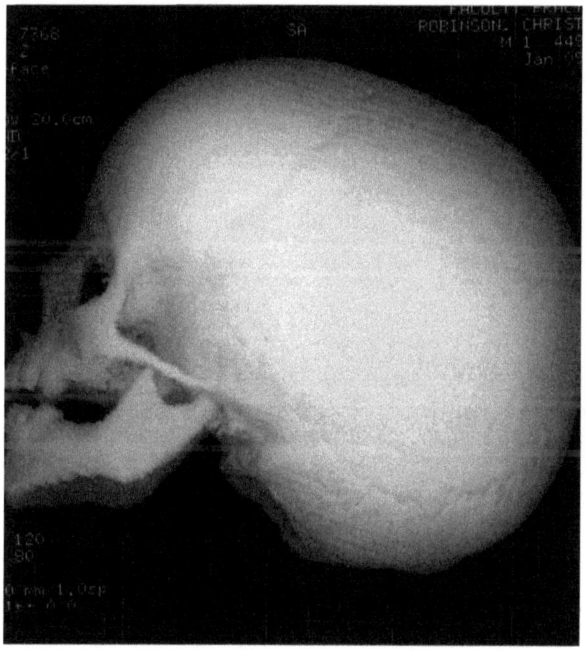

O

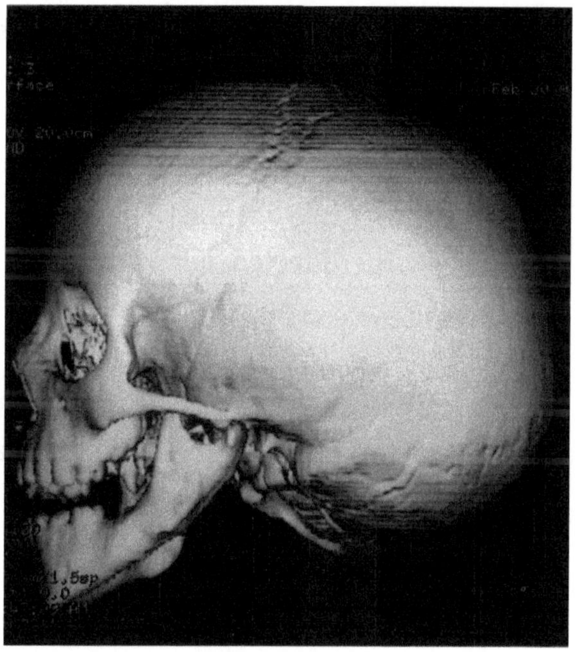

P

Case 8. S.B. was a four-and-a-half-year-old boy diagnosed with right craniofacial microsomia manifest by mild to moderate underdevelopment of the right face and partial weakness in the distribution of the right marginal mandibular branch (Figure 5.36). The maxilla and the mandible (Pruzansky I) were involved with an associated complex microtia of the right ear. The second mandibular molar tooth bud was deliberately removed at three and a half years of age in anticipation of bone distraction (21 mm). At 6 months postdistraction, the patient demonstrated a slight anterior cross bite (2–3 mm) as well as a slight occlusal cant upward. The bigonial distance had increased significantly. Correction of the chin point to the midline was also achieved.

Figure 5.36. Case 8. A four-and-a-half-year-old male with right craniofacial microsomia (Pruzansky I) who underwent unilateral mandibular distraction (21 mm).

(A) Preoperative frontal view. The chin is deviated to the affected side and there is a slight occlusal cant.

(B) Postoperative frontal view 9 months after completion of distraction. The chin is deviated to the opposite side and there is an overcorrection of the occlusal plane.

(C) Preoperative submental view.

(D) Postoperative submental view. Note the improvement in cheek contour on the affected side.

(E) Preoperative right profile.

(F) Postoperative right profile. Note the increased sagittal thrust of the mandible and the increased distance between the oral commissure and the ear remnant. The scar is well placed.

(G) Preoperative left profile.

(H) Postoperative left profile.

(I) Predistraction posteroanterior cephalogram.

(J) Postdistraction posteroanterior cephalogram. Note the increased vertical dimension of the right mandibular ramus, the restoration of the gonial angle, and the improved chin position. The volume and quality of the regenerate in the right ramus should be noted.

(K) Predistraction lateral cephalogram (oblique vector).

(L) Postdistraction lateral cephalogram. Note the sagittal thrust of the mandible in an "overcorrected" position.

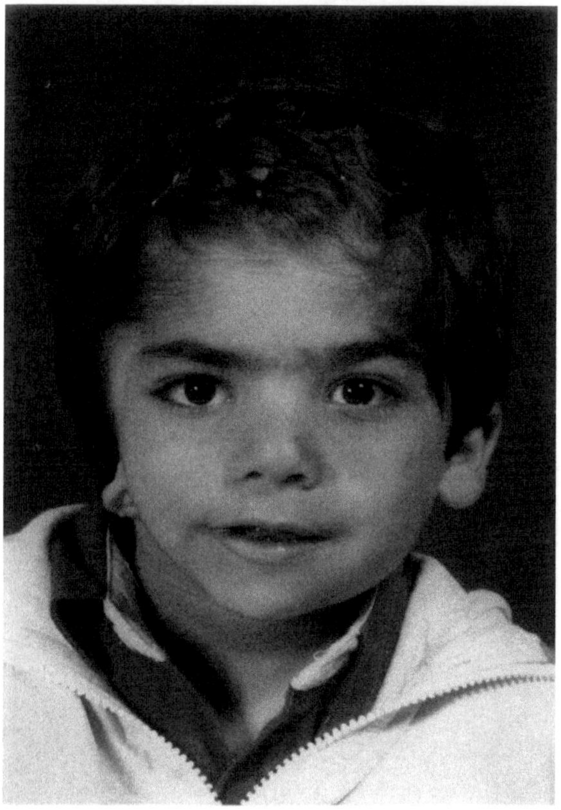

A

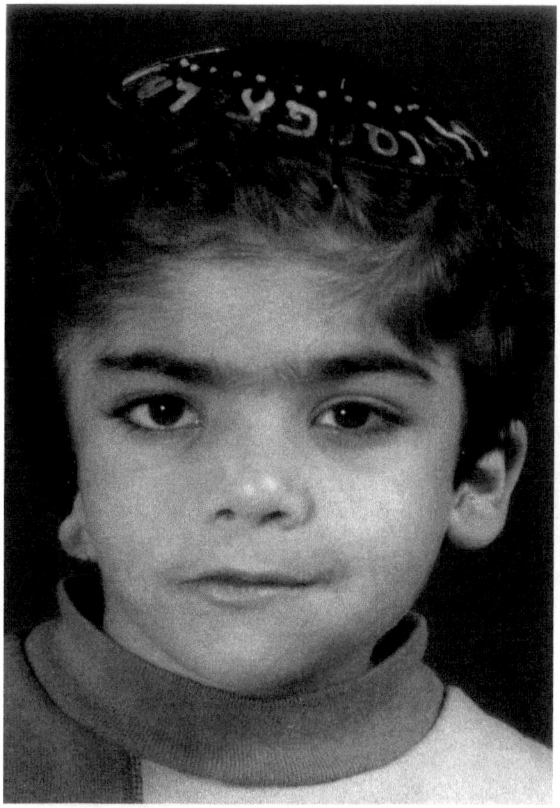

B

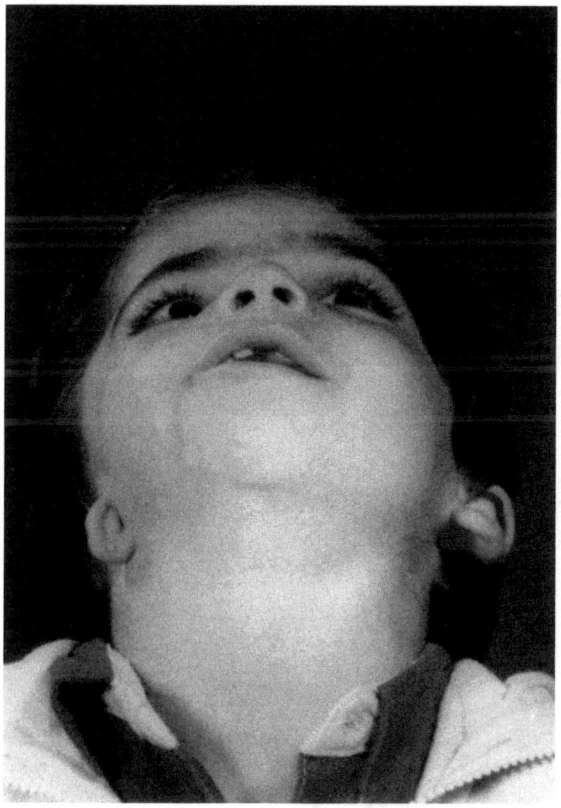

C

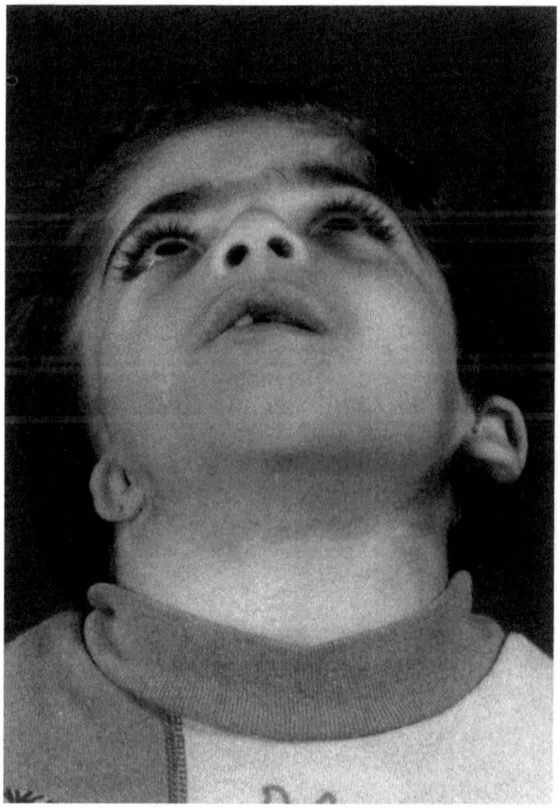

D

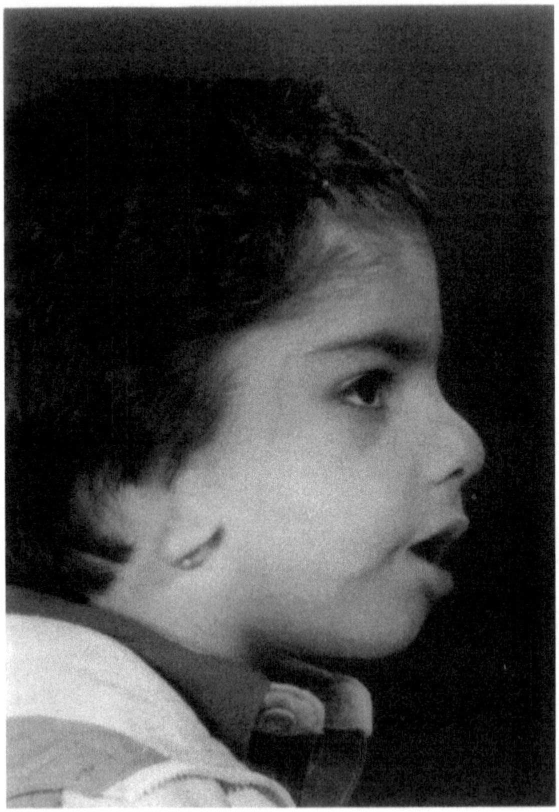

E

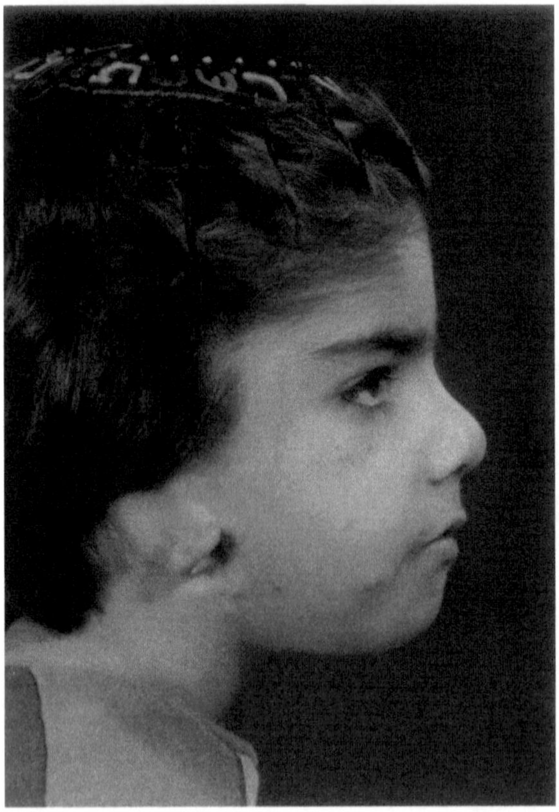

F

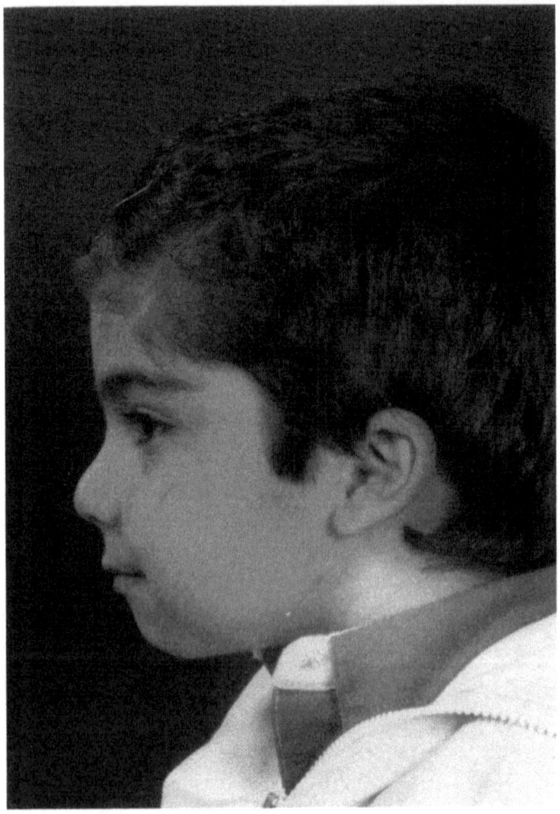

G

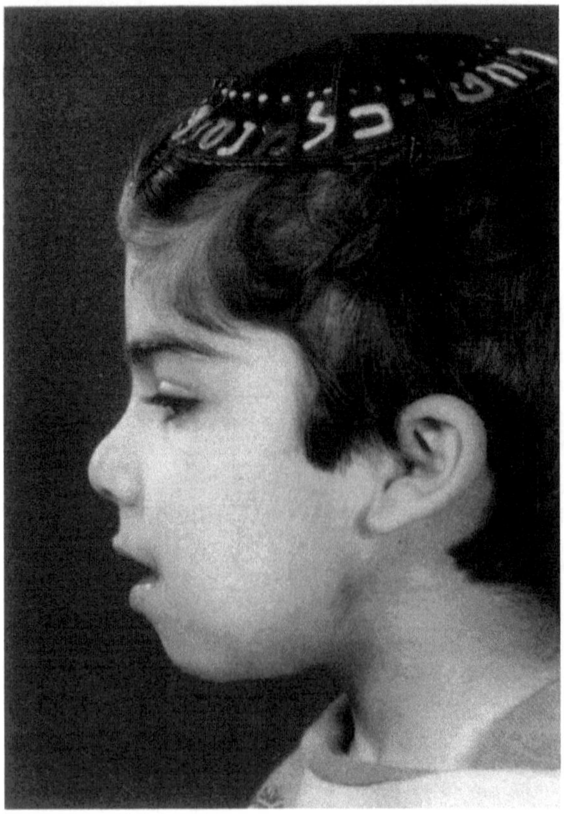

H

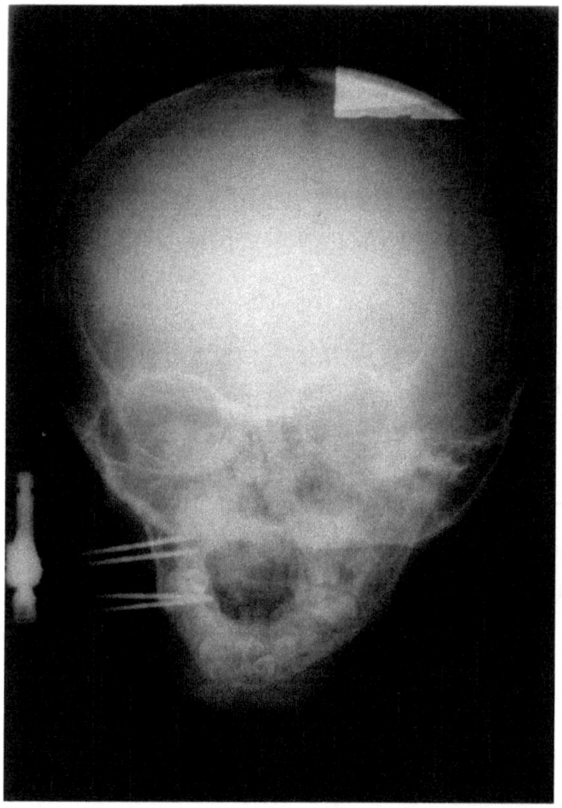

I

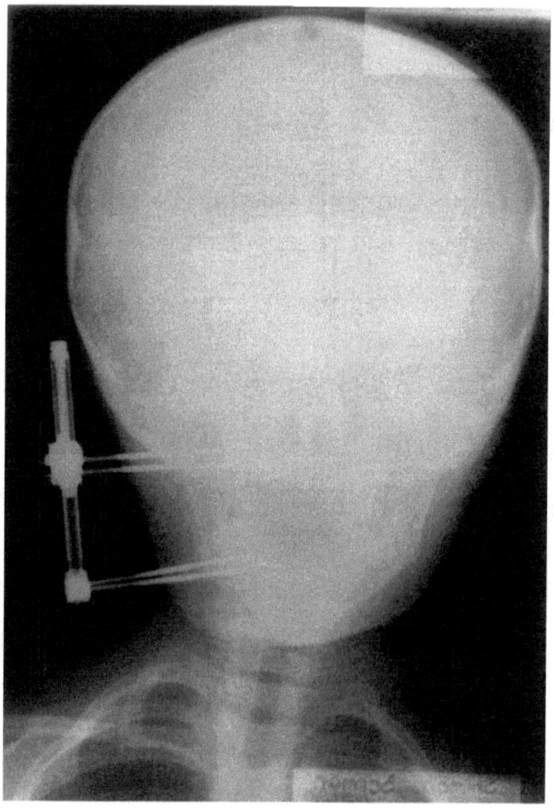

J

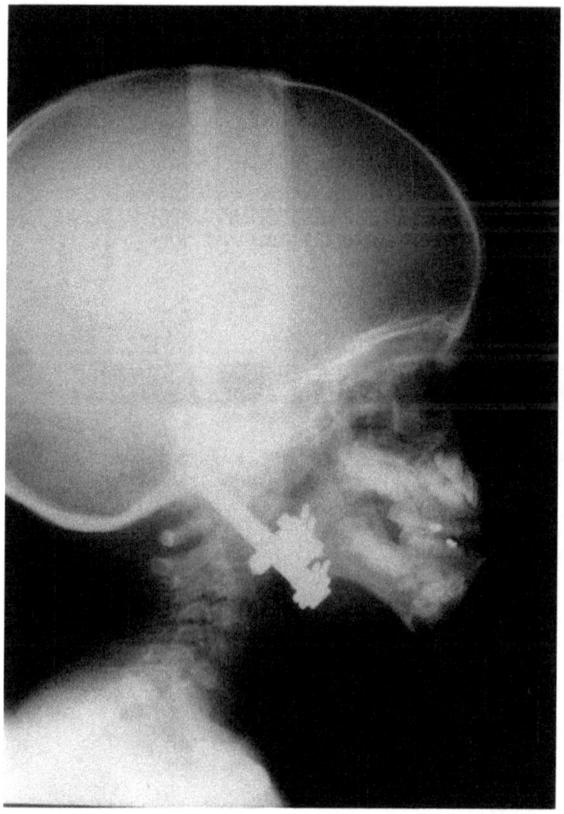

K

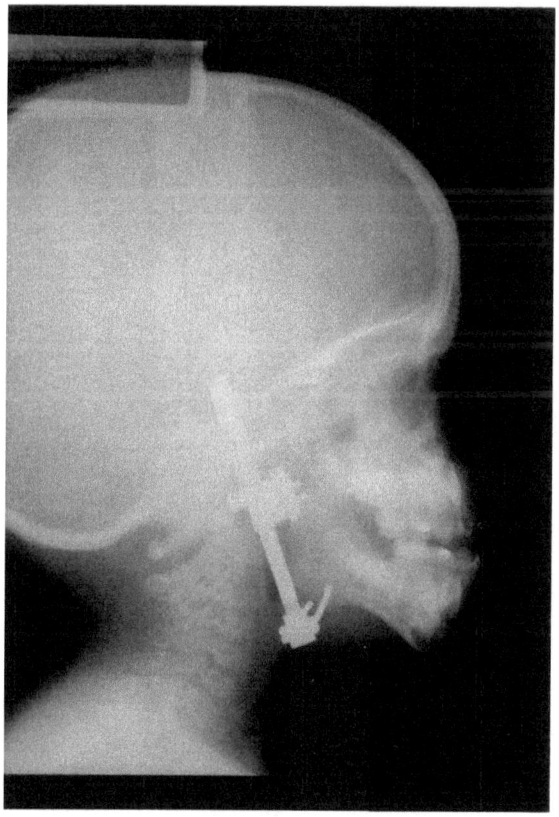

L

Figure 5.36. ***Case 8.*** *Continued*

(M) Predistraction frontal 3D CT scan. Note the hypoplasia of the right side of the mandible, the occlusal cant, and the chin deviation.

(N) Postdistraction frontal 3D CT scan. Note the open bite on the distracted side, the leveling of the occlusal plane, and the increased osseous volume in the distracted side of the mandible.

(O) Predistraction lateral 3D CT scan.

(P) Postdistraction lateral 3D CT scan. Note the increase in the size of the condyle, the increased dimensions of the mandibular ramus, the open bite on the distracted side, and the restoration of symmetry of the inferior borders of the mandibular bodies.

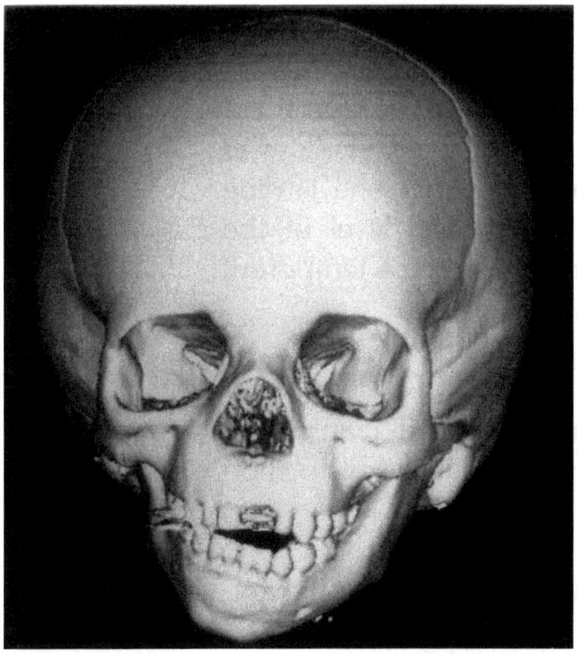

M

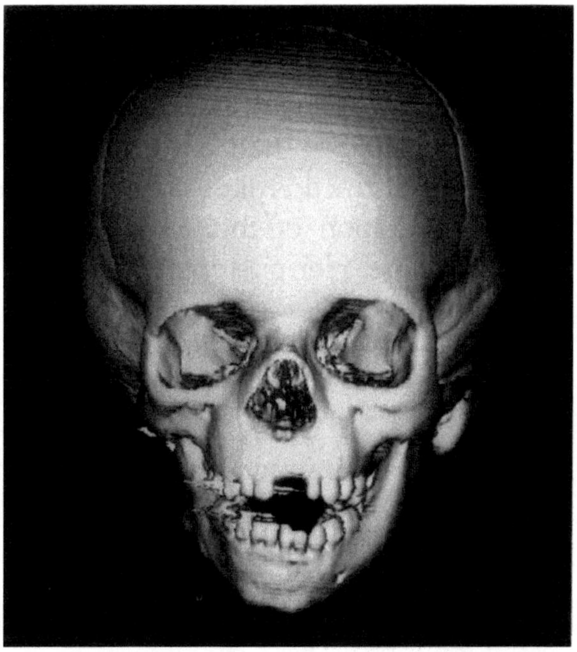

N

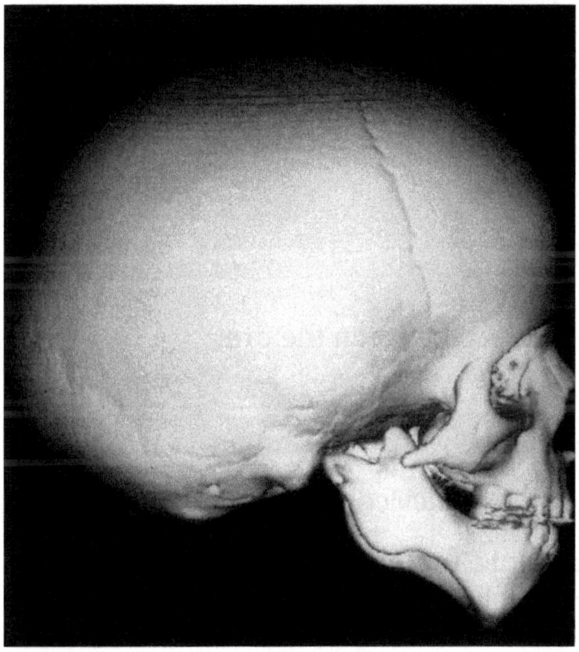

O

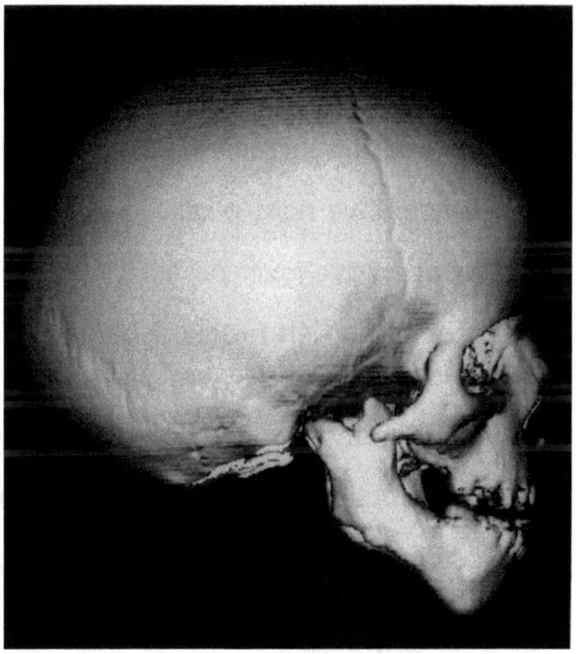

P

Case 9. I.S. was a 4-year-old girl with left craniofacial microsomia characterized by ipsilateral facial soft tissue deficiency, elevation of the oral commissure, canting of the occlusal plane, and deviation of the chin point (Figure 5.37). She had a Pruzansky I mandibular deformity. Following 22 mm of distraction (left) there was improvement in cheek and jawline contour, position of the commissure and chin point, and level of the occlusal plane. Her postoperative course was complicated by a temporary buccal palsy.

Figure 5.37. Case 9. A four-year-old female with left craniofacial microsomia (Pruzansky I) who underwent unilateral mandibular distraction (22 mm).

(A) Preoperative frontal view. Note the chin deviation, the occlusal cant, and the underdevelopment of the left cheek.

(B) Postoperative frontal view 13 months after completion of distraction. Note the increased fullness of the left cheek, the lowering of the affected oral commissure, and the improved position of the chin.

(C) Preoperative submental view.

(D) Postoperative submental view. Note the more midline contour of the chin and the increased fullness of the left cheek.

(E) Preoperative right profile.

(F) Postoperative right profile.

(G) Preoperative left profile. Note the decreased distance between the oral commissure and tragus.

(H) Postoperative left profile. The scar is well positioned.

(I) Predistraction posteroanterior cephalogram with the device in place.

(J) Postdistraction posteroanterior cephalogram. Note the improvement in the position of the chin and gonion. There has been leveling of the occlusal plane.

(K) Predistraction lateral cephalogram (vertical vector).

(L) Postdistraction lateral cephalogram.

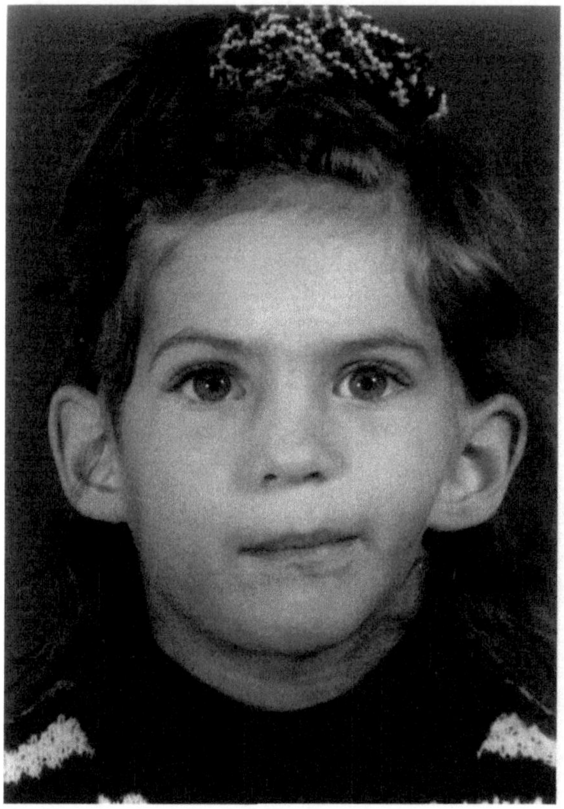

A

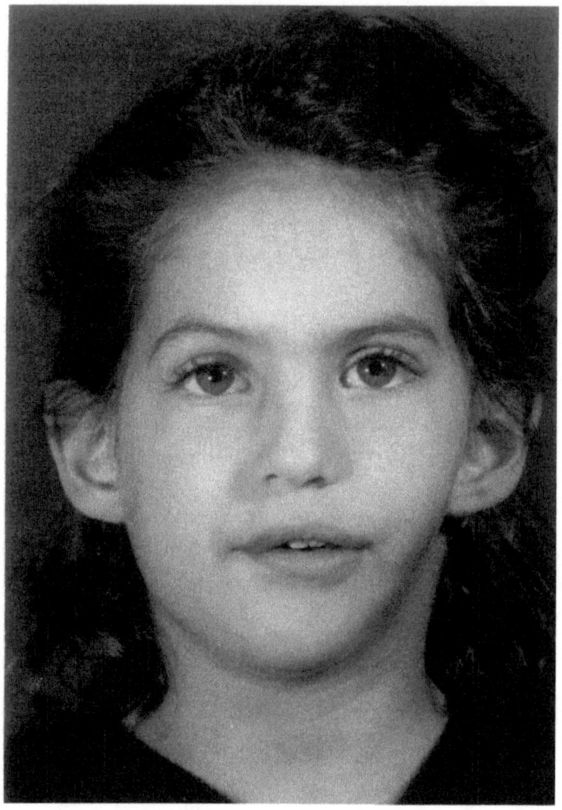

B

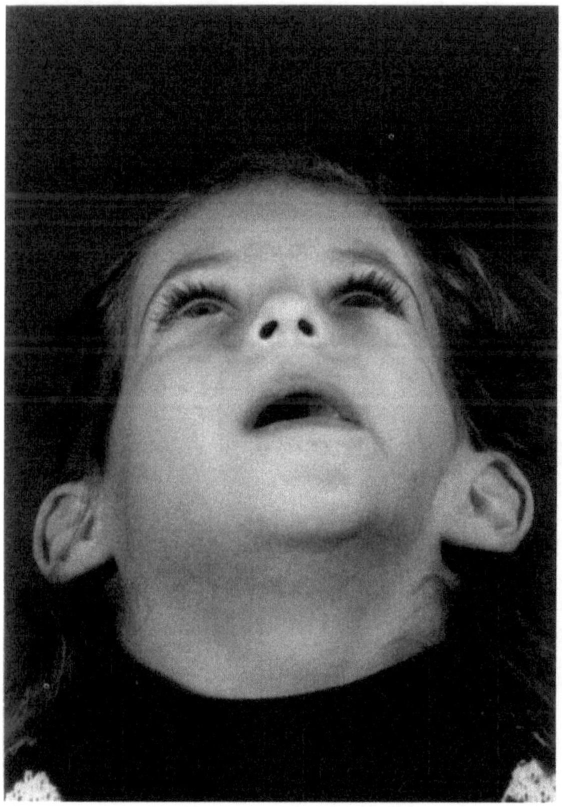

C

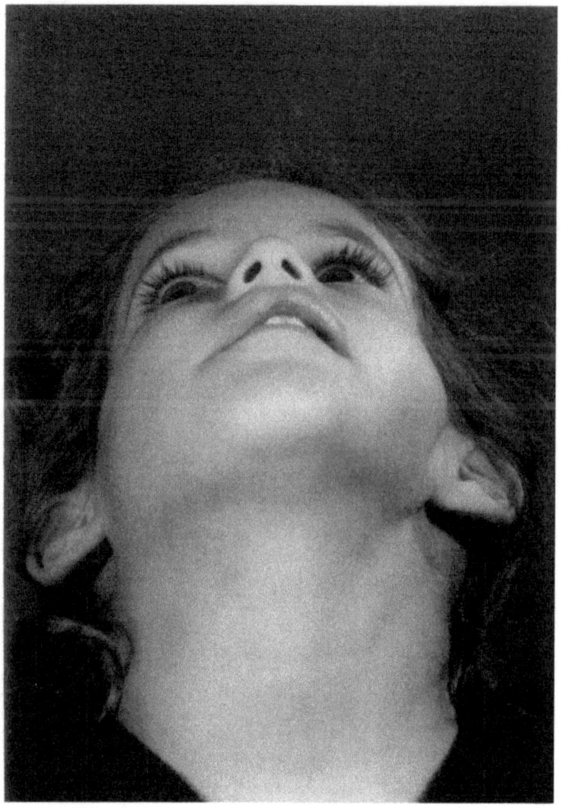

D

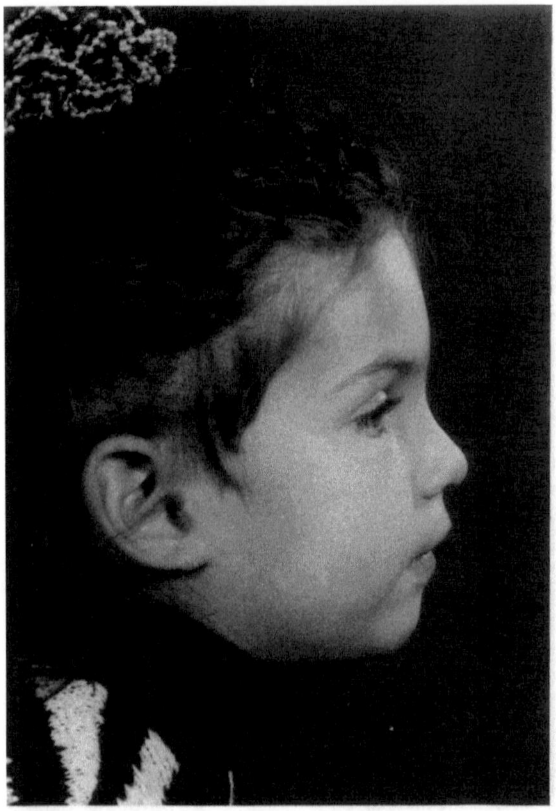

E

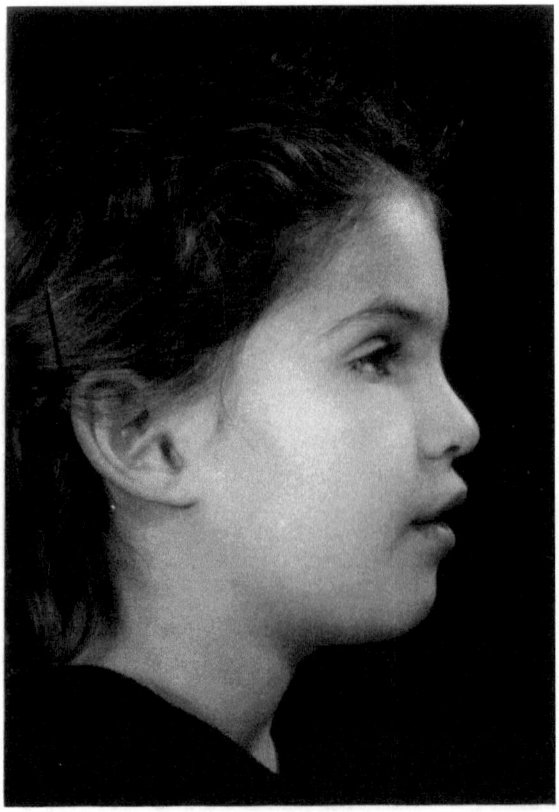

F

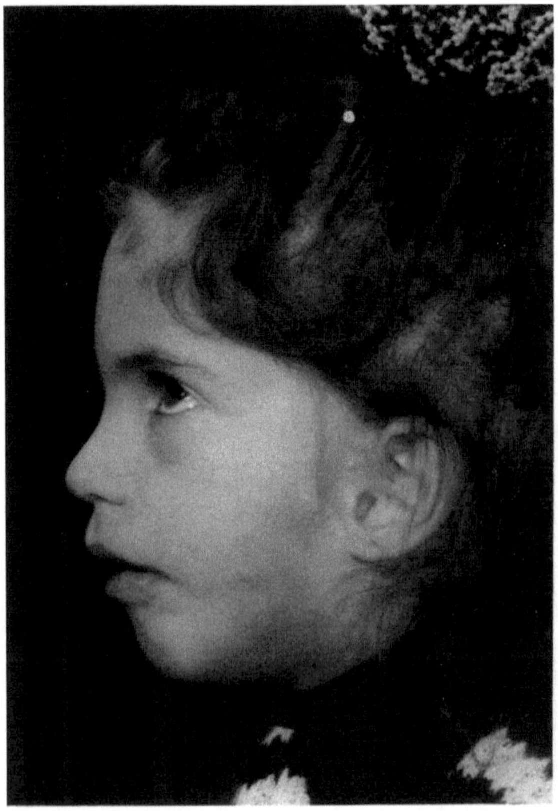

G

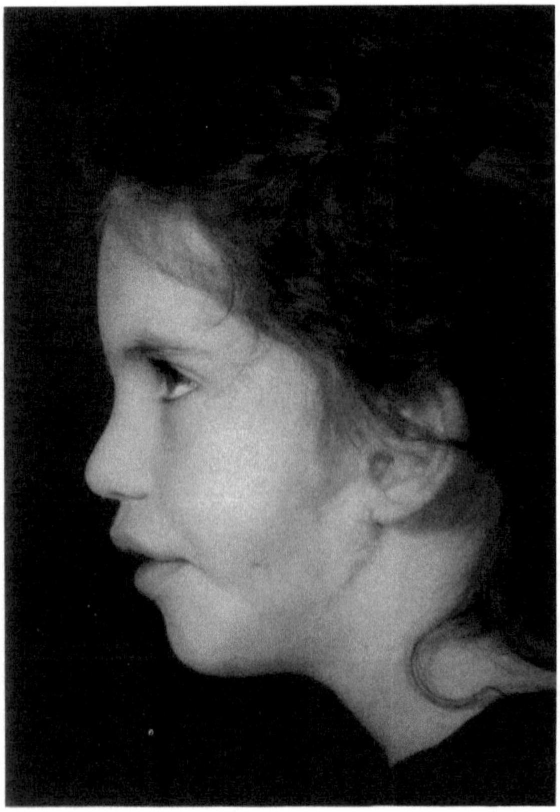

H

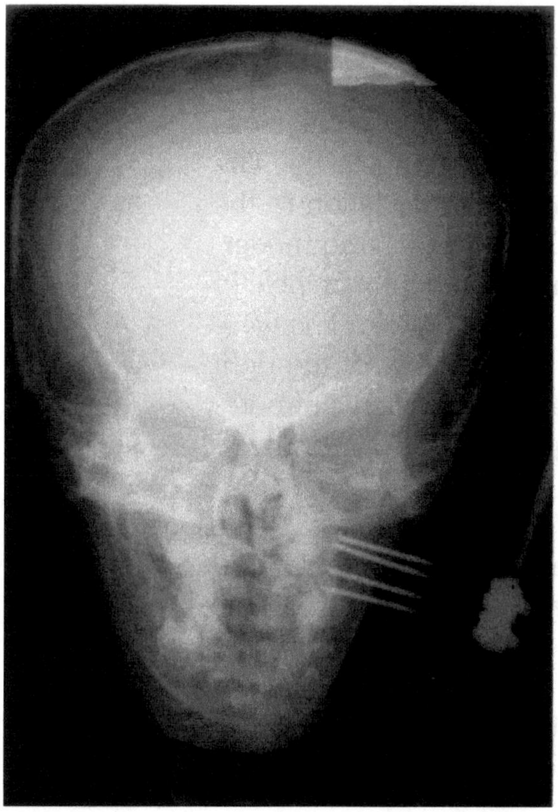

I

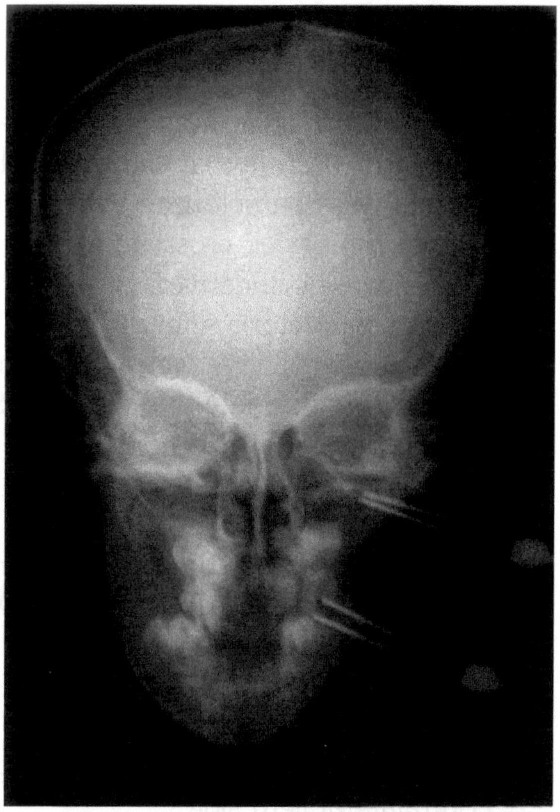

J

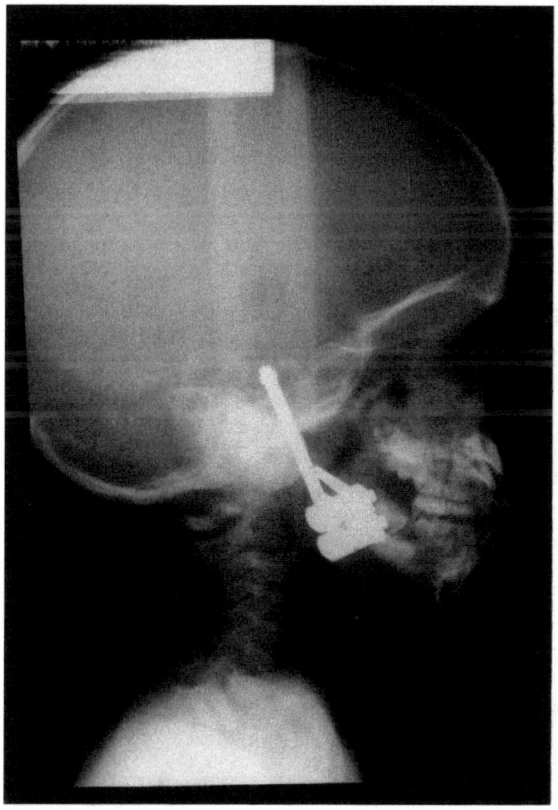

K

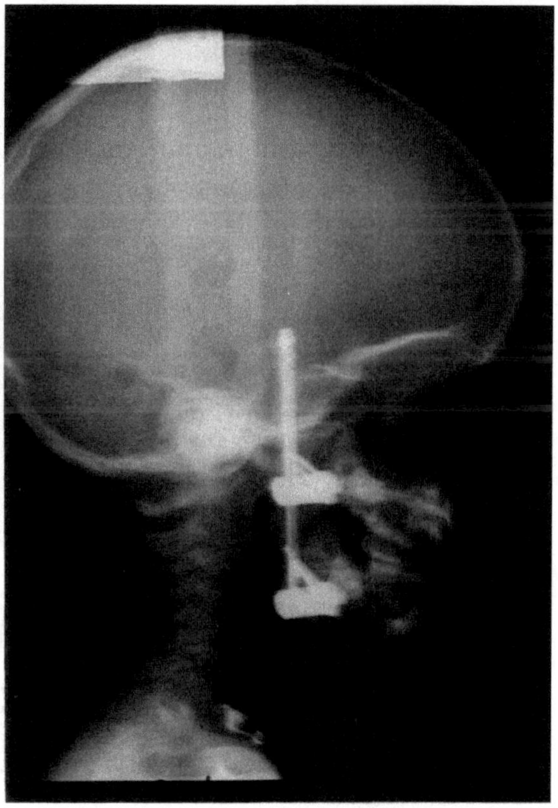

L

Case 10. J.C. was a 4-year-old girl with right craniofacial microsomia (Pruzansky IIa) with an ipsilateral microtia (Figure 5.38). The microsomia was characterized by a significant mandibular deviation to the right with a right-sided crossbite and an overjet. The chin was also moderately retrusive. She underwent unilateral distraction of the right mandible to 25 mm (vertical vector). After distraction, the chin and midincisor line were positioned at the midline with marked increase in the volume of the right mandible and a right lateral open bite. She subsequently underwent autogenous rib graft reconstruction (staged) of the right ear (Dr. C. Thorne).

Figure 5.38. Case 10. A four-year-old female with right craniofacial microsomia (Pruzansky I) who underwent unilateral distraction of the hemimandible (25 mm).

(A) Preoperative frontal view showing chin deviation and hypoplasia of the affected cheek. She has a marginal mandibular (VII) palsy on the contralateral (left) side.

(B) Postoperative frontal view 26 months after completion of distraction. Note the improvement in chin position and contour of the affected cheek.

(C) Preoperative submental view.

(D) Postoperative submental view showing improved chin position and increased cheek fullness on the affected side.

(E) Preoperative right profile.

(F) Postoperative right profile showing increased sagittal thrust of the mandible. Staged auricular reconstruction has commenced.

(G) Preoperative left profile.

(H) Postoperative left profile.

(I) Predistraction posteroanterior cephalogram.

(J) Postdistraction posteroanterior cephalogram. Note the increased vertical dimension of the right mandibular ramus.

(K) Predistraction lateral cephalogram (vertical vector).

(L) Postdistraction lateral cephalogram.

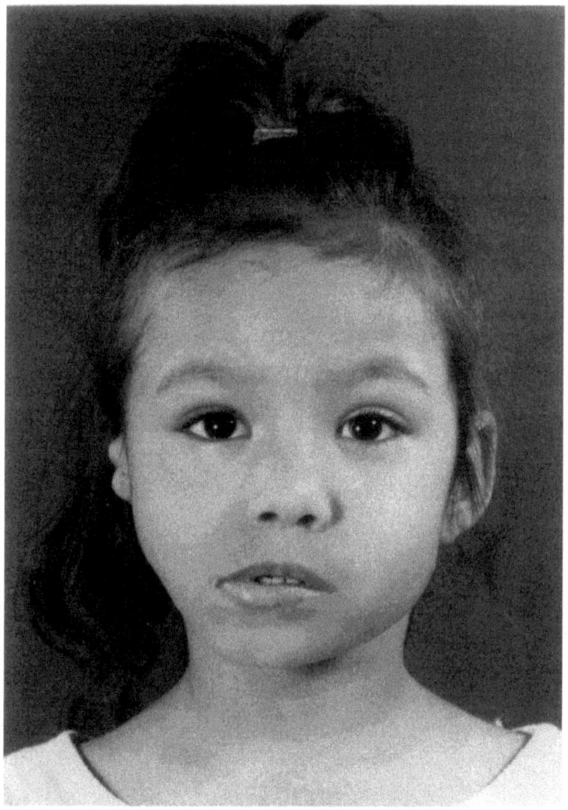

A

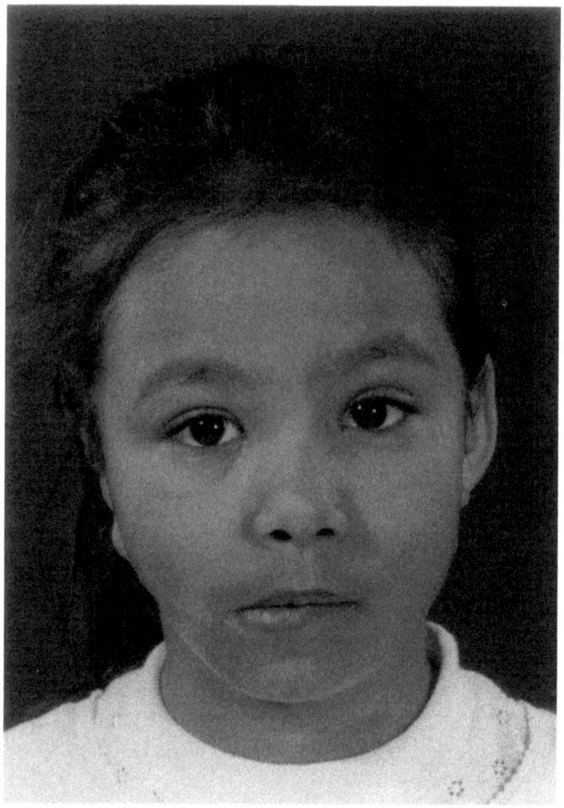

B

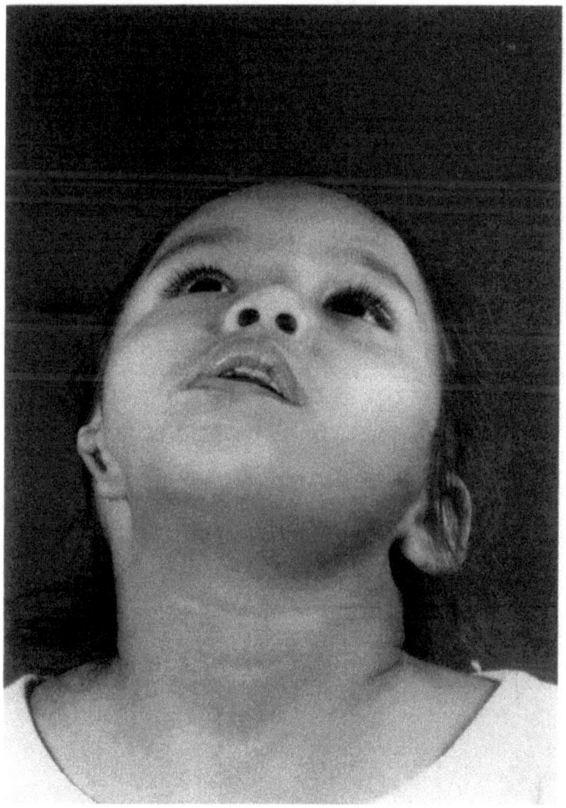

C

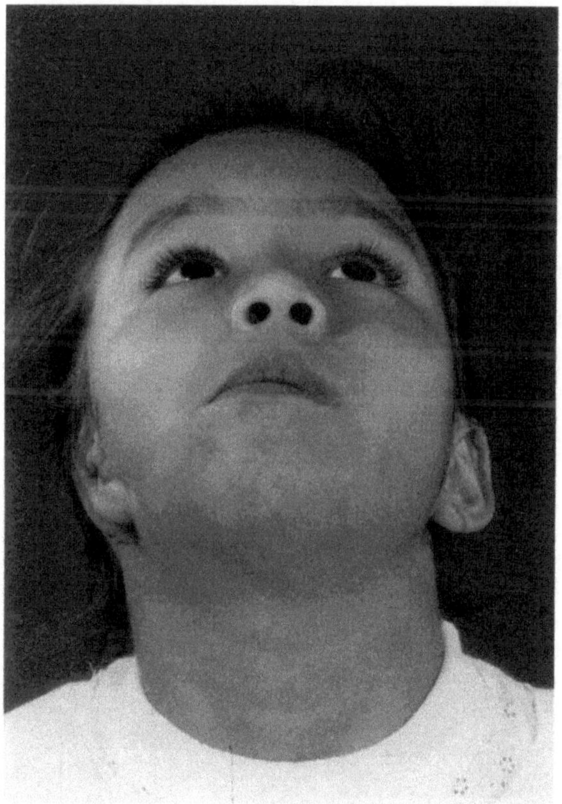

D

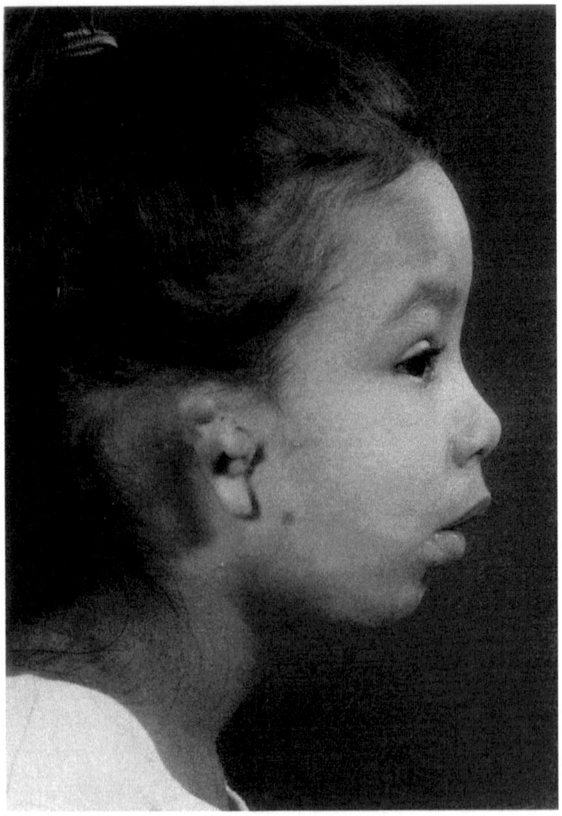

E

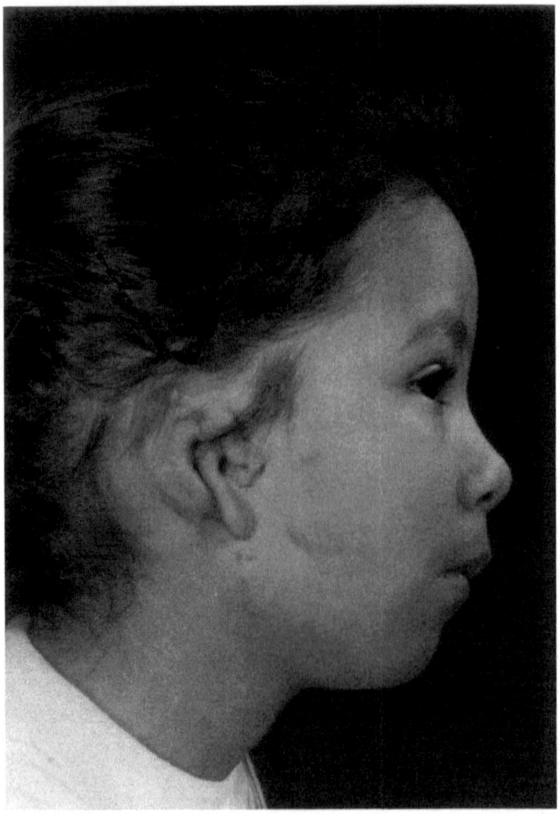

F

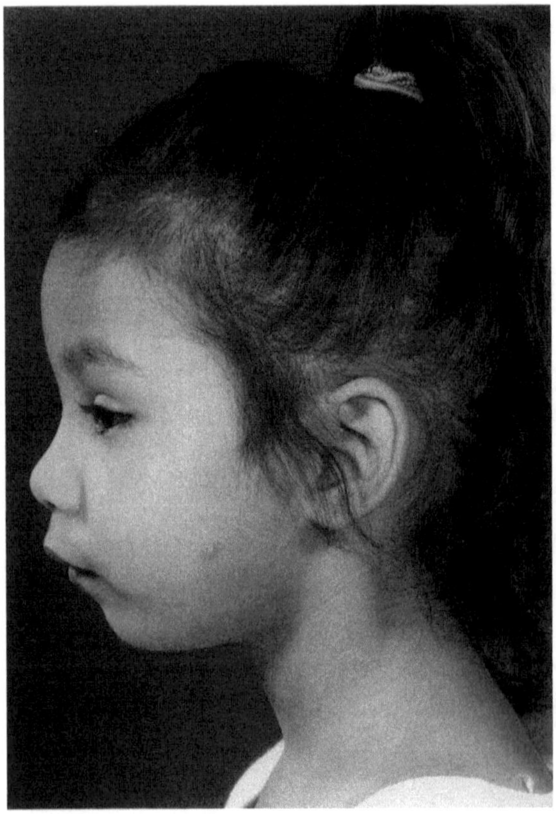

G

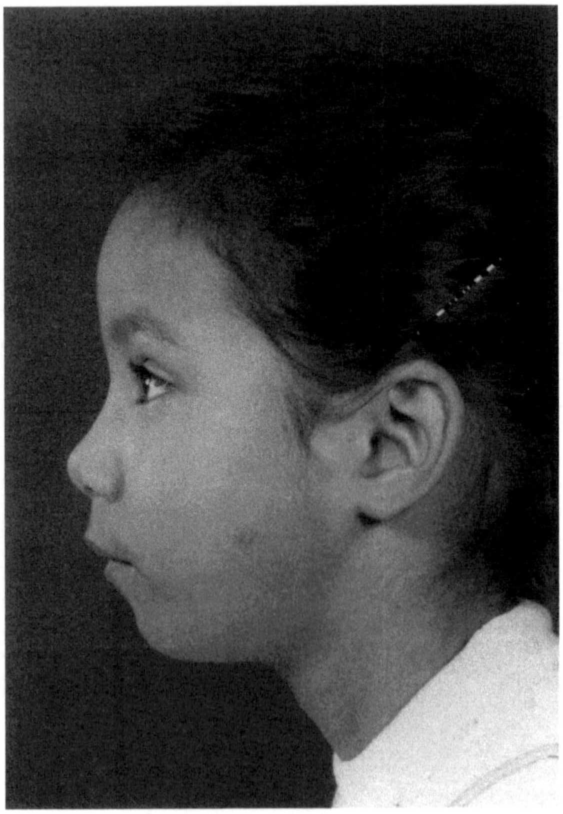

H

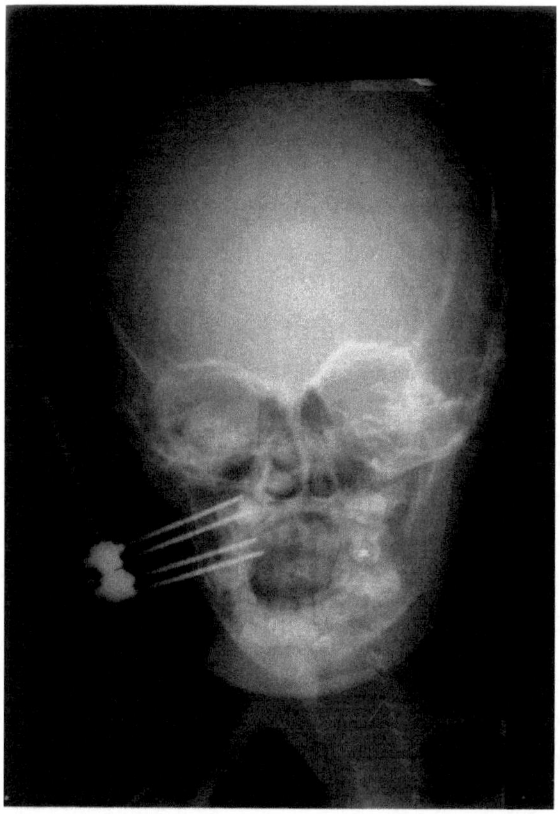

I

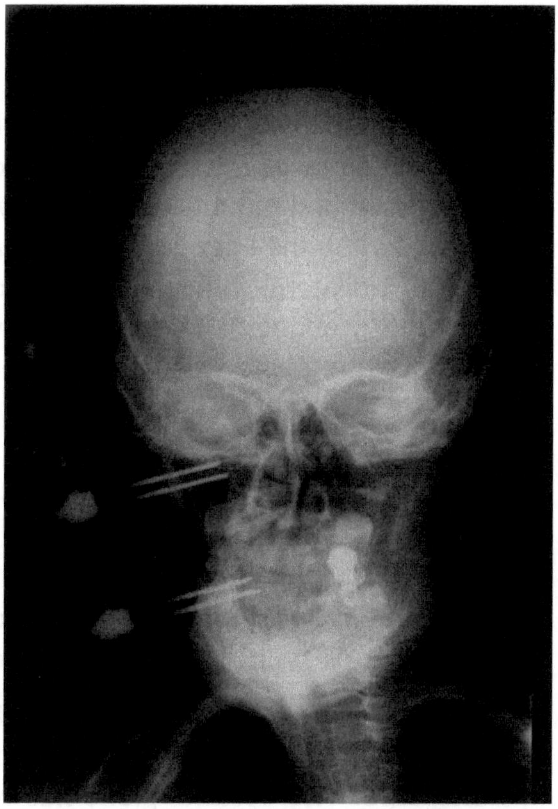

J

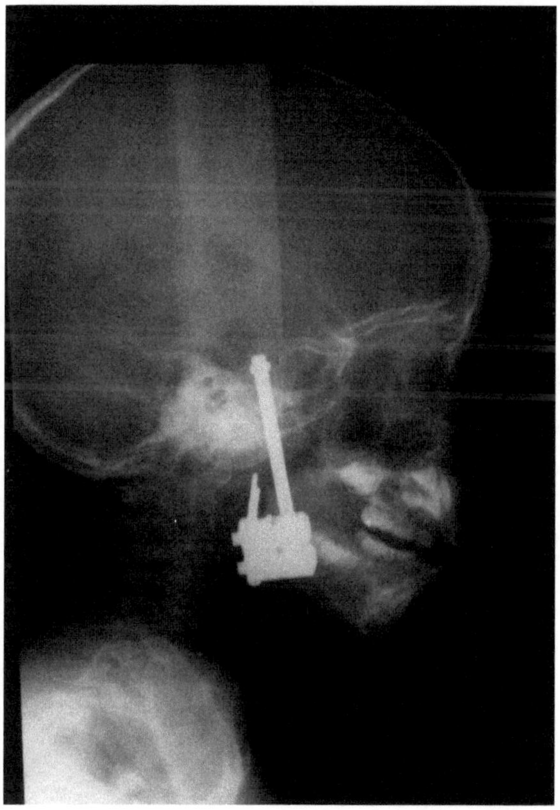

K

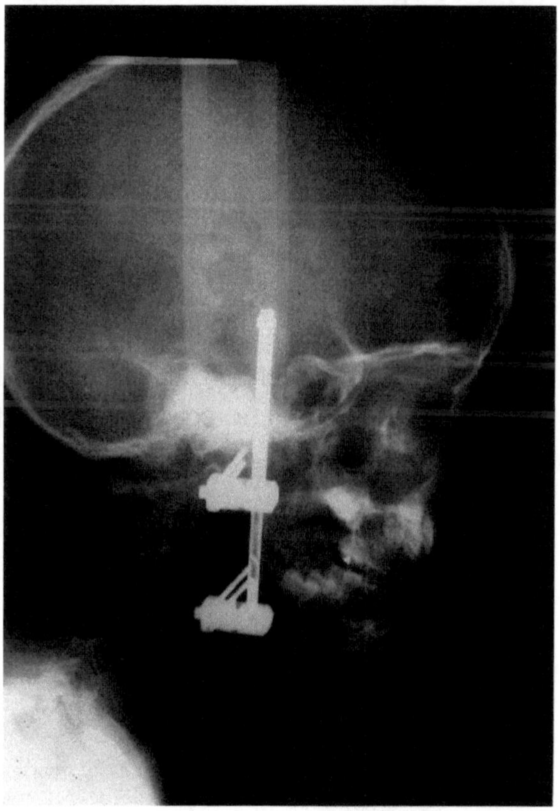

L

Case 11. R.D.S. was a two-and-a-half-year-old boy (Figure 5.39) with left-sided craniofacial microsomia characterized by deficiency of the ipsilateral soft tissue and mandible (Pruzansky I). The occlusal plane was moderately elevated on the left and the chin was deviated to the affected side. He underwent unilateral multiplanar distraction of the left mandible (23 mm linear and 80° angular). The pogonion was overcorrected to the right side and the occlusal plane was leveled.

Figure 5.39. Case 11. A two-and-a-half-year old male with left craniofacial microsomia (Pruzansky I) who underwent unilateral (multiplanar) distraction.

(A) Preoperative frontal view showing deviation of the chin, occlusal cant and hypoplasia of the affected cheek.

(B) Postoperative frontal view six months after completion of distraction. Note the improvement in the position of the chin, oral commissure and alar base. The occlusal plane has been leveled.

(C) Preoperative frontal view (occluding a tongue blade).

(D) Postoperative frontal view (occluding a tongue blade).

(E) Preoperative submental view.

(F) Postoperative submental view. Note the improved check contour on the left side.

(G) Preoperative right profile.

(H) Postoperative right profile.

(I) Preoperative left profile.

(J) Postoperative left profile. Note the increased sagittal thrust of the chin and mandible. The scars are immature.

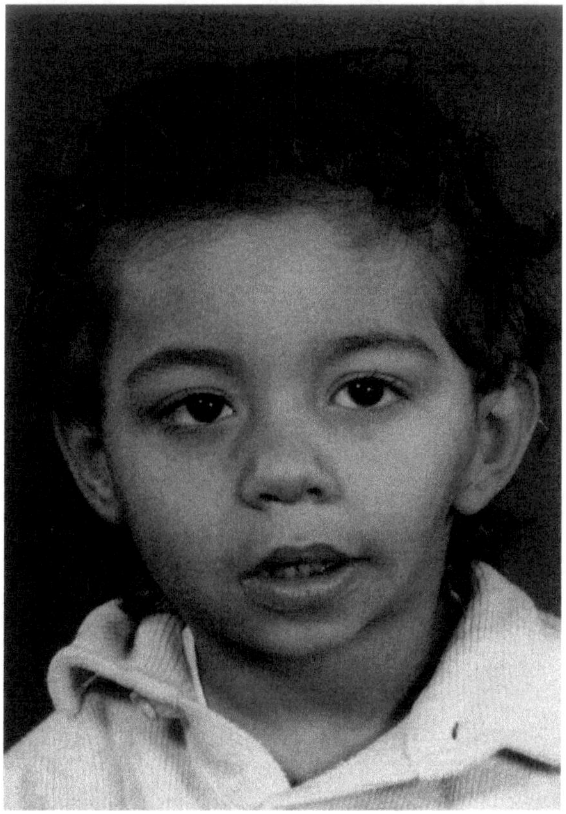

A

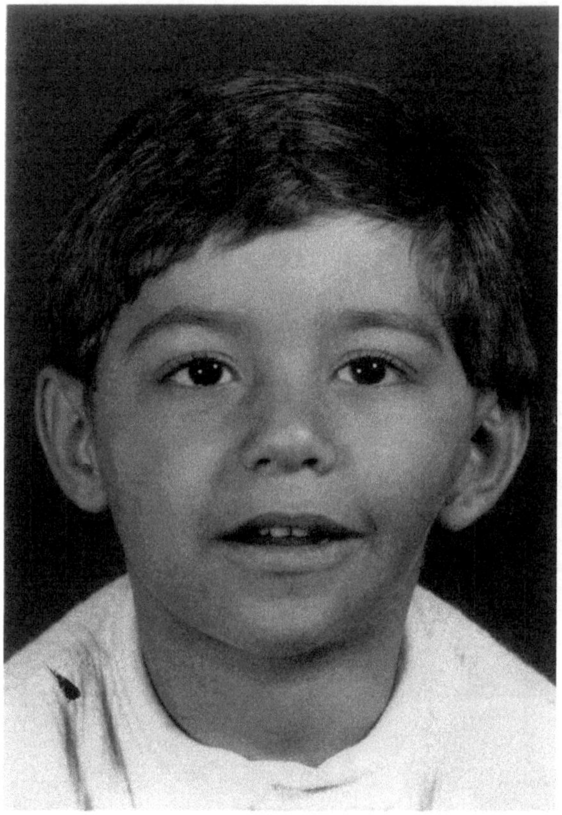

B

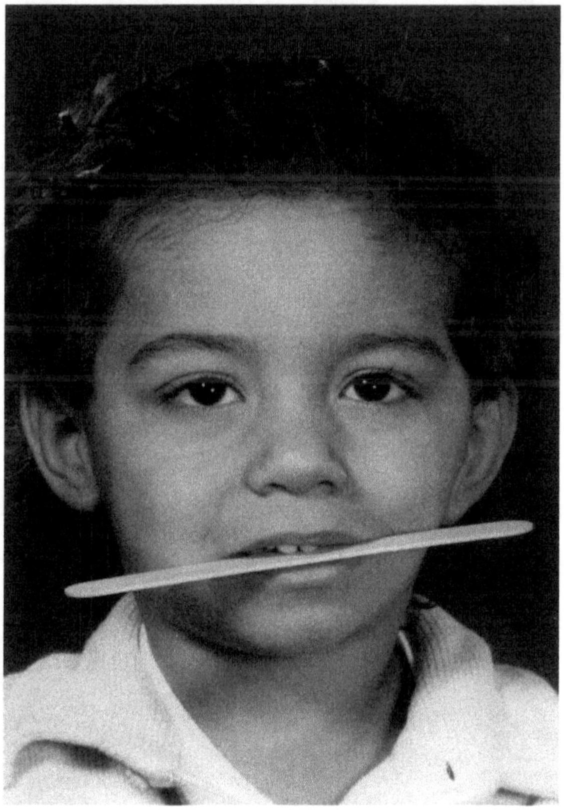

C

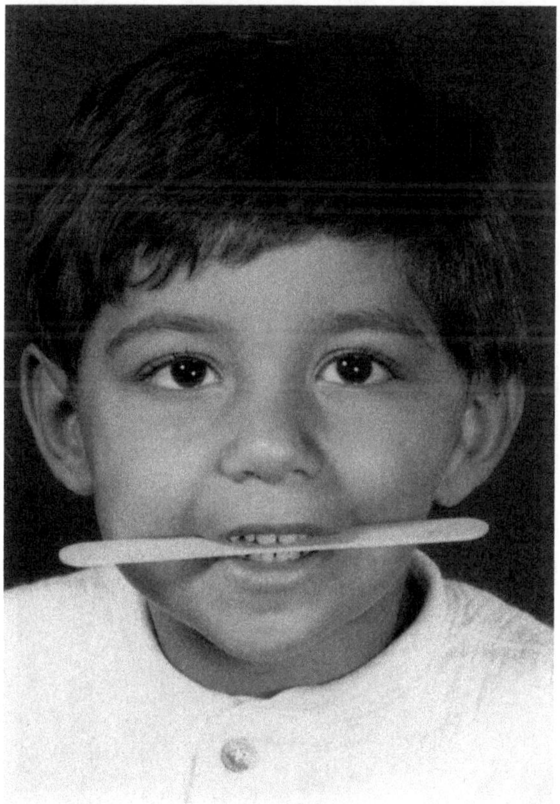

D

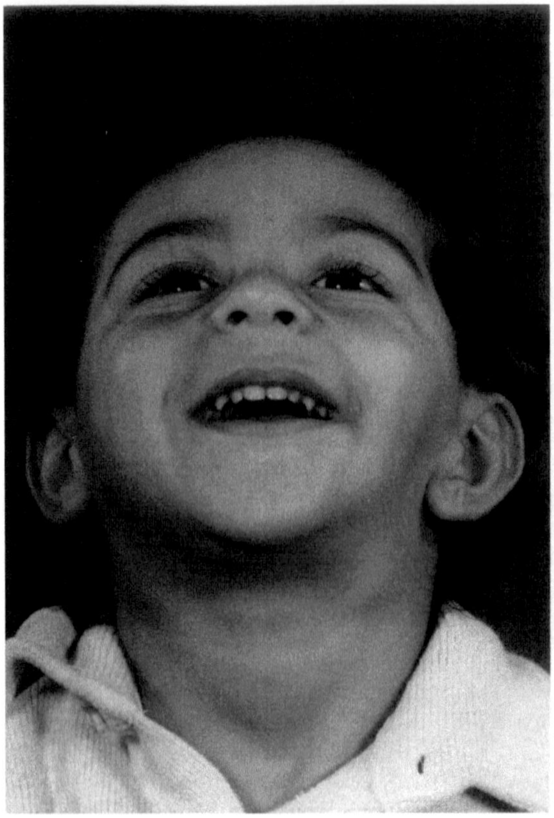

E

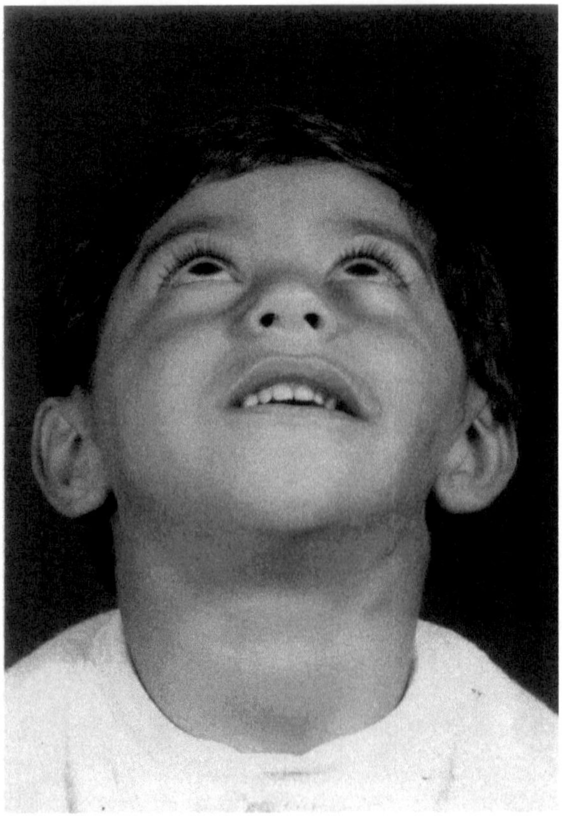

F

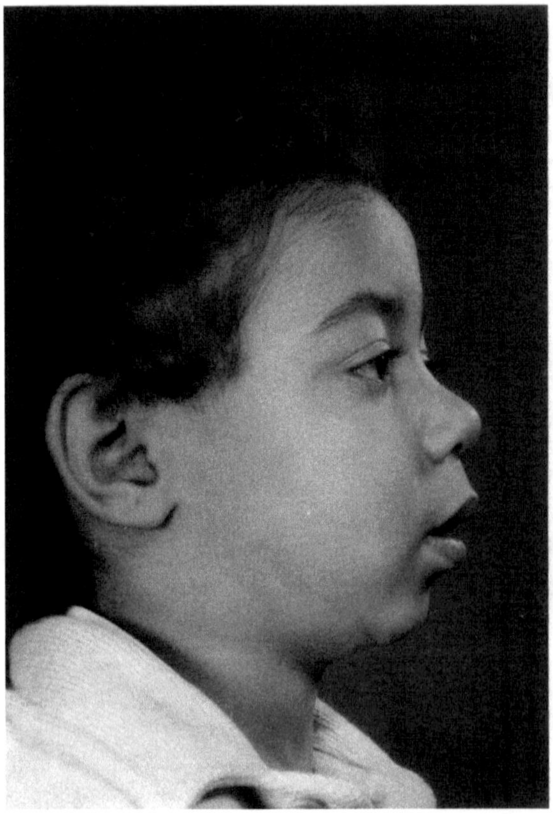

G

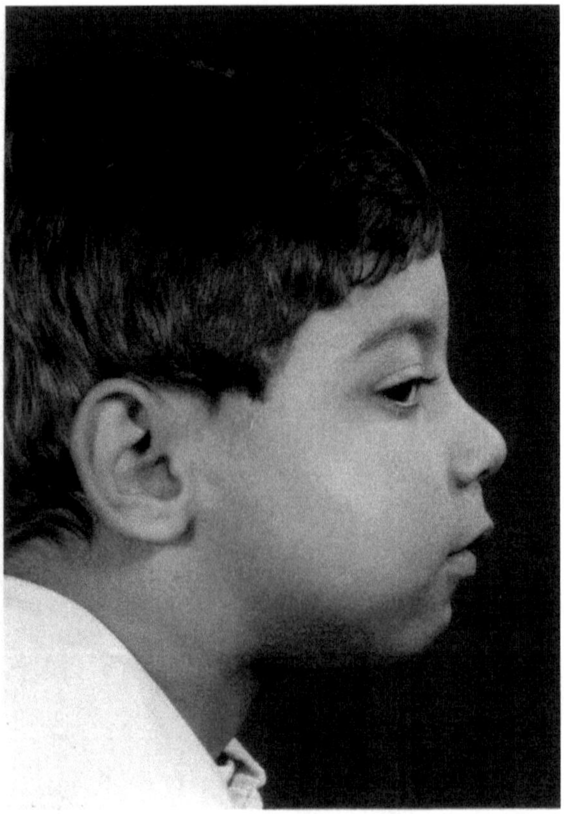

H

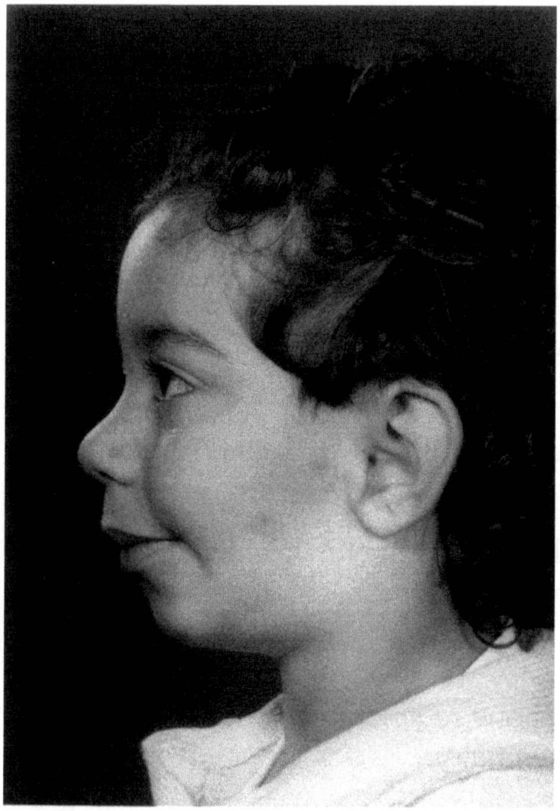

I

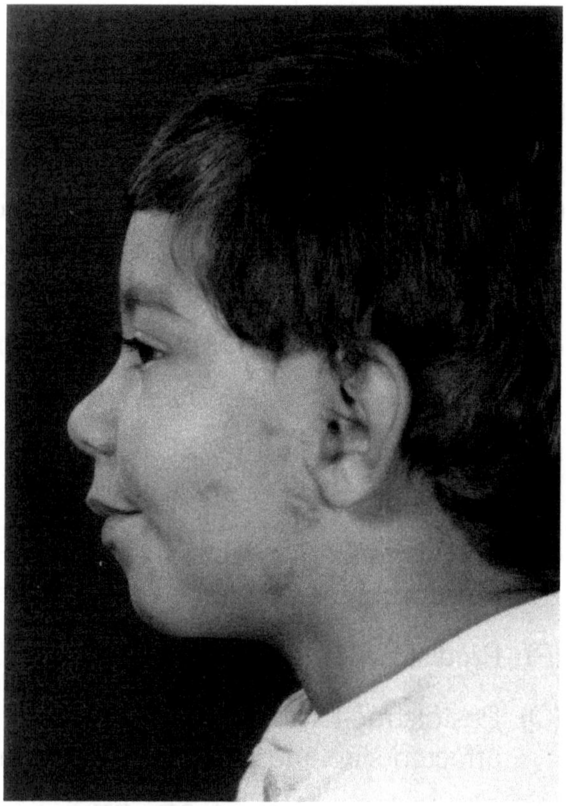

J

Figure 5.39. Case 11. *Continued*

(K) Predistraction posteroanterior cephalogram showing hypoplasia of the mandible on the affected side and deviation of the chin.

(L) Posteroanterior cephalogram at the completion of multiplanar distraction. Note the improved chin position and mandibular contour. The angle of the mandible has been reconstituted on the affected side.

(M) Postdistraction (six months) posteroanterior cephalogram (see previous legend).

(N) Predistraction frontal 3D CT scan. Note the occlusal cant and chin position.

(O) Postdistraction frontal 3D CT scan. Note the improvement in chin position, occlusal plane, and mandibular symmetry.

(P) Predistraction basilar 3D CT scan.

(Q) Postdistraction basilar 3D CT scan. Note the bony regenerate on the affected side and the improved mandibular symmetry.

(R) Predistraction lateral 3D CT scan. The hypoplasia of the affected mandibular body and ramus is apparent.

(S) Postdistraction lateral 3D CT scan. Note the improvement in shape and volume of the affected side of the mandible. Note the bony regenerate between the drill holes.

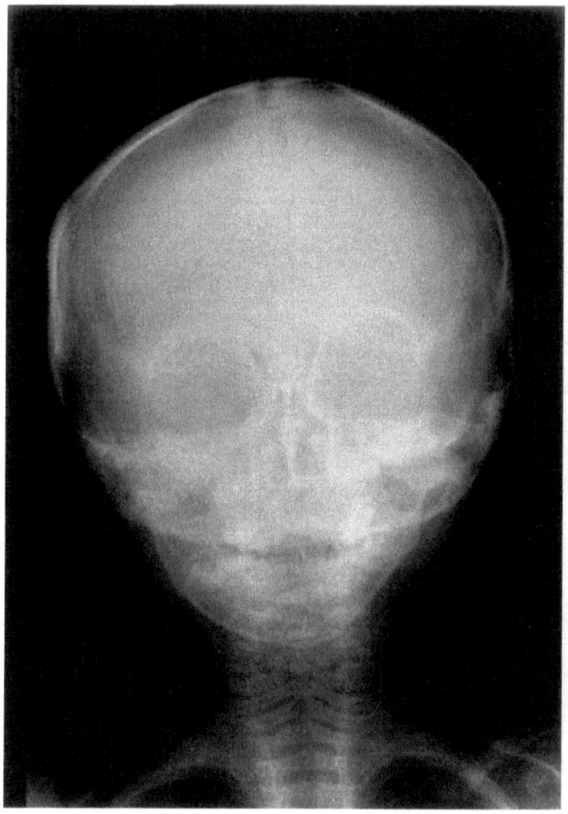

K

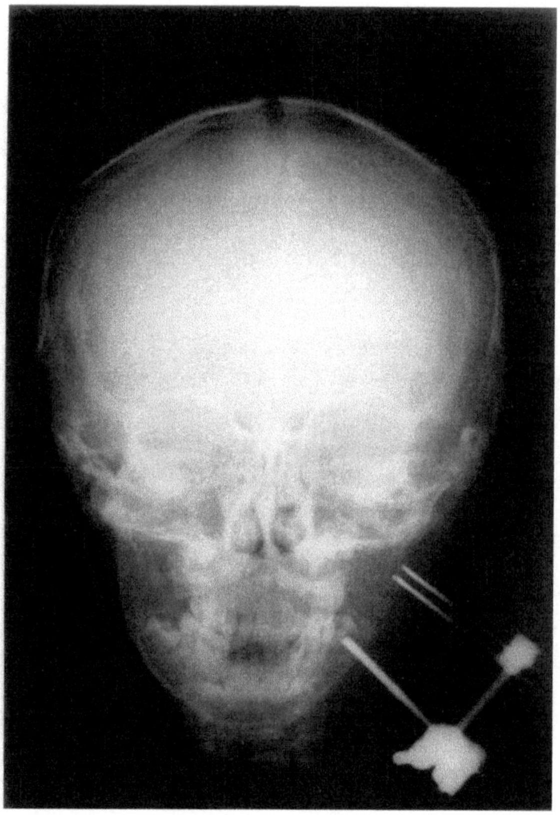

L

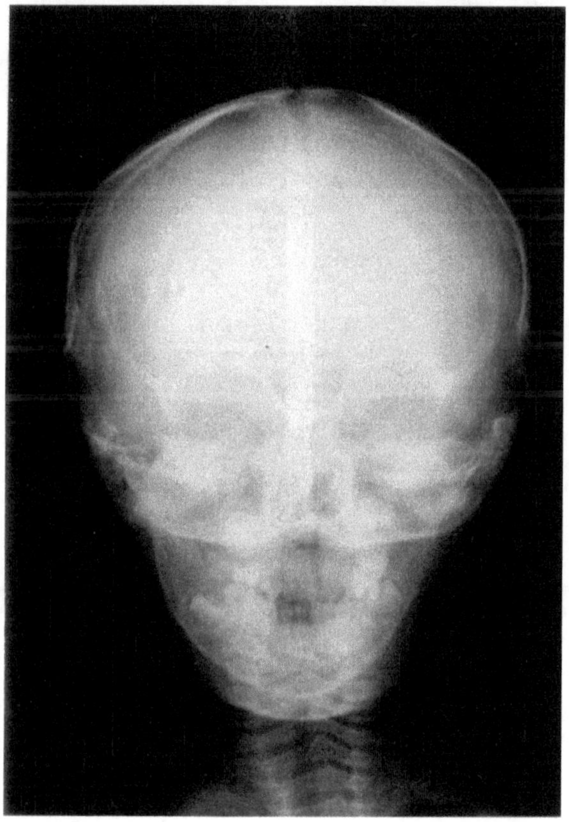

M

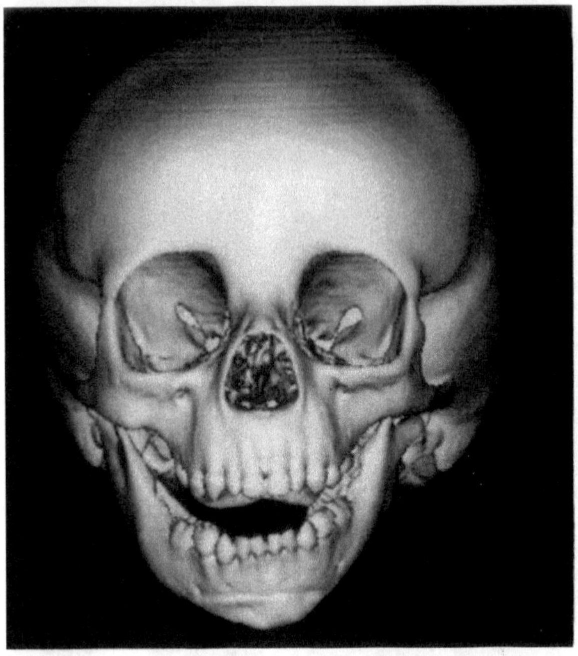

N

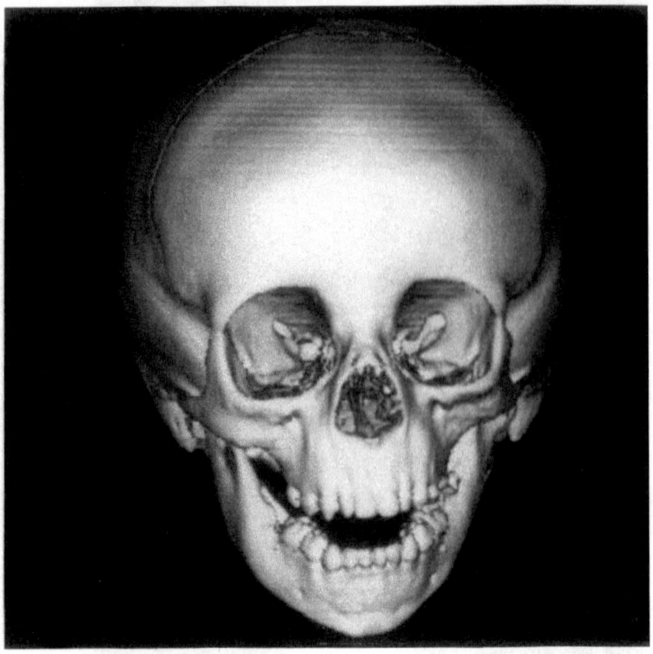

O

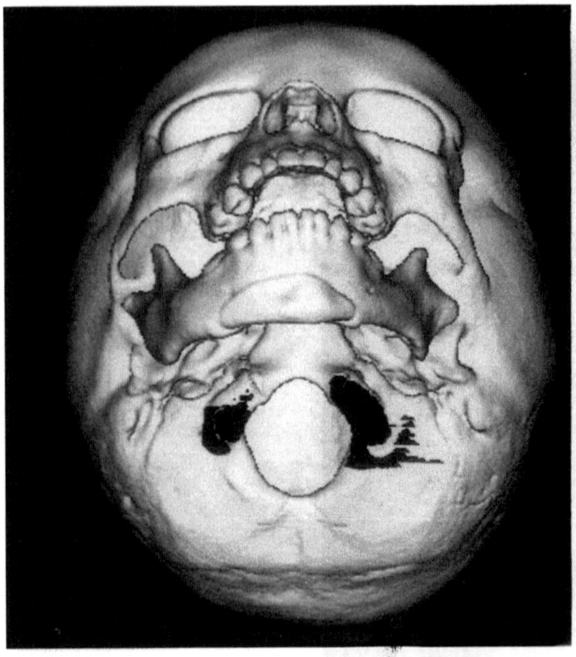

P

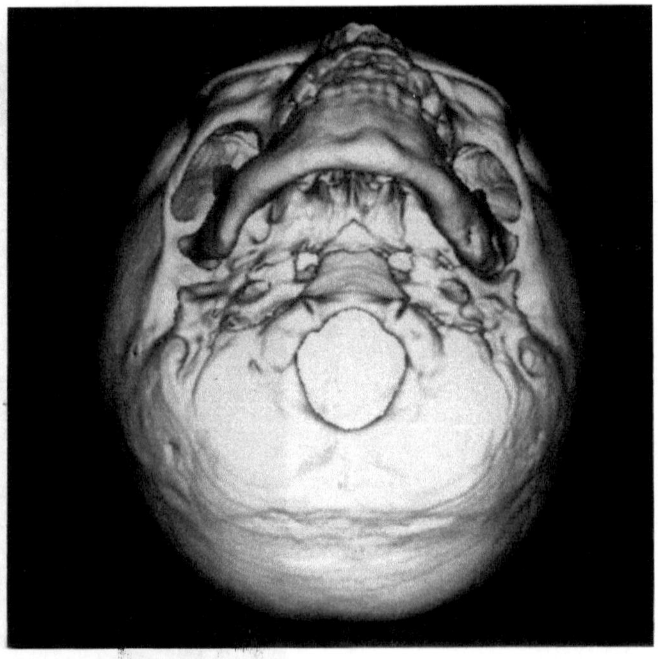

Q

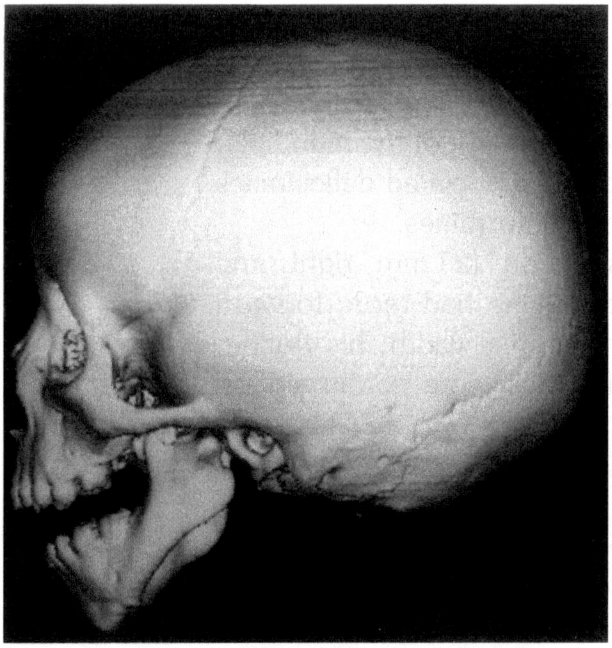

R

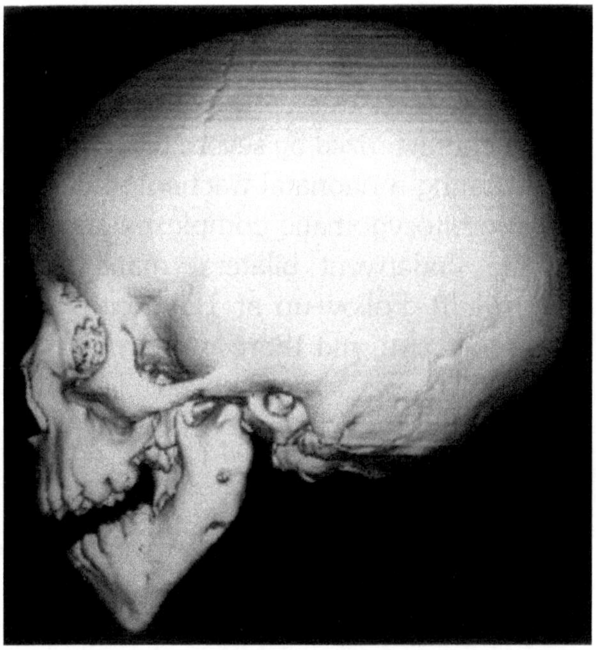

S

CASE STUDIES: BILATERAL DISTRACTION

Case 12. R.R. was a three-year-old boy (Figure 5.40) with Nager syndrome characterized by severe bilateral underdevelopment of the mandible, necessitating a neonatal tracheotomy. He also had associated deficiencies of the orbitozygomatic complexes and extremity deformities.

He underwent bilateral mandibular distraction (21 mm right and 21 mm left). Follow-up at 12 months showed that he had more forward chin projection and there was an increase in bigonial width; his tracheotomy tube was also removed. The above findings were confirmed on radiographic study (Figure 5.40).

Figure 5.40. Case 12. A three-year-old-male with Nager syndrome (Right, Pruzansky I; Left, Pruzansky I) who underwent bilateral mandibular (horizontal vector) distraction (right, 21 mm; left, 21 mm).

(A) Preoperative frontal view with tracheotomy in place. Note the severe micrognathia.

(B) Postoperative frontal view 7 months after completion of distraction and decannulation of tracheotomy. Note the increased volume and contour of the lower third of the face.

(C) Preoperative submental view.

(D) Postoperative submental view.

(E) Preoperative right profile showing the micrognathia.

(F) Postoperative right profile. The scar is well positioned.

(G) Preoperative left profile.

(H) Postoperative left profile. Note the increased projection of the chin and mandible.

(I) Predistraction posteroanterior cephalogram (devices in place).

(J) Postdistraction posteroanterior cephalogram showing the increase in the vertical dimension of the mandibular ramus on each side.

(K) Predistraction lateral cephalogram (horizontal vector).

(L) Postdistraction lateral cephalogram. Note the increased mandibular projection (relationship of the anterior occlusion) and the counterclockwise rotation of the mandible and devices.

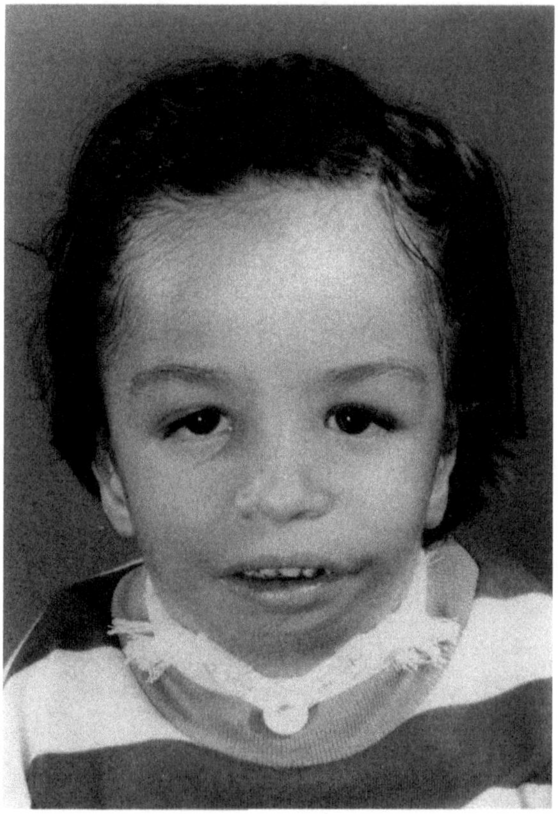

A

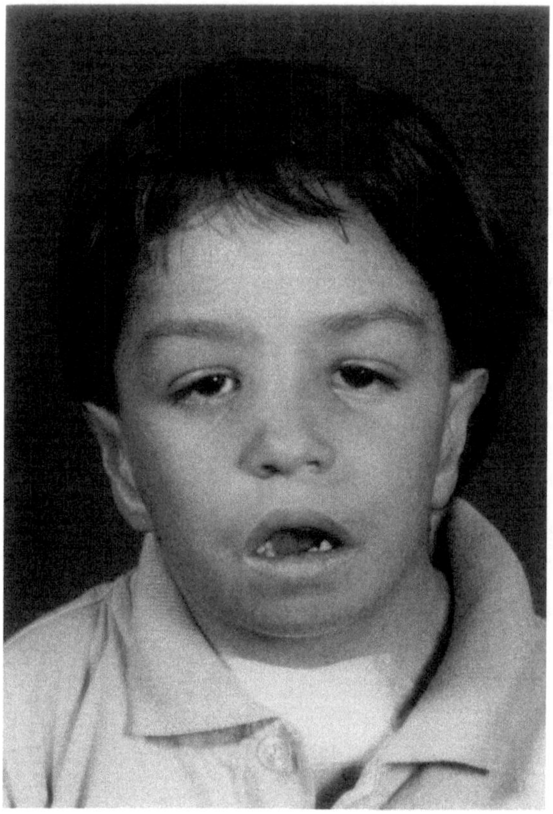

B

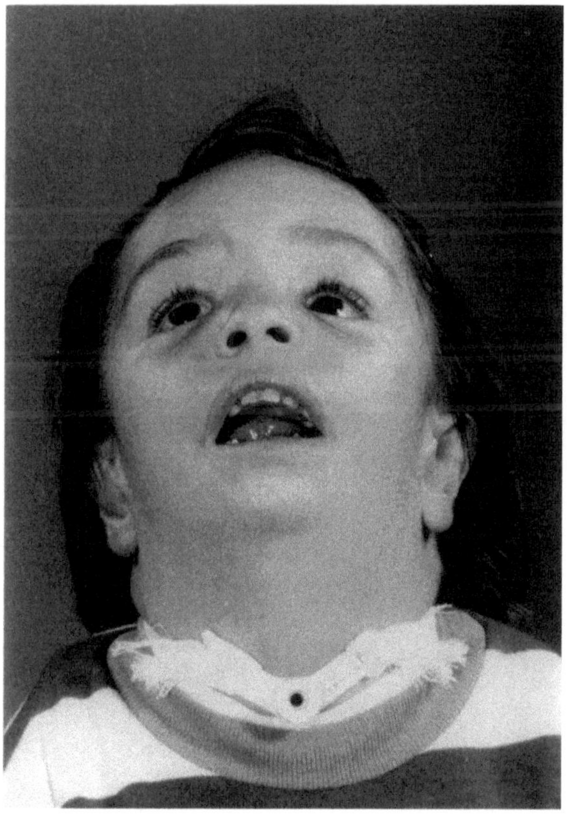

C

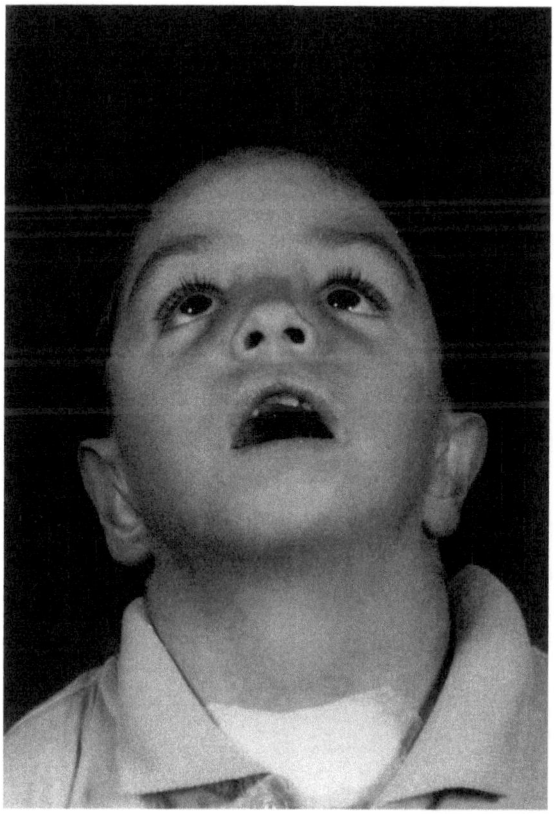

D

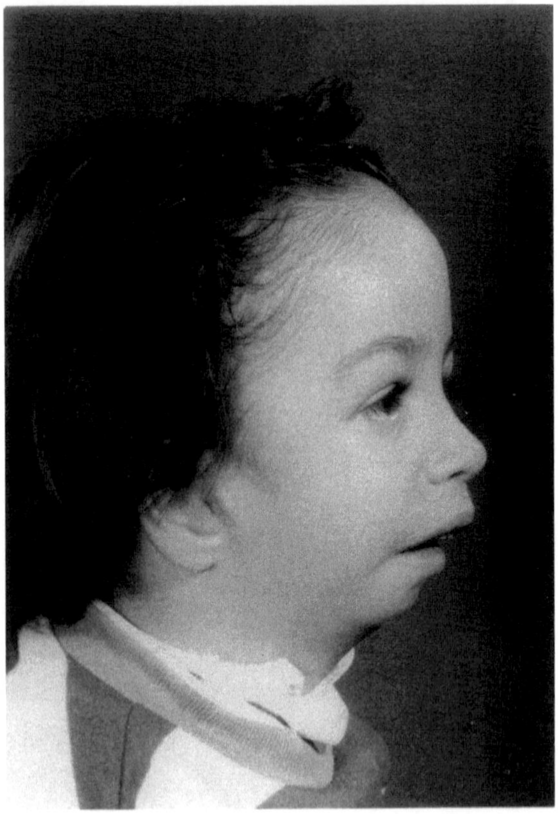

E

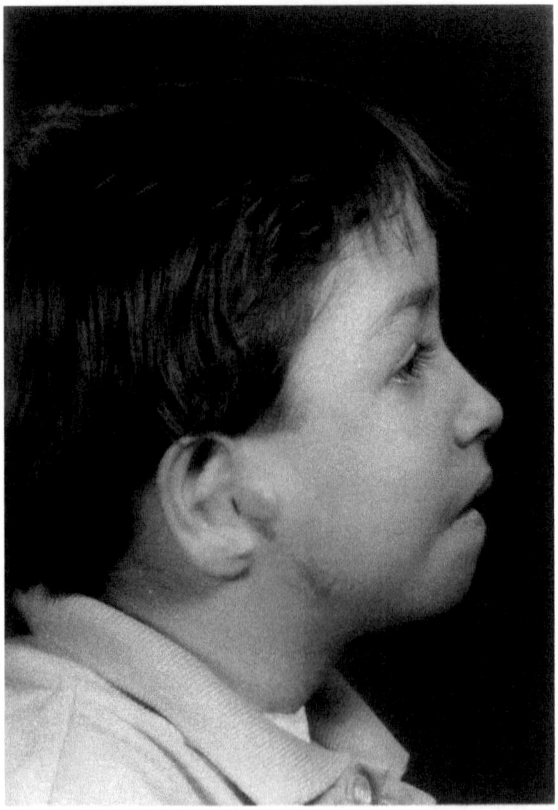

F

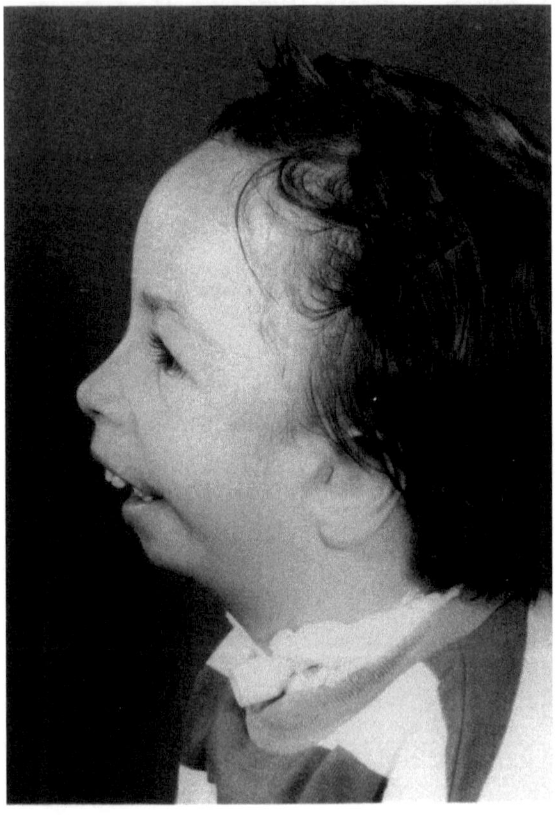

G

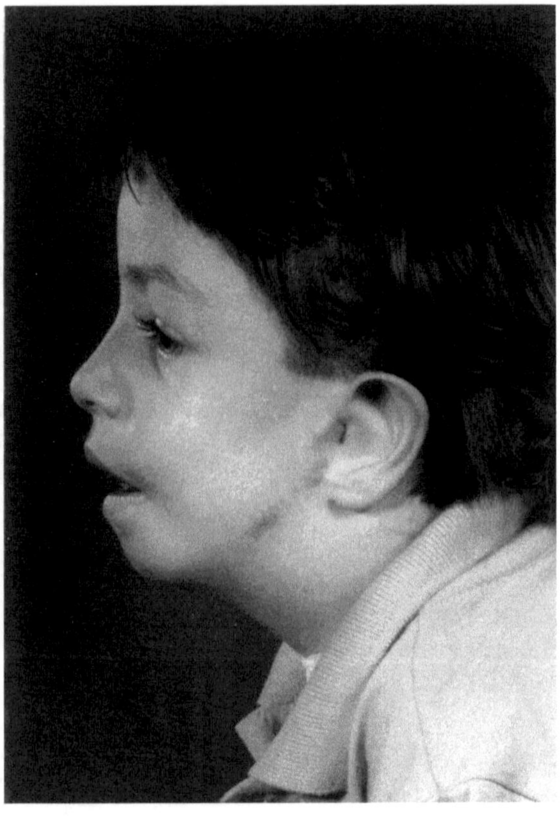

H

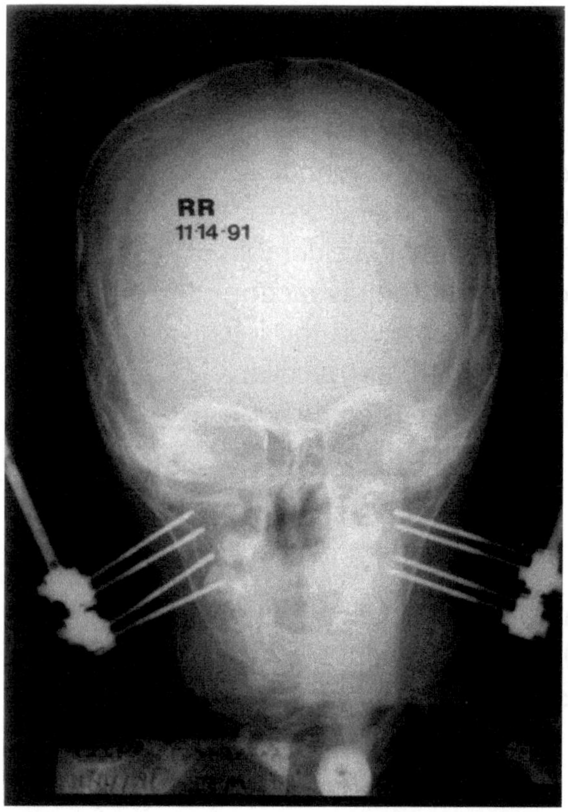

I

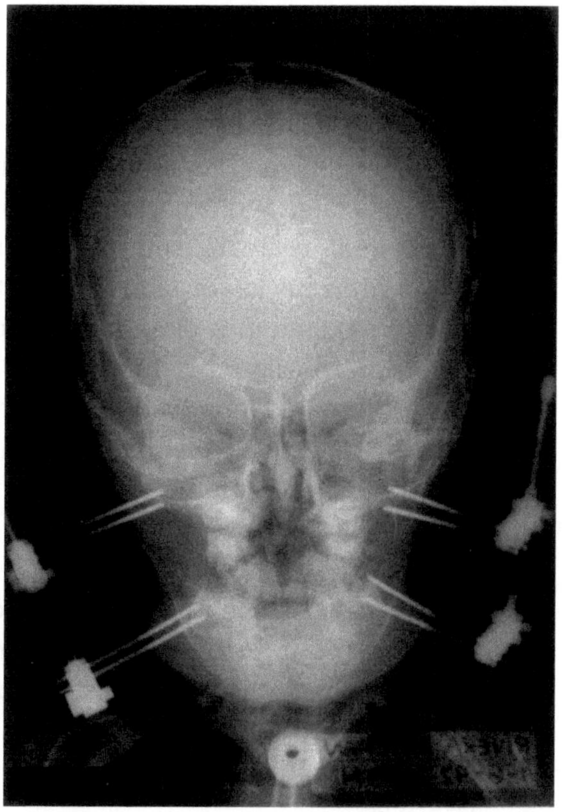

J

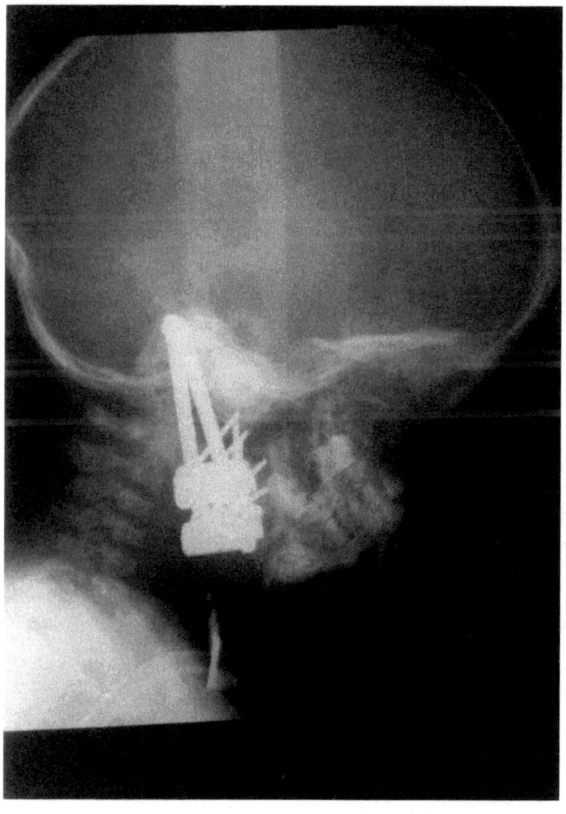

K

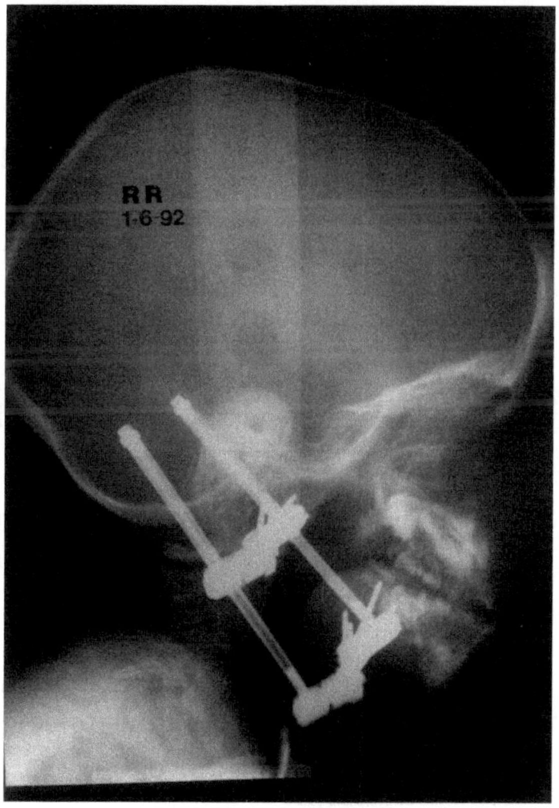

L

Case 13. C.K. was a 10-year-old boy (Figure 5.41) with a developmental micrognathia characterized by underdevelopment of the mandible, anterior cross bite, and anterior open bite. He underwent bilateral distraction (horizontal vector/28 mm right and 32 mm left) with considerable improvement in his lower facial form. It is noteworthy that the distraction deliberately resulted in a class III malocclusion and was greater on the left side in order to align his mandibular midincisor line with its maxillary counterpart. He had a resulting anterior crossbite, which persisted through his years of follow-up. His serial cephalometric studies are illustrated in Figure 5.41.

Figure 5.41. Case 13. A ten-year-old male with developmental micrognathia (right, Pruzansky I; left, Pruzansky I) who underwent bilateral mandibular (horizontal vector) distraction (right, 28 mm; left, 32 mm).

(A) Preoperative frontal view.

(B) Postoperative frontal view 21 months after completion of distraction.

(C) Preoperative submental view.

(D) Postoperative submental view.

(E) Preoperative right profile showing the severe micrognathia.

(F) Postoperative right profile showing the increased sagittal thrust of the mandible.

(G) Preoperative left profile showing the severe micrognathia.

(H) Postoperative left profile showing the increased sagittal thrust of the mandible.

(I) Predistraction posteroanterior cephalogram. Note the osteotomy on each side.

(J) Postdistraction posteroanterior cephalogram showing the increased vertical dimensions of the mandibular rami.

(K) Predistraction lateral cephalogram (horizontal vector).

(L) Postdistraction lateral cephalogram showing the expanded devices and the increased sagittal thrust of the mandible with development of an anterior crossbite.

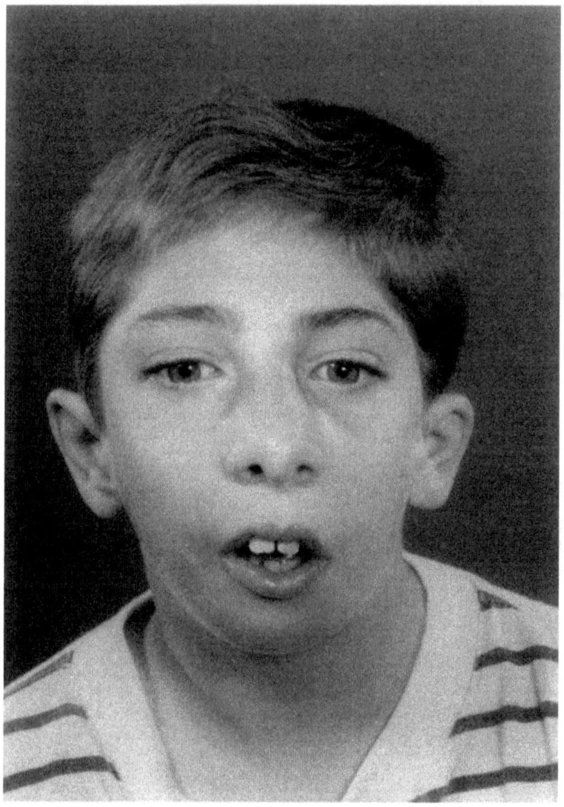

A

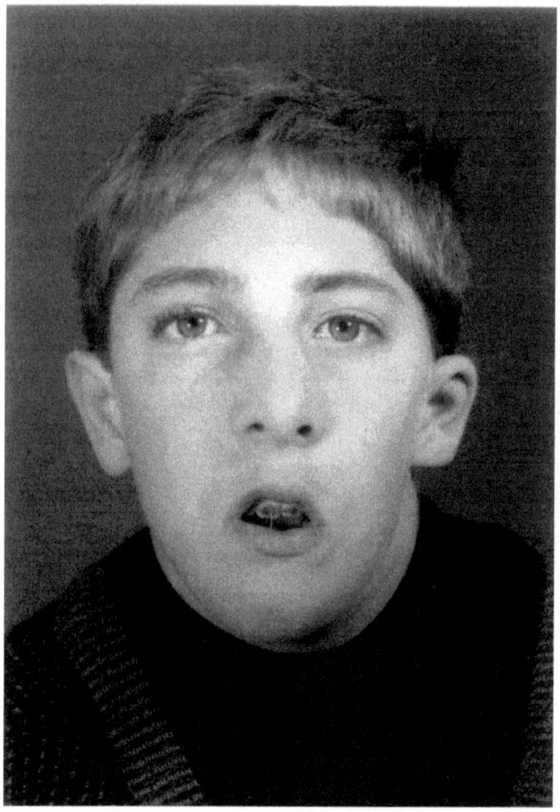

B

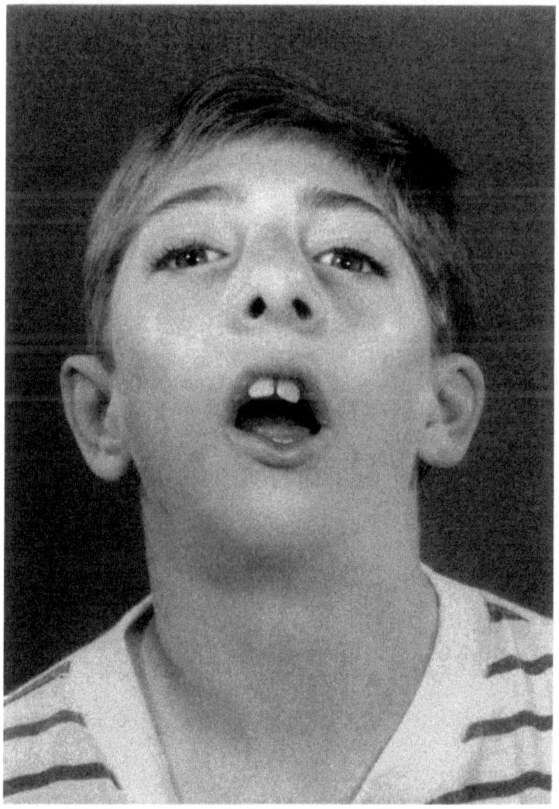

C

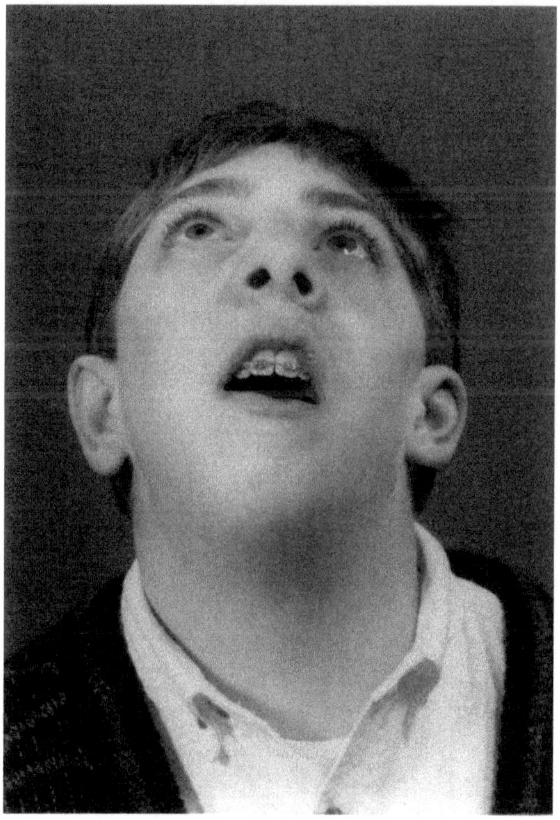

D

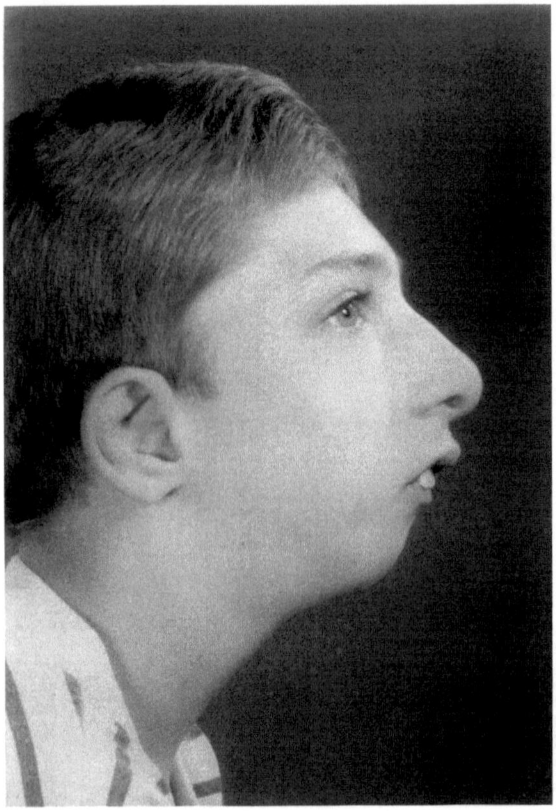

E

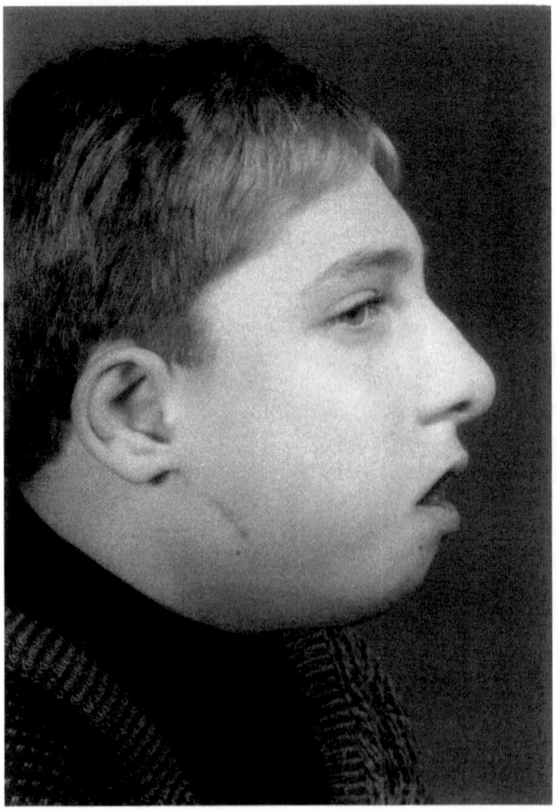

F

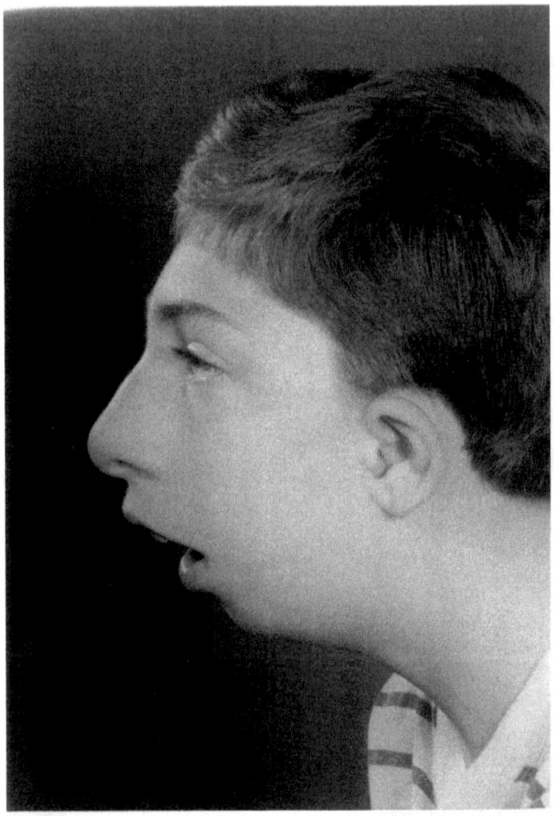

G

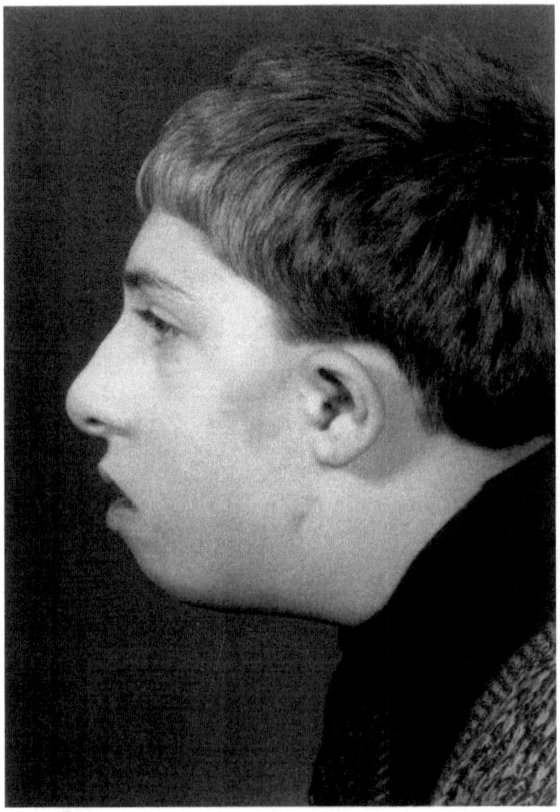

H

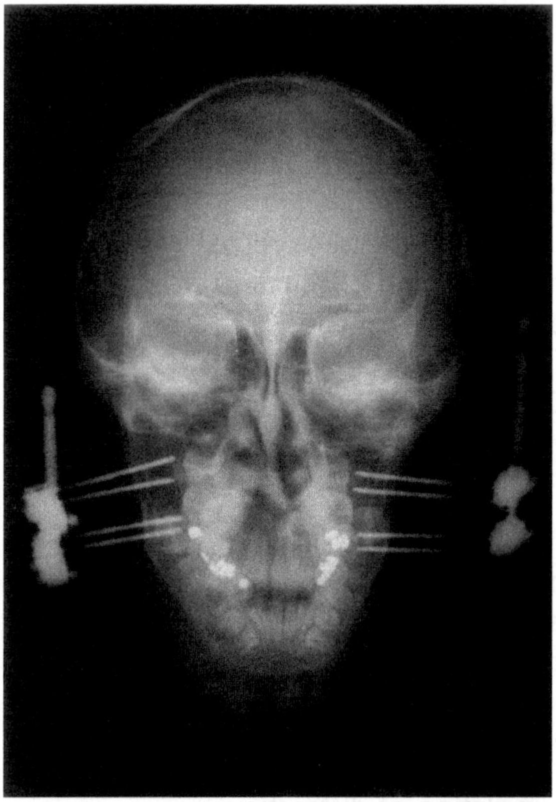

I

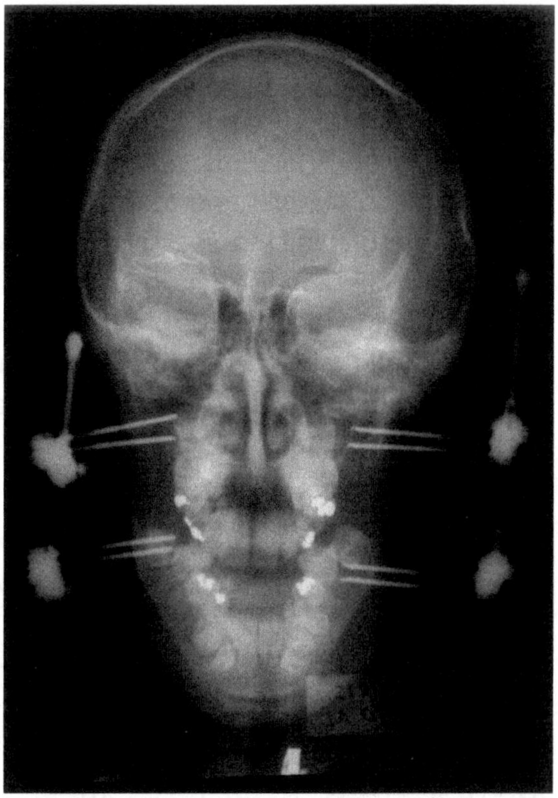

J

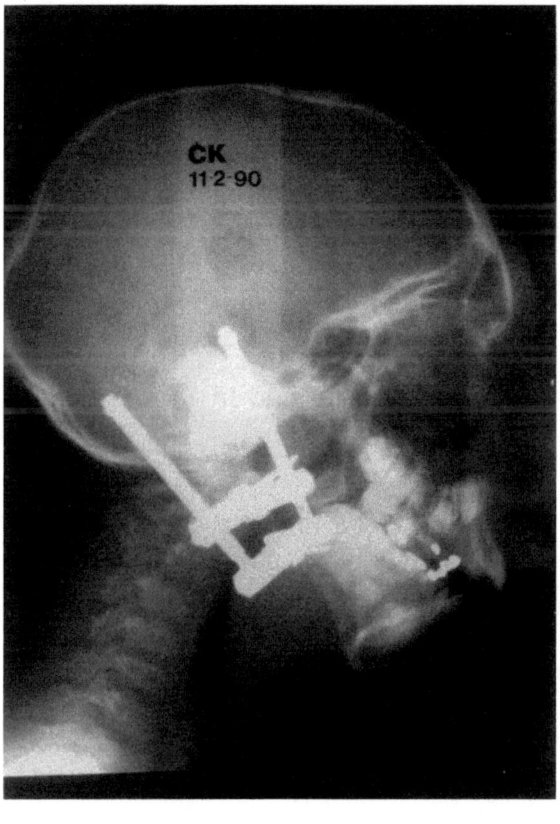

K

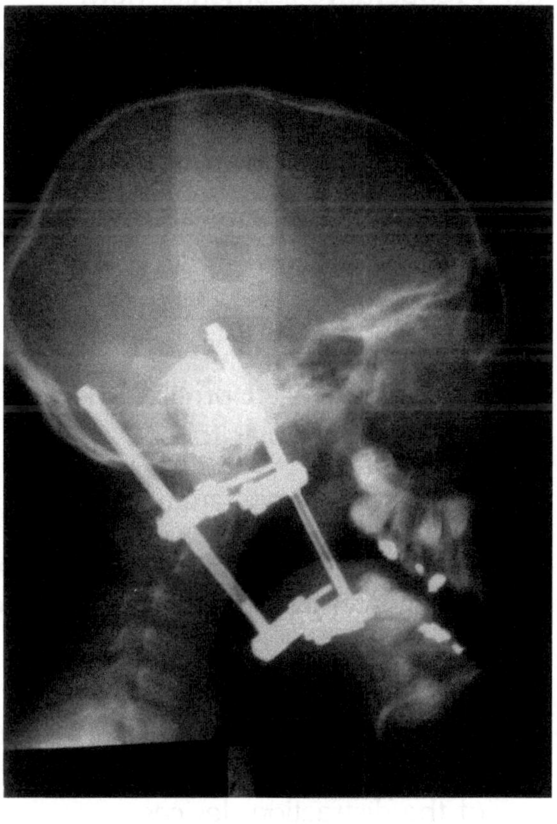

L

Case 14. J.F. was a 3-year-old boy with a development micrognathia similar to that of his father (Figure 5.42). In addition to the underdevelopment of his mandible and an anterior crossbite, there was also clefting of the midline of his chin (Tessier #30) (see also case 18). Bilateral (vertical vector) mandibular distraction was performed (29 mm right and 28 mm left) with resulting multidimensional expansion of the lower third of his face (vertical dimension of his chin, anterior thrust of his chin, and increased bigonial distance). His serial cephalometric and CT scan studies are also illustrated in Figure 5.42.

Figure 5.42. Case 14. A three-year-old male with developmental micrognathia (right, Pruzansky IIa; left, Pruzansky IIa) who underwent bilateral mandibular distraction (right, 29 mm; left, 28 mm).

(A) Preoperative frontal view showing the severe micrognathia.

(B) Postoperative frontal view 42 months after completion of distraction. Note the increase in the lower third of the face.

(C) Preoperative submental view.

(D) Postoperative submental view showing increased chin/mandible volume.

(E) Preoperative right profile.

(F) Postoperative right profile. Note the satisfactory scar position and appearance.

(G) Preoperative left profile.

(H) Postoperative left profile. The scar should preferably be positioned in the submandibular fold.

(I) Predistraction posteroanterior cephalogram.

(J) Postdistraction posteroanterior cephalogram showing the increase in the vertical dimensions of the mandibular rami.

(K) Predistraction lateral cephalogram (horizontal vectors).

(L) Postdistraction lateral cephalogram. The anterior open bite has been closed, and there has been counterclockwise rotation of the long arms of the distraction devices.

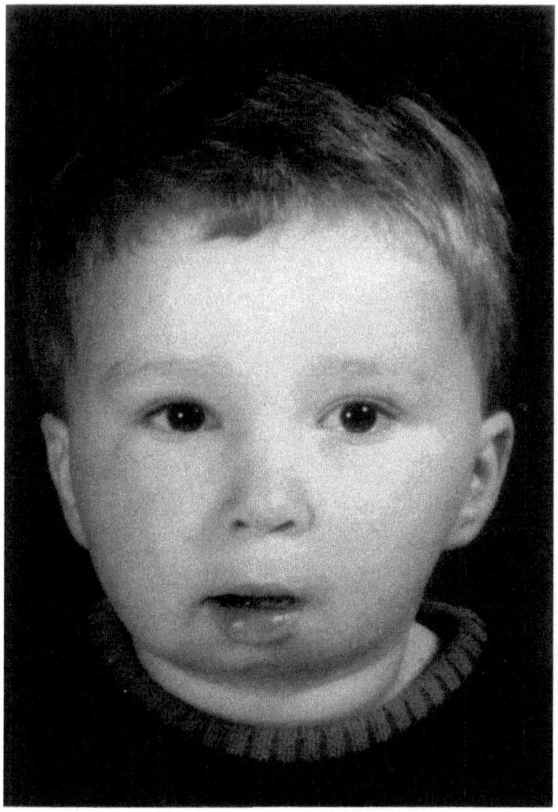

A

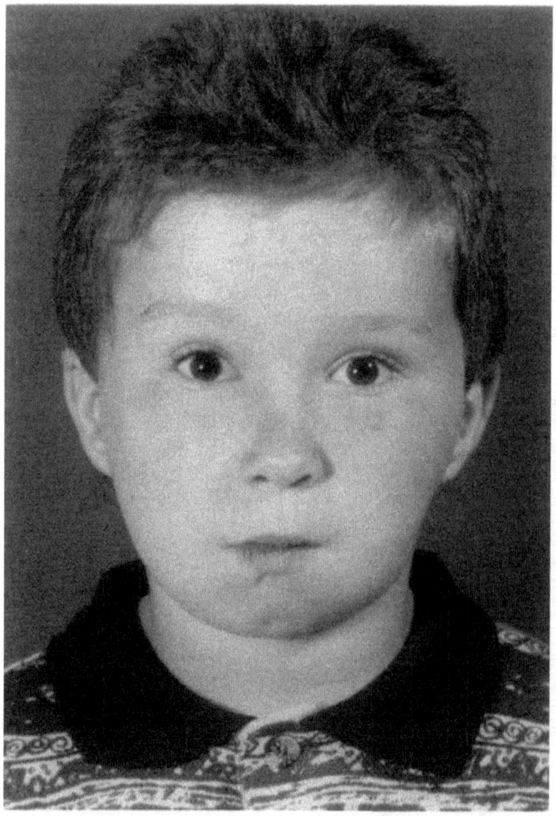

B

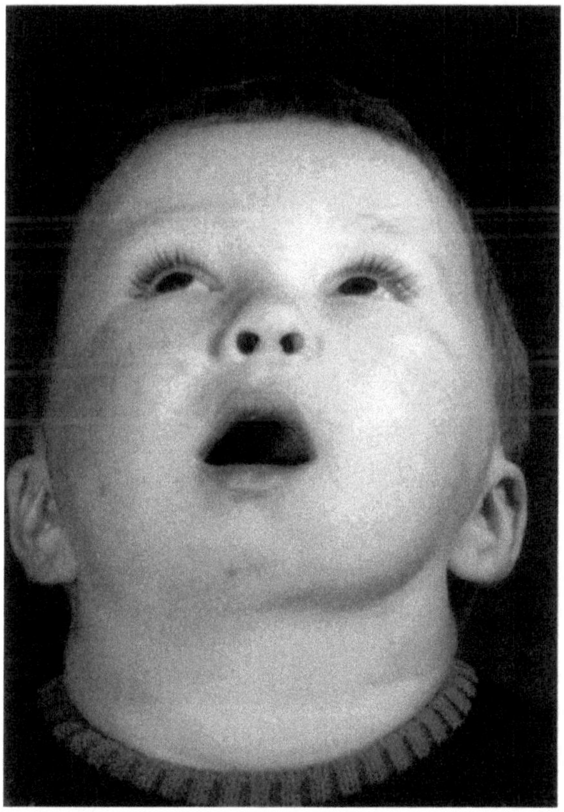

C

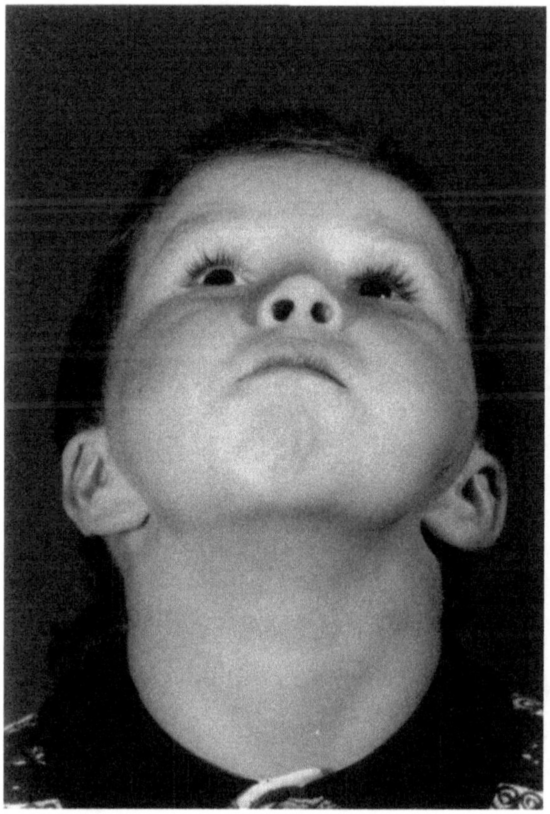

D

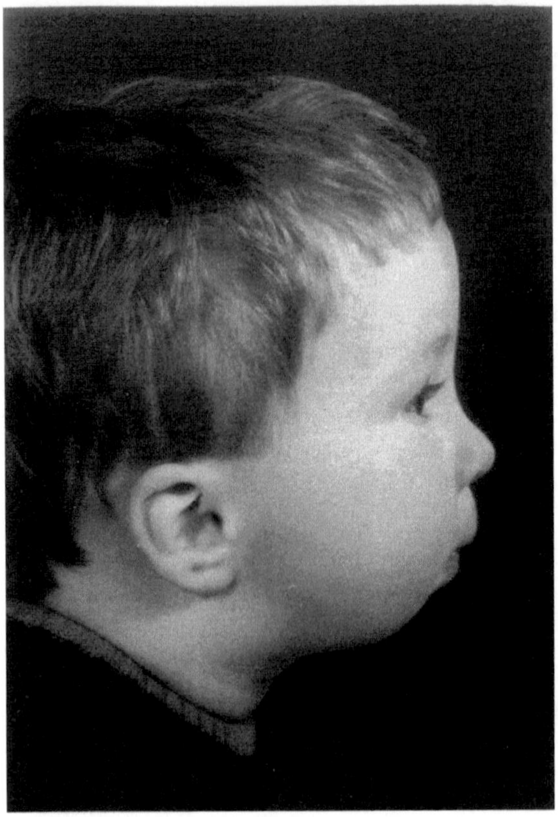

E

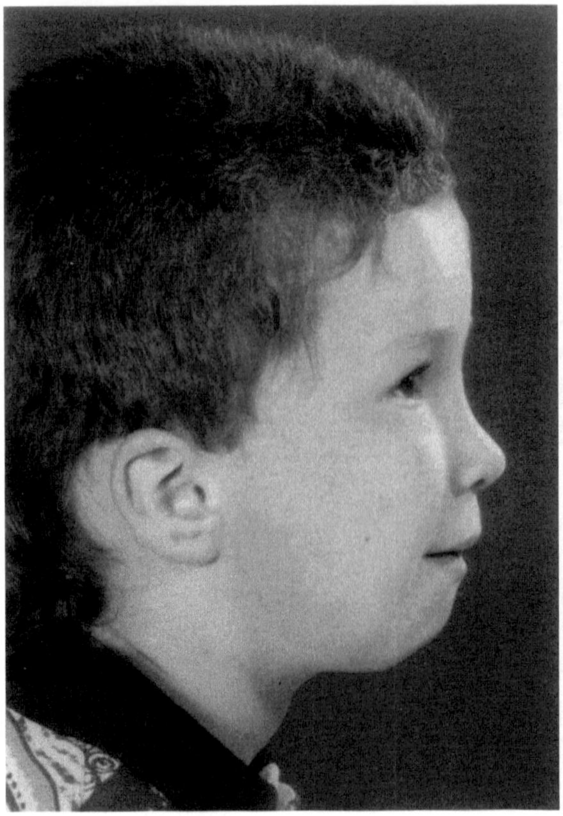

F

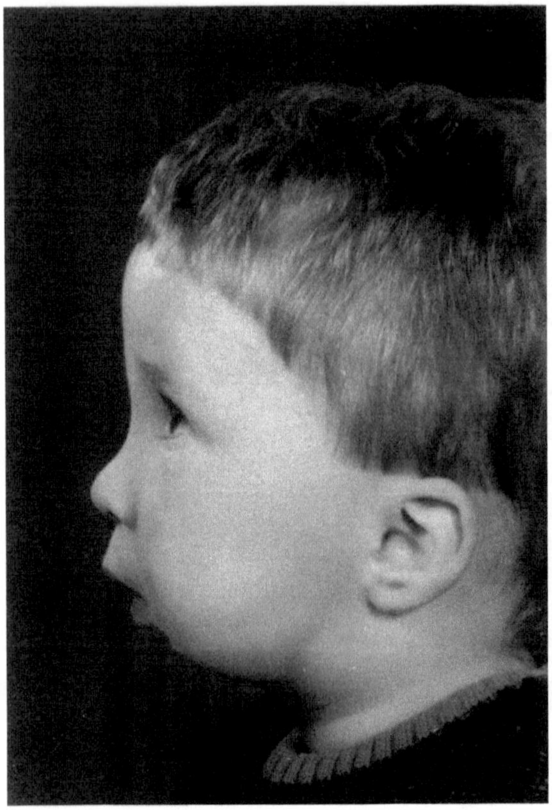

G

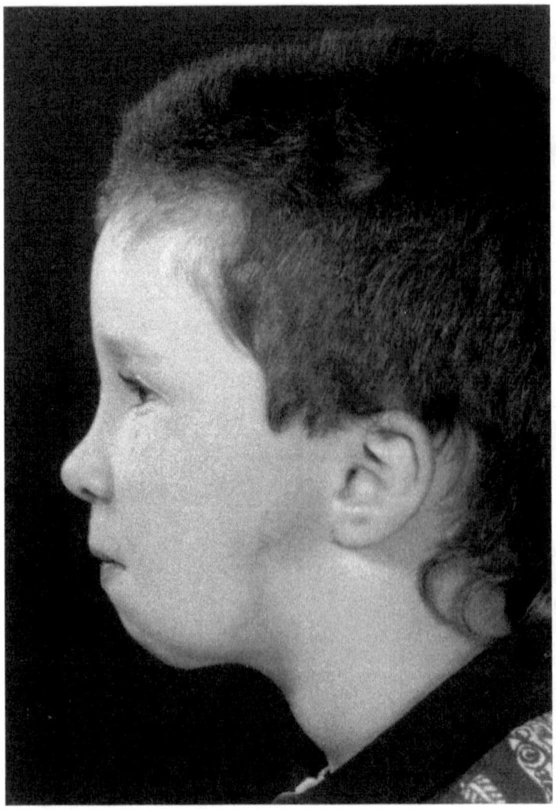

H

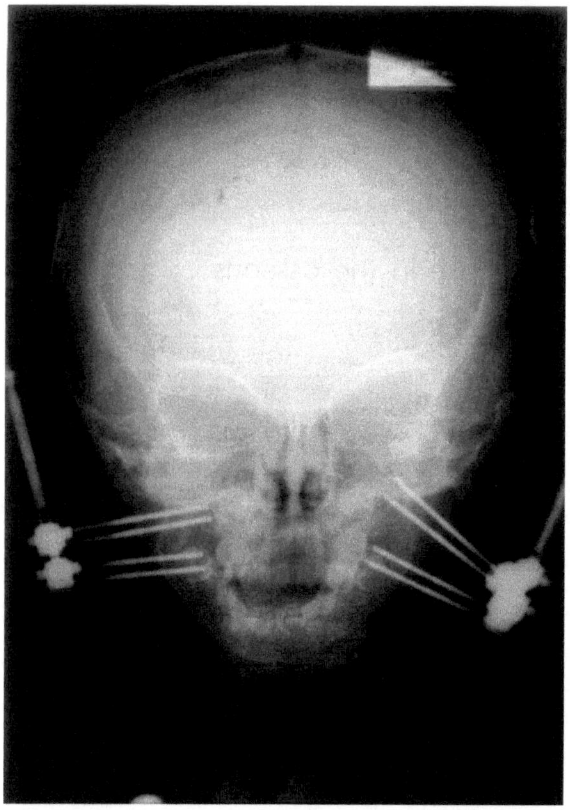

I

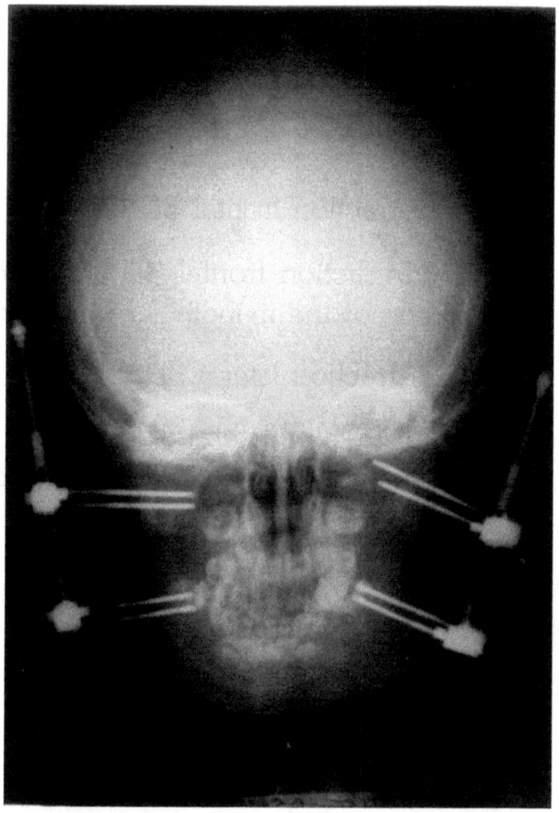

J

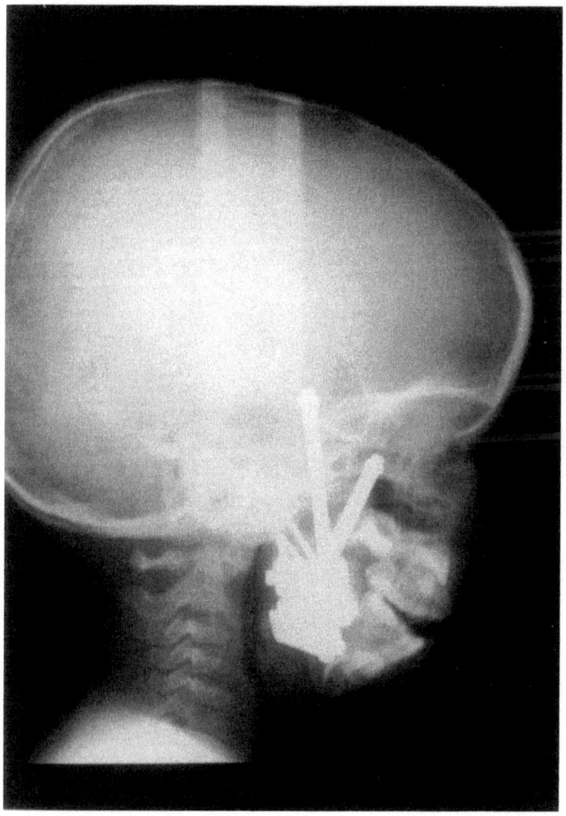

K

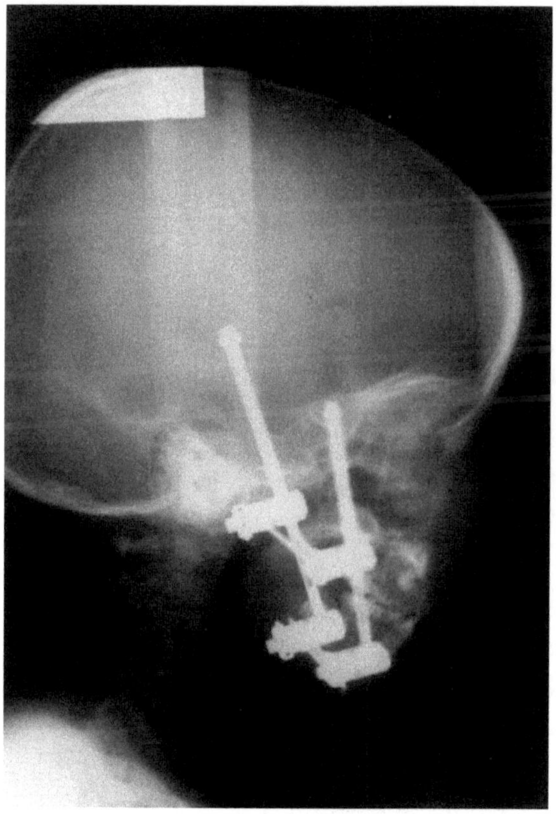

L

Figure 5.42. ***Case 14.*** *Continued*

(M) Predistraction frontal 3D CT scan.

(N) Postdistraction frontal 3D CT scan showing increase in the osseous volume of the mandibular rami and bodies.

(O) Predistraction lateral 3D CT scan.

(P) Postdistraction lateral 3D CT scan. Note the increased osseous dimensions of the mandibular rami and bodies.

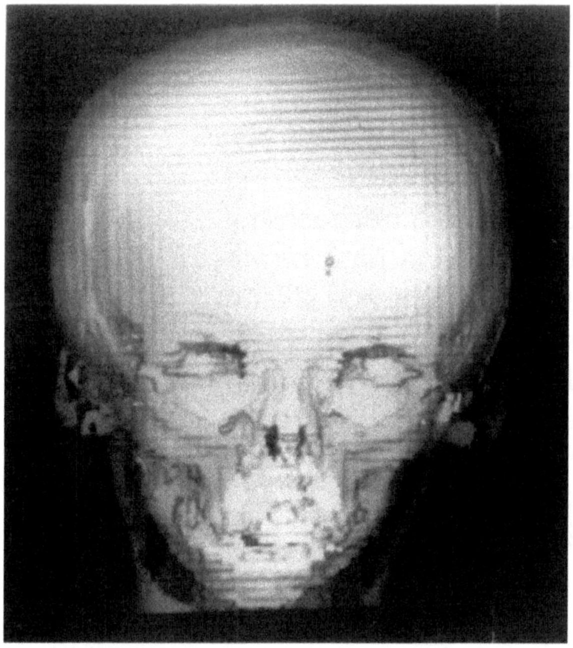

M

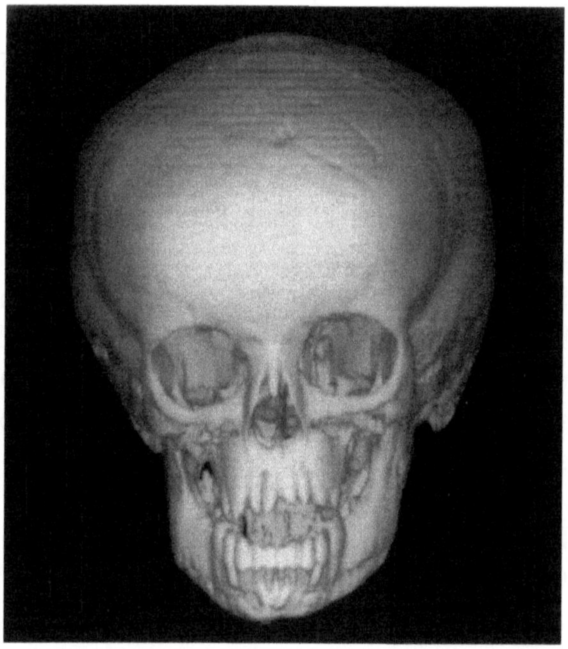

N

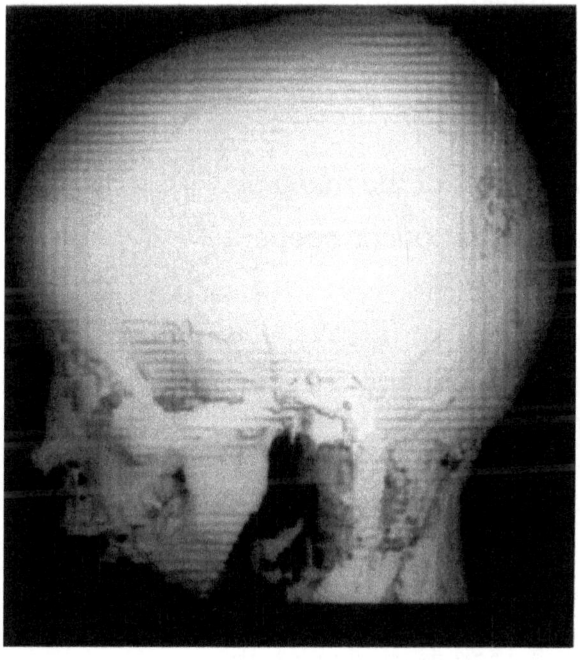

O

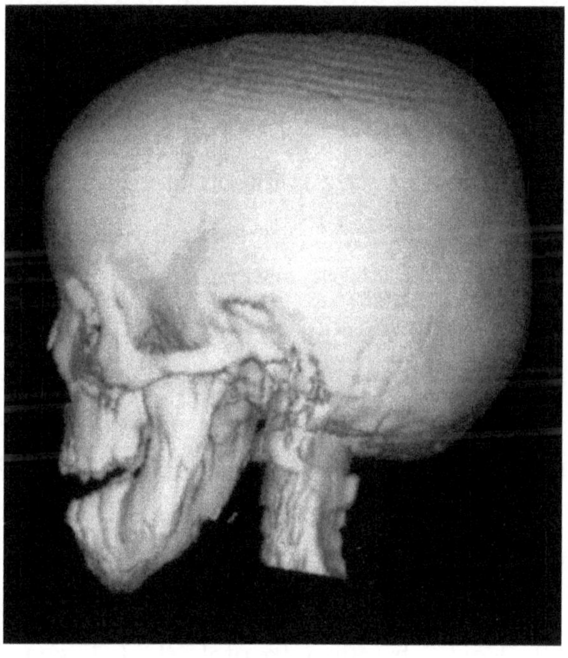

P

Case 15. J.B. was diagnosed with Treacher Collins syndrome manifest by involvement of the mandible, maxilla, and the zygomatic arches bilaterally; periorbital soft tissue hypoplasia; and clefts at the junction of the floor and the lateral wall of the orbits (Figure 5.43). The patient also demonstrated bilateral microtia (Meurman type II) and a cleft of the secondary palate. Prior to mandibular distraction he had required a tracheotomy. insertion of a gastrostomy tube and repair of a cleft of the hard palate. Bilateral mandibular distraction was completed (27 mm right and 27 mm left), and the soft palate was repaired at the time of device removal. At 36 months follow-up, significant sagittal thrust of the mandible was demonstrated and the tracheotomy tube had been removed. Periorbital reconstruction is planned.

Figure 5.43. Case 15. A four-year-old male with severe Treacher Collins who underwent bilateral mandibular distraction (right, 27 mm; left, 27 mm).

(A) Preoperative frontal view. The tracheotomy had been performed in the neonatal period.

(B) Postoperative frontal view 4 months after completion of distraction. The tracheotomy has been decannulated. Note the increase in the lower third of the face.

(C) Preoperative right profile.

(D) Postoperative right profile. Note the increased thrust of the mandible.

(E) Predistraction posteroanterior cephalogram (lack of patient cooperation). Note the osteotomy.

(F) Postdistraction posteroanterior cephalogram.

(G) Predistraction lateral cephalogram (lack of patient cooperation) showing the severe micrognathia and anterior open bite.

(H) Postdistraction lateral cephalogram showing the closure of the anterior bite and increase in the sagittal projection of the mandible.

(I) Predistraction frontal 3D CT scan showing the micrognathia and the orbitozygomatic stigmata of the Treacher Collins syndrome.

(J) Postdistraction frontal 3D CT scan. Note the increased size of the mandible.

(K) Predistraction lateral 3D CT scan showing the hypoplastic mandible and antegonial notching.

(L) Postdistraction lateral 3D CT scan showing the increase in the dimensions of the body and ramus of the mandible.

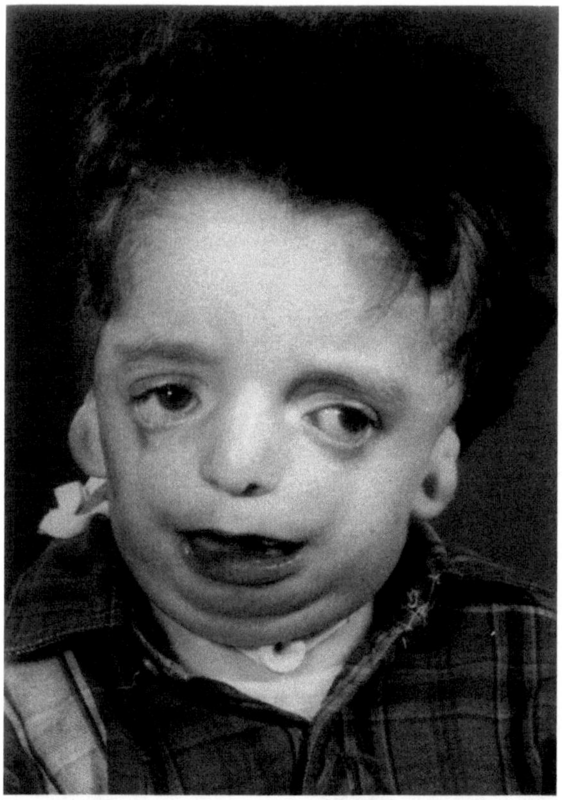

A

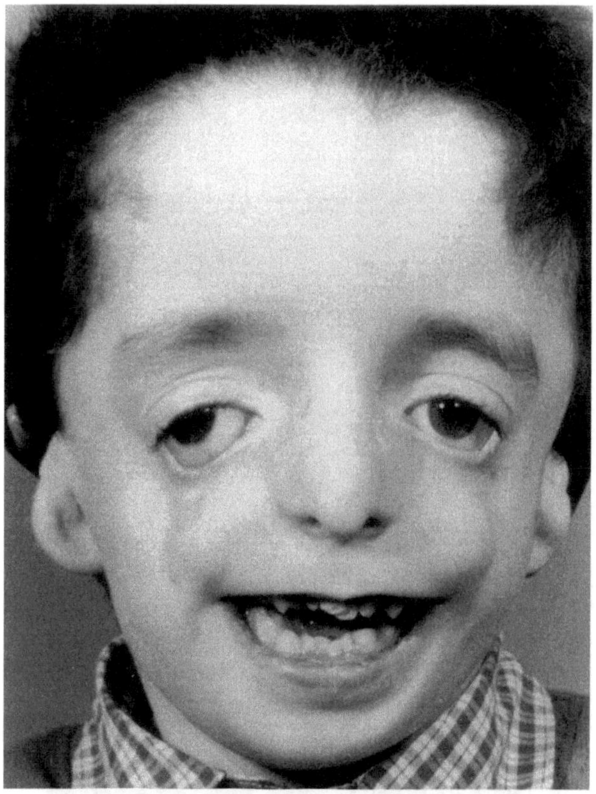

B

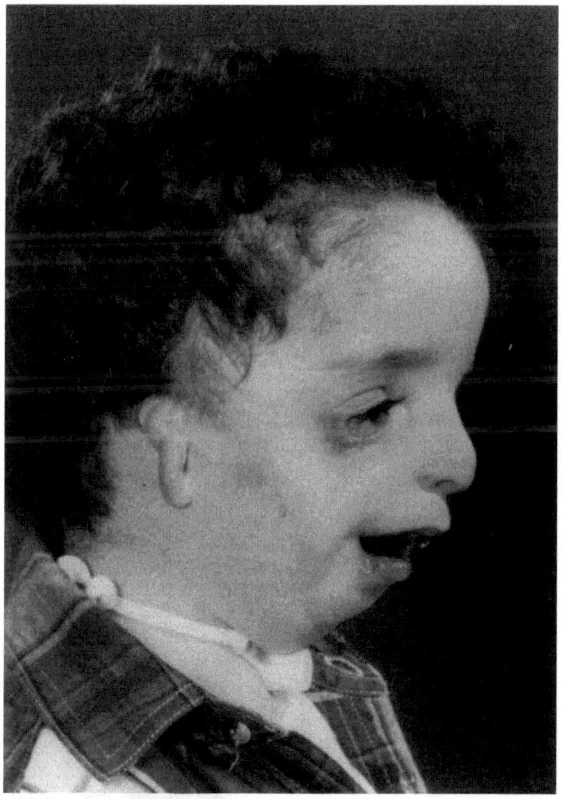

C

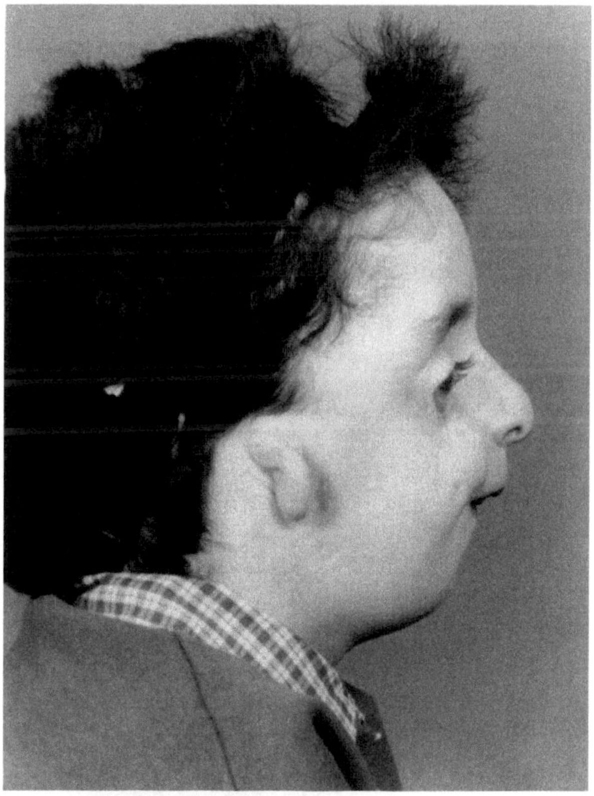

D

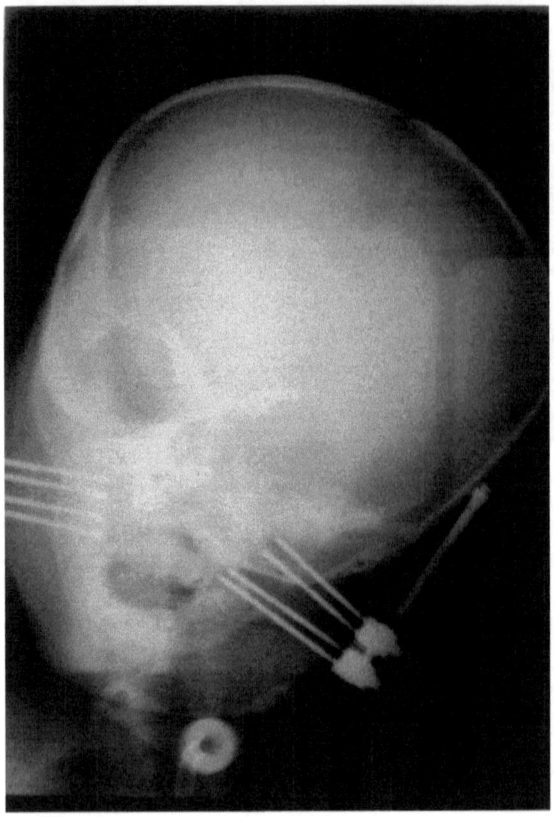

E

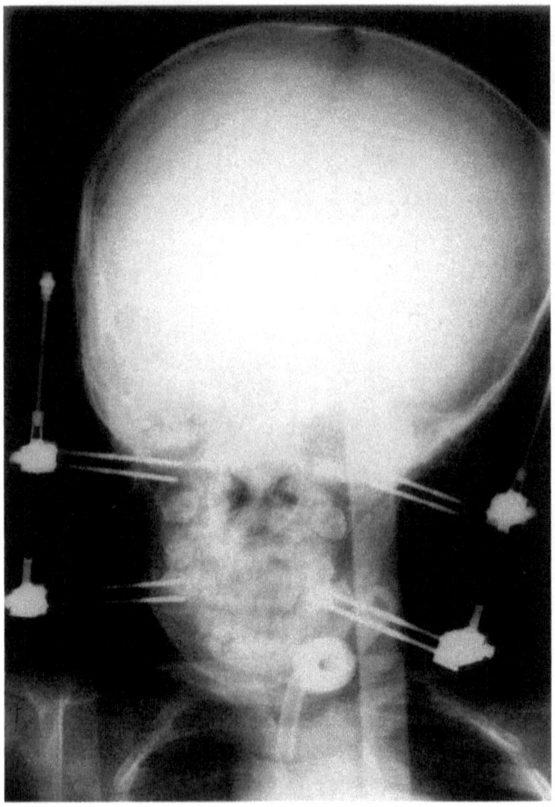

F

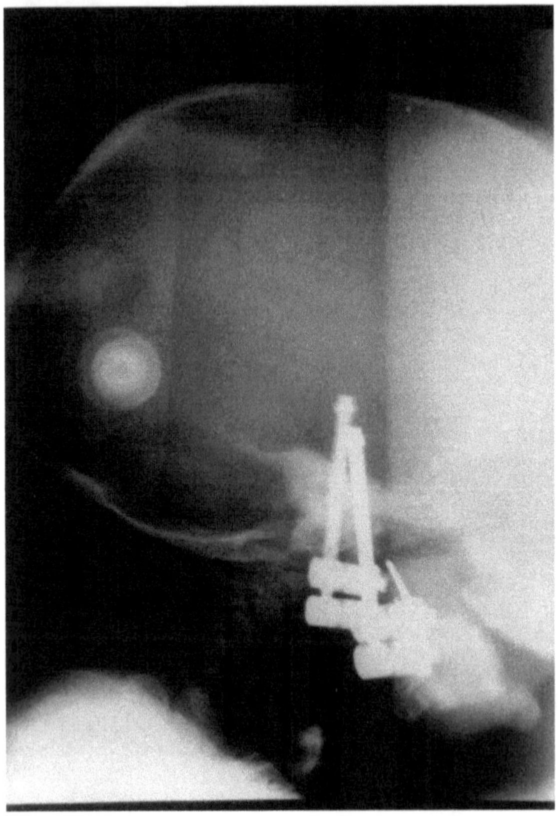

G

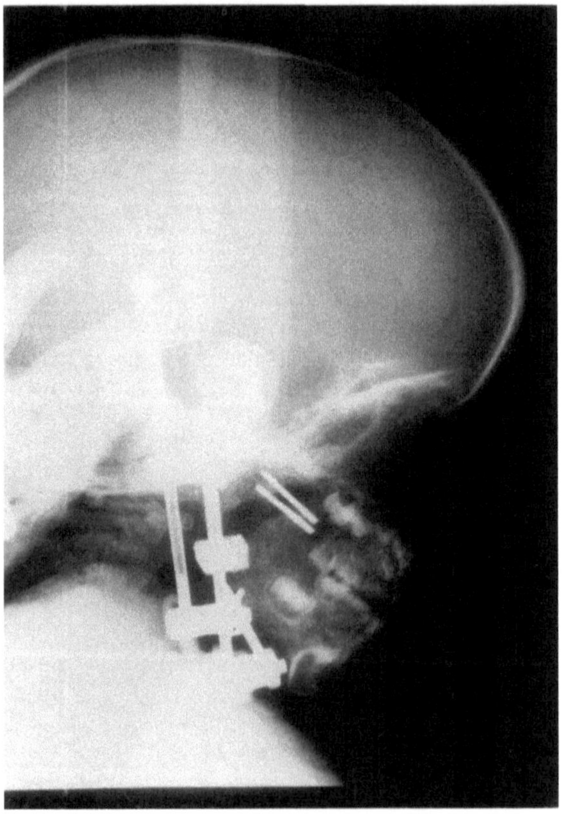

H

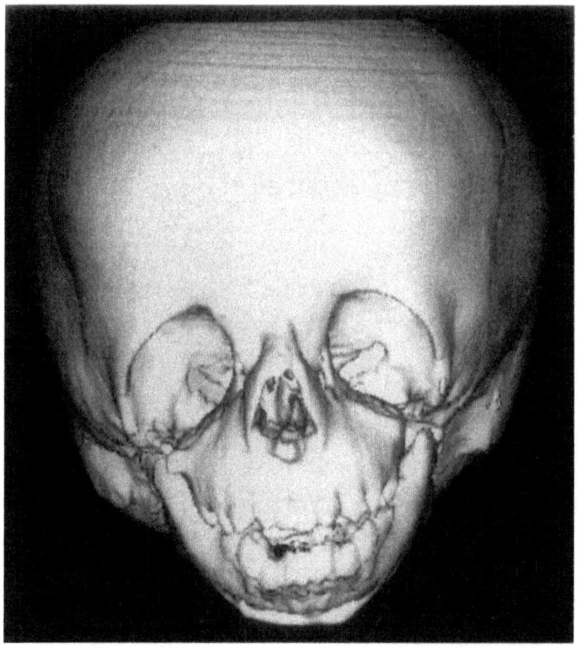

I

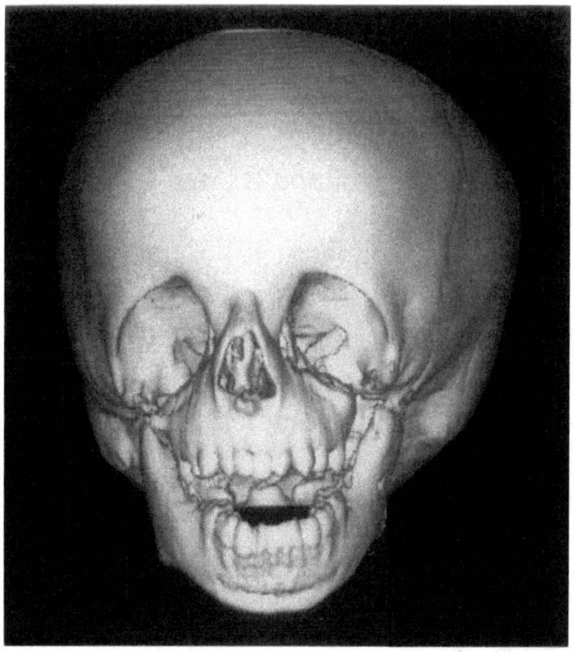

J

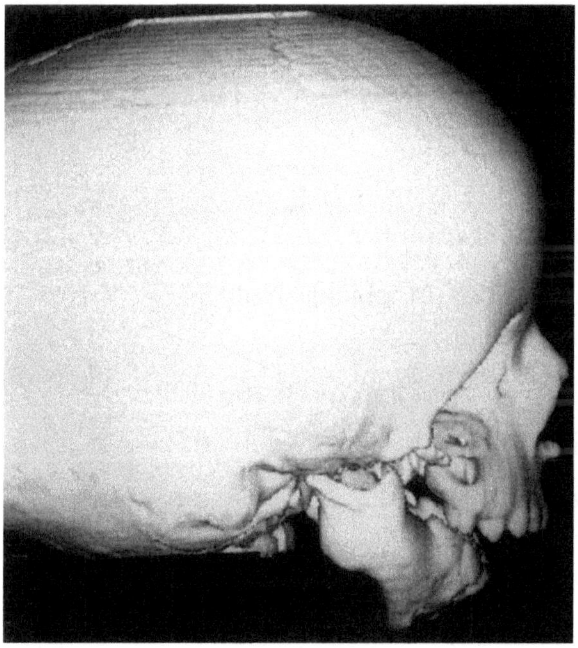

K

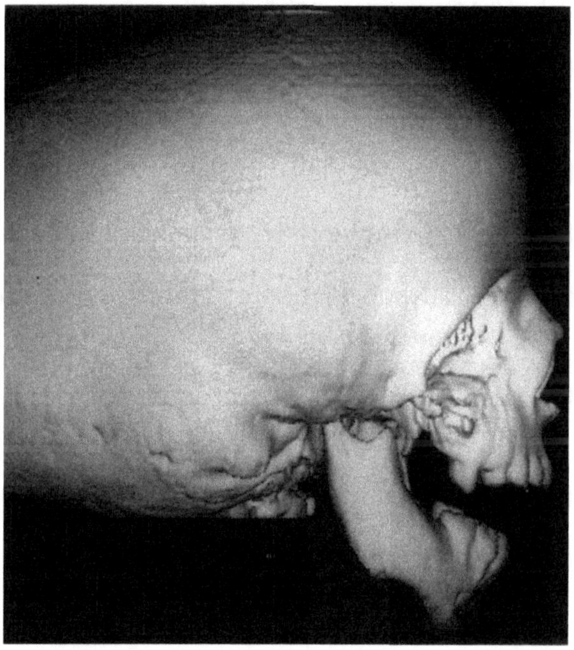

L

Case 16. M.R. was a 21-year-old male with severe bilateral craniofacial microsomia characterized by micrognathia, microgenia, and bilateral ear deformity. An otoplasty was completed at age 6, but no mandibular surgery was done (Figure 5.44). He underwent bilateral mandibular distraction (21 mm right and 21 mm left) resulting in multidimensional expansion of the lower face.

Figure 5.44. Case 16. Twenty-one-year-old male with severe bilateral craniofacial microsomia (right, Pruzansky IIa; left, Pruzansky IIa) who underwent bilateral mandibular distraction (right, 21 mm; left, 21 mm).

(A) Preoperative frontal view. Note the ear anomalies and severe hypoplasia of the chin and lower third of the face.

(B) Postoperative frontal view 8 months after completion of distraction.

(C) Preoperative submental view.

(D) Postoperative submental view.

(E) Preoperative right profile.

(F) Postoperative right profile. Note the increased sagittal thrust of the chin and mandible.

(G) Preoperative left profile.

(H) Postoperative left profile. Note the satisfactory scar.

(I) Predistraction posteroanterior cephalogram (devices in place). Note the osteotomies.

(J) Postdistraction posteroanterior cephalogram. The orientation of the right device was deliberately changed during distraction.

(K) Predistraction lateral cephalogram (horizontal vector).

(L) Postdistraction lateral cephalogram.

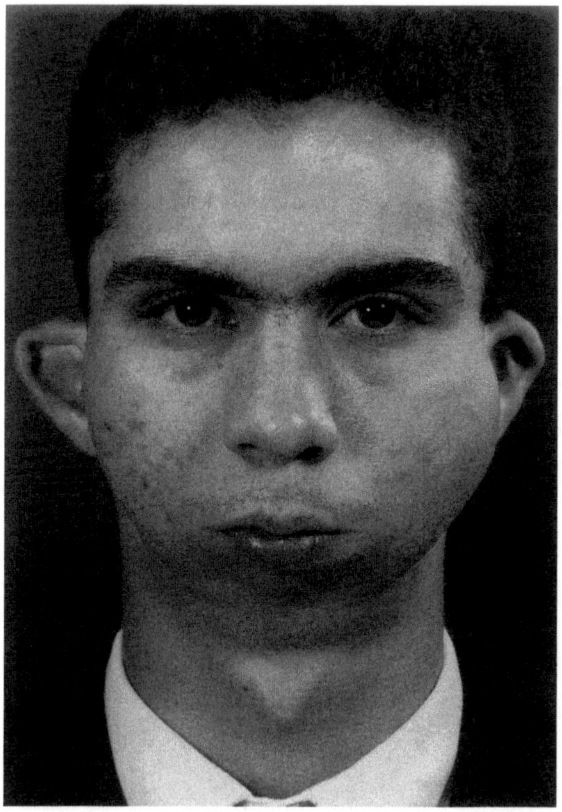

A

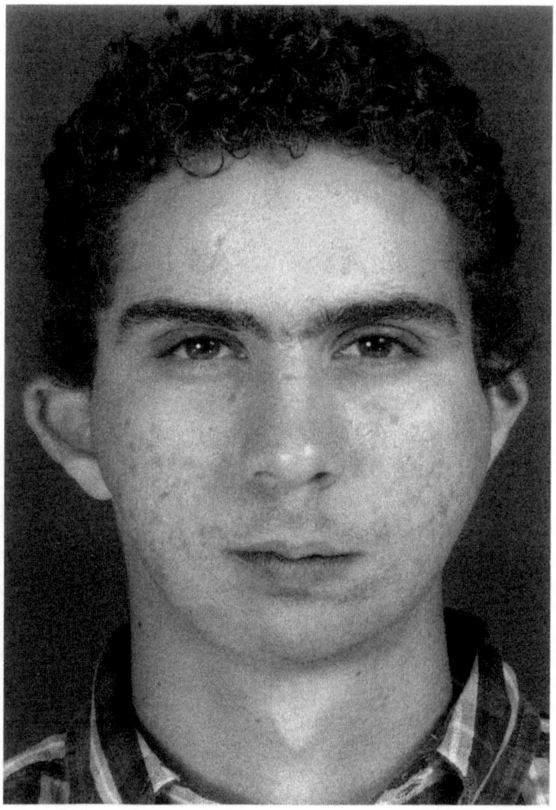

B

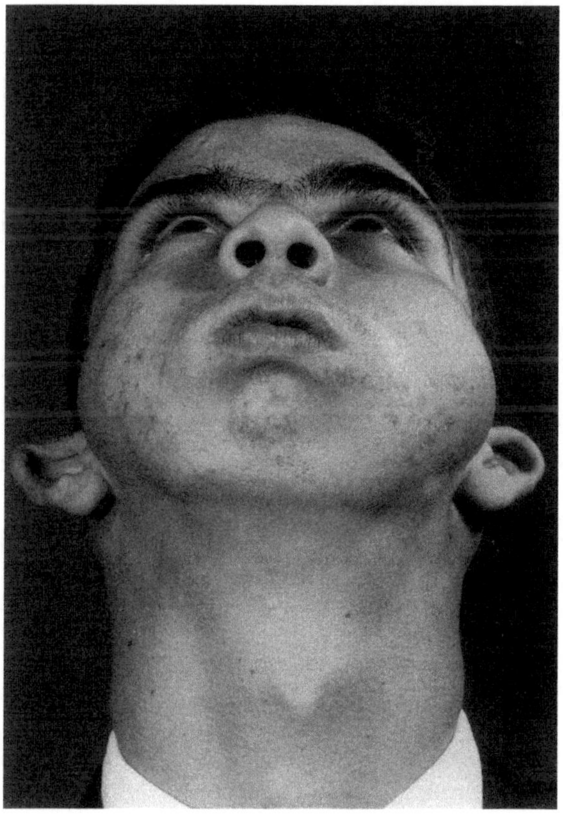

C

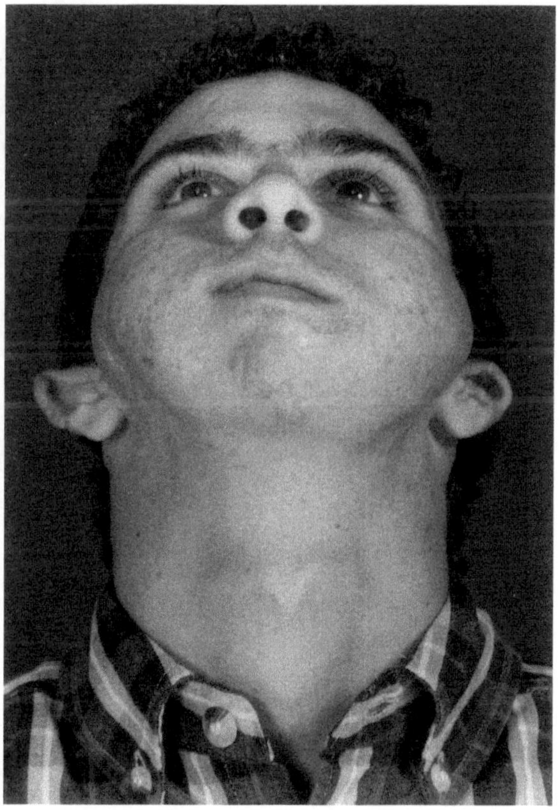

D

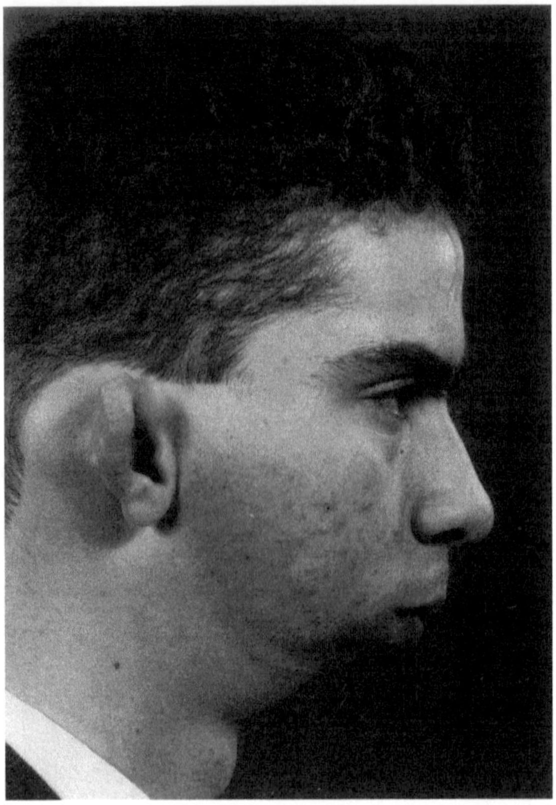

E

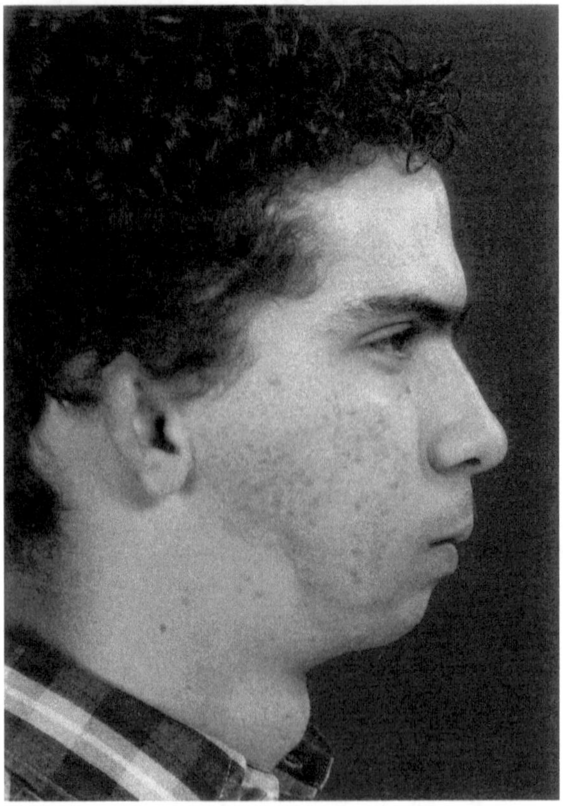

F

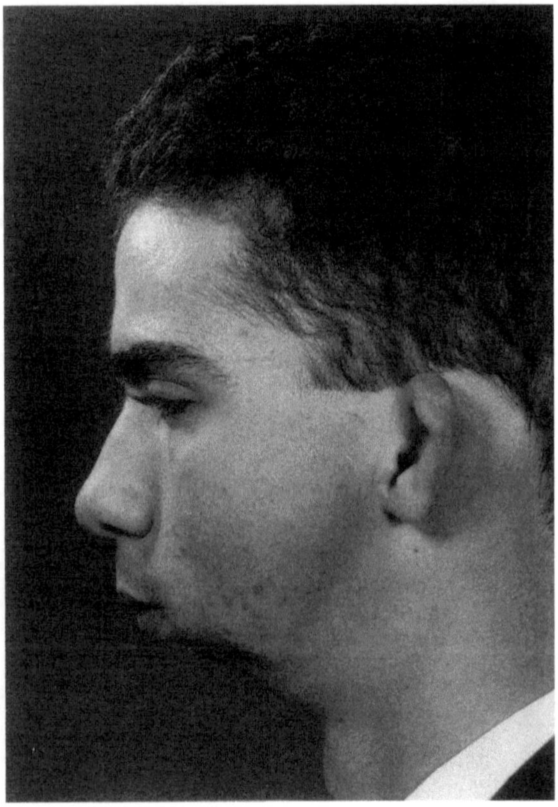

G

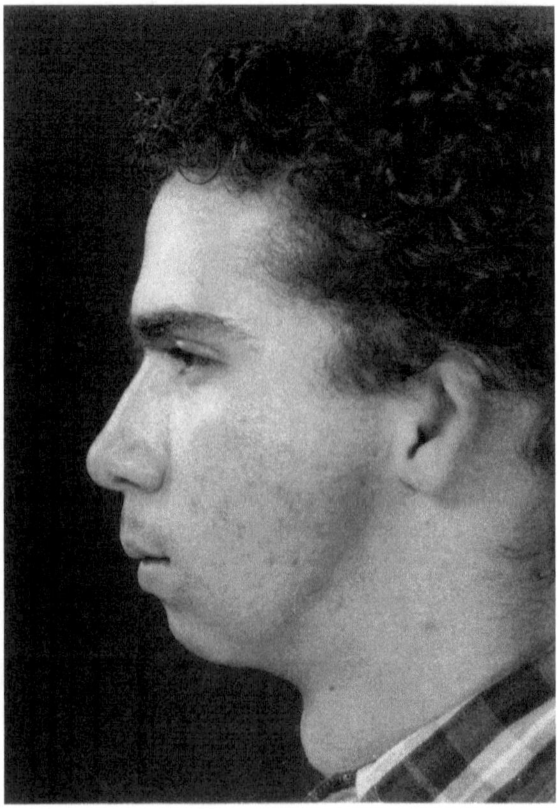

H

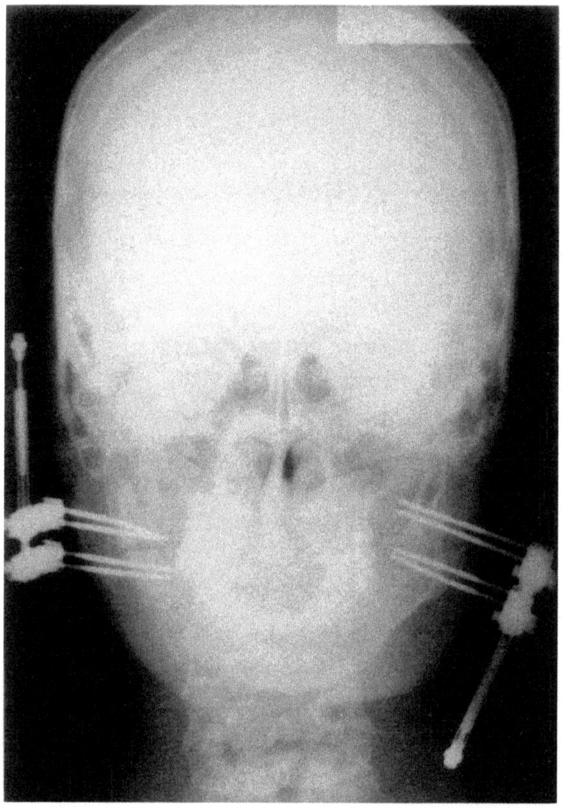

I

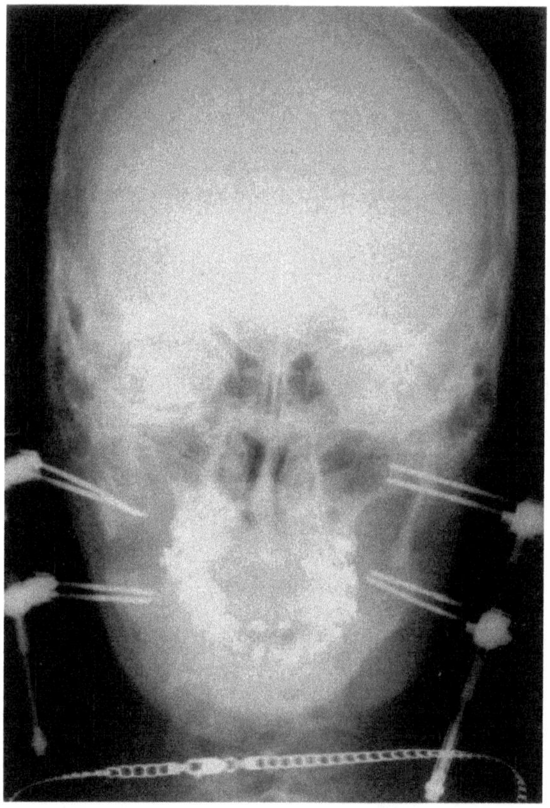

J

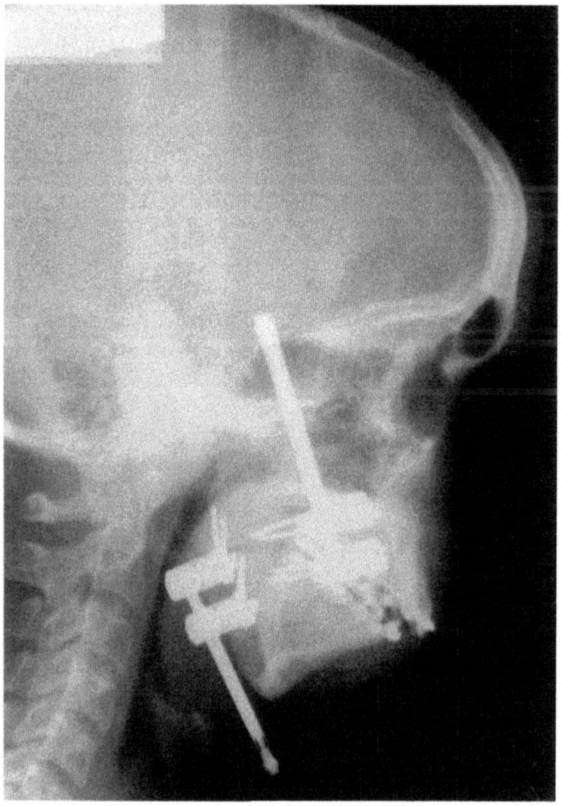

K

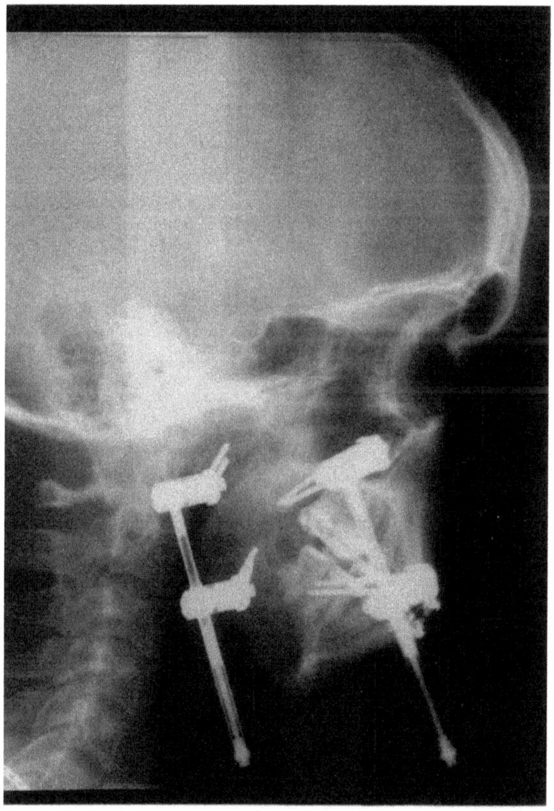

L

Figure 5.44. Case 16. *Continued*

(M) Predistraction frontal 3D CT scan.

(N) Postdistraction frontal 3D CT scan.

(O) Predistraction lateral 3D CT scan.

(P) Postdistraction lateral 3D CT scan. There has been straightening of the gonial angle and marked improvement in the occlusion.

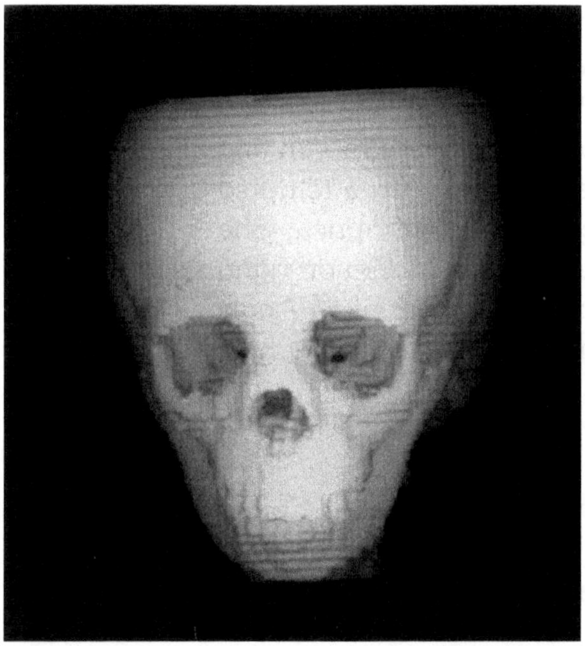

M

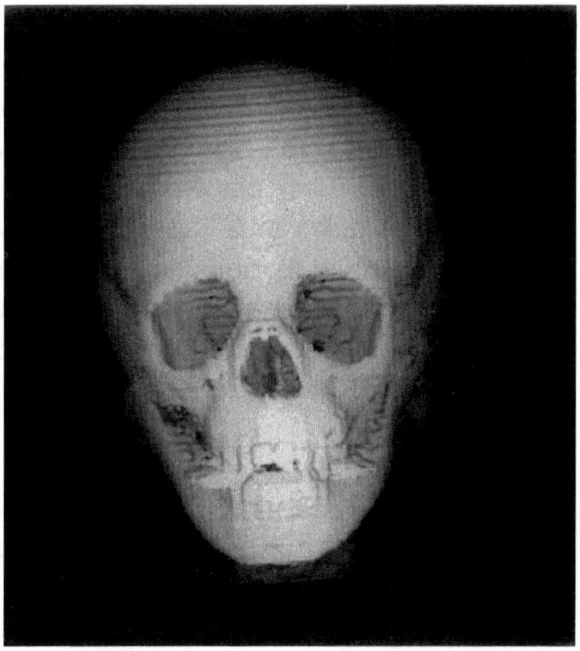

N

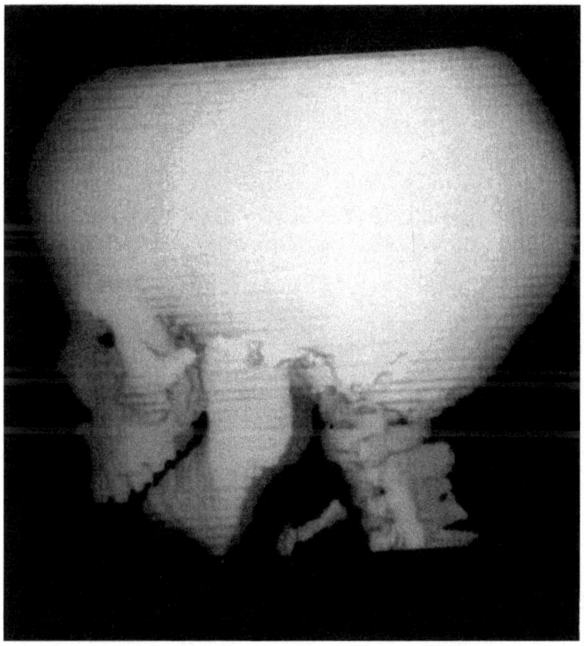

O

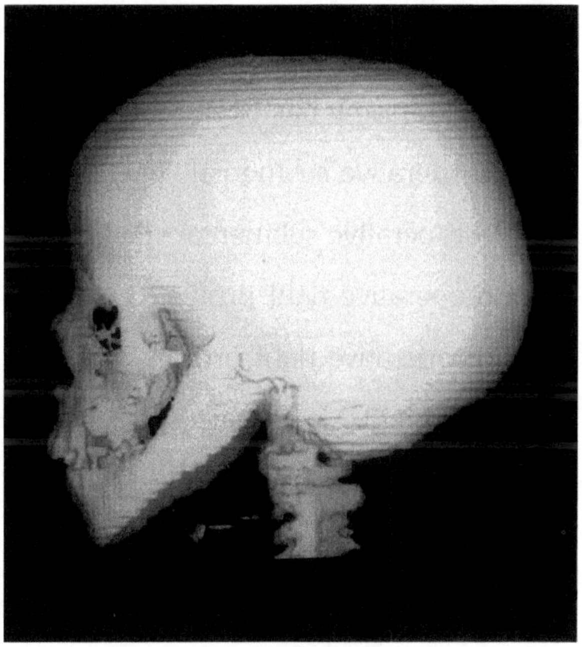

P

Case 17. D.P. was a 3-year-old girl with Treacher Collins syndrome characterized by bilateral orbitozygomatic deficiencies, eyelid colobomata, severe micrognathia (left—Pruzansky I, right—Pruzansky IIa), and bilateral microtia (Figure 5.45). She required a tracheotomy at age one month and a gastrostomy tube placement at 3 months of age. An attempted decannulation failed at 2 years of age because of persistent apnea. She underwent bilateral mandibular distraction (17 mm on left, 15 mm on right) with significant increase in the sagittal thrust and development of an Angle class III occlusion. She was subsequently decannulated (tracheal) 2 months after removal of the distraction device.

Figure 5.45. Case 17. A three-year-old female with Treacher Collins syndrome (right, Pruzansky IIa; left, Pruzansky I) who underwent bilateral mandibular distraction (right, 15 mm; left, 17 mm).

(A) Preoperative frontal view. Note the micrognathia, tracheotomy, and the auricular and orbitozygomatic stigmata of Treacher Collins syndrome.

(B) Postoperative frontal view 14 months after completion of distraction. Note the increased volume of the lower third of the face. The tracheostomy has been removed.

(C) Preoperative submental view.

(D) Postoperative submental view.

(E) Preoperative right profile.

(F) Postoperative right profile.

(G) Preoperative left profile.

(H) Postoperative left profile.

(I) Predistraction posteroanterior cephalogram.

(J) Postdistraction posteroanterior cephalogram.

(K) Predistraction lateral cephalogram (horizontal vector).

(L) Postdistraction lateral cephalogram. Note the increased sagittal thrust of the mandible.

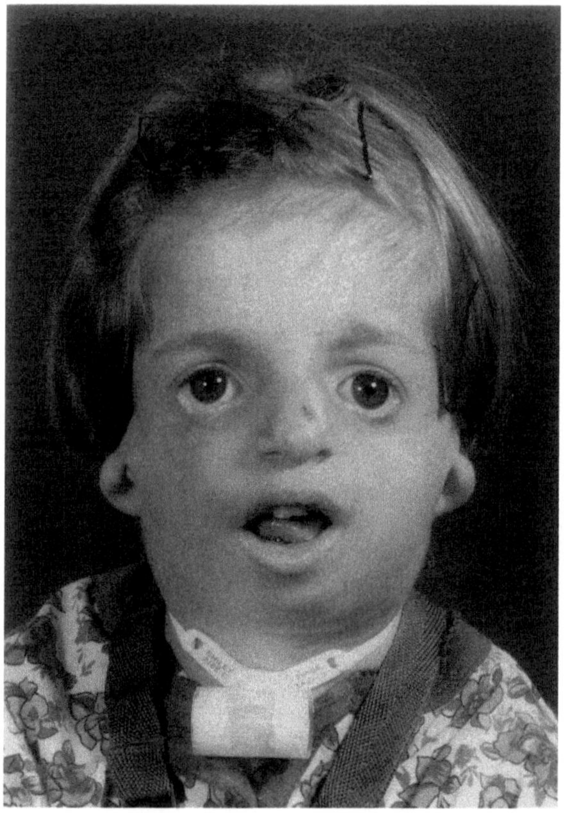

A

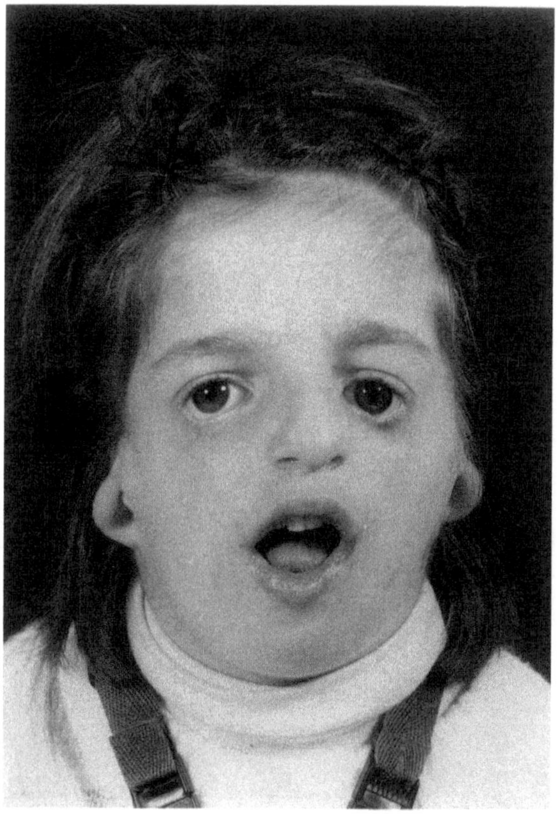

B

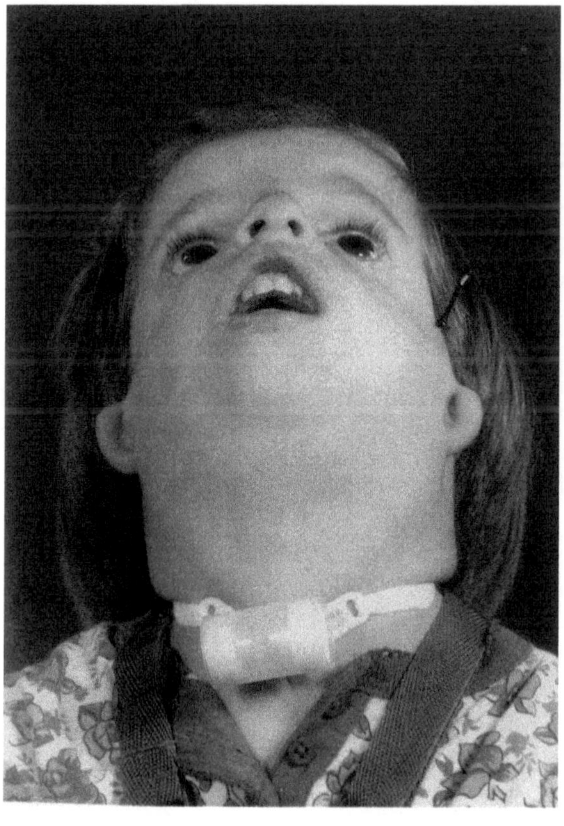

C

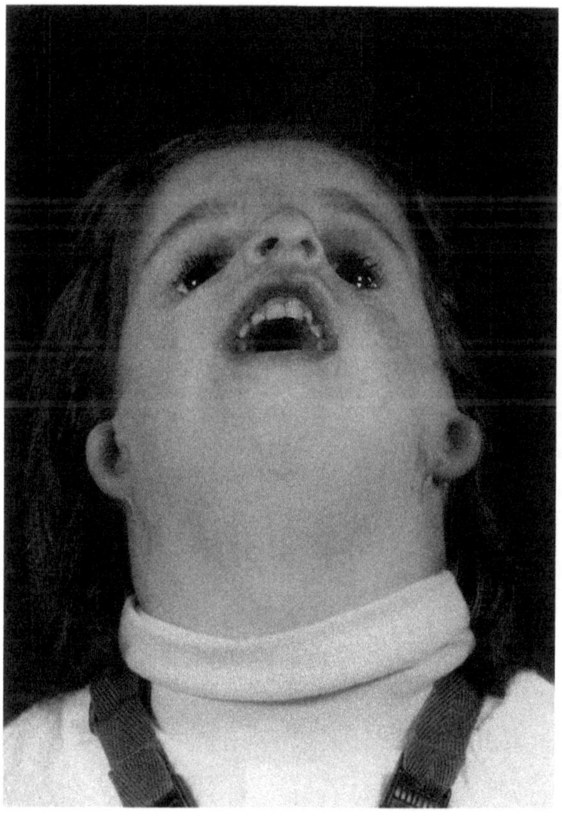

D

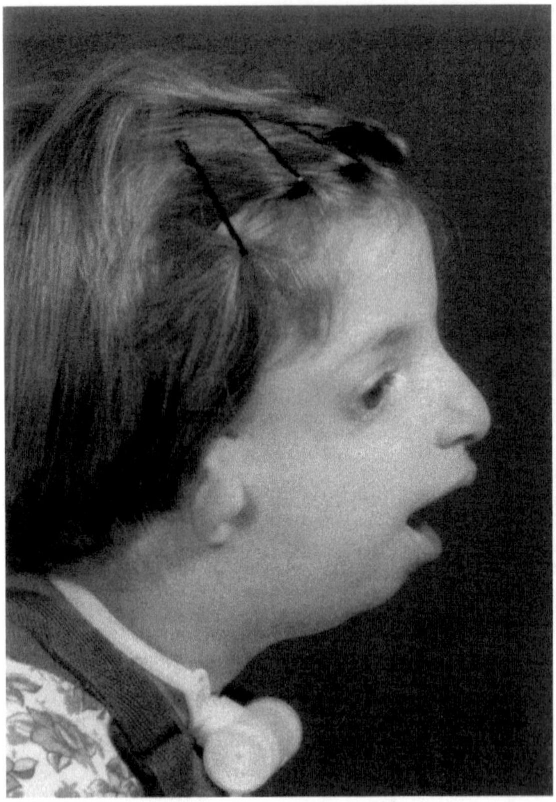

E

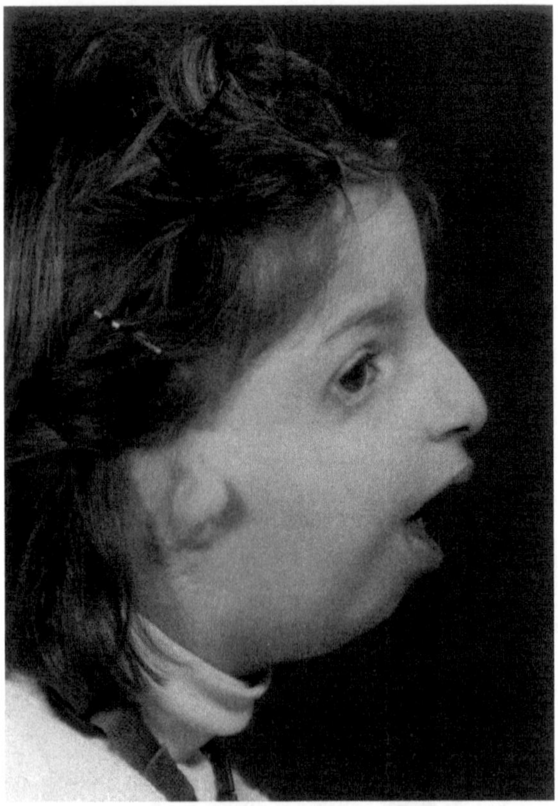

F

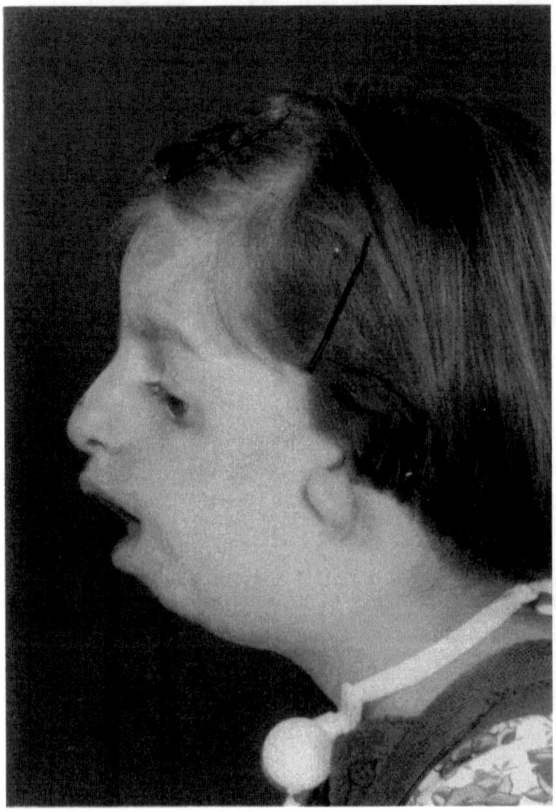

G

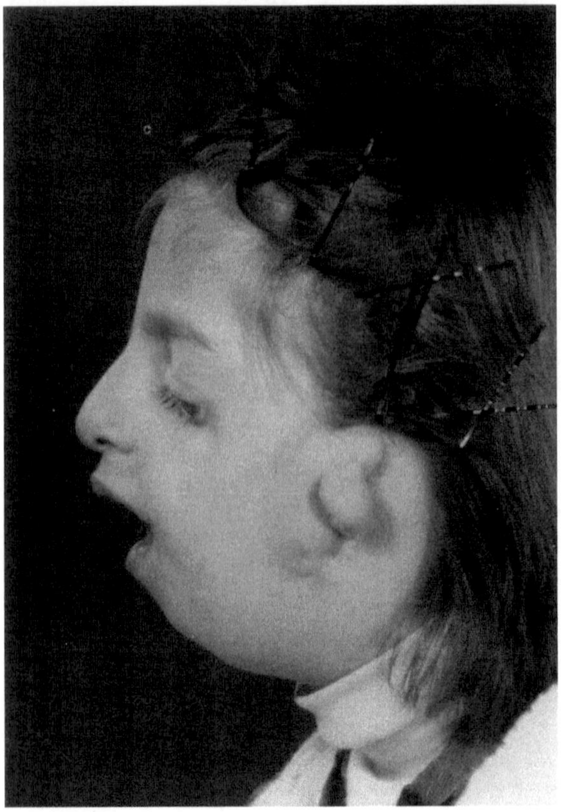

H

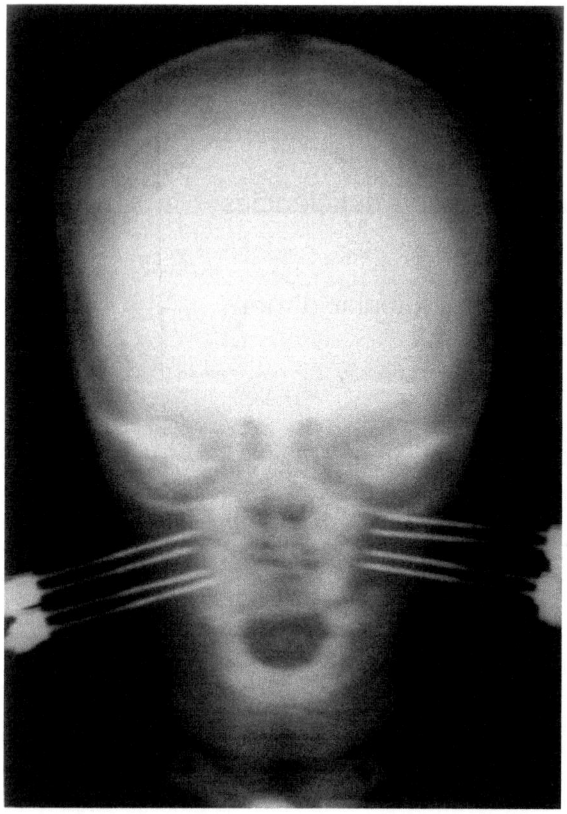

I

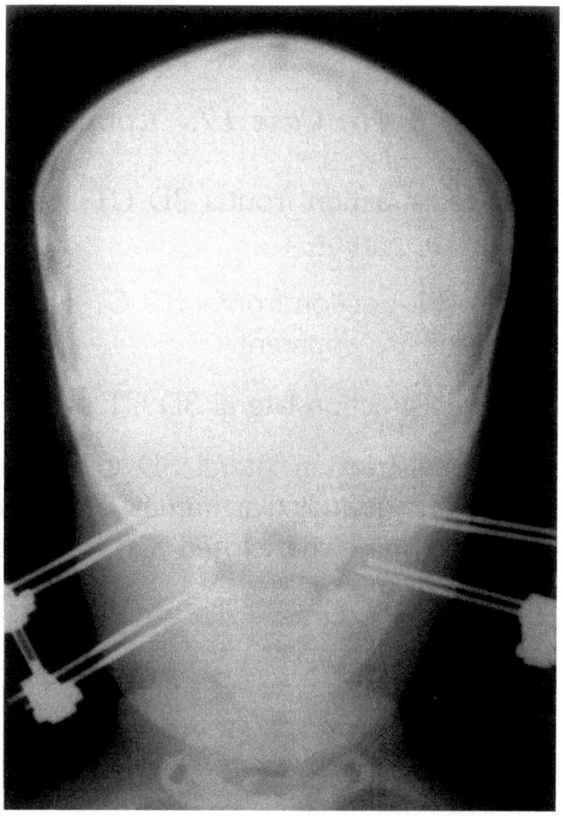

J

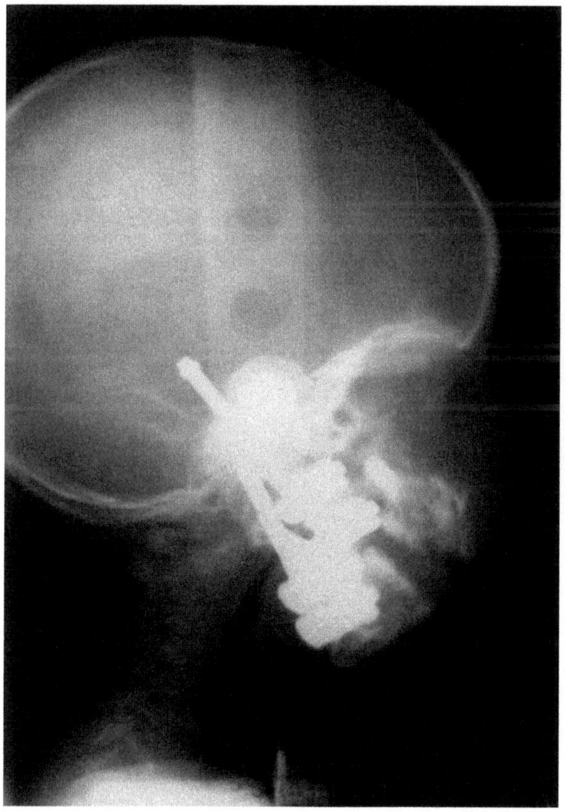

K

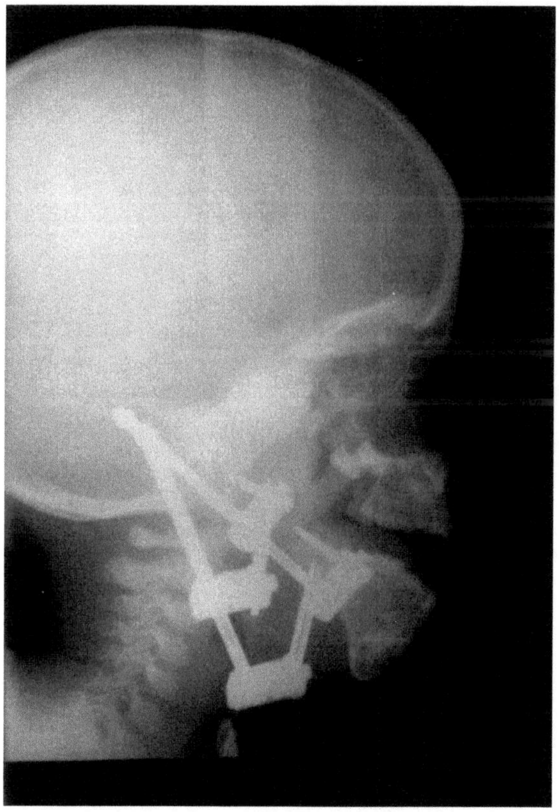

L

Figure 5.45. ***Case 17.*** *Continued*

(M) Predistraction frontal 3D CT scan. The orbitozygomatic deficiencies are apparent.

(N) Postdistraction frontal 3D CT scan. The increased mandibular dimensions are apparent.

(O) Predistraction lateral 3D CT scan.

(P) Postdistraction lateral 3D CT scan. Note the increased dimensions of the mandibular ramus and body. The anterior open bite has been somewhat closed and there is counterclockwise rotation of the mandible.

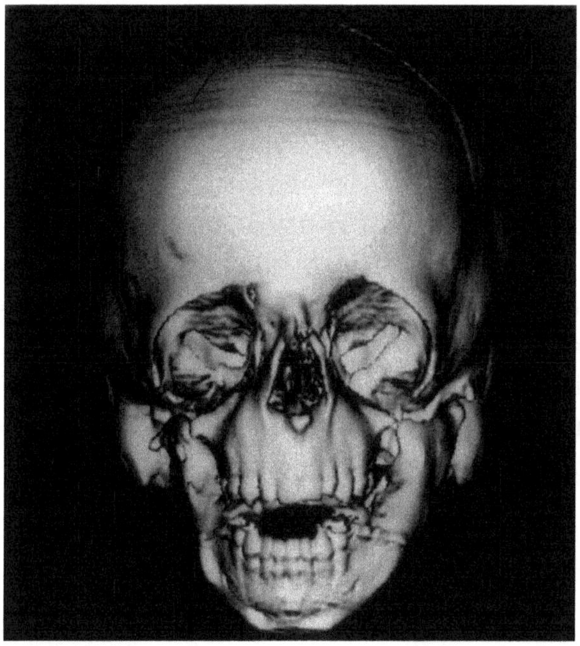

M

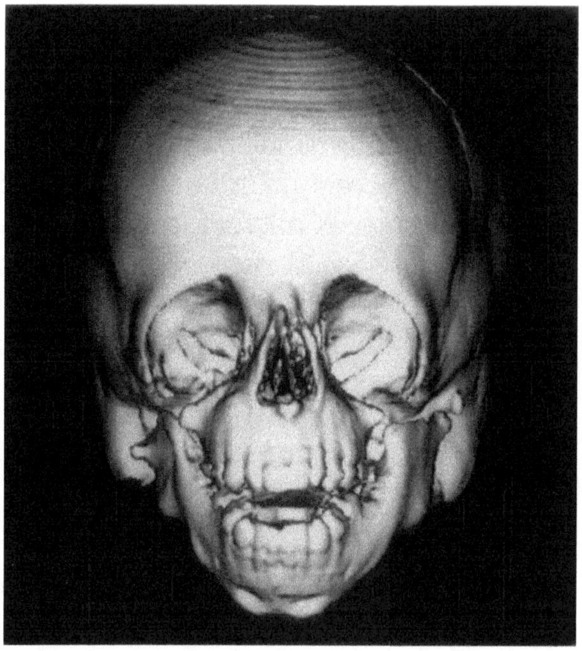

N

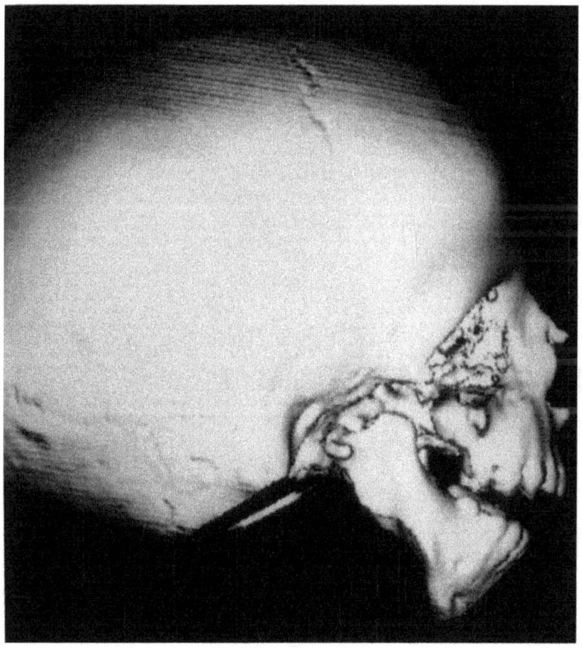

O

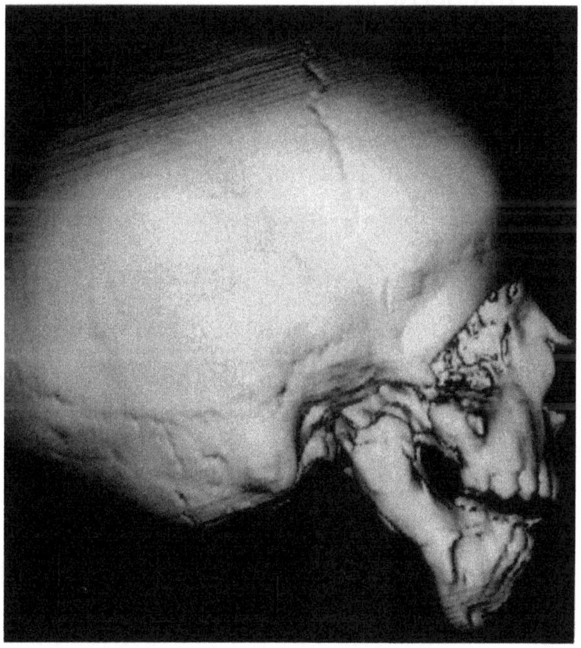

P

Case 18. M.A. was born with severe mandibular deficiency associated with clefting of his chin and ears (Figure 5.46). In the neonatal period tracheotomy and gastrotomy were emergently performed. He also had bilateral temporomandibular ankylosis. Because of his age, limited donor sites and the severity of his deformity, traditional mandibular reconstructive techniques such as microvascular fibular and iliac flaps were not possible. Accordingly, he underwent bilateral mandibular distraction (29 mm right and 27 mm left) at age 7 with considerable expansion of his mandibular complex. At the time of surgery the expansion devices were placed on his hypoplastic and retromaxillary mandible with difficulty. He subsequently underwent microvascular free flap reconstruction with the addition of soft tissue to his submental area and augmentation of his expanded mandible with a fibular free-tissue transfer.

Figure 5.46. Case 18. A seven-year-old male with severe facial clefting, bilateral mandibular deficiencies, maxillomandibular ankylosis and ankyloglossia (trifurcated) who underwent bilateral mandibular distraction (right, 29 mm; left, 27 mm).

(A) Preoperative frontal view showing severe mandibular deficiency and a tracheostomy.

(B) Postoperative frontal view 41 months after completion of distraction. The tracheostomy remains in place. Note the increased fullness of the lower third of the face which had also been augmented with a microvascular free flap (fibular onlay). He has a functioning oral sphincter.

(C) Preoperative submental view showing clefting of the chin.

(D) Postoperative submental view.

(E) Preoperative right profile showing the lack of mandibular projection.

(F) Postoperative right profile showing increased mass in the lower third of the face.

(G) Preoperative left profile.

(H) Postoperative left profile.

(I) Predistraction posteroanterior cephalogram.

(J) Postdistraction posteroanterior cephalogram showing the emergence of the mandibular remnant.

(K) Predistraction lateral cephalogram. Note that the diminutive mandible is in a retromaxillary position.

(L) Postdistraction lateral cephalogram (before device removal) showing inferior and anterior movement of the mandible. There has been counterclockwise rotation of the long arm of the distraction device.

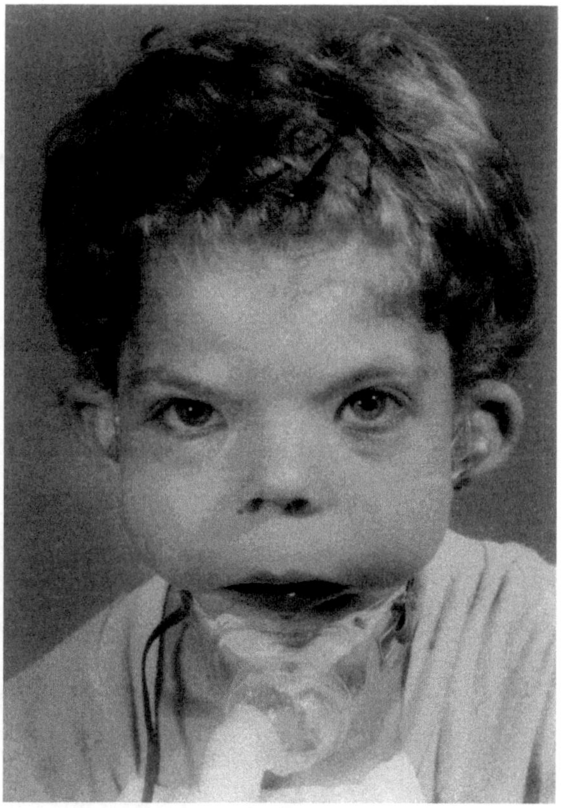

A

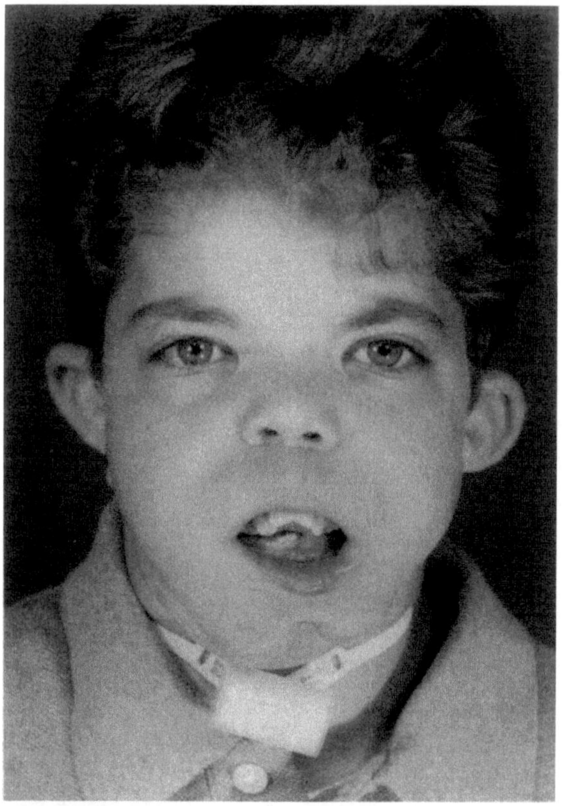

B

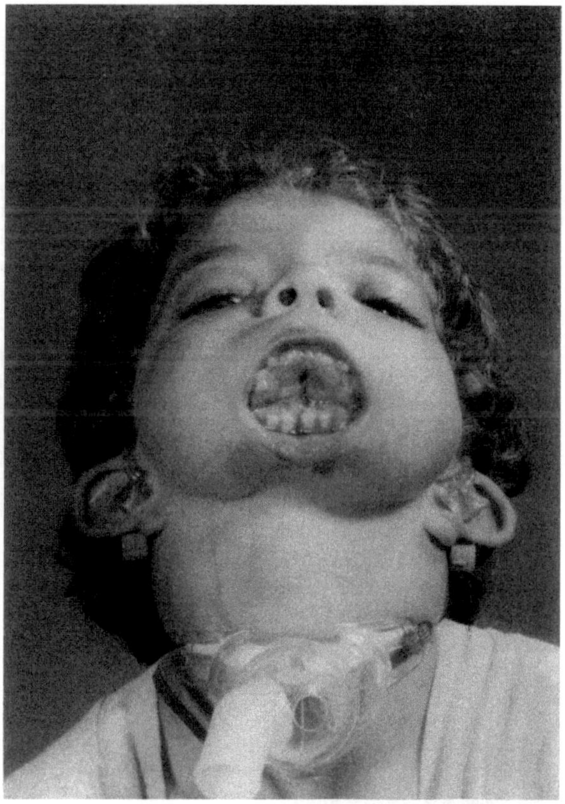

C

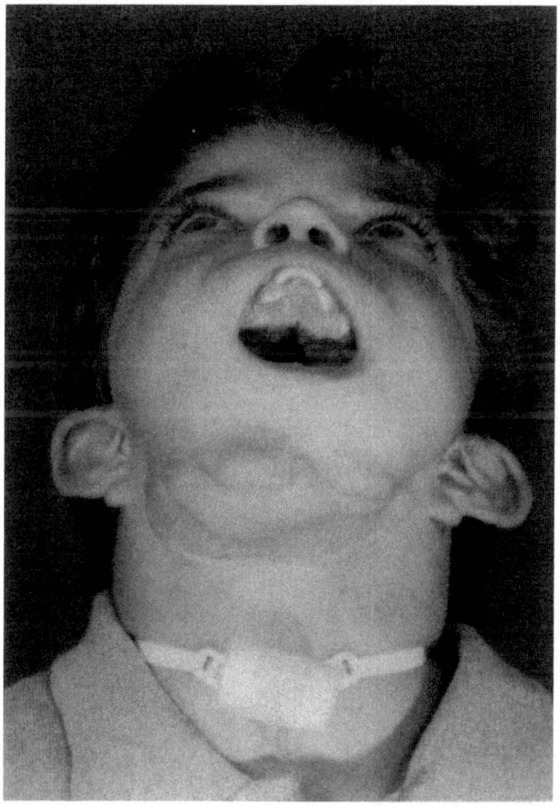

D

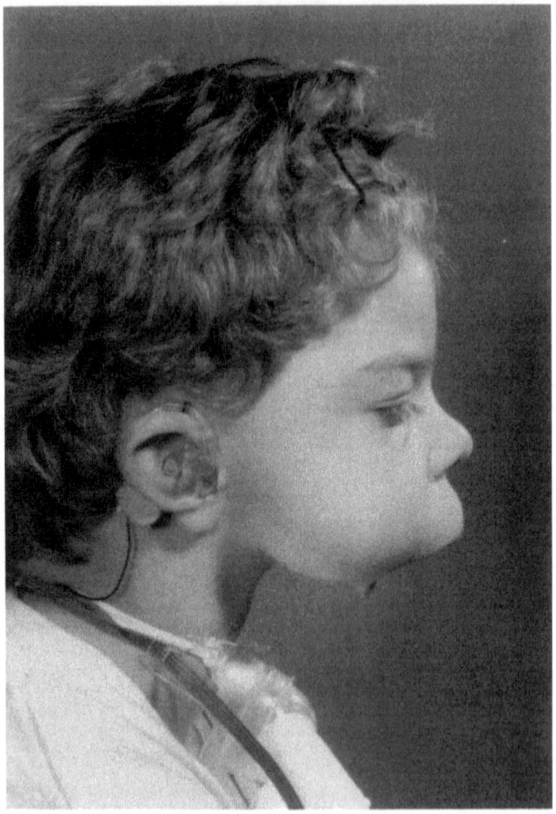

E

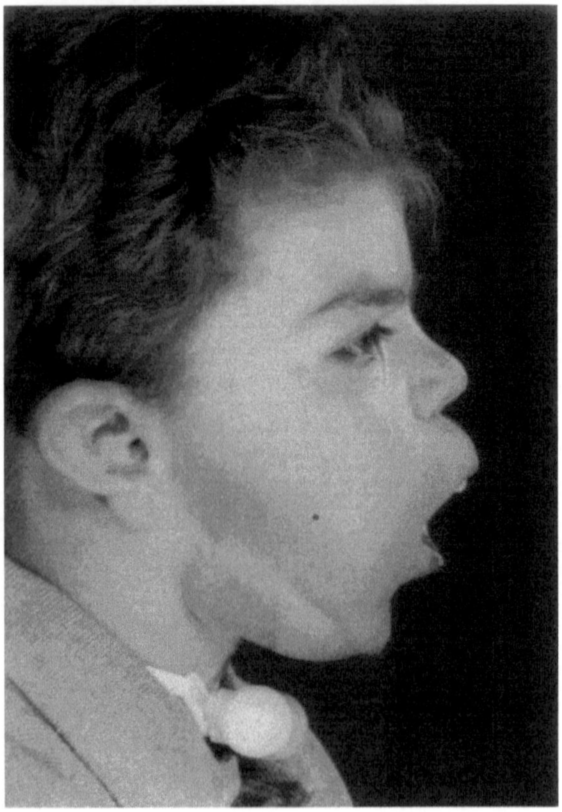

F

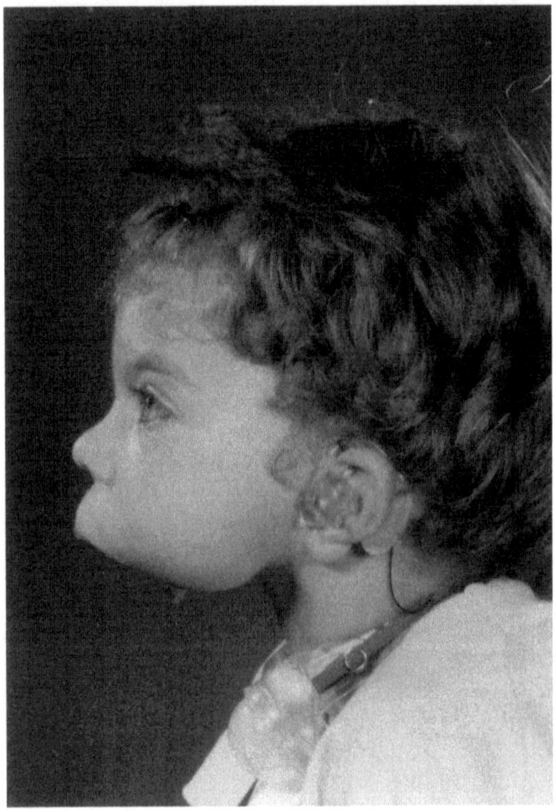

G

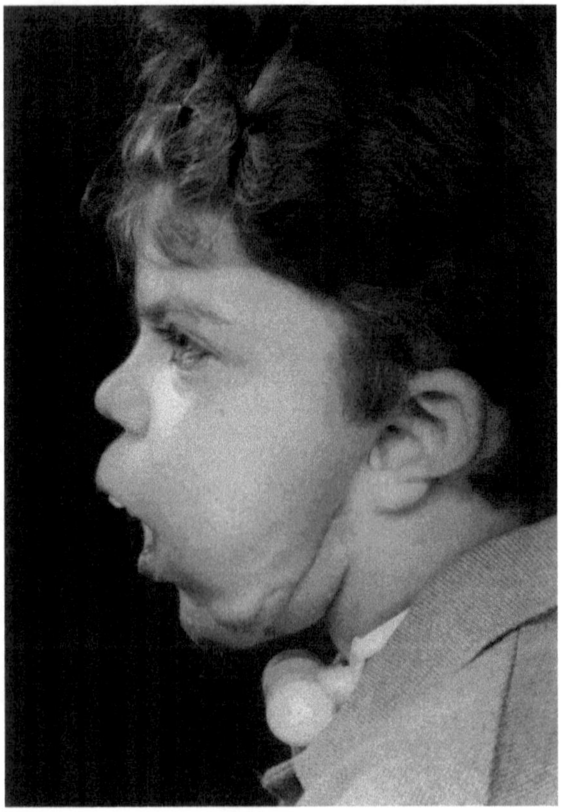

H

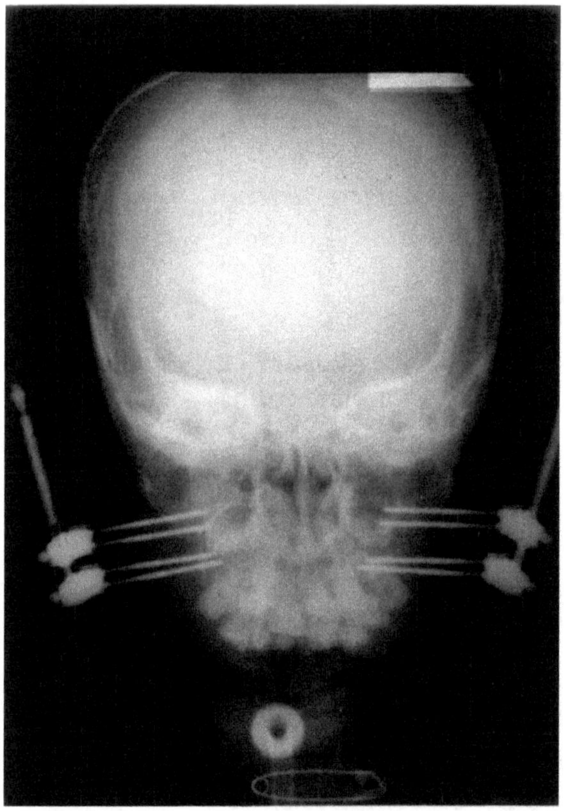

I

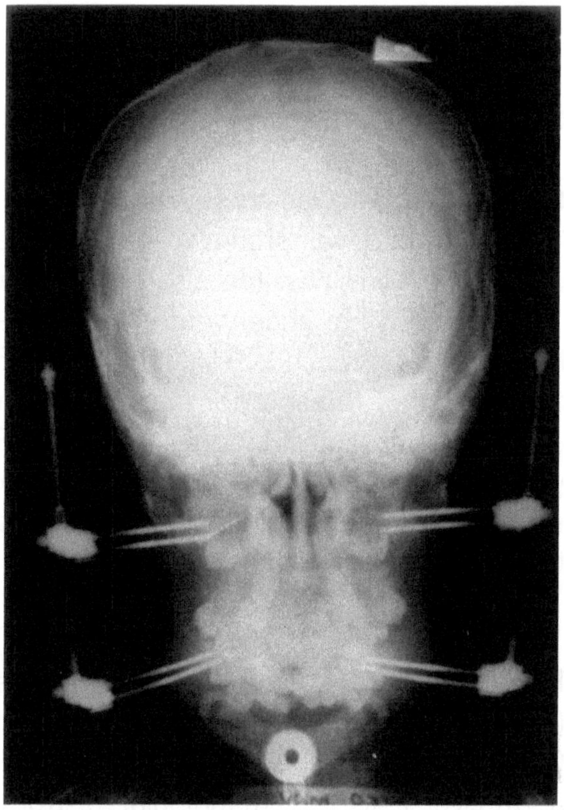

J

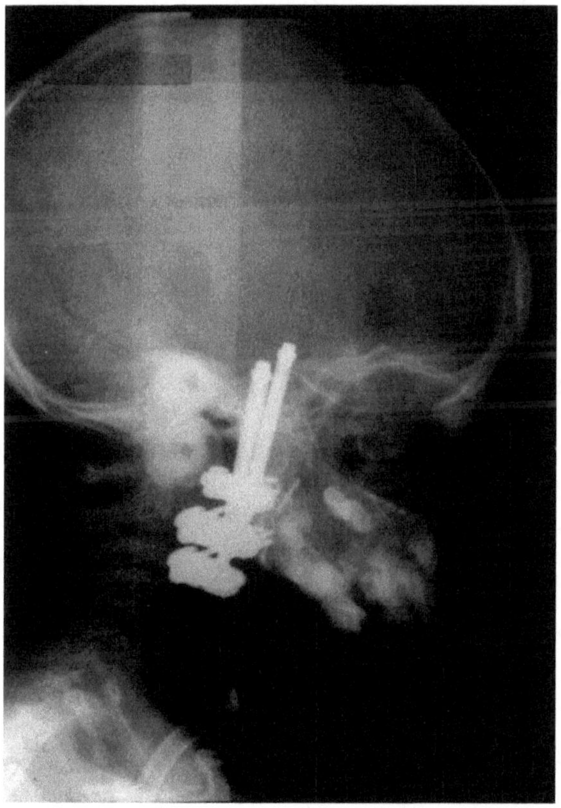

K

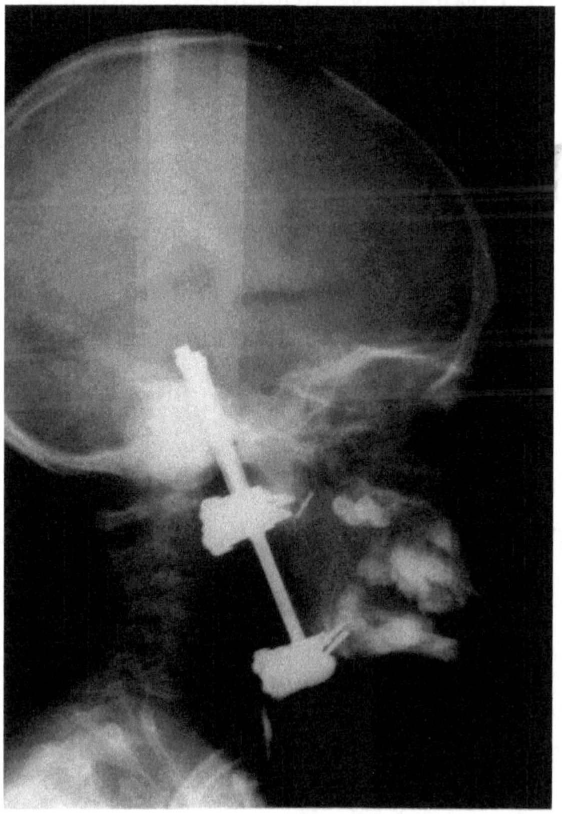

L

CASE STUDY: TRANSVERSE DISTRACTION

Case 19. C.R. was an 8-year-old male with Nager syndrome characterized by underdevelopment of his lower jaw, bilateral ear deformity, bilateral hand deformities. He also had an overjet and maxillary dentoalveolar overeruption. He underwent bilateral mandibular distraction (oblique vector/23 mm right and 23 mm left) (Figure 5.47) as well as transverse distraction (8 mm) of the anterior mandible in order to expand the mandible arch and to increase the bigonial distance. Bilateral calvarial flaps were employed to augment his zygomatic region, and a genioplasty provided additional augmentation of the chin. His skin incisions were complicated by the development of hypertrophic scars.

Figure 5.47. Case 19. An eight-year-old male with Nager syndrome (right, Pruzansky IIa; left, Pruzansky I) who underwent bilateral mandibular (oblique vector) distraction (right, 23 mm; left, 23 mm). He also underwent a transverse (8 mm) mandibular distraction (osteotomy of symphysis), a genioplasty, and cranial bone flap augmentation of the zygoma.

(A) Preoperative frontal view showing severe mandibular deficiency.

(B) Postoperative frontal view 51 months after completion of distraction showing increased mandibular volume and closure of an anterior open bite. He had also undergone orbitozygomatic reconstruction.

(C) Preoperative submental view.

(D) Postoperative submental view. Note the submental distraction scar.

(E) Preoperative right profile showing the severe micrognathia and almost straight line relationship between the upper lip and hyoid.

(F) Postoperative right profile showing the increase in mandibular volume and chin contour.

(G) Preoperative left profile.

(H) Postoperative left profile. The scar is satisfactory.

(I) Predistraction posteroanterior cephalogram (devices in place).

(J) Postdistraction posteroanterior cephalogram.

(K) Predistraction lateral cephalogram (horizontal vector).

(L) Postdistraction lateral cephalogram showing the increased mandibular volume, closure of the anterior open bite, and counterclockwise rotation of the long arm of the devices.

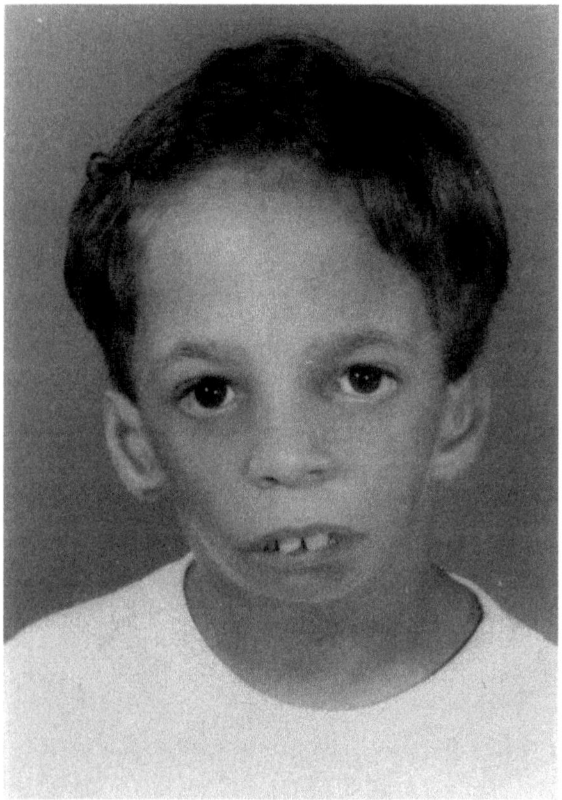

A

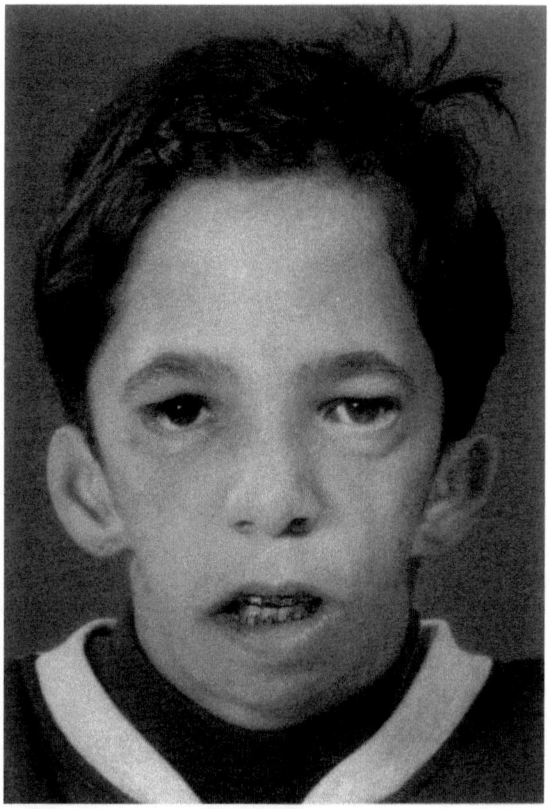

B

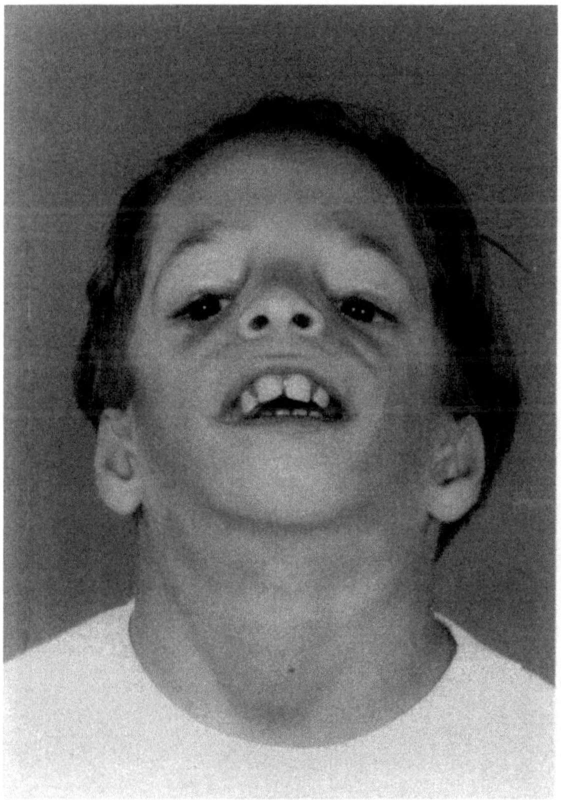

C

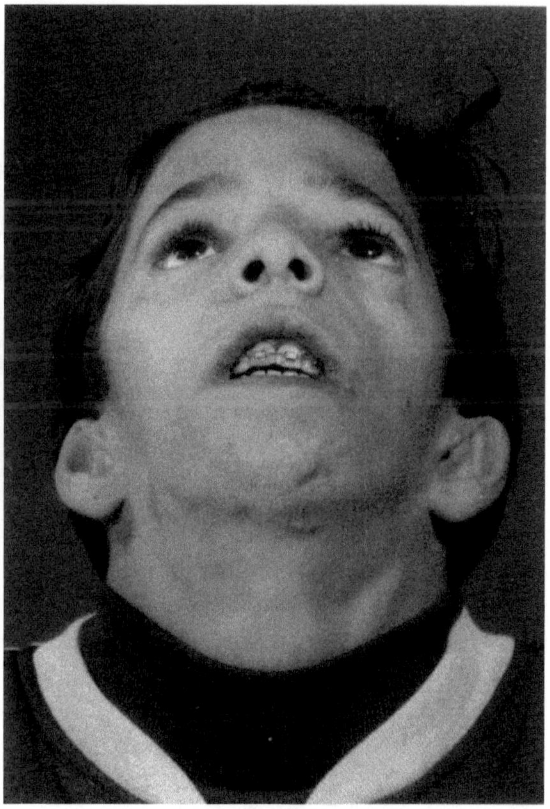

D

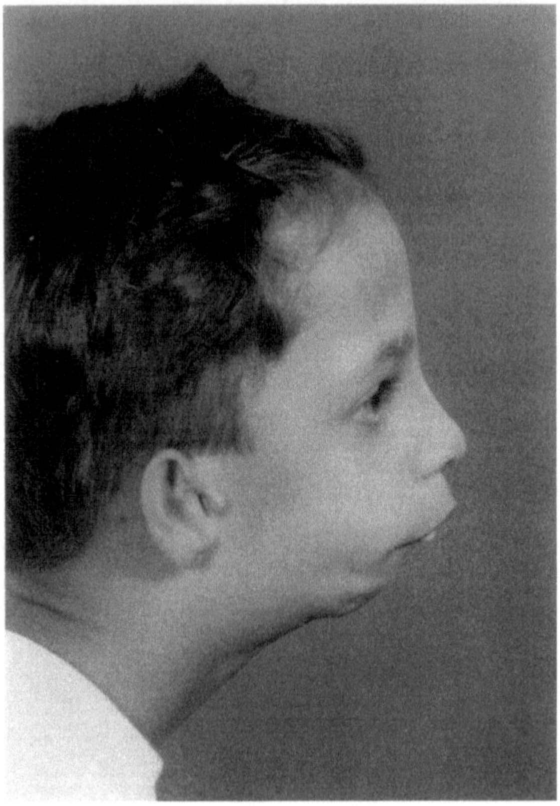

E

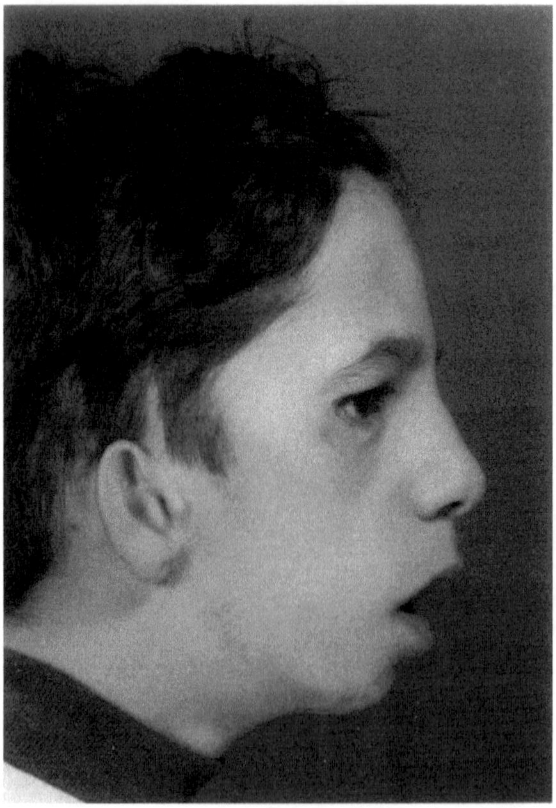

F

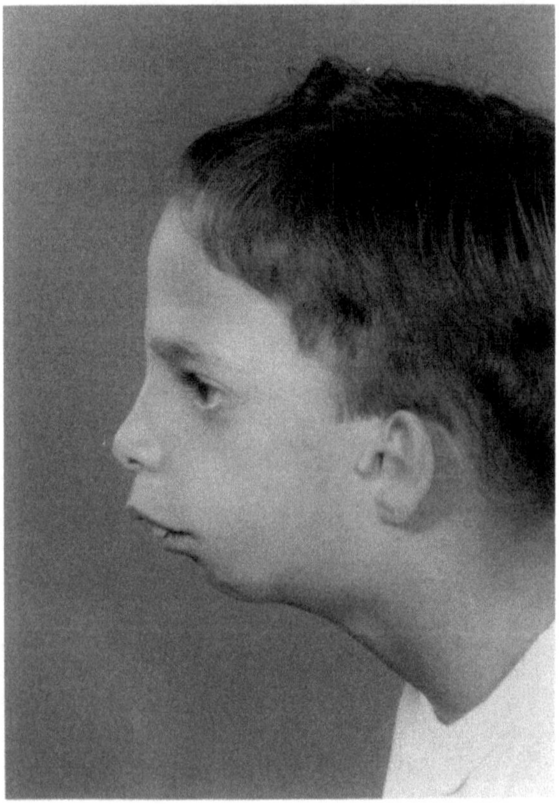

G

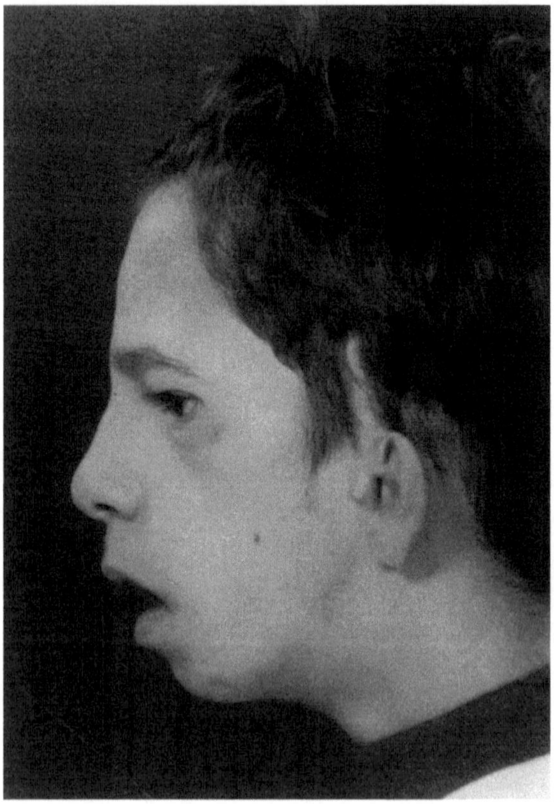

H

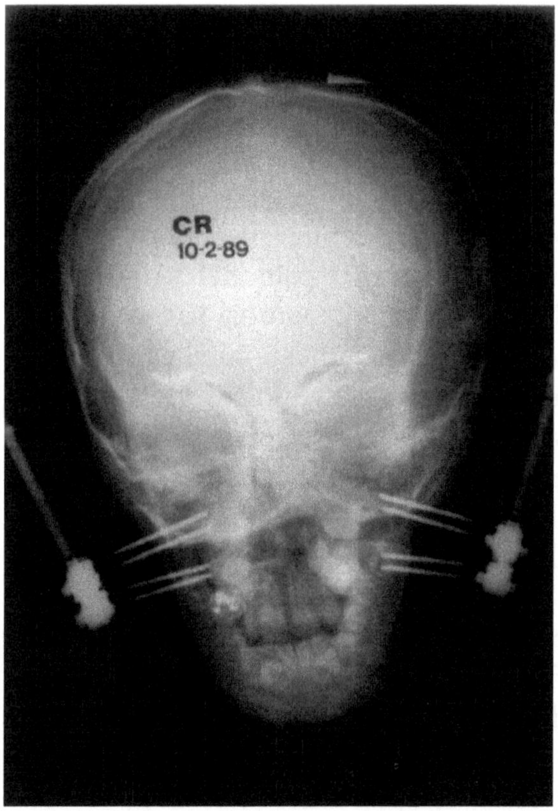

I

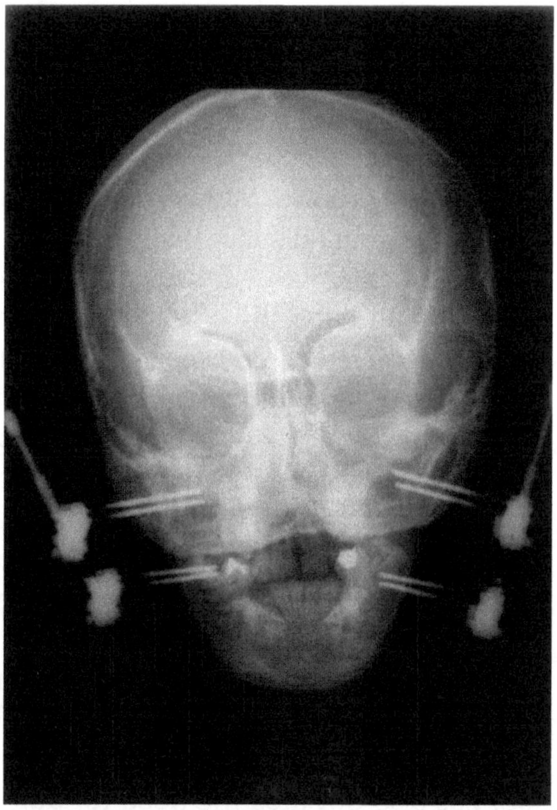

J

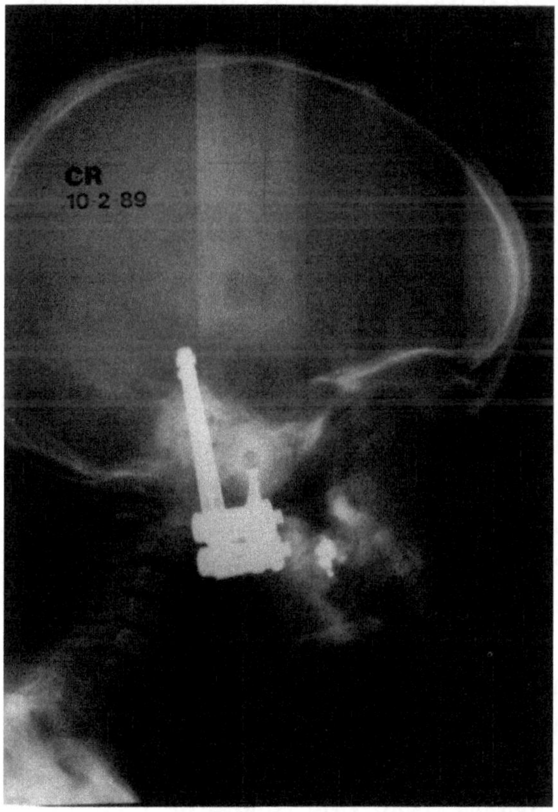

K

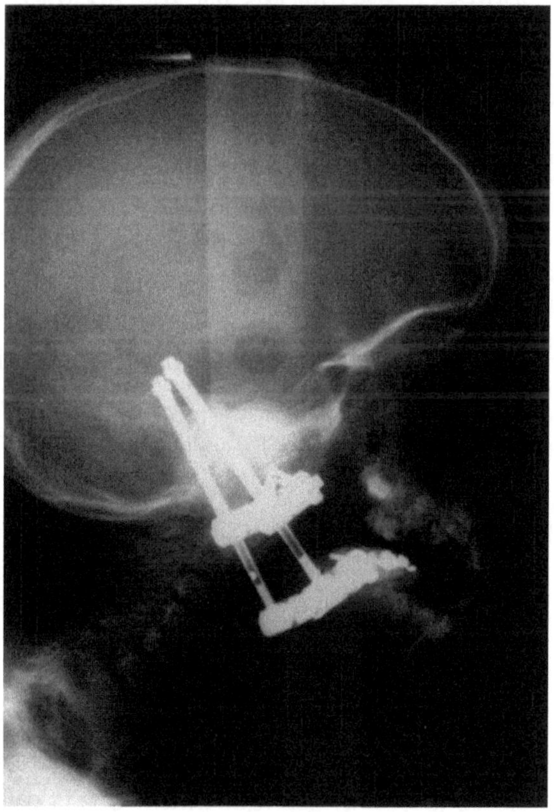

L

DISCUSSION

The current clinical study has demonstrated that mandibular distraction is a safe and effective surgical technique, findings that have also been duplicated at other centers (16–19). For patients undergoing surgical reconstruction of the hypoplastic mandible by the distraction technique, the length of hospitalization and operating time has been drastically reduced; distraction can even be performed on an outpatient or ambulatory basis. There has never been the need for a blood transfusion except for one patient with von Willebrand's disease. The technique, which can be applied at a younger age, has also obviated the need for autogenous bone grafting, as is often required in traditional orthognathic surgical procedures. It also allows for the augmentation of hypoplastic mandibles that are not amenable to traditional orthognathic mandibular advancement procedures (see Case 18).

A benefit that should also be emphasized is that there is *gradual* distraction not only of the bony skeleton but also of the associated soft tissues such as the muscles of mastication, subcutaneous tissue, and skin ("functional matrix"). Because of the expansion of the associated soft tissues and muscles, there is a resulting multidirectional expansion of the distracted mandible characterized, for example, by an increase in the bigonial distance, an increase in the vertical dimension of the chin, and the creation of a gonial angle. The secondary expansive effect on the soft tissues and muscles is also reflected in the fact that there is minimal, if any, evidence of clinical relapse. The patients have been followed up to 7 years and there is no evidence of relapse in any patient, a finding that stands in contrast to the dental/skeletal relapse observed following traditional orthognathic advancement procedures to reconstruct the hypoplastic ramus in unilateral craniofacial microsomia and to advance the mandible (ie, sagittal split osteotomy) in developmental micrognathia (20). Another factor contributing to the absence of relapse is the *gradual* (1 mm/day) rate at which the advancement/distraction is achieved. For example, in the traditional 15 mm surgical (orthognathic) mandibular advancement, wide subperiosteal undermining is required and in a single, often forceful, surgical maneuver the mandibular segment is forcibly advanced against the restrictive soft tissues. It is not surprising that the soft tissues subsequently contract from their advanced state and this factor probably represents the most important cause of clinical relapse. In contrast, in the distraction technique there are two differences: (1) both the skeletal and soft tissues are concomitantly lengthened and (2) the lengthening is achieved at a gradual rate (1 mm/day) over an interval of several weeks.

Another advantage of distraction is that it can be applied as early as 2 years of age because the technique is relatively simple and because bone grafts are not required to augment the hypoplastic ramus and body.

There has also been concern about the effects of mandibular distraction on the temporomandibular joints. In one patient with coronoid process-zygoma ankylosis following bilateral distraction, subsequent bilateral coronoidectomies were required. In this patient the osteotomies were made between the condyles and coronoid processes, resulting in impingement of the latter against the zygomatic complexes following distraction. In another patient undergoing unilateral distraction, there was nocturnal TMJ pain on the affected side, presumably secondary to bruxism. This was relieved when an occlusal splint was constructed and worn. Serial radiographic studies (21,22) conducted on this series of patients showed that the hypoplastic condylar segment improved in size and in orientation and assumed a more normal radiographic appearance (see Chapter 8). A concomitant canine laboratory study (21) of changes in the temporomandibular joints following unilateral mandibular distraction showed that there was a transient posterior condylar flattening on the ipsilateral side and posterosuperior flattening on the contralateral side. There was histologic evidence of subchondral degeneration followed by repair and remodeling, the latter resulting in a correction of the condylar flattening (see Chapter 8).

There are disadvantages of the distraction technique. The most obvious is residual cutaneous scarring, but, with careful placement of the incision, the scar can lie in the lines of minimal tension in the submandibular fold. The intraoral approach, for performance of the osteotomy and pin insertion has, however, evolved as the approach of choice because of reduction in the size of the scar. It can be anticipated that miniaturized intraoral devices will also be developed in the future.

There has also been concern about injury to the inferior alveolar nerve, a potential complication with all mandibular osteotomies. Questioning of our older patients has failed to detect any postoperative evidence of change in sensation of the lower lip. One must also question what is the status of the inferior alveolar nerve in the hypoplastic mandible of patients with unilateral craniofacial microsomia or whether there is, in reality, a functioning inferior alveolar nerve. The Mexico City technique (buccal corticotomy without disruption of the lingual cortex) represents an effort to maintain the integrity of the inferior alveolar nerve, and its authors have noted that another benefit of this technique is a bowing out of the gonial angle (see Chapter 6). Our technique, described above, makes every effort to avoid injury to the mandibular canal, and the osteotomy (lingual aspect) is completed by a "greenstick fracture."

The total treatment time approaches 3 months for reconstruction of the hypoplastic mandible by distraction, a length of treatment similar to that of traditional orthognathic mandibular surgery with intermaxillary fixation before the development of rigid skeletal fixation. However, it must be stressed that this criticism is more than offset by the reduced period of hospitalization and operating time and by the facts that there is no discomfort when the device is in place and the child is able to eat a regular (soft) diet during the period of treatment. Deglutition and distraction of the muscles of mastication have a positive influence on the resulting morphology of the bony regenerate.

In the initial laboratory and clinical studies of mandibular distraction, Ilizarov's principles of bone lengthening were applied. Yet, sufficient clinical experience with mandibular distraction has now accumulated so that these principles can be reexamined and even challenged. For example, the term corticotomy, as popularized by Ilizarov, has been abandoned by the authors in favor of the term osteotomy as there is complete disruption not only of the buccal and lingual cortices but also of the periosteum and endosteum with complete separation of the mandibular segments. It should be noted that the technique proposed by Molina and Ortiz-Monasterio (19) initially preserves the lingual cortex of the mandible, but the latter is eventually disrupted by the forces applied by the distraction device (see Chapter 6).

Following another principle enumerated by Ilizarov, we initially dissected in a supraperiosteal plane. However, it was quickly learned that distraction of the mandible could also be successful in those cases in whom the periosteum was elevated, and the same observation was made in the patients of Molina and Ortiz-Monasterio (19) and Klein and Howaldt (16) in whom dissection was routinely performed in the subperiosteal plane. Moreover, the placement of the pins and execution of the osteotomy is technically simpler when the mandible is exposed in the subperiosteal plane. It is ironic, but it appears that Ilizarov devoted his professional career to distracting enchondral bones (extremity), which are not as amenable to the technique as are the membranous bones of the craniofacial skeleton. The latter are smaller in size and have a richer blood supply. It is these anatomic characteristics that may account for the lower incidence of complications than that observed by orthopedic surgeons in distraction of the long bones of the extremities (tibia, etc.), that is, pin tract infections, loosening of the device, pain, and prolonged periods of treatment.

At this stage of development of the distraction technique, attention must be directed at precise preoperative planning that can predict and achieve posttreatment mandibular morphology that approximates the contralateral side in the unilateral deformity and normal form in the bilateral deformity. There are three variables with which the surgeon is dealing: (1) surgical technique, (2) type of distraction device, and (3) the role of the "functional matrix" (soft tissue and masticatory muscles) during and after distraction.

Surgical Technique

As discussed earlier, the authors and the Frankfurt group (16) practice a true bicortical osteotomy. In the New York technique, the final technical maneuver is disruption of the lingual cortex by a "greenstick fracture." It should be noted that the Mexico City group (19) prefers to maintain the lingual cortex (unicorticotomy), but eventually (within several days of activation) the forces generated by the device disrupt the latter. It has thus been established that in all techniques an eventual bicortical disruption (osteotomy) of the mandible into two segments is a prerequisite for successful mandibular lengthening.

In contrast to the recommendations of Ilizarov, the periosteum can be elevated on the buccal side only, a maneuver that facilitates precise pin placement and completion of the osteotomy without compromising formation of the bony regenerate.

Pin placement establishes the positioning of the distraction device, and the latter dictates, to a great extent, the vector of distraction (modified, of course, by the functioning muscles of mastication). In unilateral and bilateral mandibular deficiencies the pathology is usually located predominantly in the ascending ramus. Consequently, the goal is vertical elongation of the ramus with or without horizontal elongation of the body. In most of the unilateral cases the pins/device have been inserted along a predominantly *vertical* vector (perpendicular to the mandibular body) with a more oblique position of the device in the bilateral cases where sagittal thrust of the body and chin is also desired (*oblique* vector). A *horizontal* vector (parallel to the inferior border of the body) is used in bilateral cases in whom only anterior mandibular projection is required (see page 86). With the development and introduction of multiplanar distraction devices more flexibility will be available for control of the distraction trajectory in the vertical, sagittal, and horizontal directions. However, unidirectional devices will still be used when only vertical elongation of the ascending ramus (with leveling of the occlusal plane and oral commissure) is sought. Our longitudinal studies have also shown that, especially in bilateral cases, vertical elongation of the ramus is also associated with counterclockwise rotation of the mandible with anterior projection of the body and chin (see page 98). This type of correction will be facilitated by the newer multiplanar distraction devices, which can be manipulated in the *X*, *Y*, *Z* planes. The Mexico City group achieves this goal by making two corticotomies, placing three pins, and using a bidirectional device (see Chapter 6).

The osteotomy/corticotomy is ideally made at right angles to the distraction device, but this is often not possible because of inadequate bone stock or the presence of teeth and tooth follicles. Successful distraction can, however, be achieved even when the osteotomy cannot be made at right angles to the vectors. In essence, the osteotomy/corticotomy serves only one purpose—the creation of two mandibular segments to create a gap for distraction and formation of the bony regenerate.

A technical difficulty is posed when the ramus is so hypoplastic that it is inadequate for pin placement/osteotomy (eg, Pruzansky type III mandibular hypoplasia). There are two alternatives: (1) curettement of a tooth follicle and allowing an interval of 6 months for bony regeneration (McCarthy) before performing the distraction osteotomy and (2) preliminary bone graft reconstruction of the ramus with allowance of a suitable period for consolidation prior to performing the distraction osteotomy (19).

Distraction Device

The authors' experience was initially with a unidirectional distraction device (Howmedica). Serial radiographic studies (see page 125) have demonstrated a change in the device vector during and after active distraction, a finding that we have attributed to the role of the muscles of mastication on the newly formed bony regenerate. The introduction of a multiplanar distraction device provides more control in achieving: (1) the fundamental vertical elongation of the ramus, (2) horizontal elongation (body), and recreation of the mandibular angle with closure of the anterior open bite, and (3), transverse widening or increase in the bigonial distance.

Laboratory studies (3) and the clinical series have demonstrated a marked increase in the transverse dimension (bigonial) of the mandible, a surprising finding that we have attributed to the combined action of the distraction device and the muscles of mastication. The development of a multiplanar distraction device provides the surgeon with more control in modifying this dimension and increasing the bigonial distance.

The intraoral devices, offering the decided advantage of avoiding a cutaneous scar, will find more application in the bilateral deficiencies (micrognathia) where there is sufficient bone stock for pin placement and device application and where a horizontal vector is optimal. In the cases of unilateral distraction with severe ramal deficiency and the need for a vertical vector, the extraoral device is still preferred.

Role of the Functional Matrix

The most surprising finding has been the multidimensional type of mandibular lengthening (skeletal) that has been achieved with a unidirectional device. For example, increases in the transverse or bigonial distance, in the vertical height of the anterior mandible, in the vertical dimension of the coronoid process have been observed. It cannot be overemphasized that, while the patient uses the mandible during distraction, the masticatory muscles work on the bony regenerate and thus greatly modify ultimate mandibular morphology. Bony remodeling occurs predominantly during and after distraction while the patient is actually opening and closing the mandible during eating and talking.

Gradual distraction or lengthening not only of the skeleton but also the musculature probably accounts for the absence of relapse previously apparent after bone grafting of the ramus in unilateral craniofacial microsomia and orthognathic surgical advancement (23) for the correction of severe mandibular micrognathia.

Acknowledgments. The authors acknowledge the contributions of their colleagues at the Institute of Reconstructive Plastic Surgery of the NYU Medical Center. Patricia Chibbaro, R.N., Court B. Cutting, M.D., Arun Gosain, M.D., Nolan S. Karp, M.D., Jamie Levine, M.D., Michael T., Longaker, M.D., Richard J. Mackool, M.D., Susan McCormack, D.D.S., Douglas Roth, M.D., Norman Rowe, M.D., David Staffenberg, M.D., Charles H. Thorne, M.D., and Robert Wood, M.D.

References

1. Ilizarov GA. The tension-stress effect on the genesis and growth of tissues: 1. The influence of stability of fixation and soft-tissue preservation. *Clin Othop* 239:264, 1989.
2. Ilizarov GA. The tension-stress effect on the genesis and growth of tissues: II. The influence of the rate and frequency of distraction. *Clin Othop* 239:249, 1989.
3. Karp NS, Thorne CH, McCarthy JG, Sissons HA. Bone lengthening in the craniofacial skeleton. *Ann Plast Surg* 24:231, 1990.
4. Karp NS, McCarthy JG, Schreiber JS, Sissons HA, Thorne CH. Membranous bone lengthening: A serial histological study. *Ann Plast Surg* 29:2, 1992.

5. Snyder CC, Levine GA, Swanson HM, Browne EZ. Mandibular lengthening by gradual distraction: preliminary report. *Plast Reconstr Surg* 51:506, 1973.
6. Michieli S, Miotti B. Lengthening of mandibular body by gradual surgical-orthodontic distraction. *J Oral Surg* 35:187, 1977.
7. McCarthy JG, Schreiber J, Karp N, Thorne CH, Grayson BH. Lengthening the human mandible by gradual distraction. *Plast Reconstr Surg* 89:1, 1992.
8. McCarthy JG. The role of distraction osteogenesis in the reconstruction of the mandible in unilateral craniofacial microsomia. *Clin Plast Surg* 21:625, 1994.
9. McCarthy JG. Mandibular bone lengthening. *Operative Tech Plast Reconstr Surg* 1:99, 1994.
10. McCarthy JG, Turk AE. Distraction of the craniofacial skeleton: Mandibular reconstruction. *Adv Plast Reconstr Surg.* 12:31, 1996.
11. Meurmann Y. Congenital microtia and meatal atresia. *Arch Otolaryngol* 66:443, 1957.
12. Grayson BH, LaBatto FA, Kolber AB, McCarthy JG. Basilar multiplane cephalometric analysis. *Am J Orthod* 88:503, 1985.
13. Pruzansky S. Not all dwarfed mandibles are alike. *Birth Defects* 5:120, 1969.
14. Kaban LB, Moses MH, Mulliken JB. Surgical correction of hemifacial microsomia in the growing child. *Plast Reconstr Surg* 82:9, 1988.
15. McCarthy JG, Staffenberg DA, Wood RA, Cutting CB, Grayson BH, Thorne CH. Introduction of an intraoral bone-lengthening device. *Plast Reconstr Surg* 96:978, 1995.
16. Klein C, Howaldt HP. Correction of mandibular hypoplasia by means of bidirectional callus distraction. *J Craniofacial Surg* 7:258, 1996.
17. Diner PA, Kollar EM, Martinez H, Vazquez. Intraoral distraction for mandibular lengthening: a technical innovation. *J Cranio-Maxillo-Facial Surg* 24:92, 1996.
18. Wangerin K, Gropp H. Enoral application of Ilizarov's callus distraction of the mandible—initial clinical reports. *Int J Oral Maxillofacial Surg*. In press.
19. Ortiz-Monasterio F, Molina F. Mandibular distraction in hemifacial microsomia, operative techniques. *Operative Tech Plast Reconstr Surg* 1:105, 1994.
20. Grayson BH, McCormick S, McCarthy JG. Long-term studies after mandibular distraction. In press, 1998.
21. McCormick SV, McCarthy JG, Grayson BH, Staffenberg DA, McCormack SA. Effect of mandibular distraction on the temporomandibular joint: Part 1, Canine Study. *J Craniofacial Surg* 6:358, 1995.
22. McCormick SV, Grayson BH, McCarthy JG, Staffenberg DA. Effect of mandibular distraction on the temporomandibular joint: Part II, Clinical Study. *J Craniofacial Surg* 6:364, 1995.
23. Obwegesser HL. The indications for surgical correction of mandibular deformation by the sagittal splitting technique. *Br J Oral Surg* 1:157, 1953.

CHAPTER 6

Distraction of the Mandible

The Mexico City Experience

Fernando Molina and Fernando Ortiz Monasterio

Facial asymmetry secondary to mandibular hypoplasia is a common problem in craniofacial surgery; its correction is critical for the quality of the final esthetic result (1–7).

Mandibular hypoplasia, unilateral or bilateral, may result from disturbed embryogenesis or may represent an acquired deformity as a sequela of condylar fractures suffered at an early age with secondary ankylosis of the temporomandibular joint.

Bone lengthening or distraction osteogenesis using osteotomies and circumferential gradual distraction was described by Ilizarov in 1954 to align fractures segments of long bones and later to elongate these bones without a bone graft (8,9).

Although initially the technique was developed to lengthen the long bones, it was not until 1973 that Snyder, using an extraoral device, reported mandibular lengthening in a canine model (10), and a similar report on two dogs using an intraoral device followed from Italy (11). More recently, Karp and McCarthy reported successful membranous bone lengthening with external devices and noted that cortical bone formed in the expanded area of the mandible; histologic examination of the zone revealed a highly organized biologic process (12). McCarthy and colleagues at New York University reported their preliminary clinical results in 1992; they successfully elongated the mandible in four young patients using a bicortical osteotomy and a rigid external fixator (13).

In our group in Mexico City, since 1990 we have been performing mandibular distraction using a technique of external corticotomy and flexible unidirectional and bidirectional external devices to achieve

Table 6.1. Clinical series.

Unilateral craniofacial microsomia	132 patients
Grade I	25
Grade II-A	71
Grade II-B	36
Micrognathia	31 patients

simultaneous skeletal and soft tissue correction with mininal surgery (14,15). The treatment philosophy is to elongate and remodel the hypoplasic mandible.

During the last five years we have performed 163 mandibular corticotomies and distractions: 132 patients with unilateral craniofacial microsomia and 31 patients with micrognathia (Table 6.1).

In the unilateral group, the age ranged from 2 to 17 years; these were 82 female and 50 male patients, and the mandibular hypoplasia has been classified according to Pruzansky (16): grade I, the hypoplasia affects only the gonial angle; grade II-A, the angle and the ascending ramus are affected; grade II-B, the hypoplasia is more severe, affecting the angle, ascending ramus with a flat and rudimentary condyle; and grade III, a complete absence of the ramus and condyle. Mandibular distraction is not indicated in grade III cases.

Lateral and posteroanterior cephalograms were obtained preoperatively. Panorex views were used to compare both sides of the mandible and to identify the tooth follicles and inferior alveolar nerve, in order to avoid injury during surgery. The superimposing method of Björk (17) was used to obtain a mandibular growth prediction and assess the ideal dimension of the mandible and the growth/rotational movements (anterior and posterior) that are achieved during development.

SURGICAL TECHNIQUE

Under general anesthesia a 3-cm incision is made through the mucosa on the lateral aspect of the buccal vestibule. A subperiosteal dissection is performed exposing the gonial angle and the neighboring area of the ascending ramus. The sites of the planned external corticotomy and of the pin insertion are marked with Gentian violet, avoiding the nerve and the tooth buds.

The corticotomy is made with a side-cutting burr, beginning at the retromolar angle, cutting the medial and lateral buttresses, and extending through the lateral aspect of the mandibular angle including all of the cortex to the cancellous layer. Along the inferior aspect, the corticotomy is extended widely around the angle where the bone is thick (Figure 6.1). *Most of the*

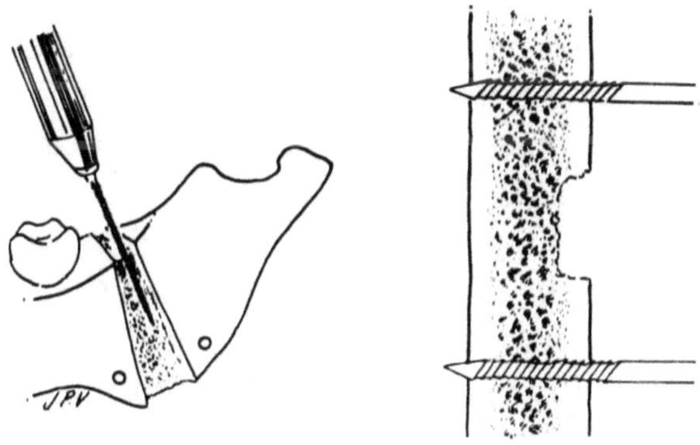

Figure 6.1. Diagram of the corticotomy extending widely around the mandibular angle but sparing the inner or lingual cortex. Cross-sectional view shows that the inner or lingual cortex remains intact. Two pins are introduced through the full thickness of the mandible.

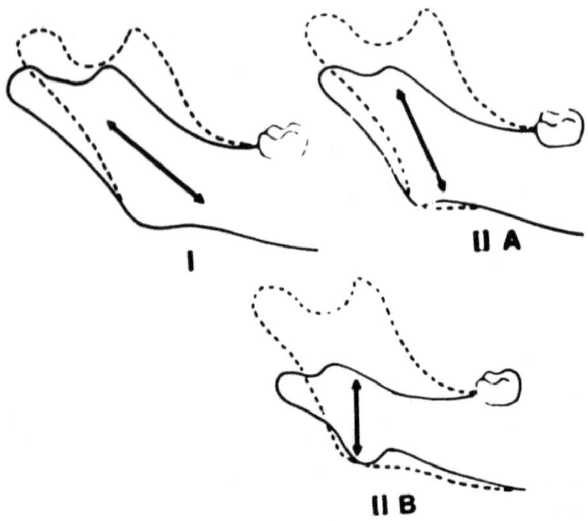

Figure 6.2. The distraction vector is different in each grade (Pruzansky) of bony hypoplasia. The arrow on the mandible angle depicts the different vectors. Note the vertical vector in grade II-B.

internal cortical layer remains intact. In fact, different zones of bone resistance are encountered, minor at the angle but major resistance at the alveolar ridge, that will be elongated differently under a perpendicular distraction vector.

The orientation of the corticotomy and the position of the pins determine the distraction vector. The distractor vector is different in each patient, depending on the grade of mandibular hypoplasia (Figure 6.2).

In patients with grade I hypoplasia (unilateral), the corticotomy extends obliquely from the posterior edge of the hypoplasic gonial angle to the retromolar angle in the alveolar ridge. The pins must be placed perpendicular to the corticotomy, obtaining an oblique vector distraction that produces a larger bone elongation in the angle and a minor bone elongation in the alveolar ridge.

In patients with grade II-A hypoplasia the distraction process must remodel and elongate the angle and the initial portion of the ascending ramus. For this reason the corticomy is placed obliquely in the junction of the angle and ramus, and the pins must be inserted in an intermediate position between a vertical and oblique vector distraction.

In patients with grade II-B hypoplasia, the corticotomy is placed horizontally in the base of the ascending ramus, and the pins must follow a vertical vector distraction in order to obtain more elongation in the hypoplastic ascending ramus.

Two stainless steel screws, 2.5 to 3.5 millimeters in diameter, are introduced percutaneously through the thickness of the mandible (bicortical) 3 to 5 mm in front of and behind the corticotomy. The diamond tip design of the pins obviates the need for previous holes drilled before their introduction in the bone. The cheek skin is pinched between the thumb and the index before introducing the second screw to allow for stretching and to minimize the length of the scar. Care must be taken to position the pins parallel to each other and facilitate their fixation to the distraction device.

The mucosa is closed with fine absorbable suture, and the distraction device is applied (Figure 6.3). This is made of two hollow plates with central perforations to allow the entrance of the mandibular pins. The two plates are joined by another stainless steel screw running free in one of them and transversing the length of the other plate, so that when it is turned, the distance between the plates is increased or decreased. The steel resistance of the

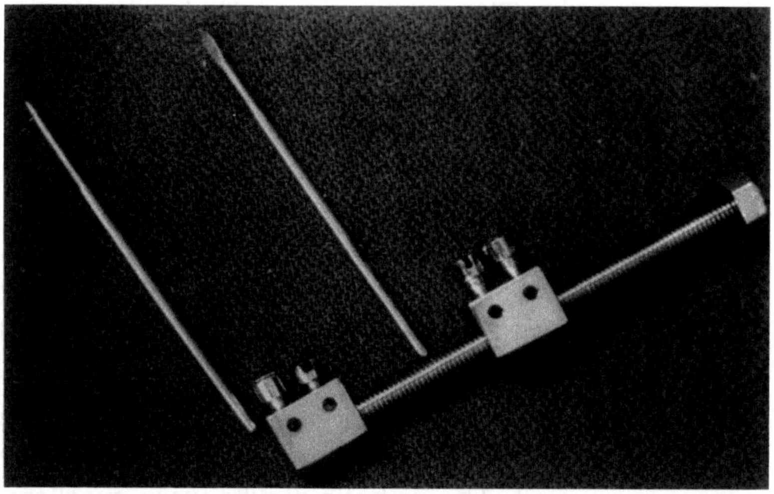

Figure 6.3. The unidirectional external device.

distractor device is softer than the pins, thus producing a flexible device that can bend under the masticatory muscle action and that externally reflects the shape of the elongated area.

Elongation is commenced on the fifth postoperative day at a rate of approximately 1 mm per day. This is done by the parents with minimal discomfort for the patient.

Elongation is usually completed in 3 to 4 weeks, and the device is left in place for an additional 6 to 8 weeks until radiographic evidence of new cortical bone formation is documented. At that time the screws are easily removed under sedation.

The patients with micrognatia (bilateral) present a different type of bone hypoplasia than do the unilateral patients. In the former group of patients the deformity is bilateral and both the mandibular body and the ascending ramus are affected. For this reason micrognathic patients require a bilateral and a bidirectional type of distraction. This concept is also true for patients with Treacher Collins, Pierre Robin, Nager, and bilateral craniofacial microsomia syndromes.

In this group two corticotomies were done: a vertically oriented one in the mandibular body and a horizontally oriented one in the ascending ramus (Figure 6.4). Three pins are used: A central one is introduced at the mandibular angle between the two corticotomies, a second into the mandibular body, and a third into the central aspect of the ascending ramus. One bidirectional device is used on each side, each one with two distraction plates to allow independent and more precise elongation of each segment, using the central pin as the fixed pivot for both of them (Figure 6.5).

Measurements of the distance between the pins and the distance of the soft-tissue structures (external canthus-buccal commissure and the inferior orbital rim-buccal commissure) are recorded weekly. Dental casts and cephalograms

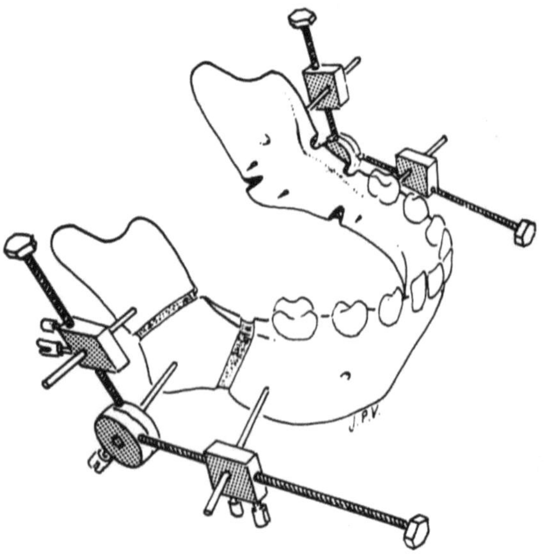

Figure 6.4. Diagram showing two corticotomies and two devices applied for bidirectional elongation. A central screw introduced at the angle serves as a pivot for independent vertical and horizontal distraction.

are obtained at the end of the distraction period and again at 6 to 8 weeks later to assess osteogenesis at the site of the corticotomy and to document occlusal changes.

The results of mandibular distraction were evaluated at the conclusion of the distraction period, at the time of removal of the device (end of the consolidation period), and subsequently every 3 months.

In patients with unilateral hypoplasia grade I, the elongation varied from 12 to 18mm (mean 16mm). The dental occlusion remained stable without evidence of posterior open bite. No active functional orthodontic appliances were used. The esthetic results were excellent; the facial symmetry was restored with descent of the oral commissure to the level of that of the contralateral side; the menton became horizontal and located at the midline.

In unilateral hypoplasia grade II-A, mandibular elongation ranged from 14 to 22mm (mean 19mm). The dental occlusion was disrupted, and a posterior open bite of 1 to 3mm was produced in half of the patients. Bite blocks and dynamic orthodontic appliances were used to maintain the elongation and to stabilize

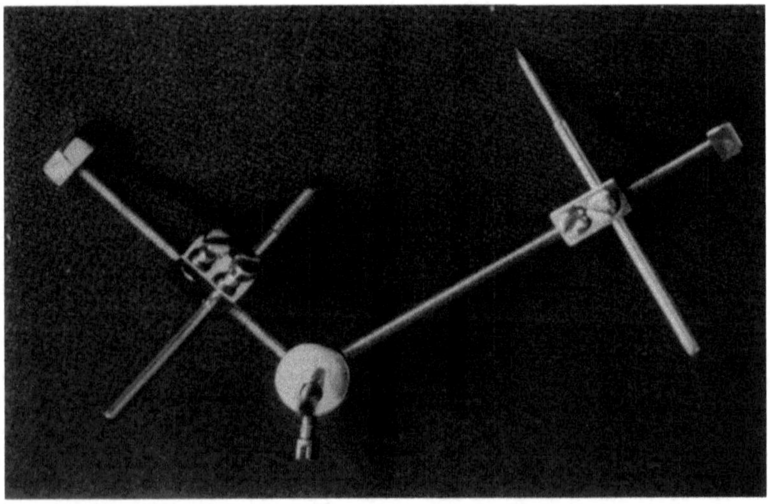

Figure 6.5. The bidirectional external device.

the occlusion (Figure 6.6A,B). The esthetic results were excellent, with restoration of facial symmetry and horizontalization of the chin and the buccal commissure (Figure 6.6C–H).

The group of patients with unilateral hypoplasia grade II-B characteristically had a stable but abnormal dental occlusion with marked deviation of the mandibular dental midline to the affected side. During distraction, bite blocks were required to maintain the posterior open bite; the blocks were gradually reduced to allow vertical descent of the maxillary dentoalveolus. Dynamic orthodontic appliances were also used in all of the patients at an early stage. After distraction, the initial occlusion was reproduced in the opposite direction on the contralateral side as a result of overcorrection. The esthetic improvement and the restoration of symmetry have also been impressive in these patients (Figure 6.7).

In the patients with micrognathia (bilateral), there was a range of 6 to 9 mm of vertical elongation of the ramus and 10 to 16 mm increase in the length of the mandibular body. The resulting dental occlusion was aceptable in most of the cases. Six of the posttraumatic cases were asymmetrical, requiring more elongation on one side, a goal that was easily achieved because the distraction was manipulated in two different directions on both sides, all independent of each other. The esthetic results were excellent with an improved gonial angle, satisfactory projection of the chin and remarkable expansion of the soft tissues of the lower face and upper neck (Figure 6.8).

Mandibular distraction has been an extremely benign experience for the patients. Morbidity is essentially limited to the presence of cutaneous scars slightly enlarged by the distraction, which have evolved satisfactorily with time, and no revisions have been necessary.

No symptoms of functional temporomandibular dysfunction have been detected. Radiographic studies have documented in the unidirectional cases that the condylar head uprighted and increased in size and volume, and, because of skeletal remodeling in the gonial angle, the condyle was laterally displaced, assuming a more medial and anatomic position that resembled the contralateral side. This change in condylar morphology occurred during the consolidation period. The contralateral or unexpanded condyle maintained its size and shape and did not show evidence of deformational changes.

Distraction osteogenesis is a technique that is becoming popular for the reconstruction of deficient mandibles and has simplified the treatment for congenital mandibular hypoplasia. It is a relatively minor surgical procedure preserving the integrity of the nerve and vascular supply. Careful planning of the corticotomy and the position of the pins produce a distraction vector that follows closely the direction of normal mandibular growth.

In all patients, vertical and sagittal mandibular elongation was obtained. During the early stages of our clinical experience it was assumed that mandibular elongation would result in the development of a posterior open bite in all patients, but this did not occur in many of the cases. This finding is the result of dentoalveolar adaptation at the maxillary

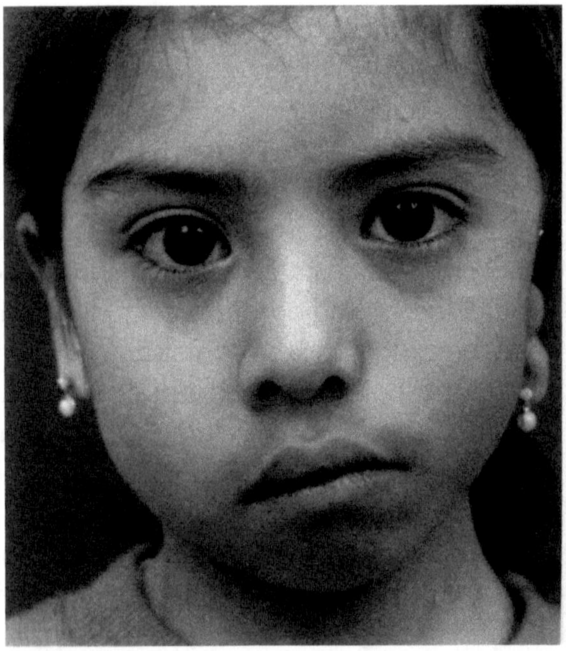

A

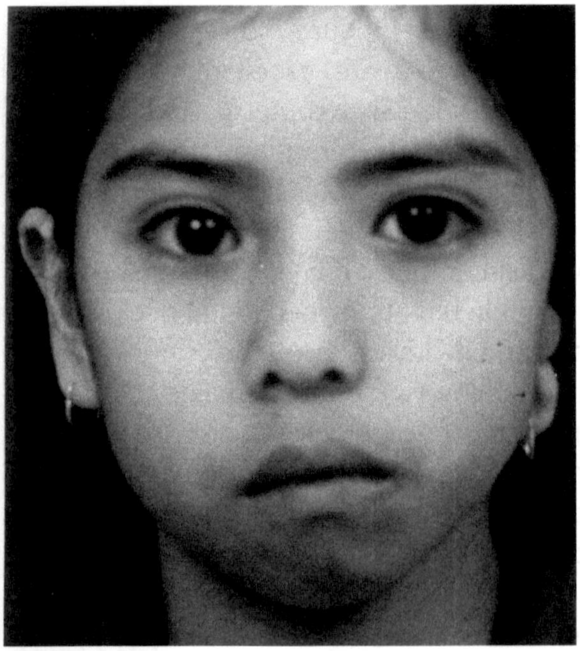

B

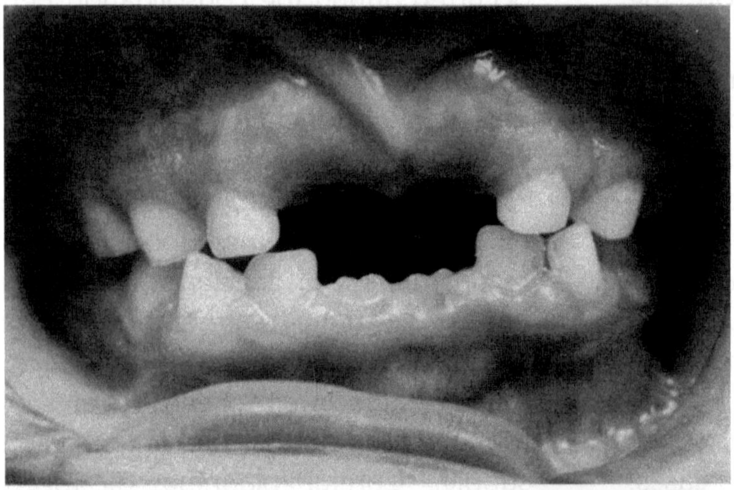

C

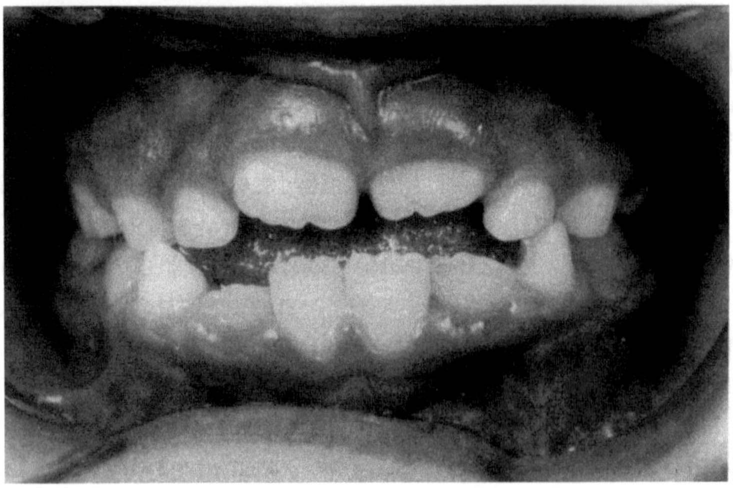

D

Figure 6.6. (A) Preoperative view of a 7-year-old girl with grade II-A unilateral craniofacial microsomia showing facial asymmetry with deviation of the buccal commissure and the chin. (B) One year after the removal of the pins showing descent of the buccal commissure and medialization of the chin. (C) Preoperative dental occlusion. (D) Postoperative view showing over-correction with displacement of the midline of the mandibular teeth to the right. (E) Preoperative posteroanterior cephalogram. Note the obliquity of the occlusal plane and the nasal floor. (F) Posteroanterior cephalogram at the end of the distraction period. There is an increase of the maxillary height on the affected side. (G) Panorex view during the distraction process. (H) Final panorex view showing elongation and remodeling of the angle and ascending ramus of the mandible.

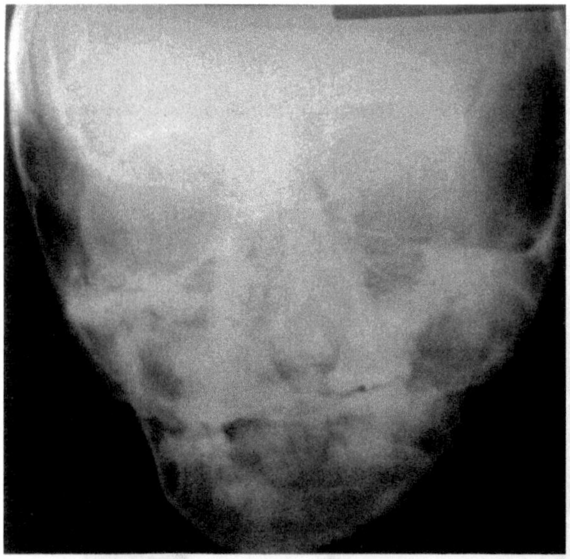
E

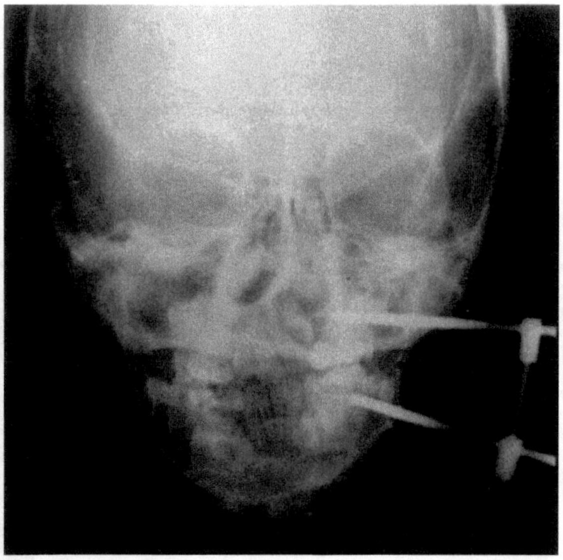
F

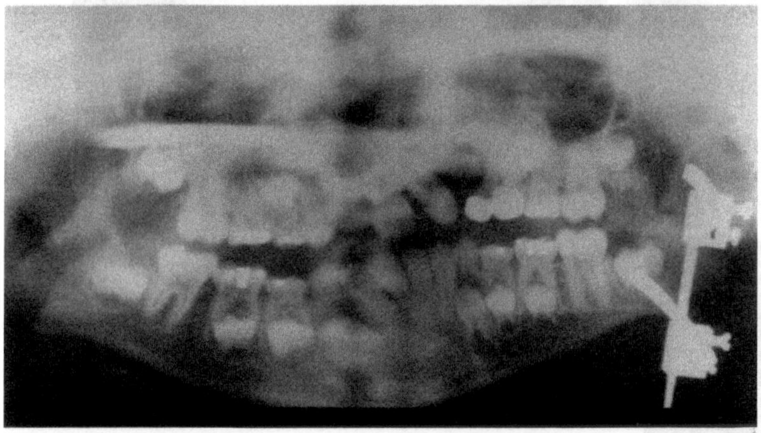
G

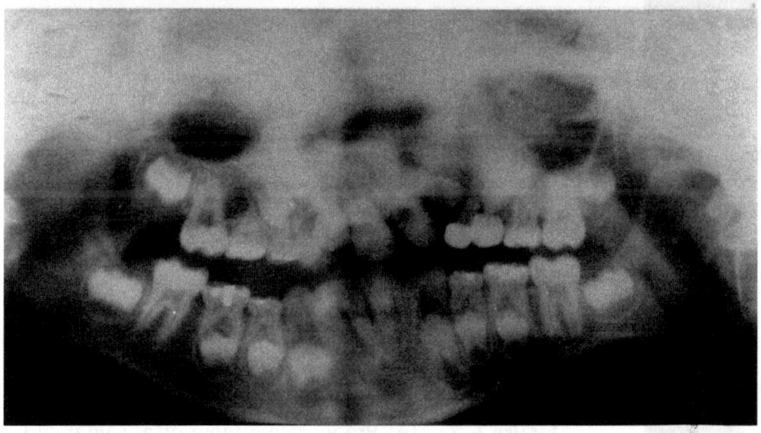
H

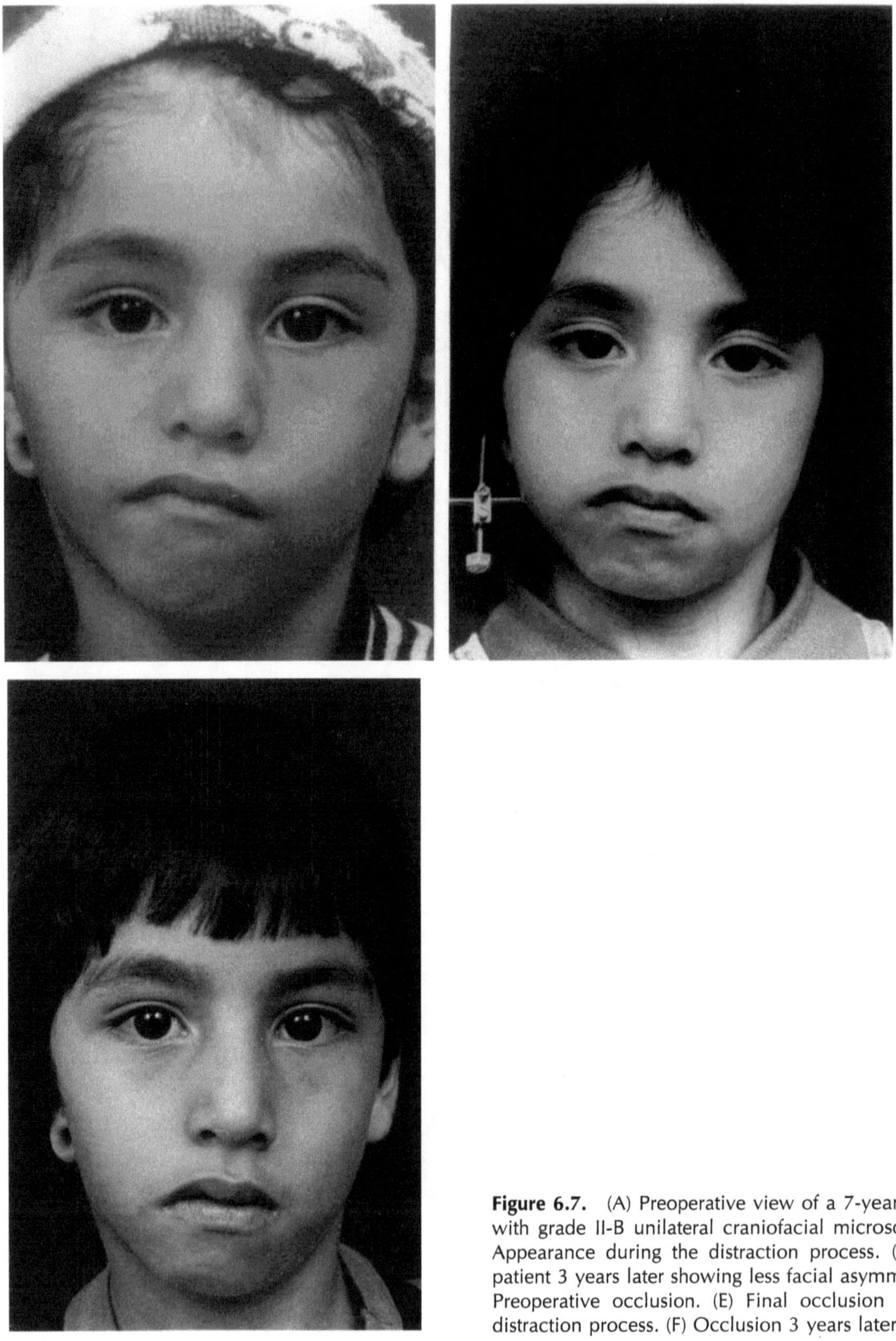

A B

C

Figure 6.7. (A) Preoperative view of a 7-year-old boy with grade II-B unilateral craniofacial microsomia. (B) Appearance during the distraction process. (C) Same patient 3 years later showing less facial asymmetry. (D) Preoperative occlusion. (E) Final occlusion after the distraction process. (F) Occlusion 3 years later.

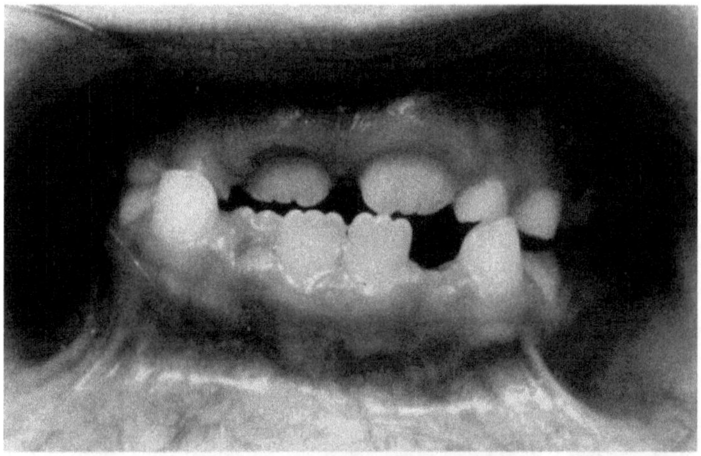

D

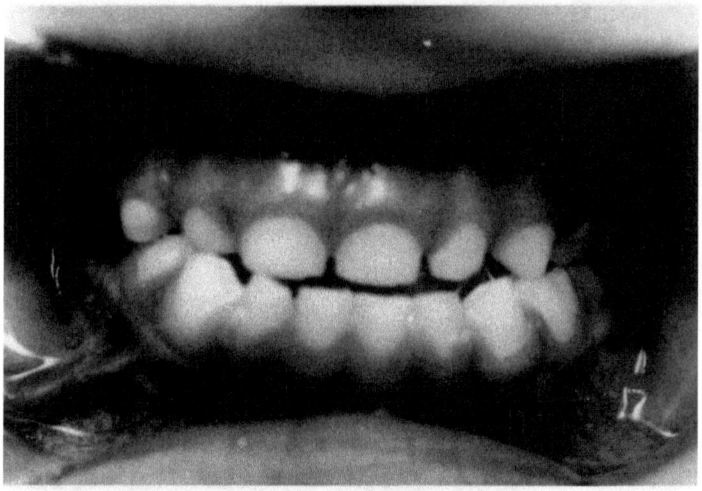

E

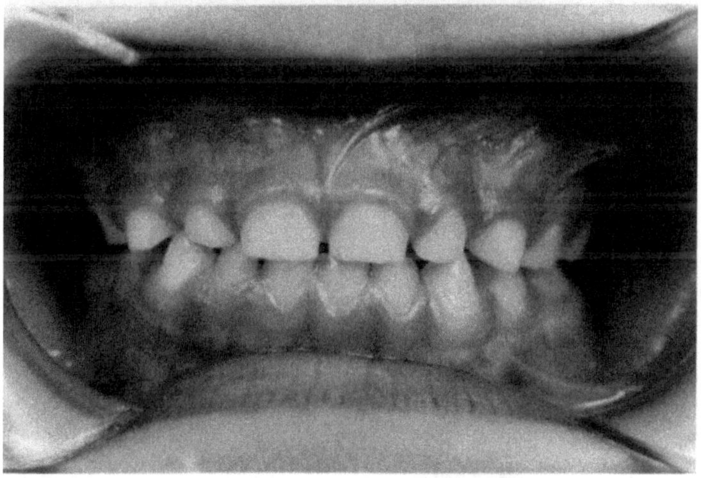

F

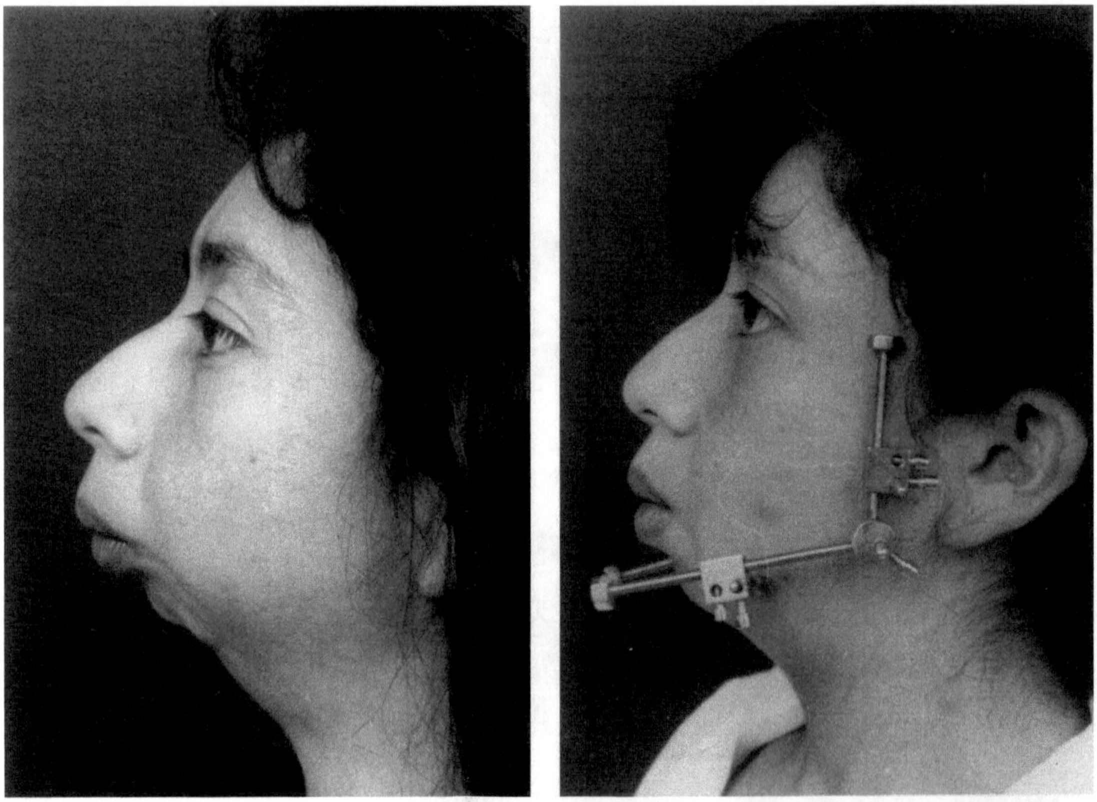

A B

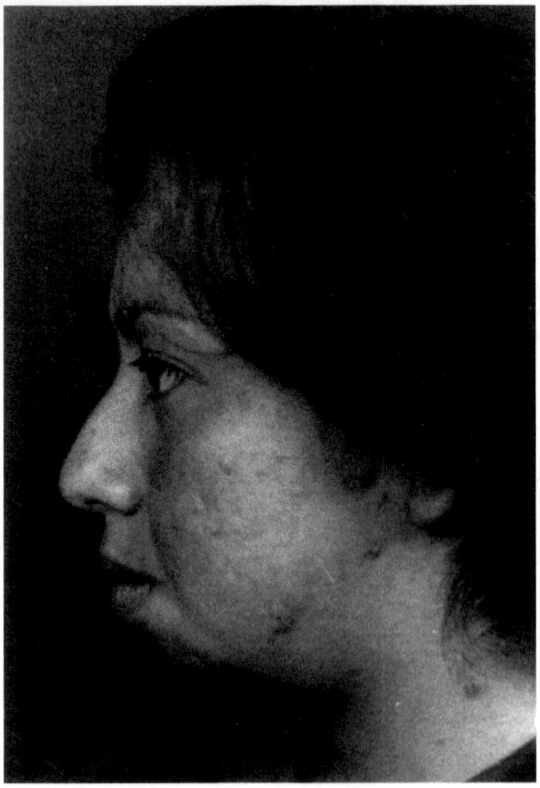

C

Figure 6.8. (A) Preoperative view of a 22-year-old female patient with congenital ankylosis and micrognathia (bilateral). (B) During the process of bidirectional and bilateral distraction. (C) Appearance one year later. Note the scars and the simultaneous soft tissue expansion and its distribution in the inferior third of the face and upper neck. (D) Preoperative panorex. (E) Panorex at the end of the distraction process showing the differential elongation obtained in the right and left mandibular bodies achieving symmetry in the mandible. (F) Panorex 18 months later. (G) Preoperative lateral cephalogrom. (H) Lateral cephalogram during the consolidation period. Note the separation between the molars; the vector of distraction in the mandibular body is parallel to the occlusal plane, thus avoiding the development of an anterior open bite. (I) Final lateral cephalogram.

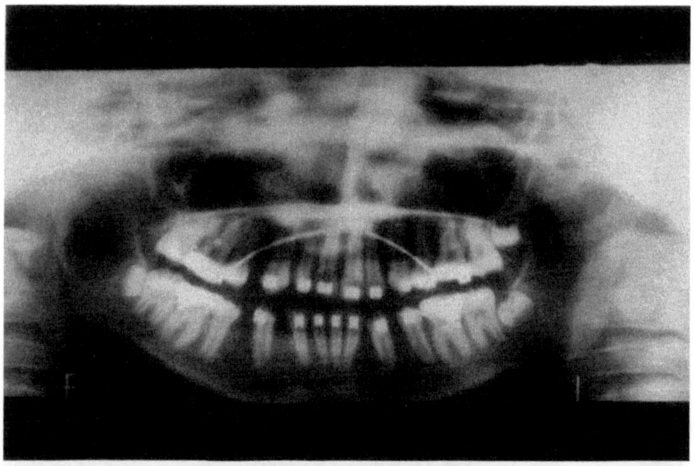

D

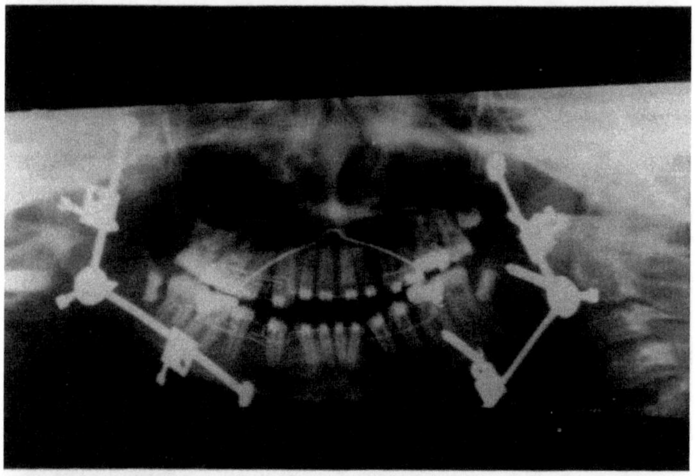

E

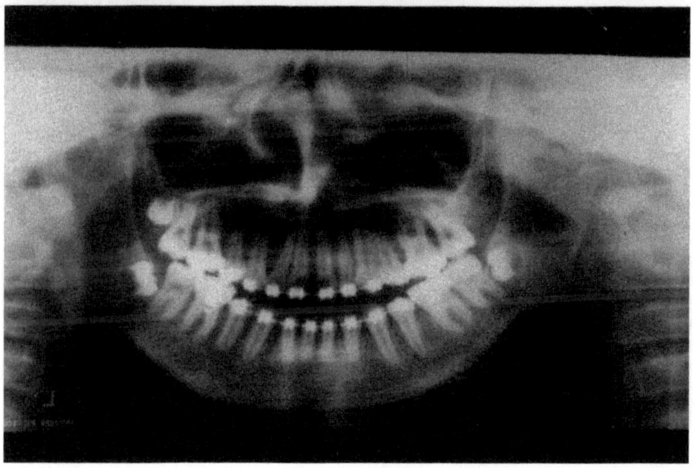

F

Figure 6.8. *Continued*

Figure 6.8. *Continued*

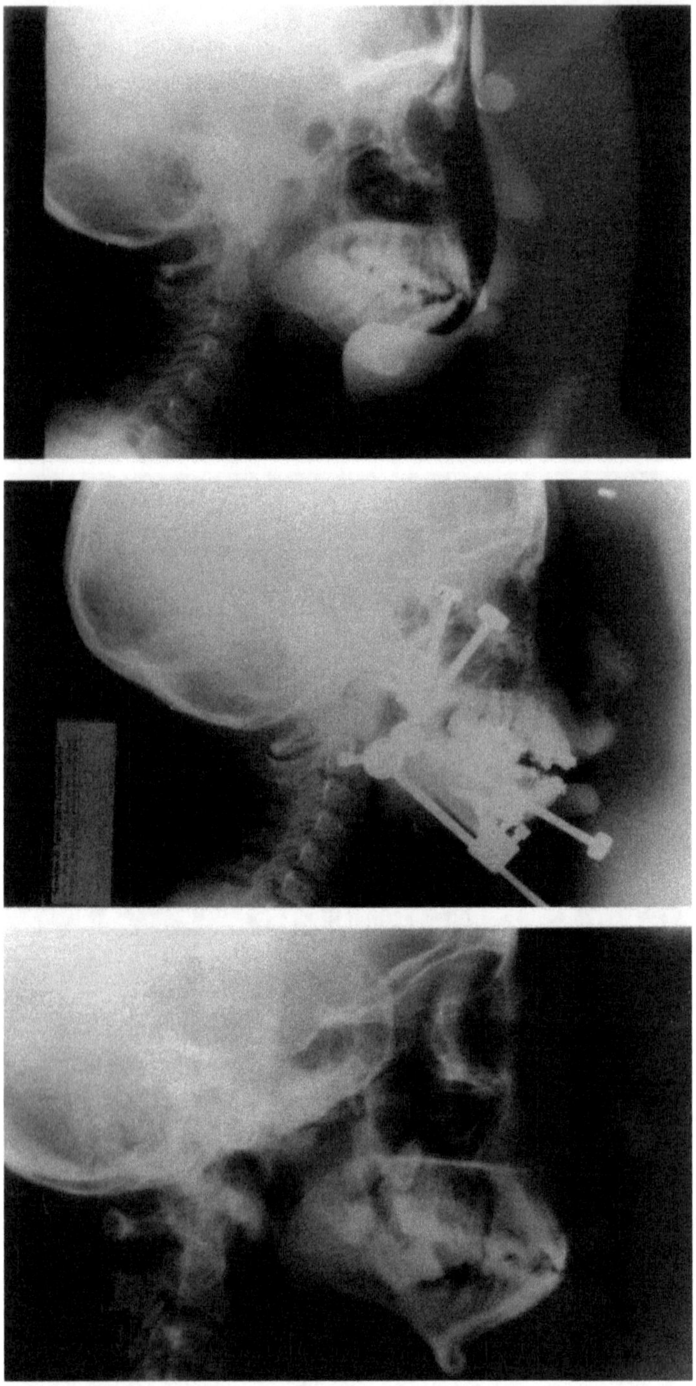

level. This type of maxillary vertical growth was documented in the cephalograms, suggesting that the maxilla had been liberated from the constricting effect of the hypoplastic mandible and the constricting soft tissues and thus proceeds to assume its normal growth potential. Murray and Mulliken have previously reported the same type of increased vertical maxillary growth after costochondral rib grafting of the hypoplastic ascending ramus (5).

An important benefit of mandibular distraction is the simultaneous expansion of the soft tissues of the face, characterized by rapid descent of the oral commissure to a normal position, the horizontalization of the chin, the increase in the distance between the oral commissure and the external canthus-inferior orbital rim, and the remarkable improvement in facial symmetry in all of the unilateral cases. In addition, there is an increase in the volume of the cheek soft tissue, a finding probably related to improved muscular morphology and function.

All of the patients with micrognathia (bilateral) presented with the typical "bird face" deformity characterized by deficient soft tissue of the lower third of the face and neck, absence of the cervicomental angle and shortened suprahyoid muscles. The overall esthetic result obtained with bilateral and bidirectional distraction has been impressive, beyond the patients' and surgeons' expectations. The neck assumes a normal contour with a well-defined angle; the muscles and soft tissues of the floor of the mouth expanded, as well as the masseter insertion and the muscle volume. The chin also assumes a more prominent position.

Gradual distraction of the mandible following corticotomies results in an increased mandibular mass and length and in simultaneous soft-tissue expansion adaptation (skin, muscles, vessels, and nerves) over a period of 8 to 12 weeks. The final elongation of the mandible results in an increase in size and change in position and shape, which is not possible with conventional orthognathic surgery as in the sagittal split osteotomy procedure.

The operation can be performed in an outpatient setting requiring only weekly visits. Futher refiniments in surgical technique and the development of other external or intraoral distraction devices will be neccessary, and a well-coordinated orthodontic-surgeon team is neccessary to obtain optimal results.

References

1. Converse JM, Horowitz SL, Coccaro PJ, Wood-Smith D. The corrective treatment of the skeletal asymmetry in hemifacial microsomia. *Plast Reconstr Surg* 52:221, 1973.
2. Kaban LB, Moses MH, Mulliken JB. Surgical correction of hemifacial microsomia in the growing child. *Plast Reconstr Surg* 82:9, 1988.
3. Iñigo F, Rojo P, Ysunza A. Aesthetic treatment of Romberg's disease: Experience with 35 cases. *Br J Plast Surg* 46:194, 1993.
4. Lauritzen C, Munro IR, Ross RB. Classification and treatment of hemifacial microsomia. *Scand J Plast Reconstr Surg* 19:33, 1985.
5. Murray JE, Mulliken JB, Kaban LB, Belfer M. Twenty-year experience in maxillocraniofacial surgery: An evaluation of early surgery on growth, function and body image. *Ann Surg* 190:320, 1979.
6. Munro IR. One stage reconstruction of the temporomandibular joint in hemifacial

microsomia. *Plast Reconstr Surg* 66:669, 1980.

7. Ortiz Monasterio F. Early mandibular and maxillary osteotomies for the correction of hemifacial microsomia. *Clin Plast Surg* November, 1982.
8. Illizarov GA, Soybelman LM, Chirkova AM. Some roentgenographic and morphologic data on bone tissue regeneration in distraction epiphysiolysis in experiment. *Orto Traumato Protol* 31:26, 1970.
9. Illizarov GA, Devyatov AA, Kamerin VK. Plastic reconstruction of longitudinal bone defects by means of compression and subsequent distraction. *Acta Chir Plast* 22:32, 1980.
10. Snyder CC, Levine GA, Swanson HM, Browne EZ. Mandibular lengthening by gradual distraction. Preliminary report. *Plast Reconstr Surg* 51:506, 1973.
11. Michieli S, Miotti B. Lengthening of mandibular body by gradual surgical orthodontic distraction. *J Oral Surg* 35:187, 1977.
12. Karp NS, Thorne CH, McCarthy JG et al. Bone lengthening in the craniofacial skeleton. *Ann Plast Surg* 24:231, 1990.
13. McCarthy JG, Schreider J, Karp N, Thorne CH, Grayson BH. Lengthening the human mandible by gradual distraction. *Plast Reconstr Surg* 89:1, 1992.
14. Molina F, Ortiz Monasterio F. Extended indications for mandibular distraction: Unilateral, bilateral and bidirectional. In: *Craniofacial Surgery 5*, Ortiz Monasterio F, editor. Bologna, Italy: Monduzzi; 1993.
15. Molina F, Ortiz Monasterio F. Mandibular elongation and remodeling by distraction: A farewell to major osteotomies. *Plast Reconstr Surg* 96:4, 825–1842, 1995.
16. Pruzansky S. Not all dwarfed mandibles are alike. *Birth Defects* 1:120, 1969.
17. Björk A, Skieller V. Normal and abnormal growth of the mandible. A synthesis of longitudinal cephalometric implant studies over a period of 25 years. *Eur J Orthod* 5:1, 1983.

CHAPTER 7

Intraoral Distraction

Cesar A. Guerrero and William H. Bell

In 1905, Codivilla (1) first reported the lengthening of the femur to correct a limb length discrepancy through osseous distraction, which was performed immediately after the fracture occurred. In 1927, Abbott (2) described lengthening in the tibia. However, the true clinical impact was not realized until the early 1950s when Ilizarov (3) began his long venture into clinical, biological, engineering, and basic science research in the fields of traumatology and orthopedics, utilizing the canine long bone as a model. These endeavors led to the discovery of general principles governing the stimulation of tissue growth and regeneration during distraction. Ilizarov designed the first scientific protocol on human bone lengthening. He demonstrated that gradual traction on living tissues created stresses that stimulated and maintained the regeneration and active growth of certain tissue structures (4). In subsequent studies (5–7), he showed that tissues subjected to slow, steady traction became metabolically activated. This phenomenon was characterized by the stimulation of both proliferative and biosynthetic cellular functions. Ilizarov noted that the quality and quantity of newly formed bone depended on a number of factors: (1) the rigidity of bone fragment fixation; (2) the degree of damage at the time of the osteotomy to the bone marrow, the periosteal soft tissues, and the nutrient artery and its branches; (3) the rate of distraction; and (4) the rhythm (frequency) of distraction.

In 1973, Snyder and colleagues (8) and, in 1977, Michieli and Miotti (9) demonstrated osseous lengthening by gradual distraction of the membranous bone of the canine mandible. They illustrated a specially fabricated tooth-borne apparatus to distract and later stabilize the mandibular segments. Their work showed the anchoring potential of mandibular teeth. In 1990, McCarthy and his group at New York University presented a study confirming the feasibility of mandibular lengthening through distraction in canine mandibles (10). Later they demonstrated cortical bone formation in the distraction gap of the mandible, as documented by radiographic, histologic, and vital dye studies (11). Constantino and his colleagues (12) reported on the experimental regeneration of bone (transport distraction) within a segmental mandibular defect in canine models.

In 1976, Bell and Epker (13) described a technique called Rapid Palatal Expansion to increase the maxillary width in cases of transverse deficiency. They placed a Haas appliance soldered to bands on the first maxillary premolars and molars to maintain the interarch width. The maxilla was mobilized by lateral osteotomies, pterygomaxillary disjunction, minimal down fracture of the maxillary segments, and a vertical osteotomy in the midline. The appliance was activated to the point where blanching of the gingival cuff tissues adjacent to the distraction site was evident. Postoperatively, the appliance was further activated approximately 1 mm every other day. Using this method, 10 mm of expansion could be obtained in 20 days.

Guerrero (14) described a mandibular symphysis osteotomy technique to widen the mandible in eleven patients who exhibited transverse mandibular deficiency (ranging from 4–7 mm). A tooth-borne appliance was used. The results revealed a stable expansion without temporomandibular joint dysfunction, periodontal problems, or evidence of malunion. Orthodontic correction of anterior crowding was also attained postoperatively. The average expansion was 5.05 mm (range: 4–7 mm).

McCarthy and associates (15) reported and popularized in 1991 a technique using an external bone lengthening device to obtain gradual distraction of the mandibles in four children with craniofacial microsomia. They used a modified external fixator with two double pin holders and a bolt at one end that allowed calibrated distraction of the pins. The patient remained in fixation for a 7-day latency period, following which the device was lengthened serially 1 mm per day for 20 consecutive days, obtaining an average augmentation of 20 mm. After the active distraction period, the patients were maintained in external fixation for an average of 9 weeks. Another important contribution was made by Molina and Ortiz-Monasterio (16), who used an external biphasic appliance for bidirectional mandibular ramus lengthening.

In 1992, Guerrero and Contasti (17) described in detail the orthodontic principles of mandibular widening through distraction osteogenesis, the clinical application and the surgical alternatives. Later in 1995, a surgical intraoral mandibular distraction technique was applied in 20 patients. This technique used either a tooth-borne or bone-borne distractor appliance to promote osseous growth in different mandibular sites (18). In addition, ten patients were treated to widen and lengthen the maxilla by maxillary osteotomies and anterior elastic traction (19). In 1996, Chin and Toth (20) described the feasibility and potential advantages of using internal devices for distraction osteogenesis in the management of maxillofacial skeletal deficiencies. Recently, Bell and his colleagues (21–22) reported on the biology of distraction osteogenesis associated with mandibular widening and the histologic changes in the temporomandibular joint after mandibular midline osteodistraction.

INTRAORAL MANDIBULAR DISTRACTION TECHNIQUES

Widening of the Symphysis or Parasymphysis Region

Lingual Tooth-Borne Appliances

The intraoral incision is made 4 to 6 mm labial to the depth of the mandibular vestibule. The dissection is directed obliquely, posteriorly, and inferiorly through the mentalis muscle until contact is made with the mandibular symphysis. The periosteum is reflected inferiorly to the lower border of the mandible, where a small channel retractor is placed. The periosteum is carefully elevated and meticulously separated, keeping in mind that much of the healing capacity in distraction originates from the periosteum. The soft tissue between the mandibular central incisors is carefully reflected superiorly to the alveolar crest with minimal detachment of the neighboring tissues. A skin hook is used to reflect the flap superiorly (Figure 7.1).

A vertical osteotomy is made through the symphyseal area with a reciprocating or oscillating saw blade, starting at the inferior border of the mandible and continuing to the interdental space between the apices of the mandibular incisors. With a straight-hand piece and a surgical burr, the cut is continued through the labial cortical plate of the mandible to the alveolar crest (Figure 7.2). The final sectioning is done with a mallet and a spatula osteotome (Figure 7.3). The forefinger should be used as a guide at all times to avoid tearing of the lingual soft tissues. Excessive pressure on the mandible should be avoided to prevent displacement of the Hyrax appliance, which is

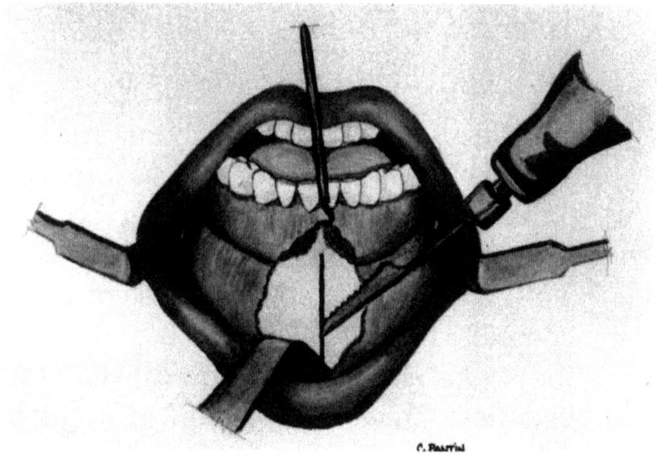

Figure 7.1. A retractor is placed in the inferior border of the mandible, and a vertical osteotomy is made with a reciprocating saw.

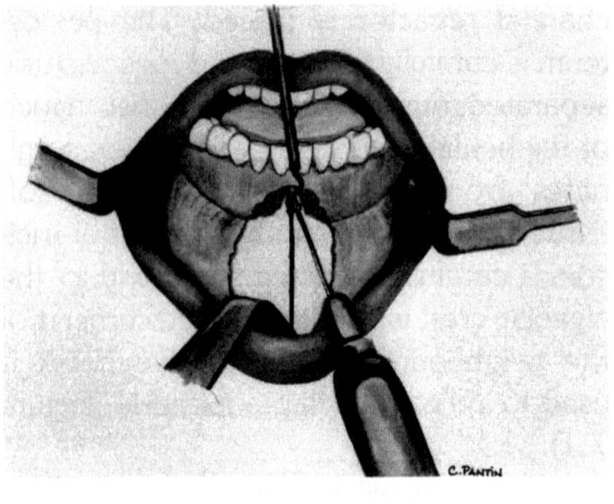

Figure 7.2. The osteotomy line is completed with a burr until the alveolar crest is reached.

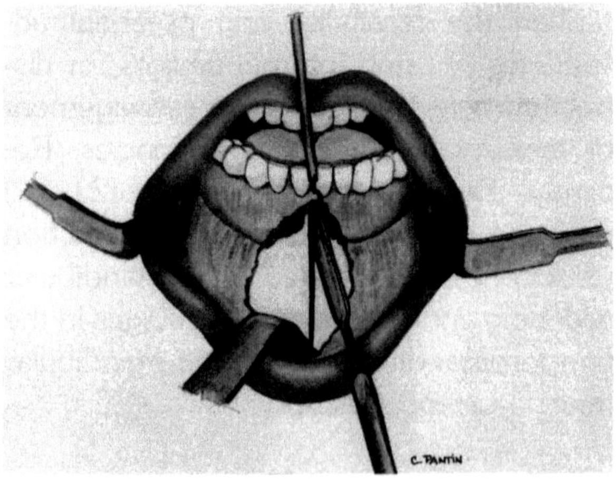

Figure 7.3. The final sectioning of the mandible is made with a spatula osteotome and a mallet.

bonded to the mandibular teeth by the orthodontist one to two days prior to surgery.

After the vertical osteotomy and sectioning of the mandible are completed, a guide pin is inserted into the Hyrax appliance. It is activated to produce immediate expansion of the mandibular arch. The activating pin possesses a security thread to avoid inadvertent displacement. Expansion should be done judiciously to achieve only a 2-mm opening. Stretching of the gingival interdental tissues will determine the amount of expansion feasible during the surgical procedure. Blanching of the interdental tissues mandates immediate cessation of the activation of the osteodistractor appliance. A layered closure of the surgical wound is made.

Buccal Bone-Borne versus Lingual Tooth-Borne Appliances

A horizontal labial flap is made with an incision 6 mm from the depth of the vestibule in the mucosa of the everted lower lip (canine to canine) through the orbicularis oris muscle. After transecting the muscle, the dissection is directed obliquely, posteriorly, and inferiorly through the mentalis muscle. The periosteum is reflected inferiorly to the lower border of the mandible, where a channel retractor is placed. The soft tissue between the mandibular central incisors is carefully reflected superiorly using a skin hook. A vertical osteotomy is made starting from the inferior portion of the mental symphysis, below the level of the incisors. The bone is sectioned using a reciprocating saw starting at the superior margin of the retracted soft tissue flap. The labial cortical plate and alveolar bone immediately below the incisor apices are sectioned with a fissure bur using copious irrigation.

After the buccal cortical osteotomy is completed, the appliance is adapted over the bone surface and fixed with four bicortical screws 10 to 12 mm in length by

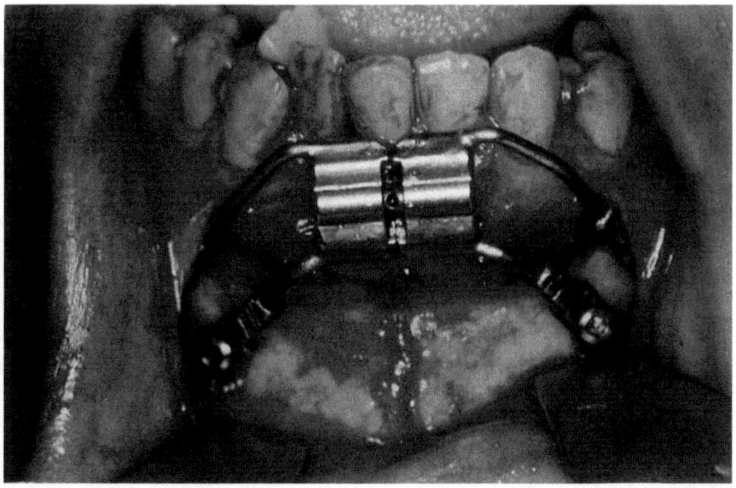

Figure 7.4. Intraoperative view of a mandibular widening in the symphyseal area with a bone-borne appliance.

2 mm in diameter (Figures 7.4 and 7.5). With the appliance in place, the lingual cortex is sectioned by malleting a spatula osteotome from the alveolar crest to the inferior border of the mandible. The appliance is turned 2 mm to assure separation of the margins of bone segments. The labial mucoperiosteal flap is repositioned, and the periosteum and the mentalis muscle are reattached to their origins with 3-0 chromic catgut sutures. The mucosa is closed with running resorbable 3-0 chromic catgut sutures.

Either the tooth-borne or bone-borne appliance will widen the mandible. The tooth-borne osteodistractor tends to widen more superiorly than at the inferior border of the mandible. The opposite is true regarding the bone-borne appliance. In either situation it is wise to have avail-

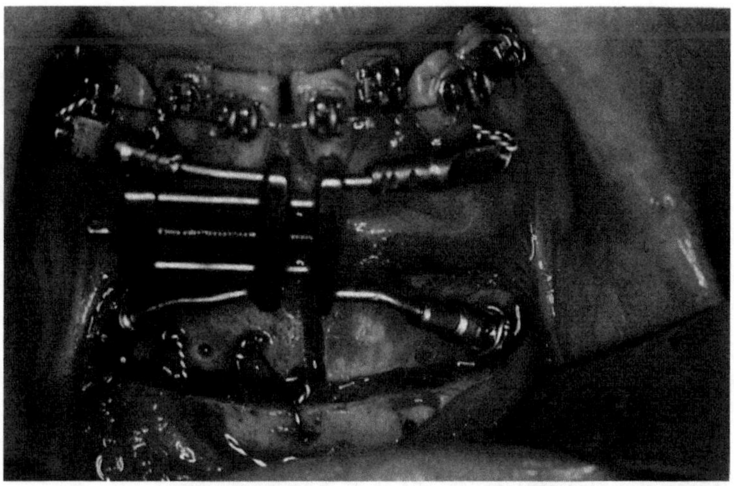

Figure 7.5. Another type of bone-borne appliance. Two o-ring ends were used to fix the upper arms with wires and resin to the mandibular canines (the root position made it impossible to place screws in that area). The distraction procedure was combined with a genioplasty. The use of the "four-wire-technique" for chin fixation allows postsurgical distraction.

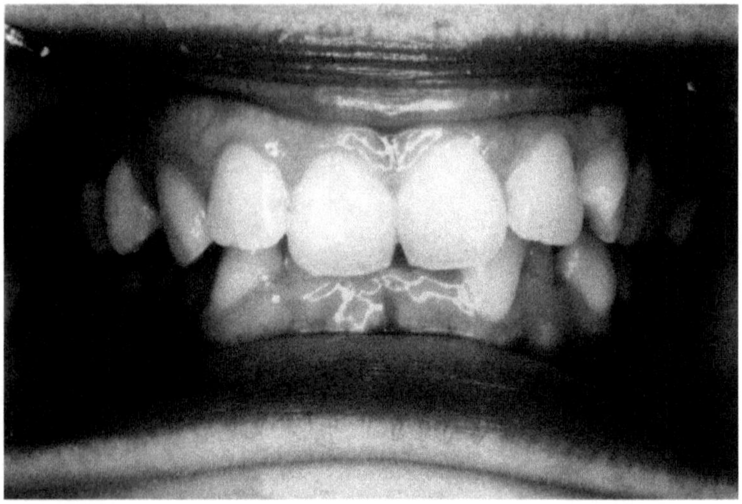

Figure 7.6. Preoperative intraoral views showing the lack of space in the mandibular arch and the consequent anterior dental crowding.

able an extra bone-borne appliance to widen the mandible in the event that the tooth borne appliance is dislocated during surgery.

Representative cases are illustrated in Figures 7.6 through 7.14.

Ramus Osteotomy Distraction

A 3-cm incision is made over the external oblique line, midway up the ascending ramus and extending inferiorly over the alveolar ridge to a position opposite the first molar. Subperiosteal tunneling dissection is performed using a periosteal elevator to expose the buccal cortex, mandibular angle, and alveolar ridge. The periosteum, muscles, and soft tissues are minimally detached in order to maintain blood supply.

With an inferior border channel retractor positioned between the second

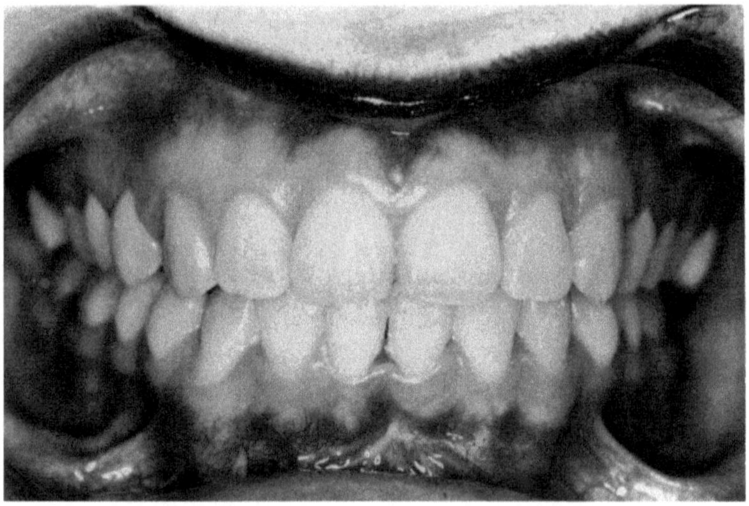

Figure 7.7. Postoperative intraoral view. An adequate occlusion can be noted after intraoral mandibular osteodistraction.

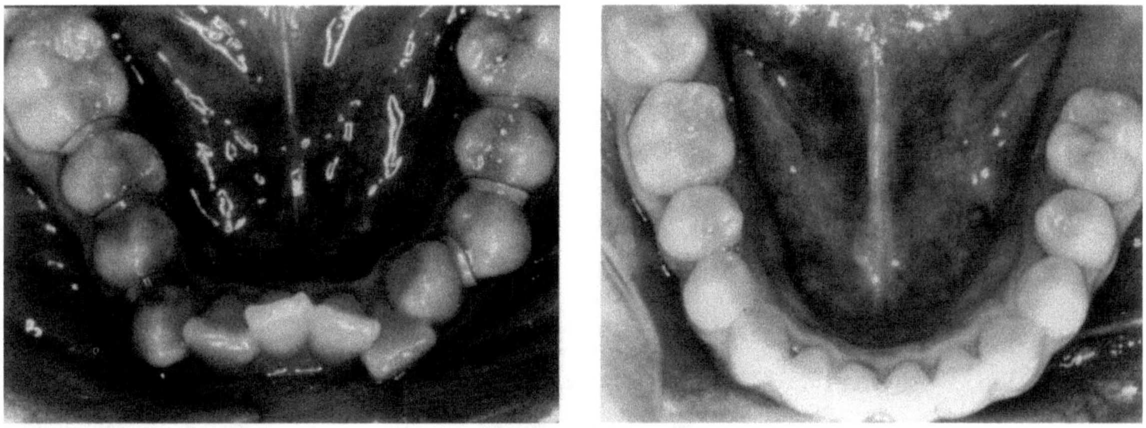

Figure 7.8. Pre- (left) and postoperative (right) occlusal views. Correction of the dental crowding, a U-shaped arch, and an optimal dental alignment were accomplished with dental extractions.

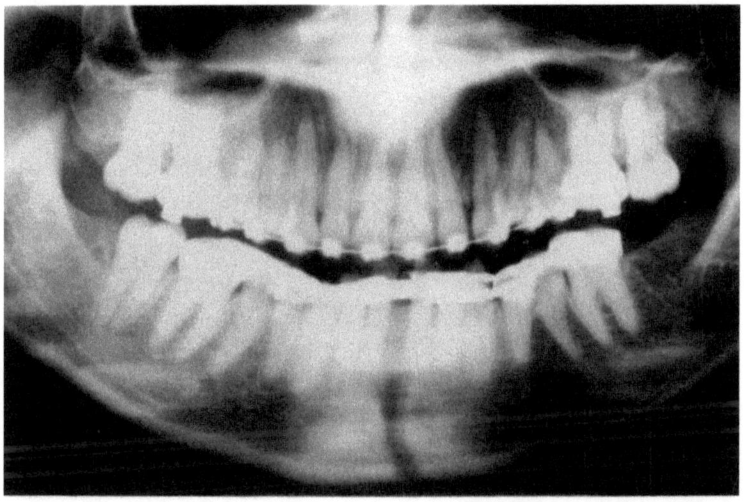

Figure 7.9. Panoramic radiograph immediately after surgery showing the vertical osteotomy in the symphyseal area along with the interdental gap.

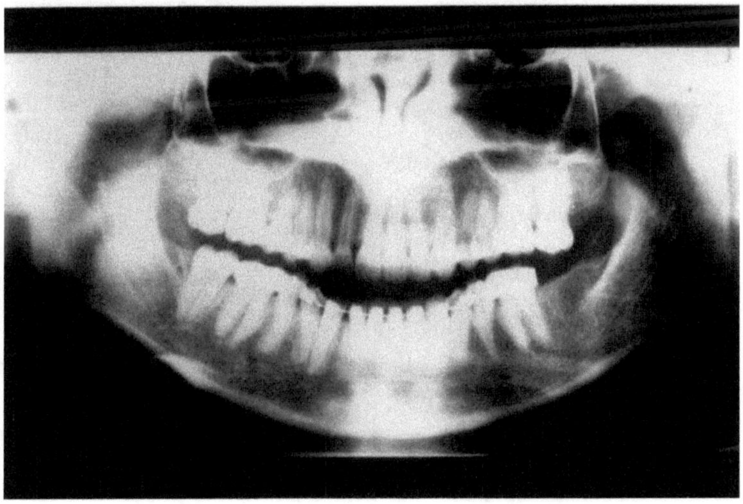

Figure 7.10. Panoramic radiograph one year after surgery showing a complete ossification at the osteotomy site.

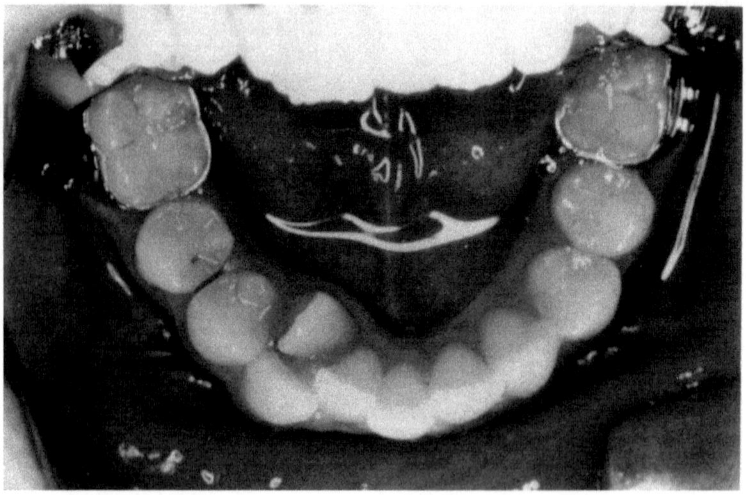

Figure 7.11. Occlusal (mandibular) view before distraction. Note the lack of space for the mandibular lateral incisor.

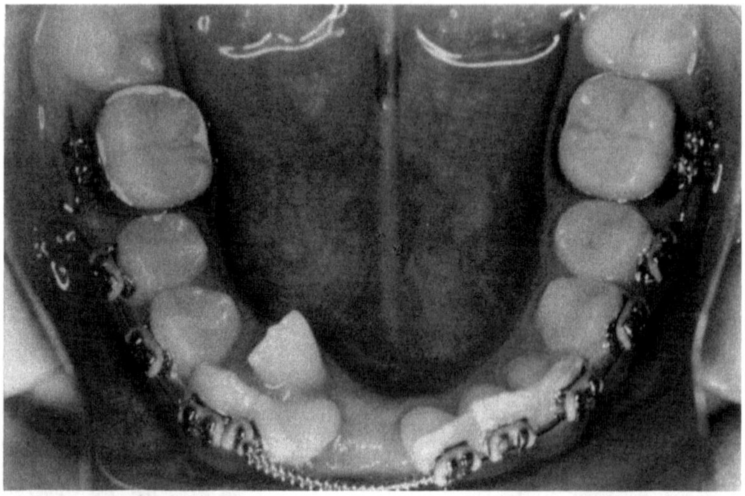

Figure 7.12. Occlusal (mandibular) view immediately after distraction. Note the gap obtained to allow an adequate alignment of the lateral incisor.

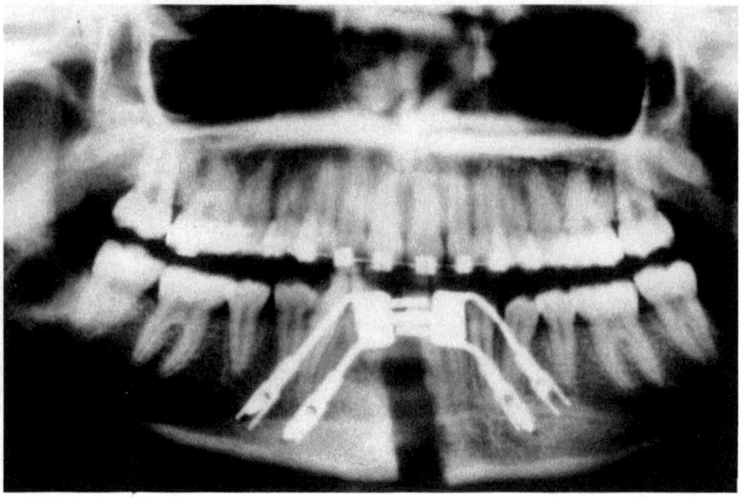

Figure 7.13. Panoramic radiograph immediately after mandibular distraction with a bone-borne appliance placed on the symphyseal area. The distraction achieved in this case was 10 mm.

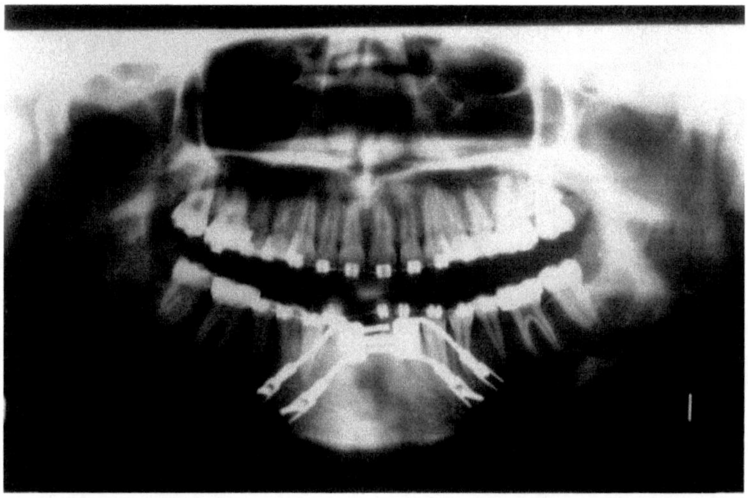

Figure 7.14. Panoramic radiograph after the stabilization period. The optimal quality of the regenerate bone can be appreciated.

and third molars, a reciprocating saw is used to etch the planned osteotomy into the mandibular surface and transect the cortical bone at the inferior mandibular border (Figure 7.15A). This is completely sectioned vertically up to a position within 3 mm from the inferior alveolar canal. The saw blade is repositioned to section the buccal cortex (Figure 7.15B). Finally the saw is reversed and the osteotomy is carried through the alveolar crest superoinferiorly (Figure 7.15C) to a point approximately 3 mm superior to the inferior alveolar canal. A periosteal elevator is used to protect the lingual periosteum and guard against lingual nerve injury. At this juncture the ramus osteotomy has been completed (Figure 7.15D), with the exception of a 5-mm section of bone posterior to the inferior alveolar nerve. All of the region is irrigated with normal saline to minimize thermal bone injury. Care is also taken to preserve the dental follicies and inferior alveolar nerve.

Lengthening is performed using a miniaturized intraoral stainless steel distractor that is sectioned and preshaped before surgery with the aid of the most current cephalometric and panotamic radiographs; only minor adaptations are usually necessary to position the device at the time of surgery. Following the osteotomy, the distraction device, consisting of a central body connected to four arms, is adapted over the mandibular surface and fixed with two posterior bicortical (7–9 mm × 2 mm) screws (Figure 7.15E). Bicortical screws are routinely used unless a tooth or nerve is subjacent to the lateral cortex; in this event monocortical bone screws are used.

The posterior arms of the appliance are positioned beneath the mucosa approximately 5 mm distal to the osteotomy. The appliance is fixed parallel to the mandibular body surface with the two bicortical screws (attachment sites of the anterior arms) placed approximately 35 mm mesial to the osteotomy. The

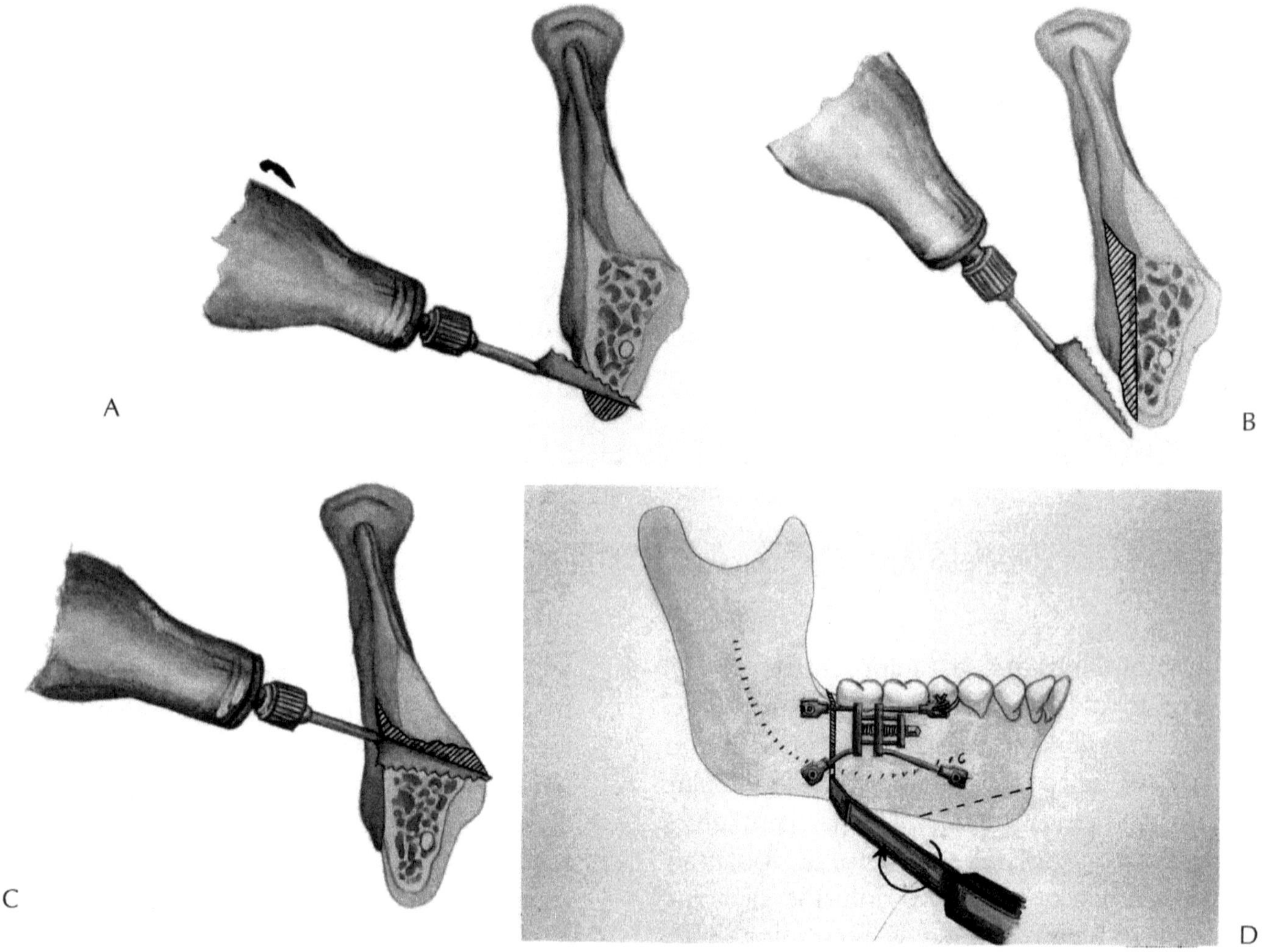

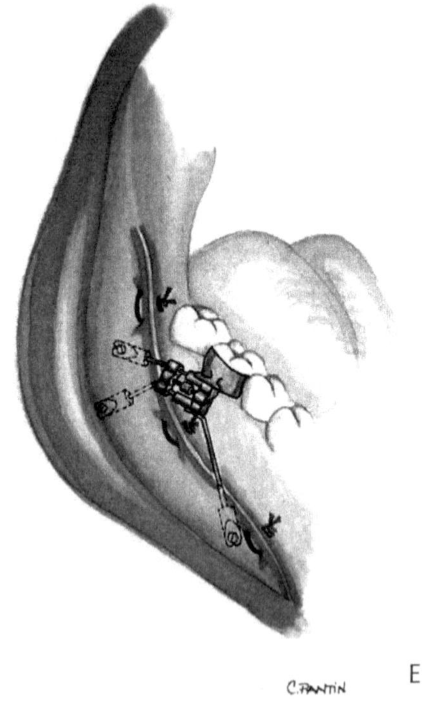

Figure 7.15. Surgical technique of ramus osteotomy-mandibular intraoral distraction. (A) The osteotomy is performed with a reciprocating saw beginning in the inferior border of the mandible. (B) The vertical ramus osteotomy is made with the reciprocating saw, which extends through the cortical bone and into the cancellous bone for several millimeters. (C) At the superior border, the saw is turned from top to bottom until it is approximately 3 mm away from the nerve. (D) The distractor is fixed in the proper position and, with a spatula osteotome, the complete separation of the bone segments is performed at the inferior border and buccal osteotomy site. (E) A suture is used to close the wound. The screw and the anterosuperior arm of the appliance are left over the mucosa, in order to allow postoperative activation of the device.

distraction device can be either a bone-borne or a hybrid bone-tooth supported appliance cemented or fixed with screws. The osteotomy of the lingual cortex is completed by lightly tapping a spatula osteotome through the inferior border (Figure 7.15D).

After the distraction device is well fixed, the ramus is completely sectioned with a straight chisel tapped lightly between the proximal and distal segments at the inferior border of the mandible. However, when both sides are to be distracted, final sectioning of the ramus is deferred until the osteotomy of the opposite side is completed. The appliance is activated to achieve a 2-mm separation of the segments.

The mucoperiosteal flap is repositioned and maintained in place by horizontal mattress sutures (Figure 7.15E). The three arms of the distractor device are positioned submucosally. The body and the anterior-superior arm are exposed to the oral vestibule to facilitate subsequent activation of the device. After the stabilization period has elapsed, the distractor is divided into two sections to facilitate its removal. The three fork-type limbs are withdrawn leaving the three screws behind, thus obviating the need for a second surgical procedure.

There are situations in which the anterior arms remain over the mucosa, and transmucosal screws will be used to fix the appliance to the underlying bone; this is particularly true in patients with deep lateral vestibules. The advantages are that the appliances are simple to clean, facilitate screw placement and permit easy removal.

Body Osteotomy-Distraction

An incision is placed in the vestibule near the external oblique ridge of the mandible. As previously noted, the periosteal dissection is kept to a minimum.

In the body osteotomy technique, the distraction device is again modified. O-Rings and interdental wires are fixed to a tooth anterior and posterior to the planned osteotomy site and stabilized with acrylic or resin. The osseous fixation is maintained by two fork-type arms and two bicortical screws. Accordingly, care must be taken to preserve the dental follicles and inferior alveolar nerve. In addition, *the metal structure of the device should be positioned parallel to the mandibular occlusal plane to allow for easy activation to achieve the planned distraction vector*. A vertical osteotomy is accomplished with the reciprocating saw to section the inferior border. The osteotomy is made with a burr in a straight handpiece. The osteotomy is completed by carefully tapping a spatula osteotome into the incompletely sectioned bone.

The distractor is activated to the point at which the interdental gingival soft tissue begins to blanch. After the elapsed latency period, the distraction rate (1 mm daily) is the same as that described in the former procedure, until the desired anatomic position is accomplished. At the end of the stabilization or consolidation period, the appliance is sectioned and removed in the same fashion as described in the ramus osteotomy technique.

Soft tissue closure is similar to the technique outlined in the section detailing the ramus osteotomy, with the exception that both the superior limbs and body of the appliance remain exposed intraorally. The subsequent removal is performed in a fashion similar to that of the ramus.

After the osteotomy, a latency period of 7 days elapses before commencing active distraction. Most importantly, the mucosa must be stretched slowly to avoid tearing and consequent periodontal wound healing problems.

The distraction of the screw is done at a rate of 1 mm a day, until the desired expansion is obtained. This is preferably performed by the surgeon or office staff instead of the patient to control the rate, rhythm, and amount of movement. A small overcorrection is indicated in the majority of patients.

After the desired distraction is obtained, cold cured acrylic is applied over the distraction device screw to minimize changes and provide appliance stability. Follow up radiographs are obtained immediately to assess the distraction gap and the position of the appliance. A monthly radiograph in the postoperative period helps to establish the duration of the stabilization period, usually between two and three months.

INTRAORAL MAXILLARY DISTRACTION TECHNIQUES

Maxillary deficiency may be present in a wide variety of clinical situations: vertical, anteroposterior, or transverse dimensions. It is frequently associated with nasal, malar, and infraorbital deficiencies. Maxillary distraction can therefore be applied in multiple ways to individualize the surgical plan based on esthetic and functional requirements.

Maxillary Widening

A Hyrax® appliance is bonded to the maxillary first or second molars and the first or second maxillary premolars bilaterally depending on the patient's presenting dentition. This is usually accomplished one to two days before surgery.

After the patient is properly sedated, local anesthetic solution with a vasoconstrictor is infiltrated into the labiobuccal vestibule, pterygomaxillary fossa, infraorbital nerves, and palatal region. A horizontal incision is made through the mucoperiosteum above the mucogingival junction, extending from the region of the maxillary first premolar of one side to the contralateral first premolar.

A horizontal osteotomy is made through the right and left lateral maxillary walls approximately 5 mm superior to the apices of teeth (the canine root serving as the reference) (Figure 7.16). It is extended from the lateral aspect of the pyriform aperture to the junction of the maxillary tuberosity and pterygoid plates. The inclination of the osteotomy from the maxillary tuberosity to the pyriform aperture (superoinferior, horizontal, or inferiosuperior) is critical and determines the ultimate vertical relationship (an increase, decrease, or no change in the vertical dimension of the maxilla). After complete mobilization of the partially downfractured maxilla is achieved by forward pressure against the maxillary tuberosities, a straight osteotome is used to separate the anterior nasal spine; a forked osteotome is tapped posteriorly approximately 30 mm to separate the nasal septum and vomer from the hard palate; the spatula osteotome is manipulated between the

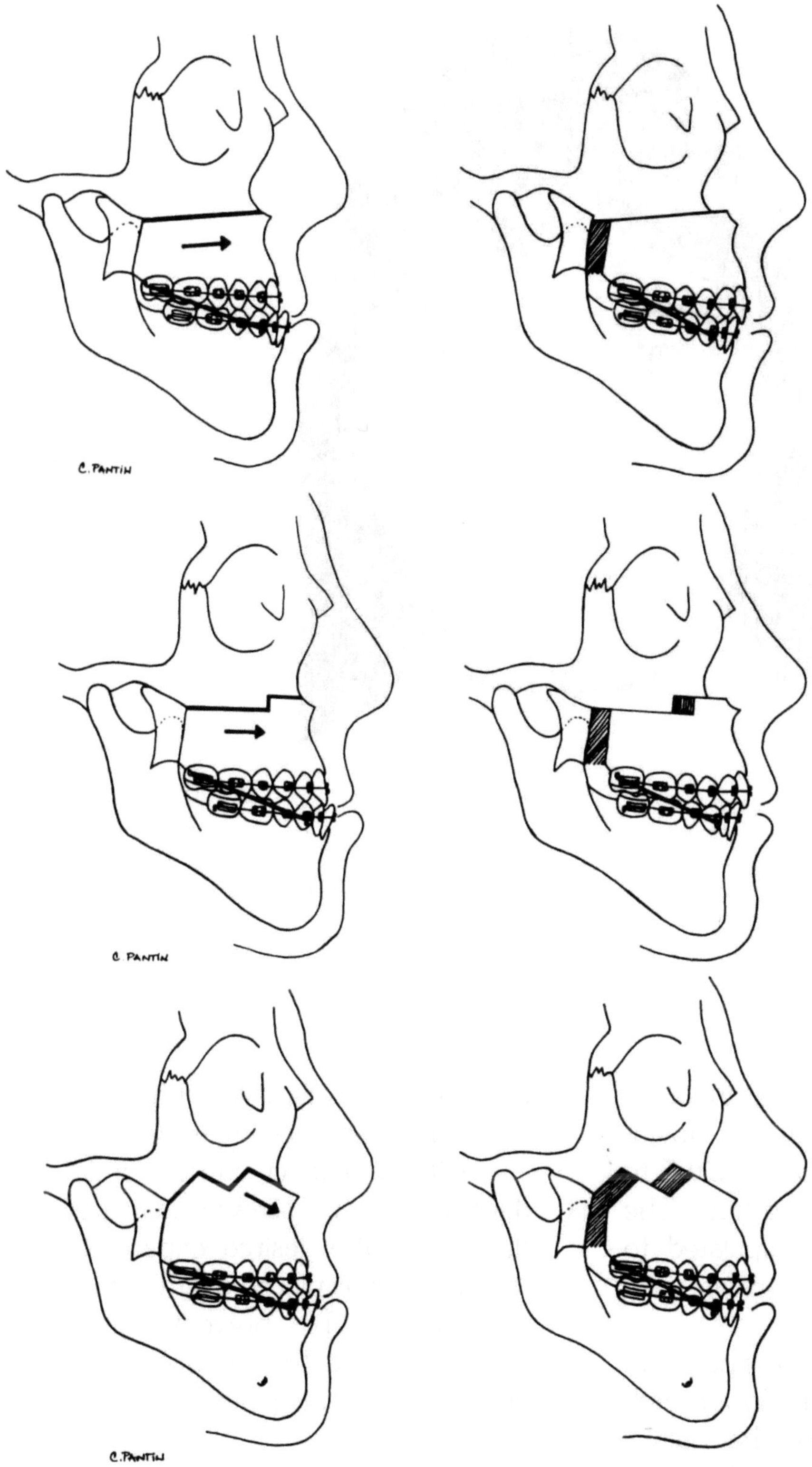

A

B

C

Figure 7.16. (A) Cephalometric prediction of an anterosuperior movement with an oblique inferosuperior osteotomy (inclination is based on individual patient requirements). (B) Cephalometric prediction of the horizontal maxillary movement with a step osteotomy (maxillary advancement). (C) Cephalometric prediction of an anteroinferior maxillary movement with M-osteotomy.

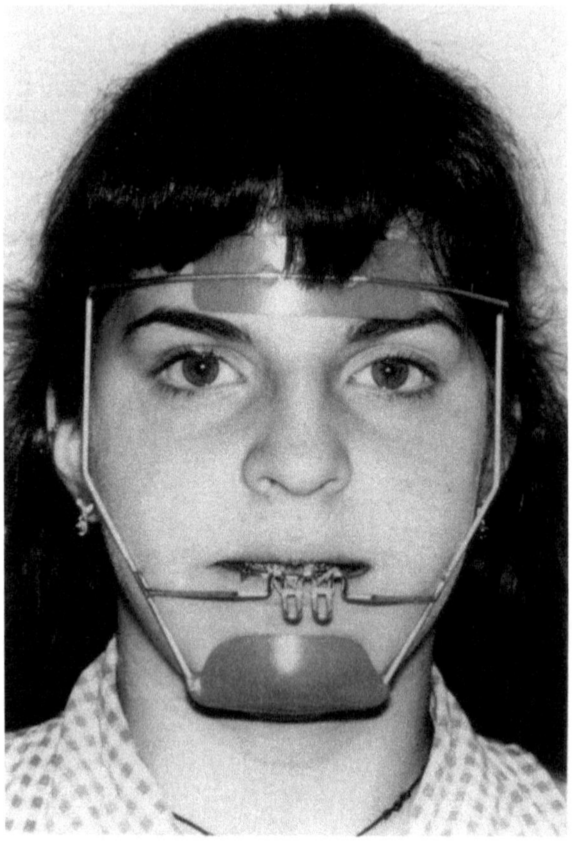

Figure 7.17. Delaire mask used by a patient with an anteroposterior maxillary deficiency, who already underwent maxillary distraction.

alveolus of the central incisors, in order to complete the osteotomy. A downfracture is performed, approximately 5 to 7 mm from the pyriform aperture. The vertical osteotomies are manipulated to complete the splitting of the palate into two halves.

At this moment, two bite-blocks are placed between the upper and lower teeth to prevent displacement of the palatal distractor. The Hyrax® is activated and the maxilla expanded 2 mm to achieve visual separation of the segments with no evidence of blanching of the gingival tissue. If tearing of the gingival cuff occurs, the expansion is immediately terminated.

After a latency period of 7 to 10 days, the Hyrax® screw is activated 1 mm daily, until the desired expansion is obtained. Resin is placed over the Hyrax® for stabilization. To prevent any further movement and to enhance appearance, an acrylic tooth is placed in the midline.

Maxillary Lengthening

Heavy orthodontic arch wires are placed before surgery to avoid extrusion of the lower anterior teeth and undesirable compensations. Hooks are soldered to the maxillary arch before surgery to facilitate appropriate elastic traction facilitated by the use of the Delaire facial mask (Figure 7.17).

The surgical procedure is performed as just described for the maxillary widening technique (see Figure 7.16).

Seven to 10 days after surgery, two 3.5-oz Class III elastics are placed from the band on the maxillary second molar extending to the mandibular canine, bilaterally. A Delaire facial mask is used after a latency period of 7 to 10 days until the majority of the planned anterior movement is obtained. It is applied for 10 to 12 daytime hours and during the night. A force of up to 2 lbs. is utilized on the facial mask. The elastics are used whenever the patient is not wearing the mask. Consequently, there is no direct detrimental force applied to the temporomandibular joints and retroinclination of the mandibular incisors is prevented. Intermaxillary elastics are changed every other day, until the desired anterior movement is obtained. At this time, bilateral light Class III elastics are utilized to maintain the new position.

Preoperative and postoperative cephalometric planning studies and panoramic radiographs are used to document skeletal and dental movement, osseous healing, and inclinations of the teeth. All patients are clinically examined and photographed. From cephalometric planning studies and analysis of the occlusion, the osteotomy design and distraction vectors are planned.

There has been no evidence of tooth devitalization. All patients showed evidence of osseous union through clinical and radiographic examination. After expansion of the maxillary arch is obtained in two dimensions, the dental arches are properly aligned and stabilized through orthodontic therapy with a Class I canine and molar occlusion (Figure 7.18).

INTRAORAL MAXILLO-MALAR DISTRACTION TECHNIQUES

Maxillary-malar deficiency is a common deformity that exhibits a true malar and infraorbital rim retrusion relative to the position of the globes. This clinical problem has been traditionally managed by major LeFort III-type osteotomies and bone grafts with extensive rigid fixation required. An alternative treatment is maxillo-malar distraction.

Surgical Technique

Under controlled hypotensive nasotracheal intubation anesthesia, the patient is placed in the supine position for application of a Dingman oral retractor. After local anesthetic solution is injected for hemostasis, an incision through the palatal mucosa is made from the first molar on one side to that on the contralateral side (around the necks of the teeth) to expose the entire palate and perform an inverted U-shaped palatal osteotomy (horseshoe shape) (Figure 7.19A). An anteroposterior distractor is placed after the complete malar-maxillary osteotomy is completed. After the Dingman retractor is removed, attention is focused on the

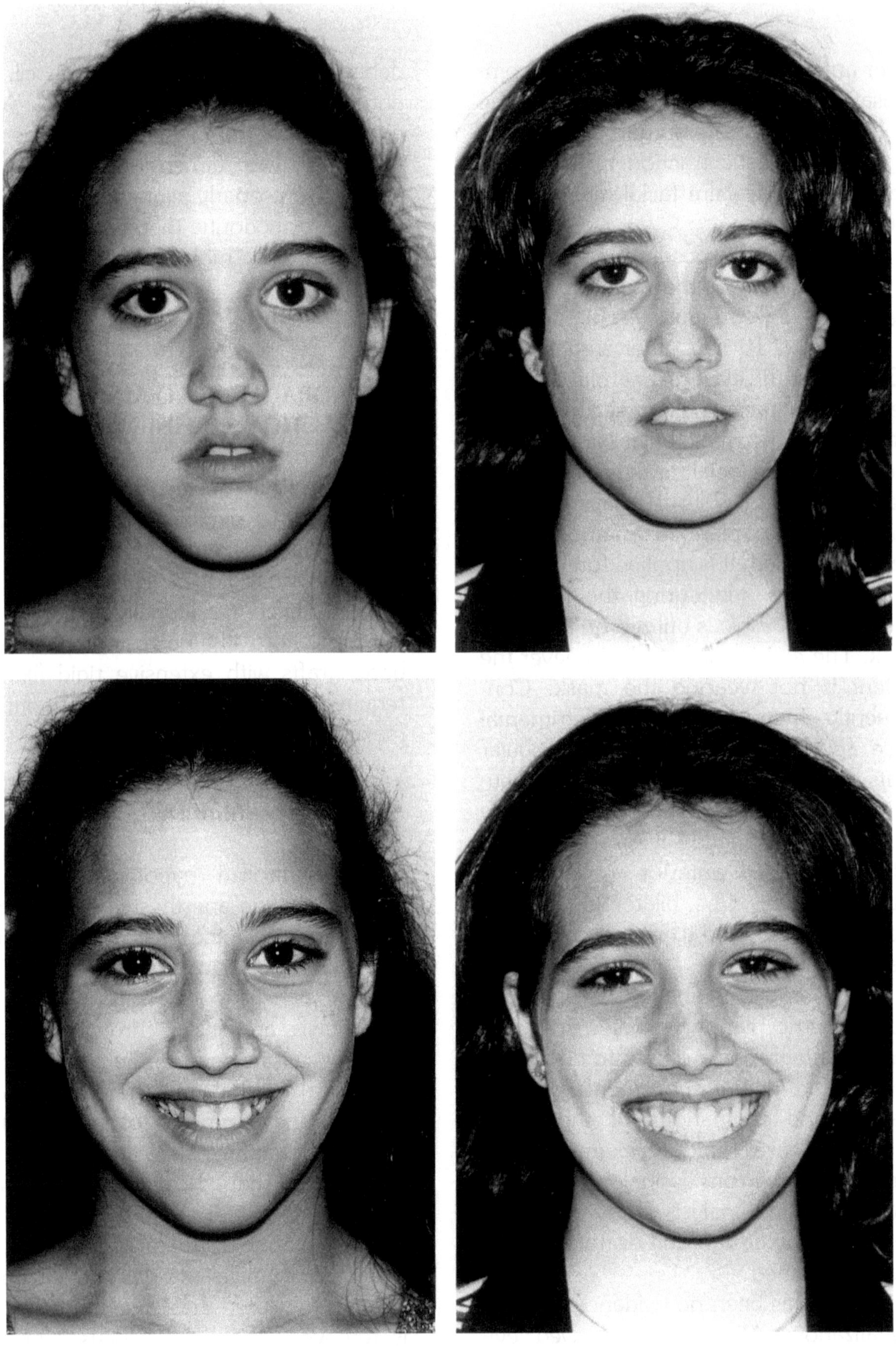

A B C D

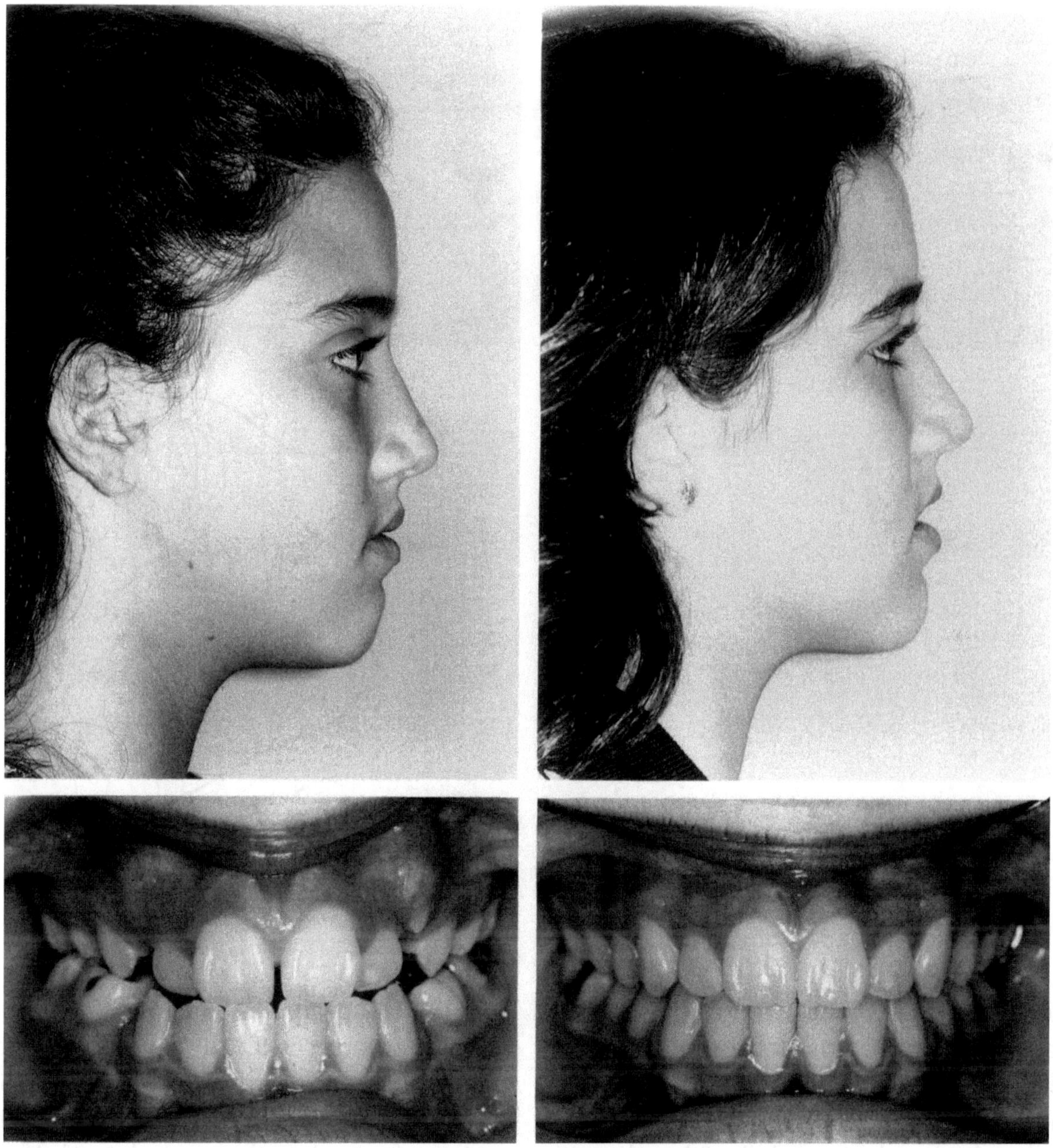

E F G H

Figure 7.18. (A) Preoperative frontal view of a patient with transverse and anteroposterior maxillary deficiency. The patient commenced the surgical-orthodontic treatment at the age of 12. (B) Postoperative frontal view four years after maxillary distraction. (C) Preoperative smiling view. (D) Postoperative smiling view. (E) Preoperative profile showing maxillary deficiency. (F) Postoperative profile. (G) Preoperative intraoral view showing the anteroposterior and transverse deficiencies. (H) Postoperative intraoral view four years after distraction. (I) Preoperative intraoral lateral view. (J) Postoperative intraoral lateral view. (K) Cephalometric analysis documenting the anterposterior movement of the maxilla (dotted lines represent post-distraction tracings).

(*Continued*)

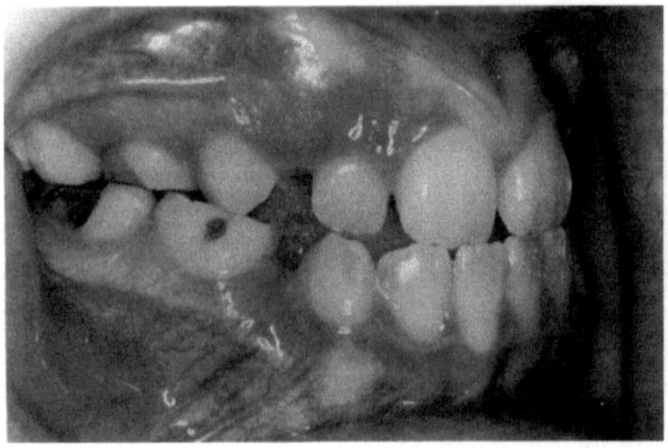

I

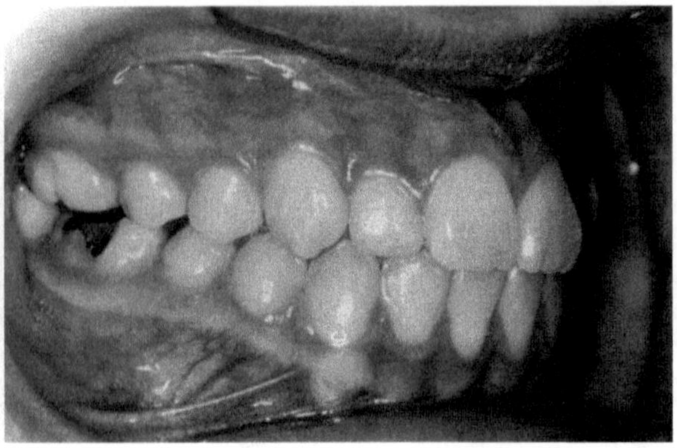

J

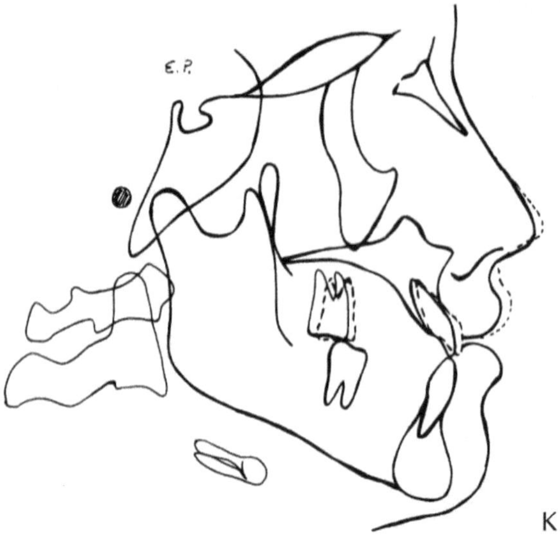

K

Figure 7.18. *Continued*

lateral maxillary wall where a 15-mm incision is made to elevate the mucoperiosteum as far as the infraorbital area and a tunnel is extended to the malar area. A straight hand piece drill with a bur is used to perform the ostetomy (Figure 7.19A).

The osteotomy design will vary according to the individual clinical situation. The osteotomy includes the malar bone divided in two (extended laterally above the infraorbital nerve and obliquely anterior to avoid the nasolacrimal duct, but as high as possible at the pyriform aperture). Posteriorly, an osteotomy is extended from the pterygomaxillary suture superior and anterior with a curved osteotome. The osteotomy reaches the posterior aspect of the zygoma. A similar osteotomy is performed on the contralateral side, taking care with the anterior soft tissue pedicle which will be the sole vascular pedicle for the anterior maxilla. The anterior flap is reflected laterally or a small vertical incision in the midline is used to separate the cartilaginous septum from the posterior bony septum, which is kept intact.

Two curved osteotomes are placed behind the maxillary tuberosities to dis-

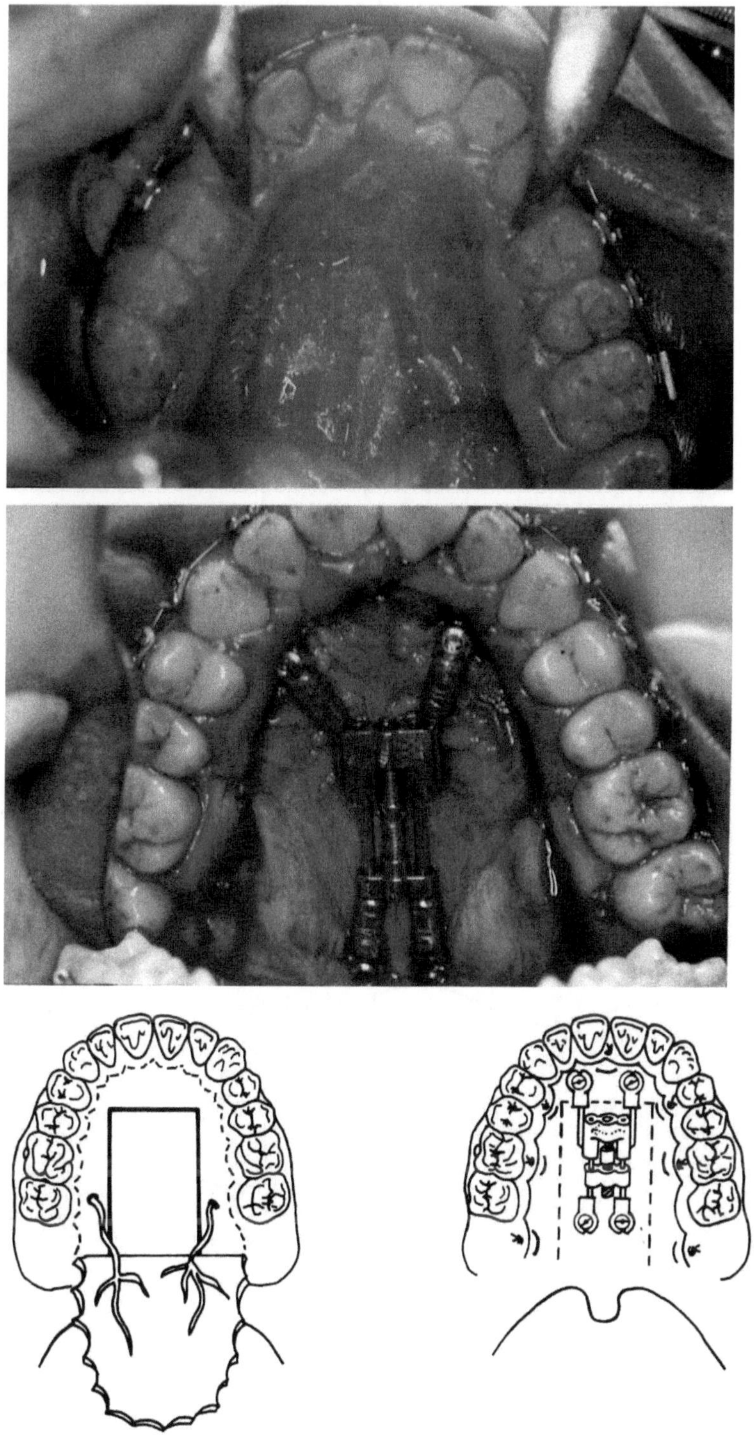
A
B
C

Figure 7.19. (A) A horseshoe incision is made from the first molar on one side to the opposite and an inverted U-shaped osteotomy is performed on the palate. (B) The distraction device is placed to control the anteroposterior movement of the maxilla. (C) Distraction device used in the palate to control anteroposterior movement of the maxilla.

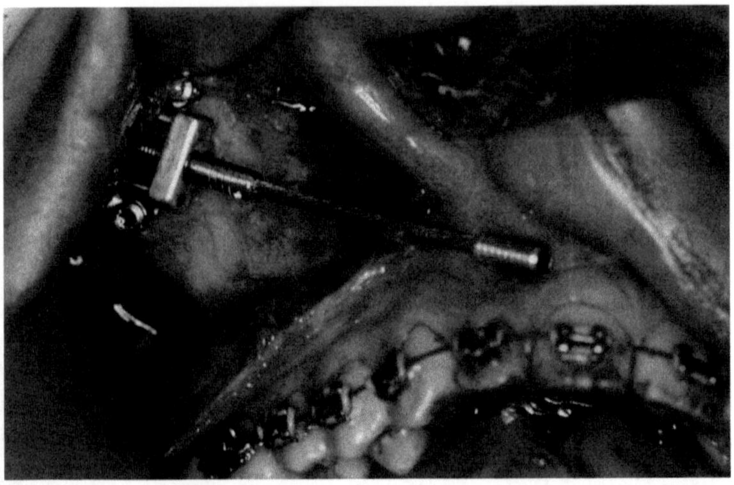

A

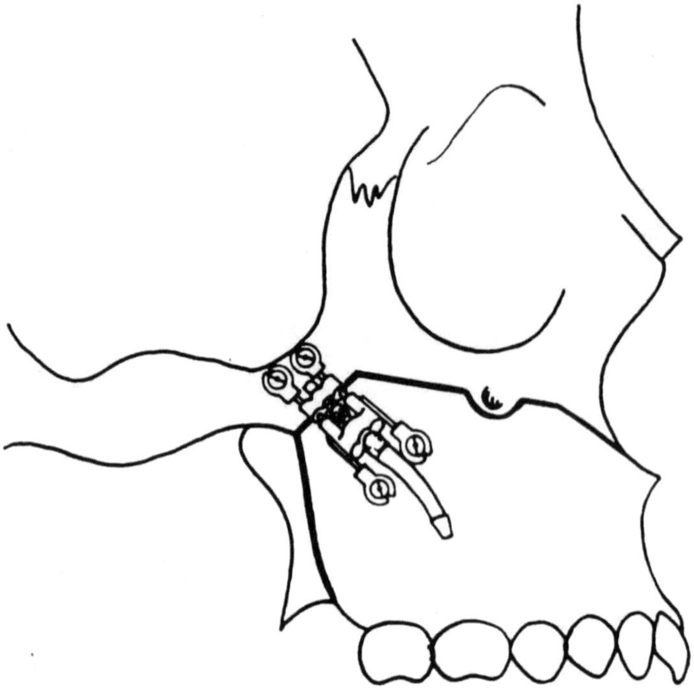

B

Figure 7.20. (A) Distraction device used for malar advancement. (B) Distraction device used in the malar region. The appliance has a conector to the oral cavity to allow postsurgical activation. The osteotomy line is designed to avoid damage to the infraorbital nerve and the nasolacrimal duct.

place the malar-maxillary complex. After it is completely mobile, the distractors are fixed. A palatal anterior positioning device is placed and secured with four (13 mm × 2 mm) screws, after the mucosa has been replaced and sutured (Figure 7.19B,C). The distractor and screws are fixed transmucosally.

One distractor is placed on either malar site; the anterior screws are secured transorally and the superoposterior ones are located with a neurosurgery trocar through the skin (Figure 7.20). A connector is attached to the activation screw head in the malar bone to activate the device in the oral cavity; the connector can be pulled and removed after the desired distraction is obtained. It is most important to place the distractor devices accurately in order to obtain proper direction of the movement; minimal variation in placement will deviate the whole maxilla vertically.

Distraction Protocol in Maxillo-Malar Lengthening

The distraction protocol is based on the clinical goal of an overcorrection of 20%; Class III elastics are indicated for 20 hours a day. After the appliances are removed three months after surgery, routine orthodontic mechanics are resumed. The palatal distractor controls the anteroposterior movement at the tooth level and limits any superoinferior movement tendency. The superior malar distractors project the infraorbital rims, malar bones, and perinasal area forward (Figure 7.21).

INTRAORAL BIFOCAL DISTRACTION MULTIPLANAR APPLIANCES

A careful cephalometric planning study is accomplished to simulate the desired post-treatment positional changes of the maxilla and mandible. In the child whose permanent teeth have not yet erupted, the planning studies may not involve immediate repositioning of the maxilla. Templates of the maxilla and mandible are made to simulate the vertical and anteroposterior positional changes. In the typical patient with mandibular deficiency (ie, anterior open bite and vertical maxillary deficiency), the initial planning simulation will be a ramus osteotomy to facilitate a vertical increase of mandibular ramus height. A simulation will be made of the necessary mandibular advancement to correct the Class II relationship and anterior open bite. The occlusal plane serves as a reference line for the planned vertical and horizontal positional changes of the mandible. By increasing the ramus height, the occlusal plane is decreased and the ramus and posterior facial height increased. The mandibular advancement is simulated by anterior repositioning of the mandibular template parallel with the desired occlusal plane.

In some cases the simulated movements create a posterior open bite. The simulations are the basis for the planned line of distraction, which parallels the occlusal plane. These complex movements can usually be best achieved by multiplanar distraction devices. A vertical increase of the ramus height combined with mandibular lengthening will be accomplished by intraoral osteodistractors. A careful study of the planned osteotomy and its relationship to erupted and unerupted teeth, the position of the mandibular canal and the quality and quantity of the bone stock is best made from radiographic analysis.

A 1.5-mm pilot hole is drilled into the proximal segment approximately 5 to 6 mm proximal to the planned osteotomy site (Figure 7.22). A second pilot hole is drilled 5 to 10 mm lateral to the first pilot hole. Care is taken to avoid injury to the inferior alveolar nerve. Transosseus screws (2 mm) are used to stabilize the plate to the ramus. Stabilization of the distal segment is accomplished in one of

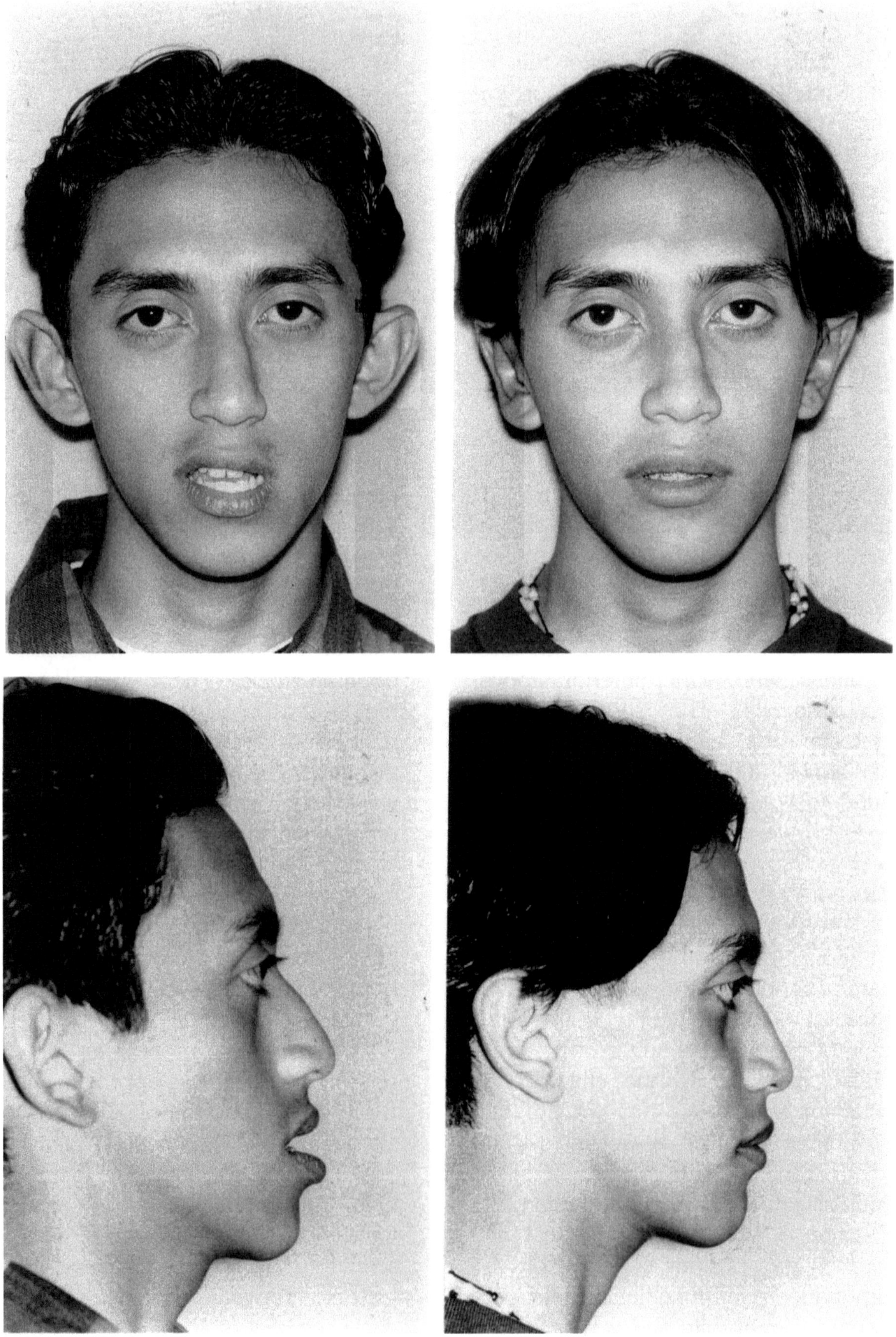

A B C D

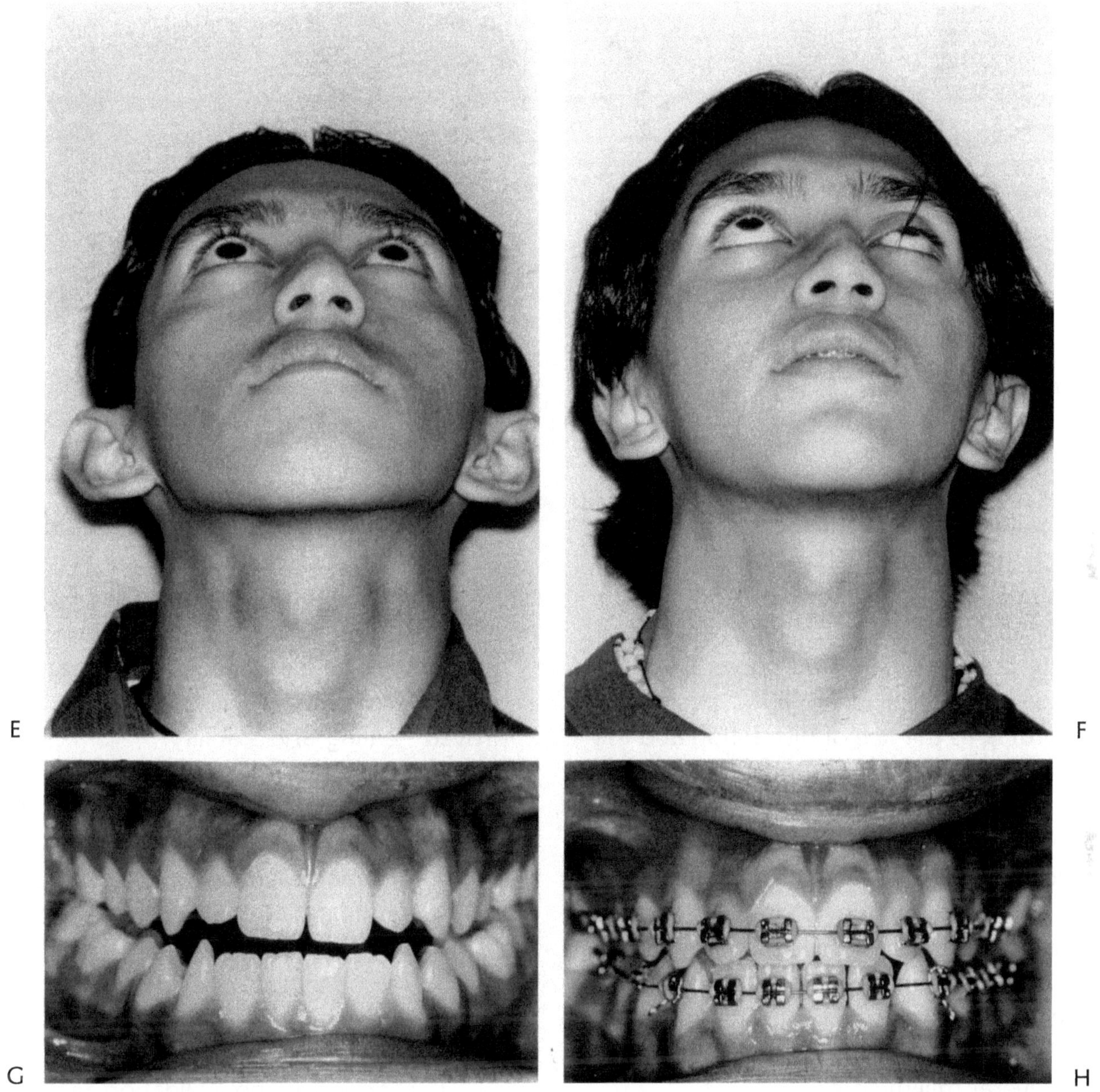

Figure 7.21. (A) Preoperative frontal view of a patient with midface hypoplasia. Note the perinasal and malar deficiencies, the anterior open bite, and the ear deformity. (B) Postoperative frontal view. The midface deficiency and the open bite were corrected by intraoral maxillo-malar distraction. (C) Preoperative profile showing the malar and midface deficiencies. Note the Class III relationship. (D) Postoperative profile. Note improvement in the malar and perinasal areas, leading to a more balanced facial profile. (E) Preoperative basilar view showing the perinasal and malar deficiencies. (F) Postoperative basilar view. (G) Preoperative occlusal view. Note the Class III maloclussion and anterior open bite. (H) Postoperative occlusal view showing correction of the Class III maloclussion and the open bite. (I) Preoperative lateral view showing the anteroposterior maxillary deficiency. (J) Postoperative occlusal lateral view after maxillo-malar distraction.

(*Continued*)

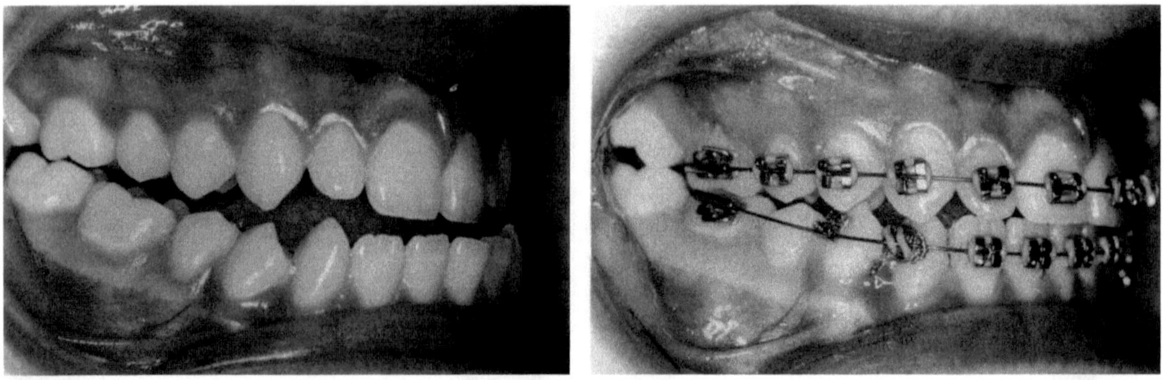

I J

Figure 7.21. *Continued*

several ways. The appliance arms and the attached fork ends should be bent and manipulated so that the arms lie as passively as possible against the mucosa opposite the site where the screws are to be placed. The appliance will be positioned according to the line of distraction and the anatomical position of the dental roots, mental nerves and inferior alveolar nerves. Separate osteotomies are made on the buccal cortex of the ramus and body. The second part of the distraction device is fixed to the mandibular body as illustrated in Figure 7.22A. After the two osteotomies are completed, the segments are mobilized and the device is activated for several millimeters.

DISCUSSION

Some clinical considerations must be emphasized in any distraction procedure. The basic surgical principles are:

1. The incisions must be limited with special attention to minimal dissection of the periosteum to facilitate optimal blood supply to the osteotomy site.

2. All osteotomies are well planned and performed under copious fluid irrigation to reduce damage to membranous bone. This principle also facilitates improved healing and stability.

3. A 7-day latency period allows for soft tissue healing and stretching in the distraction site.

4. Distractor activation is commenced at a rate of 1 mm per day (once a day).

5. A consolidation period of 45 to 90 days is required.

The period of consolidation yielding bony union depends on other variables: (1) patient age, (2) magnitude or distance of the distraction, (3) quantity and/or quality of hard and soft tissue observed at the time of surgery, (4) rate of distraction, (5) rhythm of distraction, (6) type of fixation, and (7) type of diet in the postoperative period. Bone regeneration in younger patients is relatively rapid. An extended period of stabilization is therefore warranted

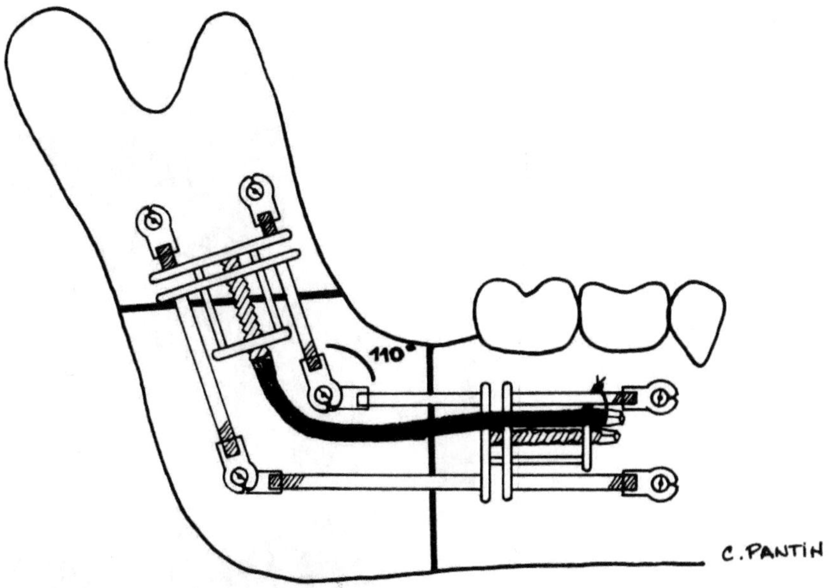

A

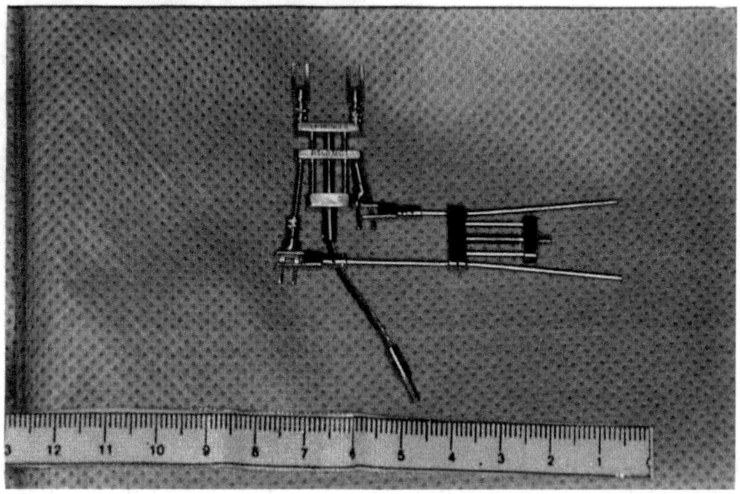

B

Figure 7.22. Intraoral biphasic distraction device used to achieve (A) vertical and (B) anteroposterior mandibular distraction. (C) The connector that is exposed to the oral cavity allows activation of the device. Osteotomies are made on the buccal cortex of the mandibular ramus and body. The vertical component of the device is placed on the ramus. (D) The second part of the distraction device is fixed to the mandibular body. After the appliance is secured with screws in the correct position, the osteotomies are completed, the segments mobilized, and the device is activated.

(*Continued*)

Figure 7.22. *Continued*

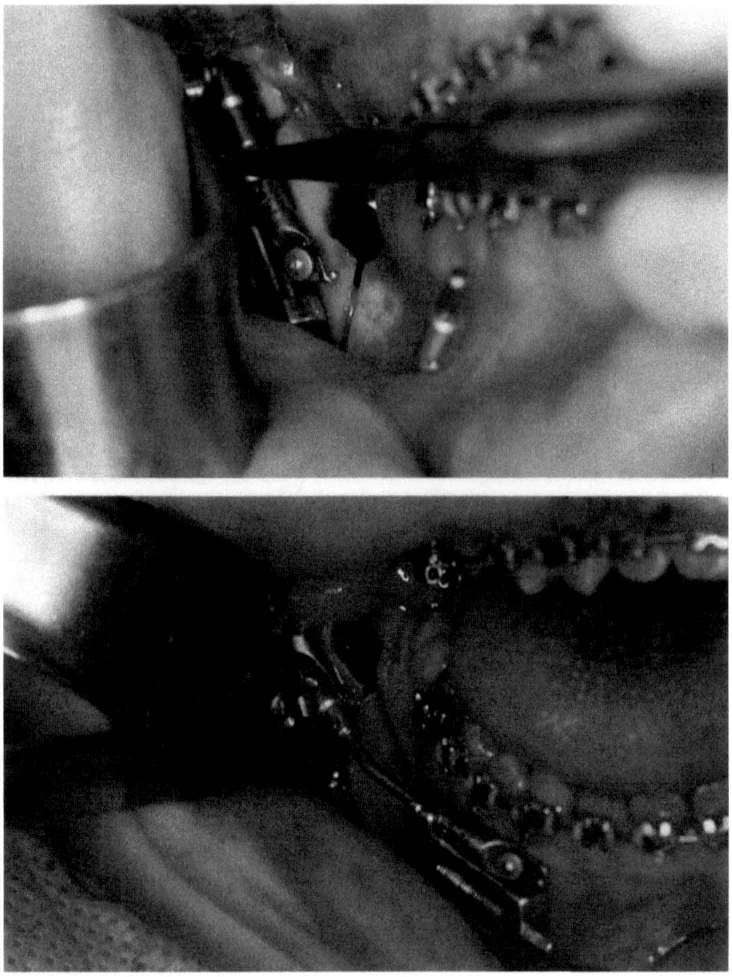

C

D

in situations where the planned distraction is large. If at the time of surgery a deficient quantity and/or quality of skeletal and soft tissue is observed, the latency period is prolonged to promote the initial bone healing phase.

Controlled distraction was performed on a 1.0mm per day basis subsequent to the 7-day latency period. Ilizarov's (7) histomorphic and biochemical studies of the elongated osseous tissue, fascia, skeletal muscle, blood vessels, nerves, and skin determined that distraction at a rate of 0.5mm per day often led to premature consolidation of the distracted bone, while a distraction rate of 2.0mm per day often resulted in detrimental changes within the elongated tissues, such as nonunion, fibrous union, and bone weakening. A distraction rate of 1.0mm per day consistently gave satisfactory results. Additional research, however, is necessary to substantiate this in the mandible and maxilla.

The amount of distraction required is estimated preoperatively based on clinical, radiographic and orthodontic evaluation. In addition to the amount of bony expansion accomplished, the nerves, as well as any associated muscles and soft tissue, will also lengthen as demonstrated by Ilizarov and others (7.22). Excessive distraction pressure may cause ischemia leading to possible tearing of the tissues, periodontal problems, malunion, fibrous union, and/or the inability for orthodontic movement of the teeth into the expanded area. Gradual distraction and meticulous surgical technique have minimized periodontal problems.

The described technique has been successful and offers many advantages. First, the technique can be performed in an outpatient setting under deep intravenous sedation. This potentially proves to be important in the modern climate of rising hospital costs. Because of the limited dissection and technique of gradual distraction, there is less postoperative morbidity, thus allowing most patients to be treated on an ambulatory basis. The need for maxillary orthognathic surgery is eliminated in many cases.

The mandibular intraoral distractor device eliminates donor site morbidity, minimizes the need for blood transfusion or prolonged fixation, prevents damage to the inferior alveolar nerve and developing dental follicles, eliminates hypertrophic facial scars, and yields a high rate of patient compliance. Injury to the neurovascular bundle is prevented by carefully planned osteotomies and screw placement. No long-term reported neurosensory injury in our patients substantiates the benefit of 2-mm diameter monocortical screw placement in the body and/or ramus as opposed to bicortical pins as described by McCarthy and others (15). In addition, monocortical screws minimize the possibility of injury to developing dental follicles. In other sites, when feasible, bicortical screws are used. The intraoral device, compared to external fixators, provides for an enhanced patient acceptance and reduces potential negative psychosocial effects.

The concern for temporomandibular dysfunction originating from distraction, especially when the goal was to gain transverse width, are minimal as compared with changes arising from other orthognathic surgical procedures. Pre- and postoperative evaluation of condylar angulation by submental vertex radiographs revealed minimal lateral rotation. The greatest geometric change observed was only four degrees, after a symphyseal distraction. Injury to intraoral lingual anatomy by the metal structure of the Hyrax® was an initial concern in cases dealing with symphysis distraction. This was rectified by fabricating an appliance with the hardware placed as anteriorly as possible to prevent damage to the lingual frenum, tongue, and salivary structures and, at the same time, to control the distraction vector.

In maxillary distraction, it is important to use the proper distraction appliances. Originally, Bell and Epker (13) used a Haas appliance, which was tooth borne. In order not to violate the principle of adequate blood supply, the authors believe that a totally tooth borne appliance (the Hyrax®) is warranted. The method, in which the Hyrax® appliance is secured to the maxilla, may vary and depends on the dentition which is present. The patient may present with missing or compromised teeth, thereby preventing banding of the appliance to those areas. A variety of methods have been used to attach the device; the goal is to anchor the Hyrax® to a molar and a premolar bilaterally. The appliance is completely tooth borne, therefore preventing injury to the soft tissues of the palate.

Undesirable inclinations of teeth have not occurred. If they occur, they can be corrected by postoperative orthodontic treatment. The Hyrax® can be opened to a maximum of 13 mm. After desired distraction is achieved, resin is placed over the screw to fix it, and the Hyrax® is left in place for three months to prevent relapse. If the resulting space is obvious, an acrylic tooth can be placed temporarily in the area. After three months of healing, the acrylic is progressively stripped in a mesial-lateral direction, as orthodontic forces are used to realign the segments.

The elastic traction can successfully advance and vertically alter the maxillary position. The Delaire facial mask (24) and 3.5-oz. heavy elastics are placed in a Class III tension pattern from the maxillary second molar to the mandibular canine bilaterally in order to achieve forward and vertical movement. Two elastics are placed on each side for the first five days. They are changed daily to account for loss of tension as a result of loss of stretch. After the fifth day, the elastics are changed every other day, thus slowing the anterior movement and allowing for bony fill in the distraction site. Finally, after the final advancement is accomplished, one 3.5-oz. elastic is placed bilaterally in a box Class III tension patern to prevent relapse. In our series of patients, the authors correlated movements in the vertical vector, either upward or downward, depending on the direction of the osteotomy design. The results have not shown extensive movements, but this is the result of patient selection. The maxilla will advance along the osteotomy lines. As the patient functions while wearing the heavy elastics, there is movement of the maxillary segments along these lines. There has been a tendency for the transverse dimensions of the maxilla to relapse slightly while the maxilla is been advanced. This phenomenon is compensated by using adequate force vectors of the elastics.

All treatment plans are developed in conjunction with an orthodontist. Individual needs to be considered are: (1) position of the teeth in the line of the osteotomy, (2) history of orthodontic therapy, (3) esthetics of the interdental gap, (4) postoperative orthodontic therapy, (5) and management of the reciprocal forces. The orthodontist should achieve satisfactory dental alignment and root divergence at the planned osteotomy site before surgery and ensure that sufficient alveolar bone remains intact on both sides of the proposed distraction site. Minimal orthodontic movements are made before surgery. However, with a planned Hyrax® fixation to a premolar or molar that is extremely rotated or tipped, the tooth should be uprighted prior to inserting the distractor. No preoperative dental compensations should be made at the orthodontic appointment unless the appliance is constructed immediately before surgery. This will eliminate any possibility of relapse. For the esthetics of the interdental gap, a bracket is bonded to an acrylic tooth similar in color and shape to the patient's natural teeth and ligated to an arch wire bracket. After approximately

2 to 3 months, light forces are applied to the teeth to close the space. The width of the acrylic tooth is reduced as the teeth are approximated. The teeth are subsequently aligned and leveled in the usual manner.

As with all surgical procedures, unique situations arise that mandate special consideration. First, one must consider the physical limitations of the custom-made distractor. In clinical situations in which the deficiency is greater than the largest possible expansion for that device, an immediate second-stage distraction appliance may be used and distraction continued before consolidation of the expanded bone occurs.

The second consideration deals with the inadvertent or spontaneous loosening or dislodgment of an orthodontic band in the tooth-borne appliance. The remedy is to ligate the band to the outer cortex of the basilar mandibular bone by utilizing a wire ligature. Another method has been the placement of a circumandibular wire incorporating the band.

The third consideration deals with attaining the total planned distraction in the surgical stage, when no further expansion is necessary. This is categorized as an intermediate distraction. It is limited, however, to widening or lengthening of only 3 or 4 mm. Our experience with this technique has been to stabilize the Hyrax® appliance with acrylic followed by plate and screw placement at the inferior border of the mandible. The distraction device is maintained in place 3 to 5 weeks, before resuming orthodontic therapy. The bone-borne appliance of variable length has overcome most of these difficulties.

References

1. Codivilla A. On the means of lengthening in the lower limbs, the muscles and tissues which are shortened through deformity. *Am J Orthop Surg* 2:353, 1905.
2. Abbott LC. The operative lengthening of the tibia and fibula. *J Bone Joint Surg* 9:128, 1927.
3. Ilizarov GA. A method of uniting bones in fractures and an apparatus to implement this method. USSR Autorship Certificate 98471, filed 1952.
4. Ilizarov GA, Leyav VI. The course of compact bone reparative regeneration in distraction osteosynthesis under different conditions of bone fragment fixation and experimental study. *Exp Khir Anest* 14:3, 1969.
5. Ilizarov GA. Basic principles of transosseous compression and distraction osteosynthesis. *Ortop Travmatol Protez* 32(11):7, 1971.
6. Ilizarov GA, Schreiner AA, Imerlishvili IA, Bakhlykov YN, Onirkova AM, Marterl II. On the problem of improving osteogenesis conditions in limb lengthening. In: *Abstracts of First International Symposium on Experimental and Clinical Aspects of Transosseous Osteosynthesis.* Kurgan, U.S.S.R., Sept. 1983, pp 20–22.
7. Ilizarov GA. The principles of the Ilizarov method. *Bull Hosp Joint Dis Orthop Inst* 48:1, 1988.
8. Snyder CC, Levine GA, Swanson HM, Brownw EZ Jr. Mandibular lengthening by gradual distraction: Preliminary report. *Plast Reconstr Surg* 51:506, 1973.
9. Michieli S, Miotti B. Lengthening of mandibular body by gradual surgical-orthodontic distraction. *J Oral Surg* 35:187, 1977.
10. Karp NS, Thorne CHM, McCarthy JG, Sissons, H. A bone lengthening in the craniofacial skeleton. *Ann Plast Surg* 24:231, 1990.
11. Karp NS, McCarthy JG, Sissons HA, Schreiber JS, Thorne, CHM. Mandibular bone lengthening: A serial histologic study. *Ann Plast Surg* 29:2, 1992.
12. Constantino PD, Shybut G, Fiedeman CD et al. Segmental mandibular regeneration by dis-

traction osteogenesis. An experimental study. *Arch Otolaryngol Head Neck Surg* 116: 535, 1990.

13. Bell WH, Epker BN. Surgical orthodontic expansion of the maxilla. *Am J Orthod* 70:517, 1976.
14. Guerrero C. Rapid Mandibular Expansion. *Rev Venez Ortod* 1:48, 1990.
15. McCarthy JG, Schreiber J, Karp N et al. Lengthening the human mandible by gradual distraction. *Plast Reconstr Surg* 89:1, 1992.
16. Molina F, Ortiz-Monasterio F. Mandibular elongation and remodeling by distraction: A farewell to major osteotomies. *Plast Reconstr Surg*, 96:825, 1995.
17. Guerrero C, Contasti G. Transverse Mandibular Deficiency. In: Bell WH (ed.), *Modern Practice in Orthognathic and Reconstructive Surgery*. Vol. 3. Philadelphia: WB Saunders, 1992: p. 2383.
18. Guerrero C, Bell WH, Flores A, Modugno VL, Contasti G, Rodríguez AM, Meza L. Distracción Osteogénica Mandibular Intraoral. *Odontol al Día* 10:116, 1995.
19. Guerrero C, Bell WH, Contasti G, Rodríguez A, Gulino D, Vasquez Z. Distración Osteogénica maxilar Intraoral. *Odontol al Día* 11: 203, 1995.
20. Chin M, Toth BA. Distraction osteogenesis in maxillofacial surgery using internal devices: Review of five cases. *J Oral Maxillofac Surg* 54:45, 1996.
21. Bell WH, Harper RP, Gonzalez M, Cherkashin AM, Samchukov ML. Distraction osteogenesis to widen the mandible. *Br J Oral Maxillofac Surg* 35:11, 1997.
22. Harper RP, Bell WH, Browne R, Cherkashin AM, Samchukov ML. Reactive changes in the temporomandibular joint after mandibular midline osteodistraccion. *Br J Oral Maxillofac Surg* 35:20, 1997.
23. Block MS, Brister GK. Use of distraction osteogenesis for maxillary advancement: Preliminary results. *J Oral Maxillof Surg* 52: 282, 1994.
24. Delaire JP, Verdon J, Lumineau A et al. Quelques resultats des tractions extra-orales appui fronto-mentonier dans de tractment orthopedique des malformations maxillomandibulaires de Class III et des sequelles osseuses des fente labiomaxillaires. *Rev Stomatol Chir Maxillofac* 73:633, 1972.

CHAPTER 8

THE EFFECT OF DISTRACTION ON THE TEMPOROMANDIBULAR JOINT

Suzanne U. Stucki-McCormick

The temporomandibular joint (TMJ) is the articulation of the mandibular condyle with the glenoid fossa of the temporal bone (Figure 8.1A). It is a diarthroidal joint with unique characteristics. Unlike the other articulations of the human musculsoskeketal system, the surfaces of the TMJ are covered by fibrocartilage, rather than hyaline cartilage. The temporomandibular joint is diarthroidal, with a biconcave disc dividing the joint into upper and lower compartments. The disc is made of fibrous connective tissue held in place by ligaments attached to the condylar head laterally. The disc is also confluent anteriorly with the lateral pterygoid muscle as it is attached to the neck of the condyle. The retrodiscal tissue has a rich neurovascular supply and attaches the disc to the posterior tubercle of the temporal bone.

Upon opening, the condylar head undergoes an initial rotational movement within the glenoid fossa. With increased mouth opening, the condyle follows a translational movement as it glides down the glenoid fossa onto the articular eminence. The combination of rotational and translational motion classifies the TMJ as a ginglymus diarthroidal joint (1). The disc also moves and translates with the condylar head during opening, producing a disc-condyle complex (Figure 8.1B). The mandible is unique because during function both joints (right and left sides) must act together to produce a bilateral diarthrosis (2). The TMJ is also the only joint to have a rigid endpoint of closure, produced as a consequence of the teeth contacting (3).

The temporomandibular joint develops embryologically from tissues that are responsible for the formation of the exter-

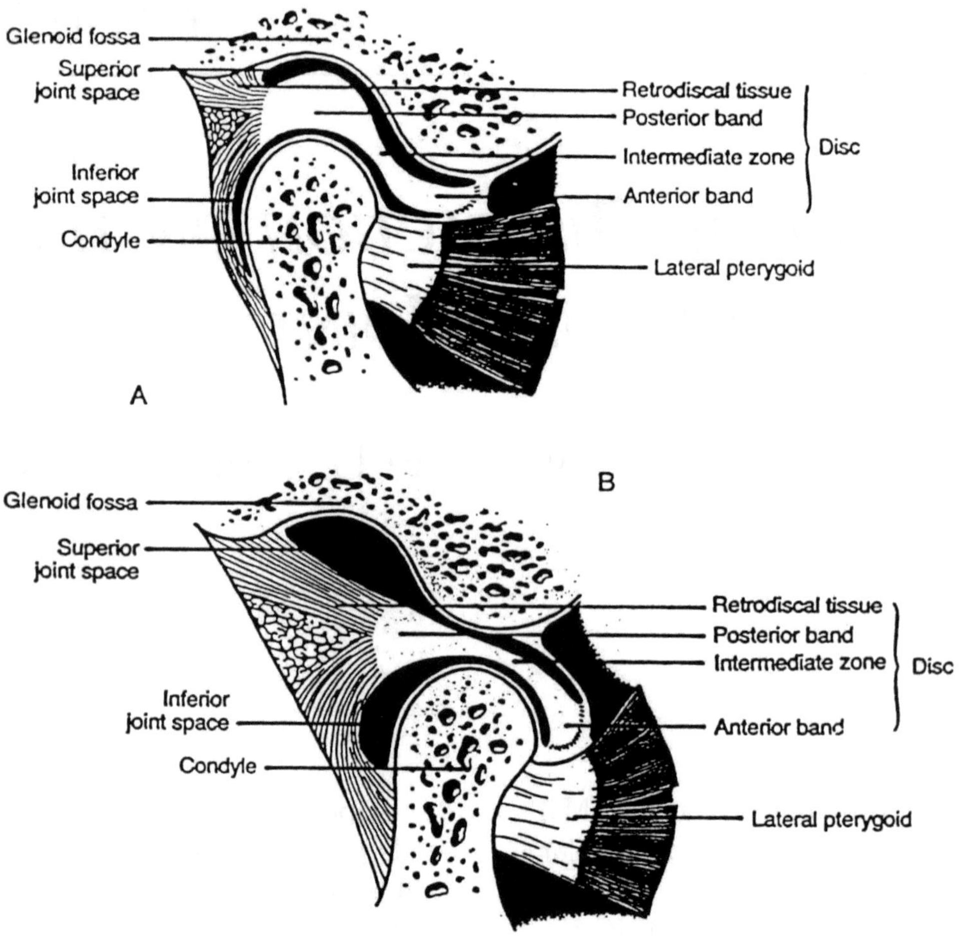

Figure 8.1. The temporomandibular joint is the articulation of the condyle in the glenoid fossa. This joint space is divided into two compartments by an intervening disc (A). Upon opening, the disc advances as the condyle is translated down the articular eminence (B). Reproduced with permission from Kaplan A and Assael L, eds. *Temporomandibular Disorders Diagnosis and Treatment* Philadelphia: WB Saunders, 1991: p. 3.

nal ear and muscles of mastication (3,4). Consequently, congenital malformations that manifest themselves as microtia and micrognathia often involve the temporomandibular joint. The expression of the TMJ pathology may be mild, as seen in patients with Treacher Collins syndrome, Pierre Robin syndrome, and Crouzon syndrome. In these conditions, the condyle and glenoid fossa are present with only restricted movement of the disc-condyle complex. Conversely, the temporomandibular articulation may be severely displaced or totally absent, as seen in patients with unilateral craniofacial microsomia. The morphologic presentation of the temporomandibular articulation is one of the parameters on which the current classification of the severity of craniofacial microsomia is based. Pruzansky classified the deficient mandible in patients with unilateral craniofacial microsomia as Type I, II, or III based on the size and shape of the condyle and ramus of the mandible (5); the classification was later modified by Mulliken and Kaban by further dividing the Type II patients into Type IIA and B (Figure 8.2) (6):

Type I: Hypoplastic condyle with a short ramus. The temporomandibular articulation is well formed with reduced rotation and translation of the disc-condyle complex.

Type II: Malformed condyle with a short, abnormally shaped ramus. Type II can be further subdivided into Type IIA and B depending on the morphology of the TMJ region. In Type IIA, the condyle is malformed and hypoplastic, but the condylar fossa relationship is maintained with the glenoid fossa in a position in the temporal bone similar to that of the contralateral side. Patients open with rotation and some translational movement of the disc-condyle complex. In Type IIB, the condyle is small, misshaped, and displaced outside the sagittal plane of the contralateral TMJ complex. The latter patients open with restricted, hinge-like motion of the mandible on the affected side.

Type III: The condyle, ramus and glenoid fossa are absent. There is hinge-like motion of the pseudo-articulation of the malformed condyle-ramus to the cranial base.

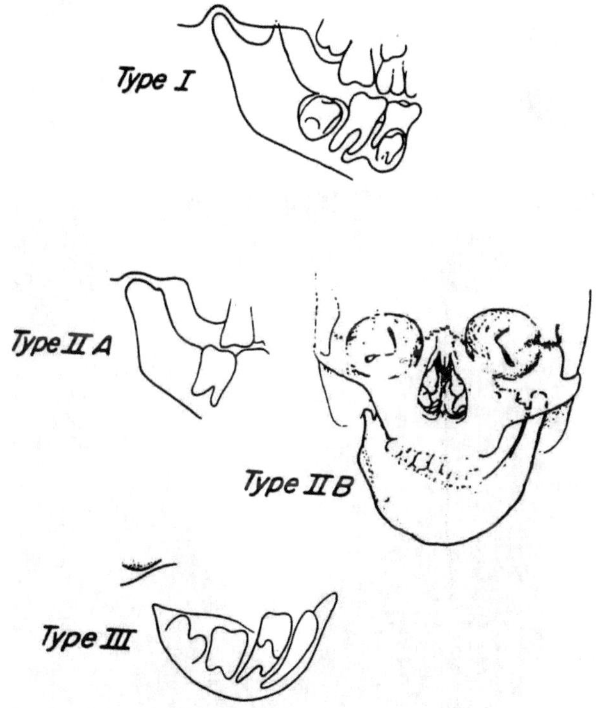

Figure 8.2. The mandible and condyle can be classified according to the severity of the dysmorphology of patients with craniofacial microsomia (see text for details). Reproduced with permission from Kaban LB, Moses MH, Mulliken JB: Surgical correction of hemifacial microsomia in the growing child. *Plast Reconstr Surg* 82:9, 1988.

Regardless of the congenital malformation, patients in whom the TMJ region is affected will open their mouths with deviation of the chin point toward the affected side. In severe cases, the involved articulation is restricted with the mandibular motion best described as a lateral shift toward the affected side, with the contralateral condyle undergoing rotation with translation (Figure 8.3).

Treatment considerations for patients with unilateral craniofacial microsomia are based on the severity of the deformity (6–8). For Type I cases, functional orthodontic appliances are advocated for young patients (3–6 years old) in an attempt to stimulate growth (9). If this is unsuccessful, orthognathic surgery is required to correct the maxillary cant and reposition the mandible. For patients with

Figure 8.3. Patients deviate their chin points toward the affected side (A) when the mandibular condyle is restricted or affected (B).

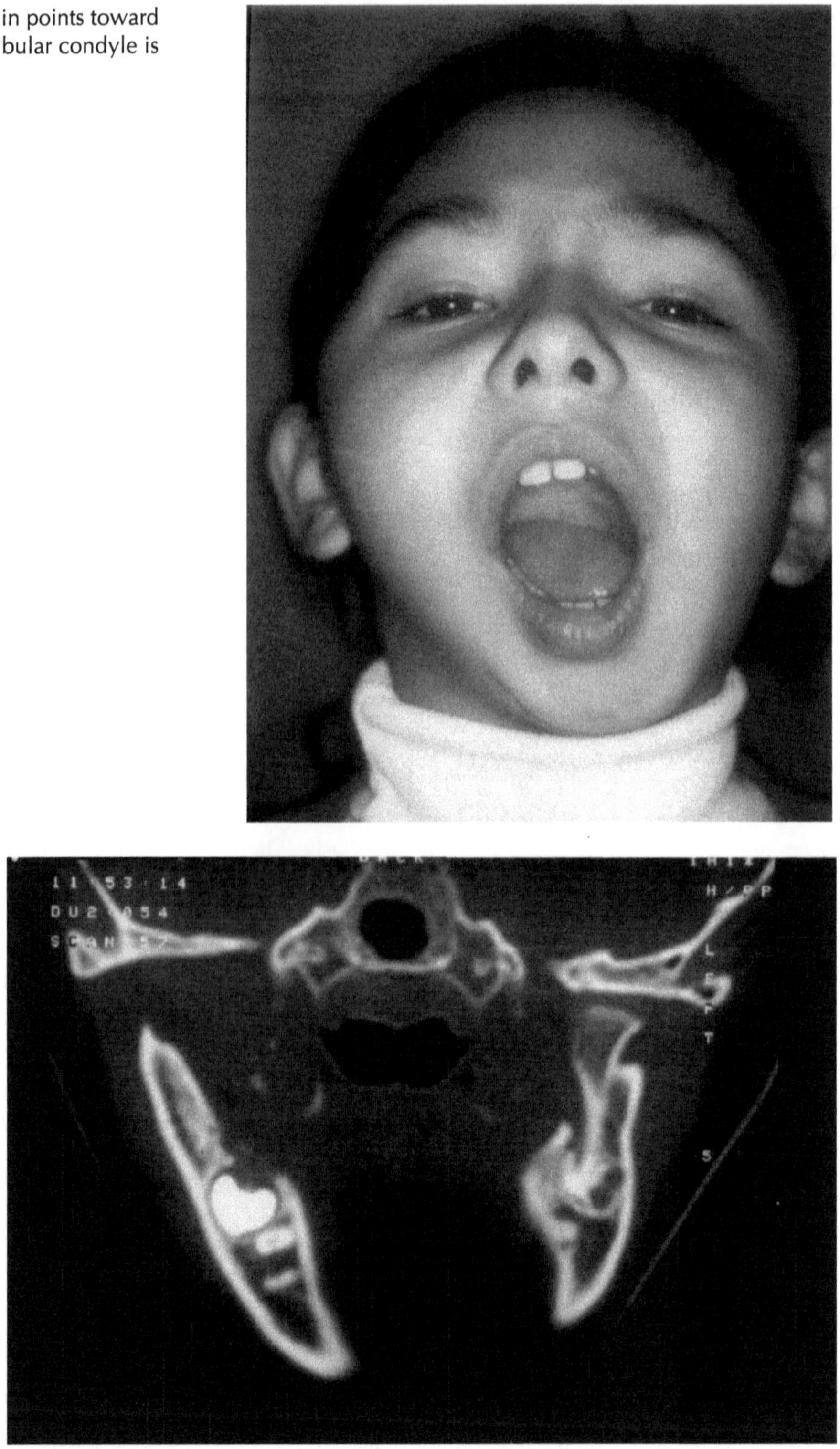

A

B

Type IIA deformities, the misshaped condyle is thought to be functional and thus can be used in the mandibular reconstruction. The mandible is corrected in three planes of space, with a vertical ramus osteotomy producing elongation and rotation of the affected side. Simultaneous ramal surgery may be required on the contralateral side, as well as maxillary osteotomies. For Type IIB and Type III cases, the condyle is thought to be nonfunctional, and total construction of the condyle, glenoid fossa, and ramus is advocated. Numerous autogenous donor sources, including iliac crest, calvarium, metatarsal, scapula, clavicle, and costochondral rib, have been utilized (6–8, 10–14). To date, the costochondral region has been the donor site of choice. While these grafts have been used successfully to treat and reconstruct the hypoplastic condyles and mandibles, the techniques fail to achieve desired esthetic goals and multiple complications have been reported (15–17). Overgrowth of the transplanted graft has also been noted, especially during the patient's pubertal growth spurt. This phenomenon results in rapid unilateral growth of the transplanted tissue with a secondary facial asymmetry of the contralateral side.

Distraction osteogenesis techniques have been recently used to reconstruct the micrognathic mandible (18–25). Distraction osteogenesis has been employed to correct the mandibular hypoplasia in both unilateral and bilateral cases. In addition to generating new bone, augmentation of the adjacent skin and soft tissue has been observed (21). It was initially thought that distraction osteogenesis would correct the mandibular ramal deformity and provide adequate bone stock should secondary condylar surgical reconstruction be required. Two clinical and one animal model studies were performed to evaluate the effect of osteodistraction on the temporomandibular joint (26–28).

CLINICAL STUDIES

Ten patients with craniofacial abnormalities were enrolled in the first clinical study. All patients had undergone mandibular lengthening procedures via distraction osteogenesis using the McCarthy technique (18–20). An osteotomy was made in the angle of the deficient mandible, and an extraoral expansion appliance was applied. Five patients underwent unilateral distraction, and five patients bilateral distraction (Table 8.1). The devices were advanced 0.5 mm twice a day in the unilateral cases until the pogonion was positioned across the midsagittal plane. The mandibles were then held in fixation for 8 weeks until a cortical outline could be seen on cephalometric evaluation.

Serial radiographs, including panoramic roentgenogram, posteroanterior and lateral cephalograms, and three-dimensional computed tomographic (CT) scans were obtained preoperatively, immediately after surgery, 6 and 12 months postoperatively. Yearly follow-up radiographs were obtained thereafter.

Comparison of the radiographs and the acetate tracings revealed that the ipsilateral condyle of the unilaterally distracted mandible had uprighted and increased in volume (Figure 8.4). By one

Table 8.1. Description of patient population undergoing distraction osteogenesis utilizing the McCarthy technique.

Patient	Diagnosis	Distraction	Vector	Follow-up years
1 (JD)	Goldenhaar	Unilateral	Horizontal	5
2 (AQ)	Craniofacial microsomia	Unilateral	Vertical	5
3 (JCR)	Nagers	Bilateral	Horizontal	5
4 (CR)	Craniofacial microsomia	Unilateral	Oblique	5
5 (PF)	Treacher Collins	Bilateral	Horizontal	5
6 (RP)	Craniofacial microsomia	Unilateral	Oblique	4
7 (JF)	Micrognathia	Bilateral	Oblique (R) Vertical (L)	4
8 (RR)	Nagers	Bilateral	Horizontal	3
9 (MP)	Craniofacial microsomia	Unilateral	Oblique	3
10 (TD)	Micrognathia	Bilateral	Vertical	2

year, the affected condyle resembled that of the unoperated side. The contralateral unoperated condyle did not show deformational changes. In the bilaterally distracted cases, the two condylar heads increased in size and volume, becoming more upright and symmetrical. Evaluation of yearly radiographs revealed that volumetric and positional gains made in the condylar head and neck region were maintained long term (up to 5 years) (Figure 8.5). In the unilateral cases, the condyle of the ipsilateral or operated side grew at a rate comparable to that of the unoperated side. In the bilaterally distracted cases, the two condylar heads grew similarly over time and remained relatively symmetric (Figure 8.6).

A second clinical study was also undertaken. Forty patients were enrolled in the study (Table 8.2). All patients had undergone unidirectional or bidirectional distraction according to the Molina technique (21,22,28). All patients had corticotomies performed at the area of bone deficiency (angle, ramus, or both), and a semirigid distraction device was placed. The unilaterally distracted mandibles were expanded 0.5 mm twice a day until the pogonion was positioned across the midline. The mandibles were maintained in fixation until a cortical outline could be radiographically demonstrated (6–8 weeks). Serial radiographs including panoramic roentgenogram, cephalograms (posteroanterior and lateral), and computed tomographic (CT) scan images were obtained preoperatively, immediately after surgery, 6 months postoperatively and yearly thereafter.

Comparison of the radiographs and the acetate tracings revealed similar findings. Following distraction the condyle of the ipsilateral side increased in size and volume to resemble that of the contralateral, or unoperated side (Figure 8.7). The condylar uprighting occurred during the period of postdistraction fixation, when functional remodeling of the mandible has

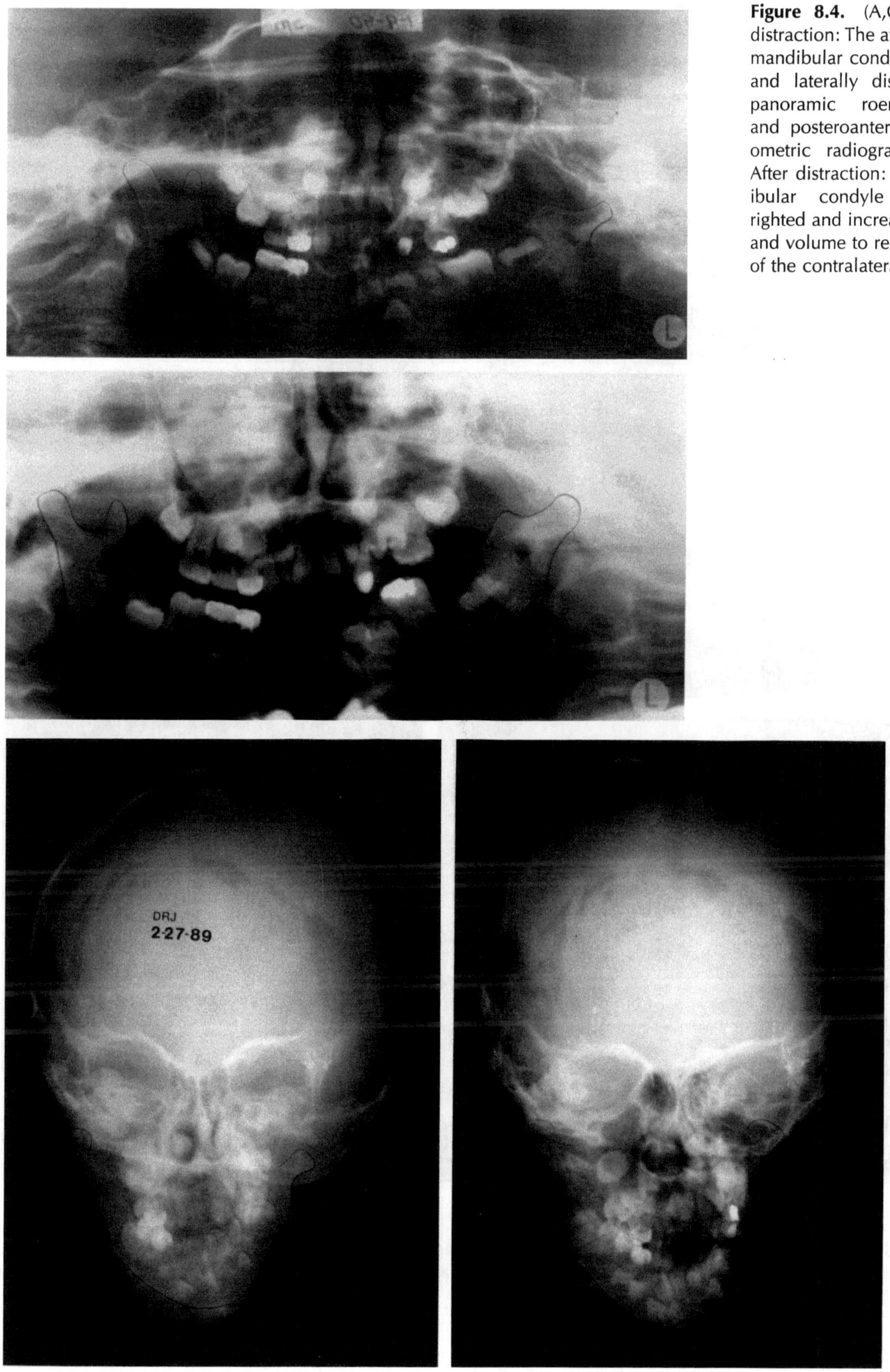

A B C D

Figure 8.4. (A,C) Prior to distraction: The affected (left) mandibular condyle is small and laterally displaced on panoramic roentgenogram and posteroanterior cephalometric radiographs. (B,D) After distraction: The mandibular condyle has uprighted and increased in size and volume to resemble that of the contralateral side.

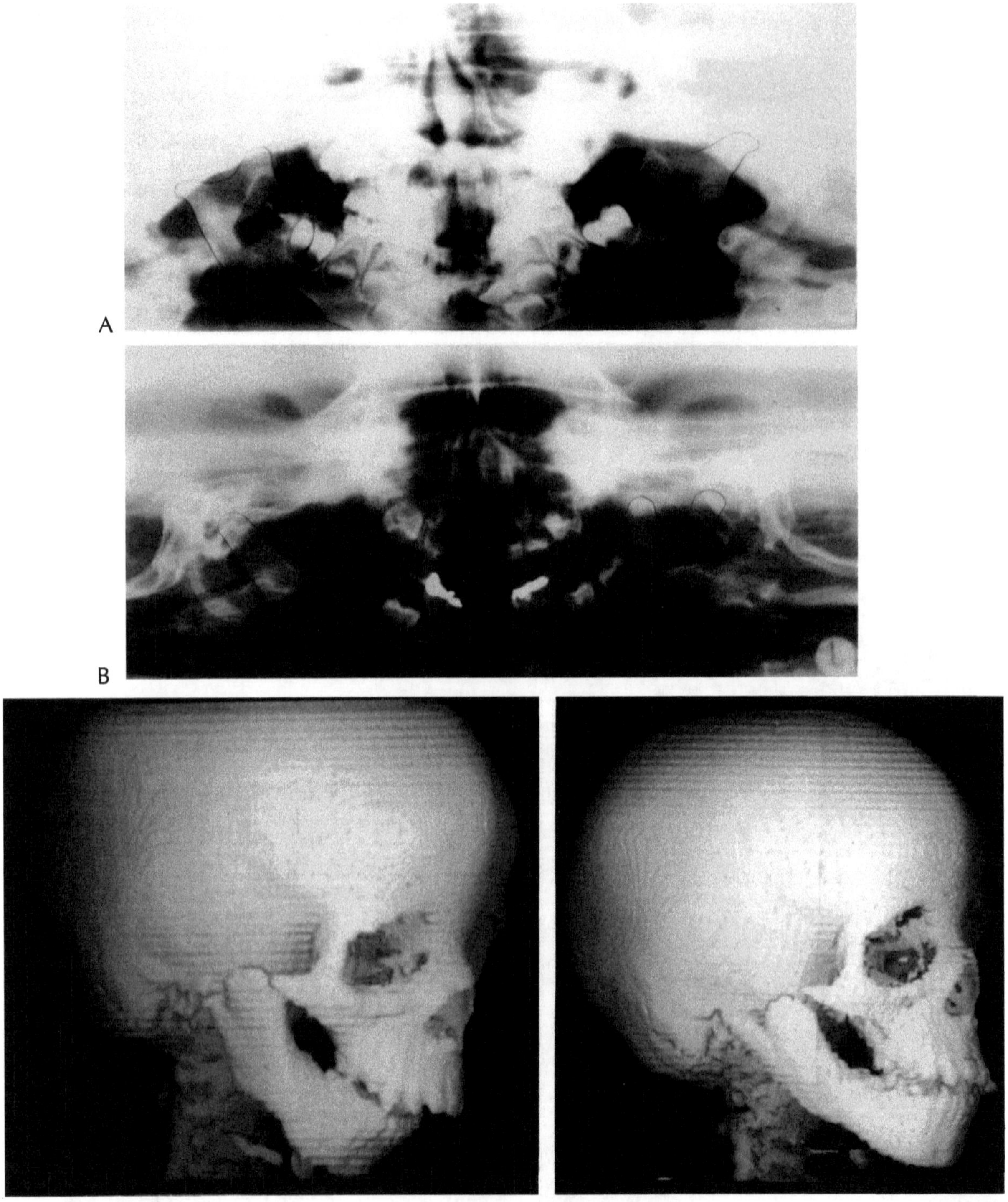

Figure 8.5. (A,C) Predistraction (bilateral case): Both condyles appear flat and dysmorphic on the panoramic and 3D CT scans. (B,D) Postdistraction: The condyles have increased in size and volume to resemble those of the unaffected condyles.

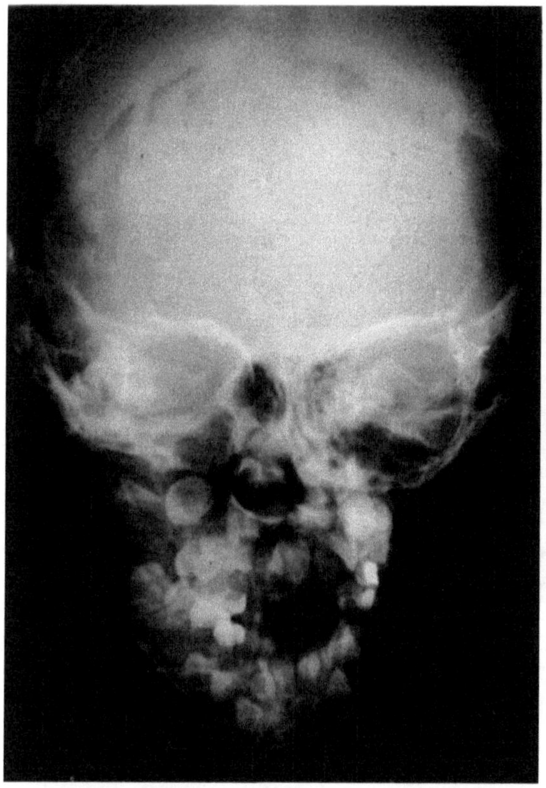

Figure 8.6. The postdistraction condylar changes noted using the McCarthy technique have been found to be stable on this 5-year follow-up radiograph.

been reported to occur (21). In the bilateral cases, the two condylar heads increased in size and volume to resemble unaffected condyles. Evaluation of long-term radiographs (4 years) also showed maintenance of the gains made in the temporomandibular joint, with comparable growth over time (Figure 8.8).

Distraction osteogenesis has been found to be a successful treatment alternative for patients with congenitally deficient mandibles. A secondary benefit appears to occur at the level of the temporomandibular joint. To date, none of the patients treated has required autogenous grafting procedures to reconstruct the originally deficient mandibular condyles. It appears that the condylar changes occur in response to the local forces applied by the distraction device to the surgical site. Although the condylar head is not a growth site, it does act as a growth center that responds to the functional loads placed

Table 8.2. Patients undergoing distraction osteogenesis utilizing the Molina technique.

Patient no.	Deformity	Expansion
20	Mandibular microsomia: Craniofacial microsomia Goldenhaar syndrome	Unilateral Unidirectional
8	Mandibular microsomia: Craniofacial microsomia, Goldenhaar syndrome	Unilateral Bidirectional
5	Mandibular microsomia: Craniofacial microsomia, Goldenhaar syndrome	Bilateral Bidirectional
5	Treacher Collins syndrome	Bilateral Bidirectional
2	Mandibular ankylosis	Bilateral Bidirectional

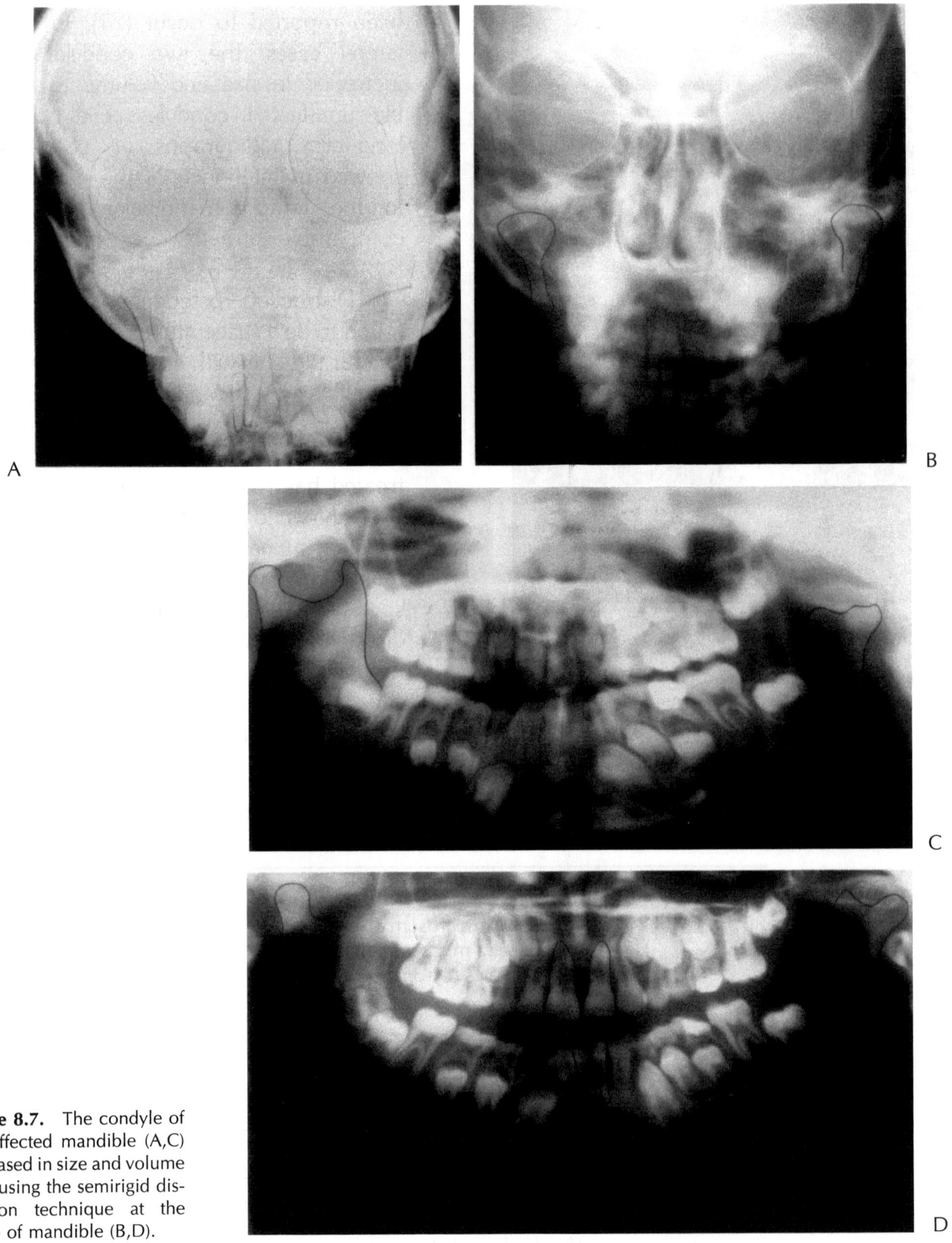

Figure 8.7. The condyle of the affected mandible (A,C) increased in size and volume after using the semirigid distraction technique at the angle of mandible (B,D).

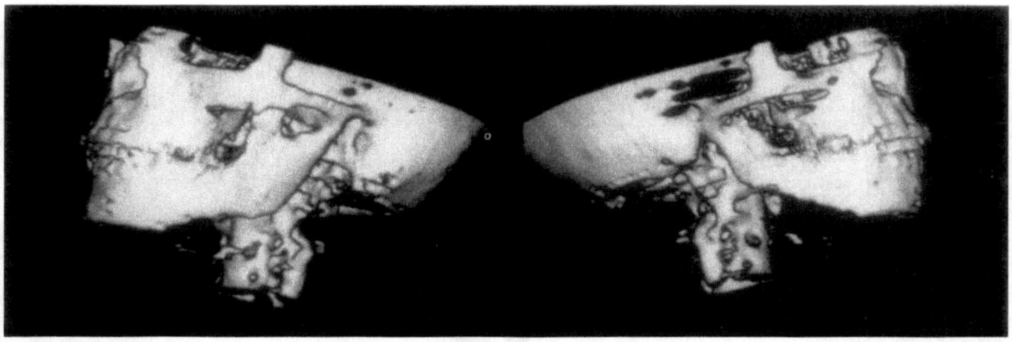

Figure 8.8. The postdistraction condylar changes were noted to be stable long term using the Molina technique as noted on this 4-year follow-up radiograph.

upon it. As such, mandibular growth occurs in a downward and forward direction by the apposition of bone on the posterior aspect of the mandible and resorption of bone on the anterior surface of the ramus (Figure 8.9) (29). In addition, the condylar head undergoes bony deposition in response to the downward and forward pull

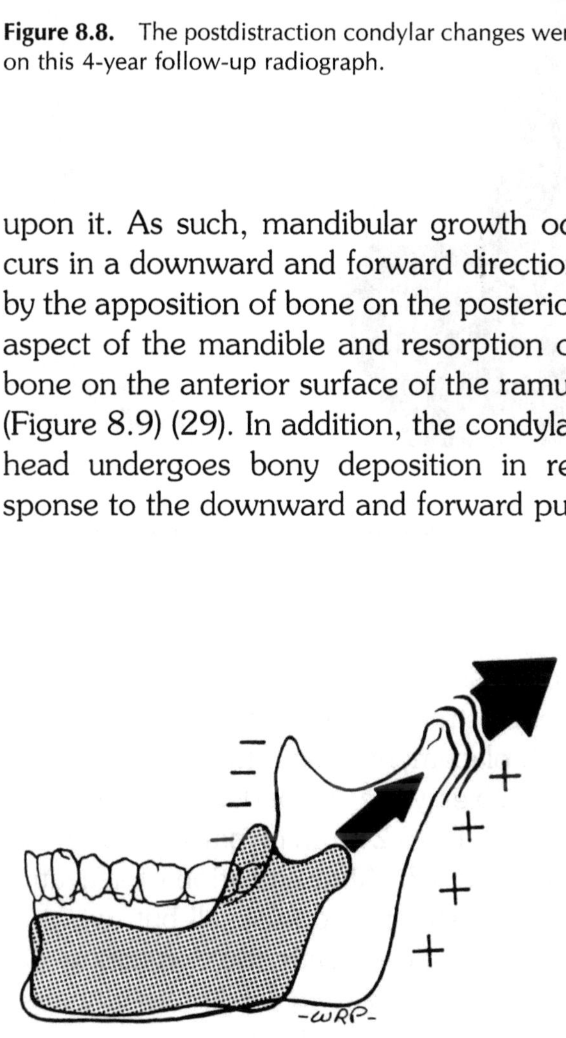

Figure 8.9. The mandibular condyle is influential for mandibular growth because the mandible grows in a downward and forward direction as a consequence of bone deposition at the level of the mandibular condyle. Reproduced with permission from Enlow DH, ed. *Handbook of Facial Growth*, 2nd Edition. Philadelphia: WB Saunders, 1982: p. 27.

exerted by the masticatory and suprahyoid musculature. Unlike conventional grafting techniques, distraction osteogenesis allows the patients to function by opening and closing their mouths during the period of active bone lengthening (Figure 8.10). It is conceivable that the force of the distraction appliance may act to enhance the soft tissue matrix which allows for the functional remodeling noted in the temporomandibular joint. It is consequently imperative that patients are encouraged to open and close their mouths during the period of active distraction and, more importantly, during the period of postdistraction fixation, during which time functional remodeling is most effective.

CANINE STUDY

In addition to the two clinical studies, a canine study (26) was undertaken. The potential effect of the compressive nature of the distraction device was investigated. Several authors have reported that exces-

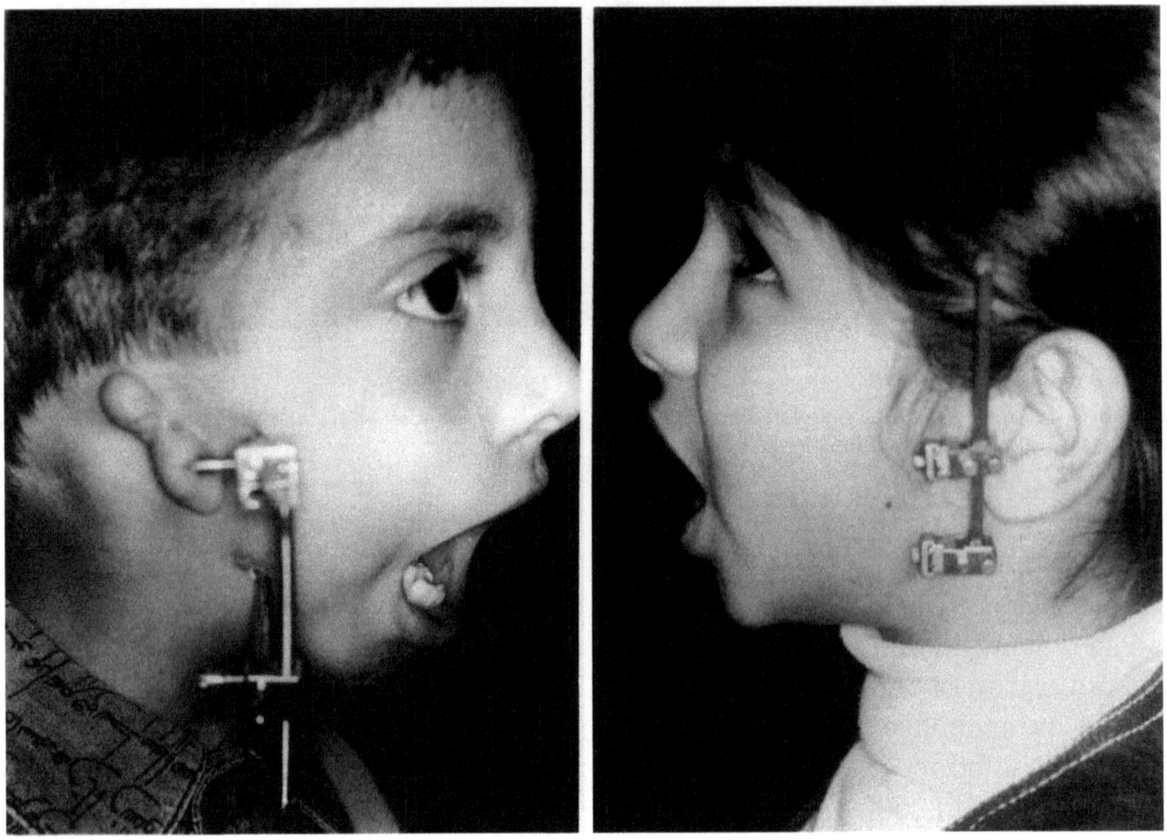
A B

Figure 8.10. During the period of active distraction, patients are encouraged to open and close their mouths regardless of the type of distraction device used: semirigid (A) or rigid (B).

sive compression of the temporomandibular joint may lead to condylar resorption, as noted in the case of patients who have undergone orthognathic mandibular advancement surgery with immediate and severe superior repositioning of the proximal segment (Figure 8.11) (29,30). Although the distraction device advances the mandible locally in a downward and forward direction, this force could also be potentially transmitted in a posterior direction to the condyle. A histologic study was therefore undertaken to evaluate this effect using a canine model.

Eleven mongrel dogs were included in this study (Table 8.3). Ten dogs underwent a mandibular osteotomy procedure with placement of an intraoral device. The mandibles were expanded 1 mm per day either fully to 20 mm or partially to 10 mm (Figure 8.12). After cessation of activation of the distraction device, all but two dogs were sacrificed, with the remaining two dogs held in fixation for an additional 10 weeks prior to sacrifice.

Cephalograms (lateral and ventrodorsal) and three dimensional computed tomographic (CT) scan images were obtained prior to sacrifice. The temporomandibular joint region was harvested en bloc bilaterally, snap frozen in liquid nitro-

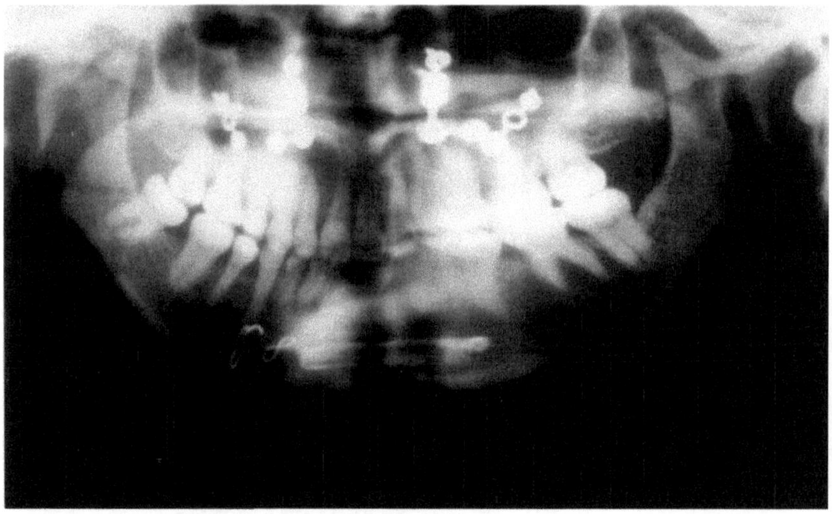

Figure 8.11. Compression of the mandibular condyle has been associated with idiopathic condylar resorption as observed in this patient who underwent several orthognathic surgical procedures.

Table 8.3. Distraction osteogenesis and harvesting protocol for the canine study.

Dogs	Expansion	Harvest
1,2	20 mm	30 days
3	0 mm (sham control)	30 days
4,5	20 mm	20 days
6,10	10 mm	10 days
11	Unoperated control	30 days

gen, and 3-mm macroscopic gross sections were prepared. Serial photographs were made prior to the specimens being processed for histologic evaluation.

Examination of the sections revealed no gross deformational change of the condylar head and neck region or the glenoid fossa (Figure 8.13).

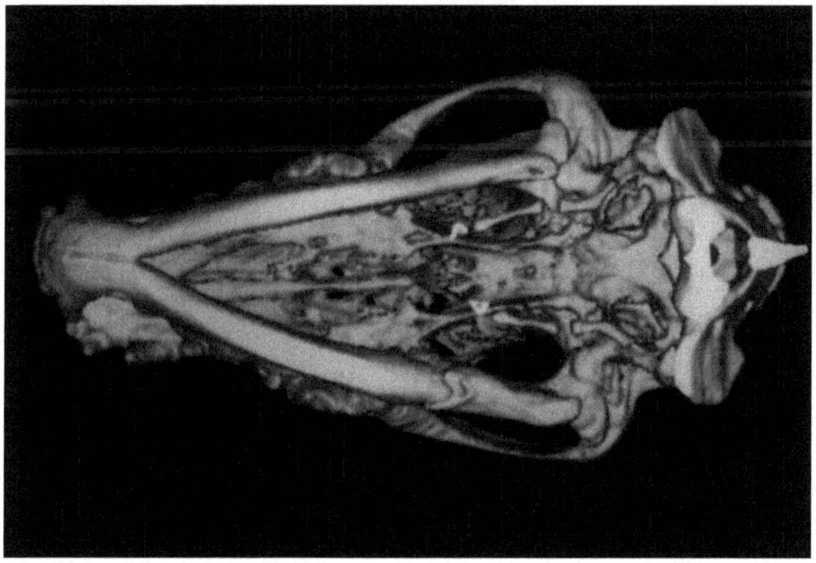

Figure 8.12. Basilar 3D CT scan of a unilaterally distracted canine mandible. No gross bony changes are apparent at the level of the mandibular condyle on 3D CT scan images. Note the laterognathia produced as a consequence of distraction of the right mandibular angle region.

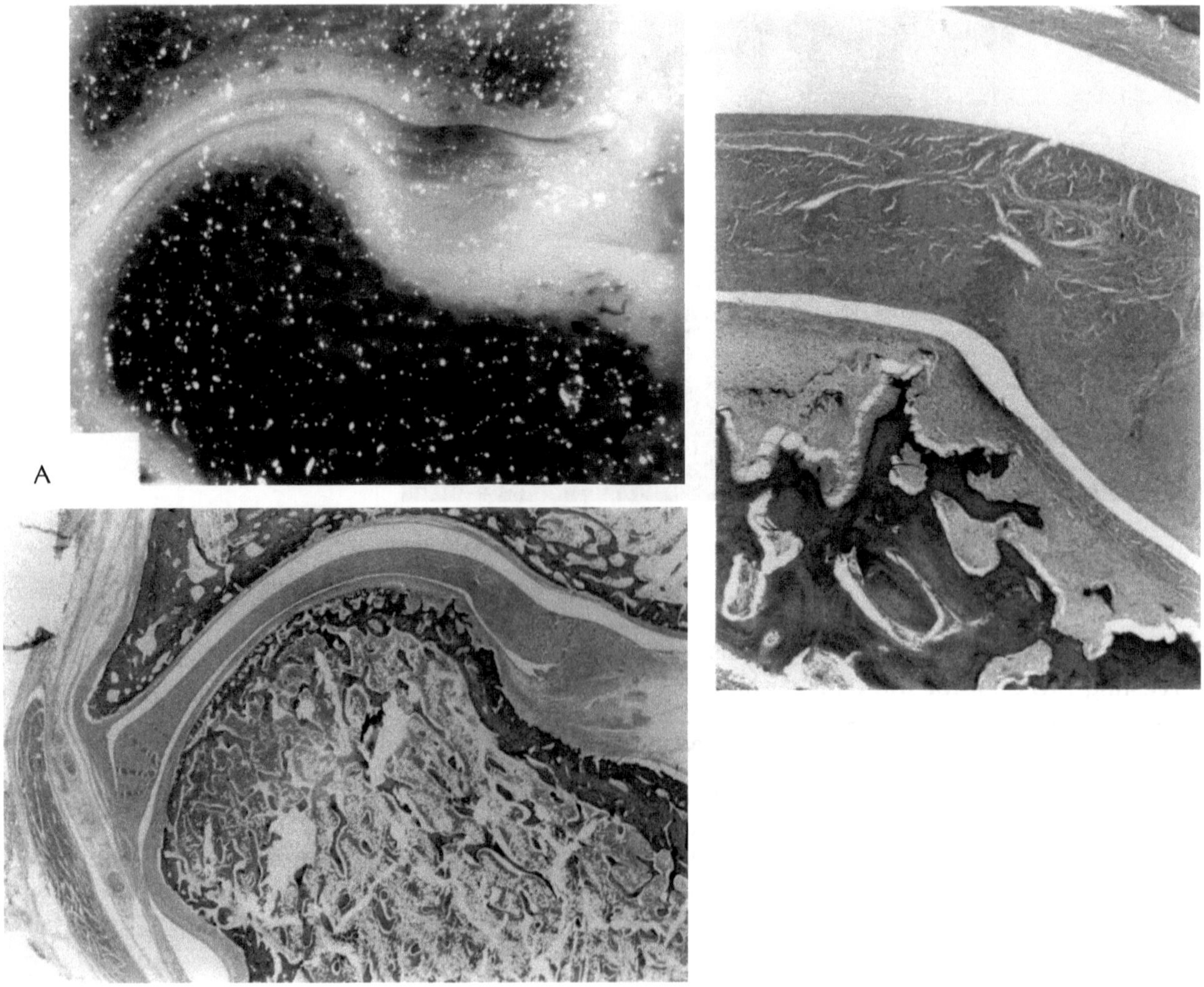
A
B
C

Figure 8.13. (A) The normal disc-condyle relationship was maintained on the distracted (10 mm) side of the canine mandible as noted on this 15× magnification of a macroscopic section. (B) Flattening of the posterior surface of the mandibular condyle is apparent on the corresponding 15× magnification of the mandible distracted 20 mm. (C) Anterior "lipping" was noted on the 30× magnification of the same specimen.

The normal disc-condyle relationship was maintained on examination of the macroscopic sections. Flattening of the posterior surface of the ipsilateral distracted condyle was observed. Flattening of the posterosuperior condylar surface was observed on the contralateral or unoperated side (Figure 8.14). These effects were minimal in mandibles distracted partially to 10 mm but more apparent in mandibles distracted maximally to 20 mm. These findings are significant in that the canine model represents a nonphysiologic or pathologic condition: an obvious crossbite was produced during the distraction procedure (see Figure 8.12). Although the animals were fed a soft diet, the laterognathia could only accentuate the nonphysiologic condition within the temporomandibular joint. Consequently, the observation that only mild bony changes (that underwent reparative processes) were seen represents significant positive or encouraging findings.

Histologic evaluation of the specimens revealed thinning of the condylar cartilage associated with the areas of flattening. These regions also displayed

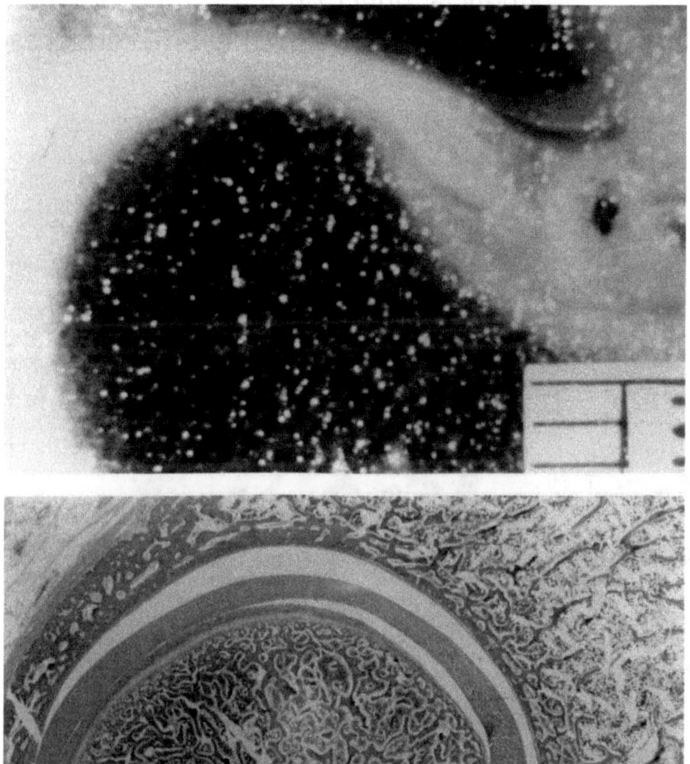
A

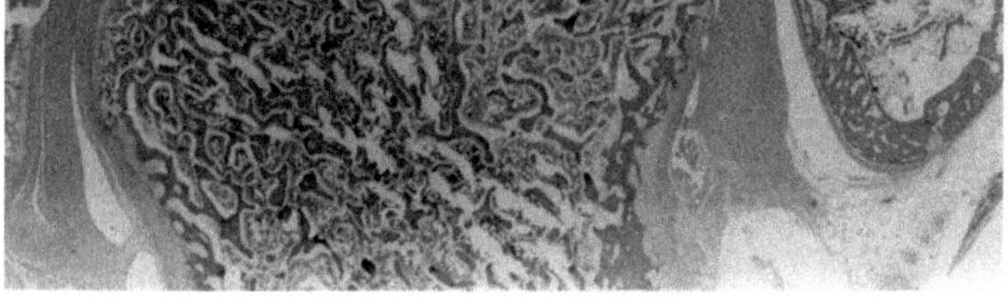
B

Figure 8.14. Flattening of the posterosuperior condylar surface is noted on the contralateral canine condyle distracted 20 mm. (A) Macroscopic 15×. (B) Histologic view 15×.

hyperplastic chondrocytes with bone deposition in a posterior and anterior "lipping" fashion. These observations were more pronounced in those mandibles distracted to 20 mm. Two animals were held in fixation for 10 weeks after active distraction (prior to harvesting). In these animals, flattening of the posterosuperior surface of the contralateral condylar head was noted. On histologic study, reparative processes were noted with remodeling of the subchondral region (Figure 8.15) and resolution of the bony lipping. No evidence of vascular necrosis, microfracture or cystic degeneration was noted. These finding are consistent with those reported for a sheep model (31). In this study distraction osteogenesis was performed in the mandible in seventeen growing sheep. Histologic evaluation of the temporomandibular region showed only mild bony changes, without evidence of degenerative changes, which were reversible with time.

The temporomandibular joint is a complex articulation often involved in congenital micrognathia. To date, treatment alternatives have included osteotomies to correct the malocclusion and facial asymmetries or total joint reconstruction with autogenous grafts. Distraction osteogenesis provides for a new treatment modality. Although primarily used to regenerate skeletal and soft tissues in local areas of deficiency, distraction osteogenesis appears to have a secondary beneficial effect on the temporomandibular joint region. In the unilateral cases,

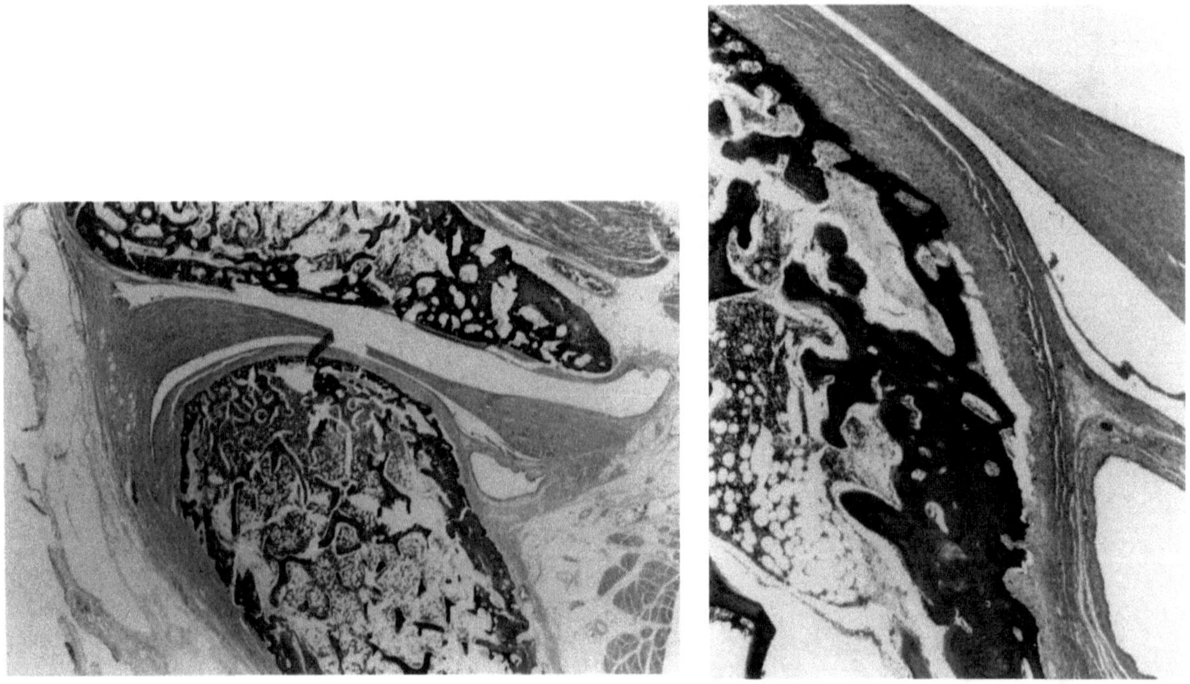

Figure 8.15. Condylar repair and remodeling is noted on the condyle distracted 20 mm and held in neutral fixation for 10 m weeks. (A) 15× magnification. (B) 30× magnification.

the skeletal structures of the affected TMJ upright in size and increase in volume. The contralateral unoperated side shows no apparent deleterious changes at the level of the temporomandibular joint. In bilaterally affected and distracted cases, both condylar heads increase in size and volume and become symmetric in appearance. These positive gains are maintained long term. To date, patients with severe mandibular hypoplasia and agenesis of the temporomandibular joint (Type III) have not been treated with distraction osteogenesis techniques. Reconstruction of these cases may involve distraction techniques, which allow for functional remodeling during the treatment period.

CONSTRUCTION OF A NEOCONDYLE

The concept of functional remodeling can be applied to the construction of a new temporomandibular articulation as well. Ilizarov described the use of *transport* distraction for the regeneration of new osseous and soft tissues within a discontinuity defect (32–34). This technique has been recently applied to the reconstruction of mandibular discontinuity defects (35–38). A transport disc (1.0–1.5 cm in diameter) is surgically created by making an osteotomy in the proximal end of the distal segment, adjacent to the discontinuity defect (Figure 8.16). Following the Ilizarov principles, the transport disc is advanced through the discontinuity defect by an external fixator. As it is advanced, new bone and soft tissues are generated between the transport disc and the proximal end of the original bone stump. In addition, advancing the transport disc through the soft tissues of the discontinuity defect produces a fibrocartilaginous cap along the leading edge of the transport disc. The fibrocartilaginous cap must be removed to allow for union of the transport disc to the docking site. It

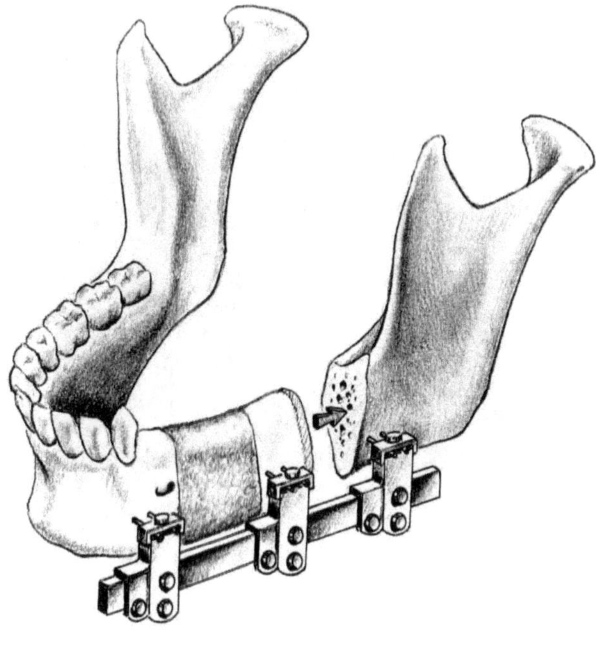

Figure 8.16. A 1.5-cm transport disc is surgically created in the distal end of the proximal segment adjacent to the discontinuity defect in the body of the mandible. An external distractor is applied and utilized to advance the transport disc through the discontinuity defect, generating new bone in its wake. Additionally, the leading edge becomes enveloped by a fibrocartilaginous cap.

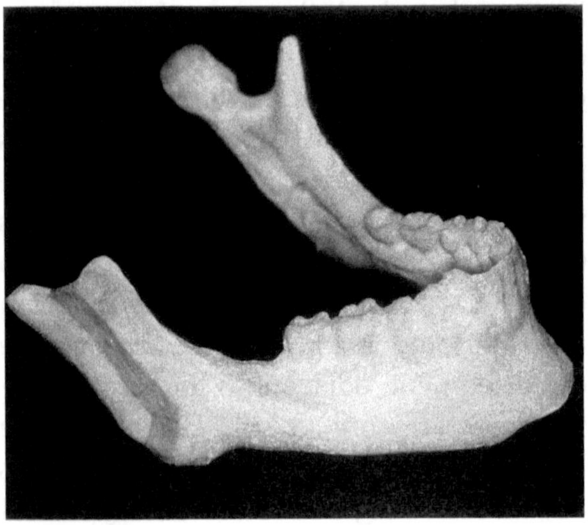

Figure 8.17. A reverse L osteotomy is created extending from the sigmoid notch to a position 1.5 cm above the inferior border of the mandible.

was the concept of the formation of a fibrocartilaginous cap on the leading edge of the transport disc which is clinically utilized in the construction of a new temporomandibular articulation.

A reverse L osteotomy is created from the sigmoid notch, posterior to the path of the inferior alveolar nerve, to a position 1.5 cm above the gonial angle (Figure 8.17). The distraction device is applied with the trajectory of distraction oriented vertically, to transport the ramal segment superiorly, until contact is made with the glenoid fossa. The distraction process is initiated 5 days postsurgically and it proceeds at the rate of 1.0 mm per day until contact is made with the glenoid fossa. The contact is verified radiographically with panoramic roentgenograms and cephalograms (Figure 8.18). Patients will note a slight preauricular sensation when the transport disc reaches the glenoid fossa docking site. Patients are encouraged to open and close their mouths and maintain a soft diet during the period of active distraction and postdistraction osteogenesis. The masticatory activity allows for functional remodeling of the transport disc to form a neocondyle.

This technique has been used to treat patients with degenerative joint disease secondary to tumor and bony ankylosis (39). One patient with Histiocytosis X of the mandibular condyle underwent local tumor resection but continued to display condylar degeneration (Figure 8.19). She

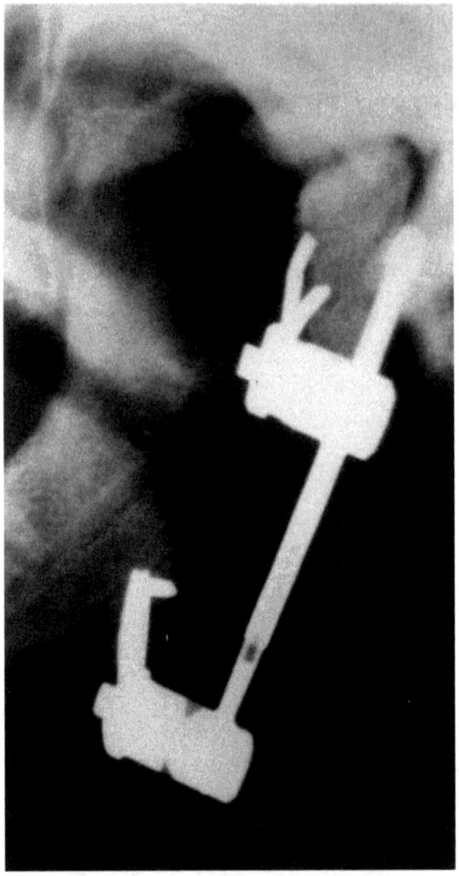

Figure 8.18. Contact of the transport disc with the glenoid fossa is verified radiographically as in this panoramic reontenogram.

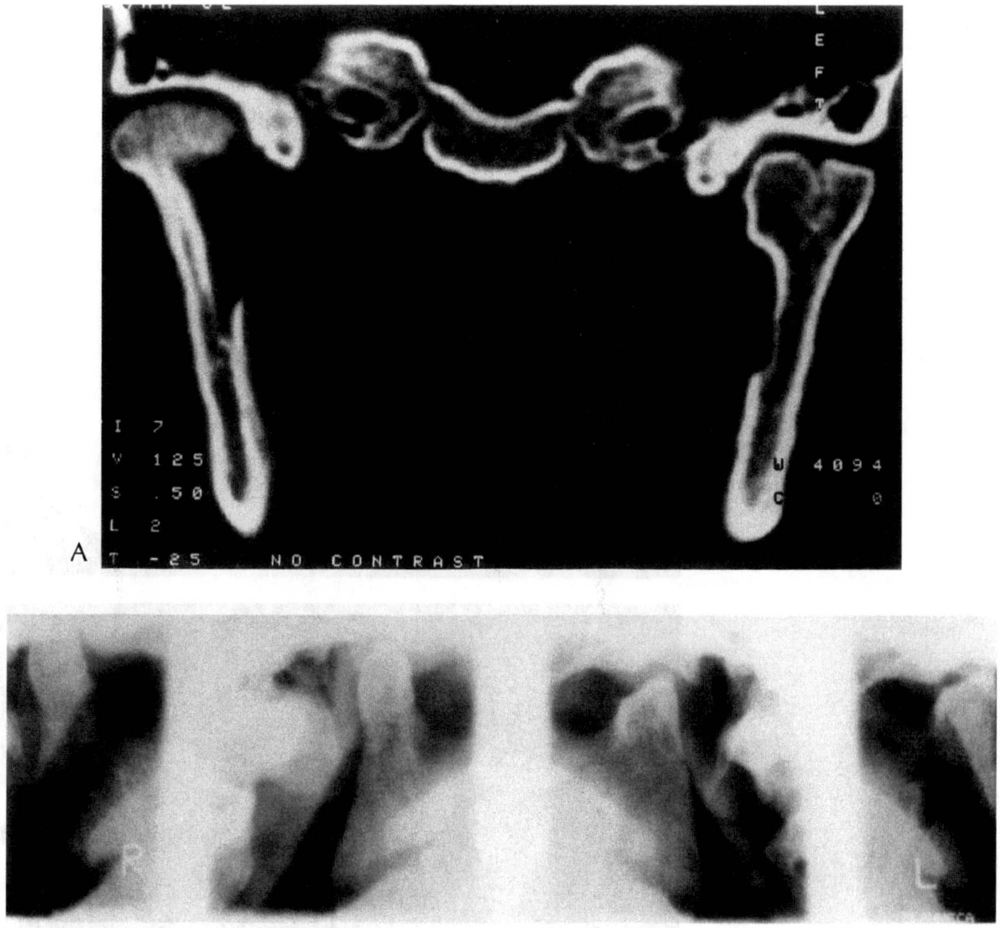

Figure 8.19. A patient with Histiocytosis X of the mandibular condyle underwent tumor resection with resultant continued condylar degeneration (A) and limited mouth opening (B), as noted on the panoramic and TMJ roentenograms.

had limited painful mouth opening and loss of vertical ramal height due to condylar degeneration. Transport distraction was utilized to reconstruct the joint articulation and to correct the facial asymmetry. Via an intraoral approach, a reverse L osteotomy was created and the external distractor was applied. The transport segment was advanced superiorly until contact was made with the glenoid fossa. The segment was then further distracted to restore the lost ramal height and to correct the facial asymmetry. The segment was held in fixation (6 weeks) until a cortical outline was radiographically observed. Postdistraction, the degenerated condylar head was found to have remodeled to produce a neocondyle, with a new cortical layer (Figure 8.20). An intervening pseudodisc was produced as evidenced by the postdistraction MRI scan (Figure 8.21). Additionally, the patient was able to open her mouth widely and masticate a regular diet.

Transport distraction was also utilized to reconstruct the condylar articulation of

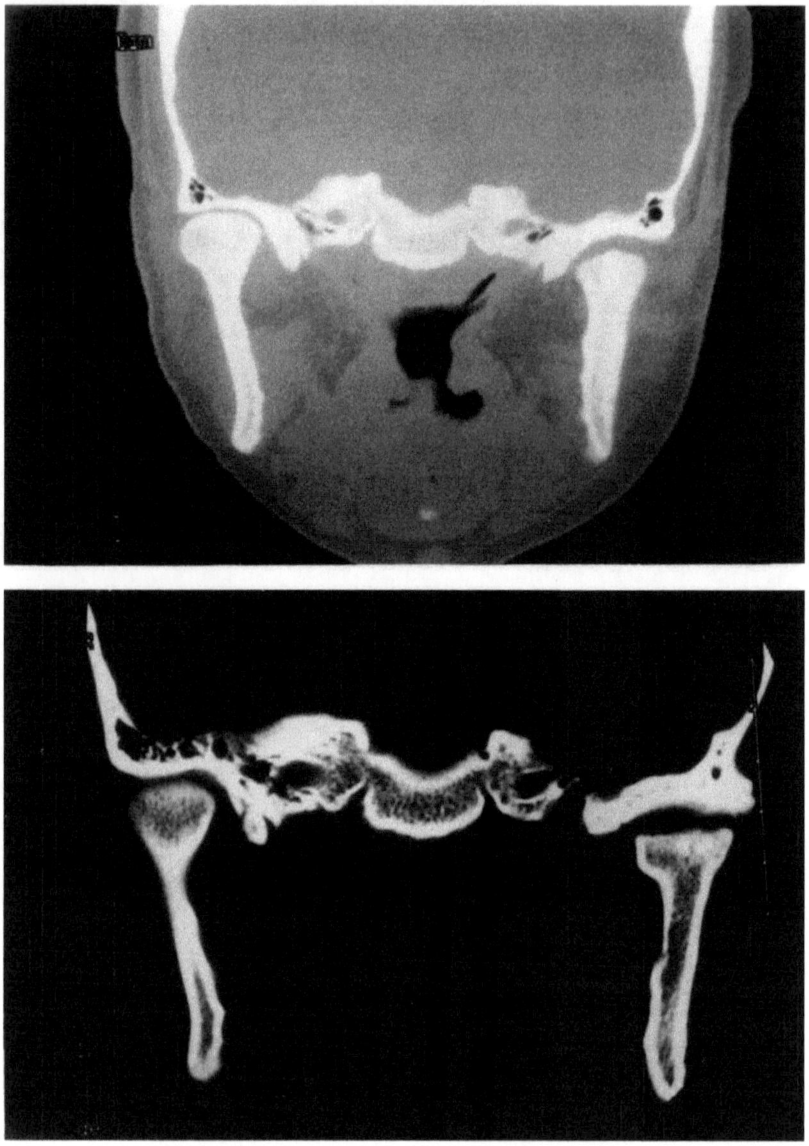

A

B

Figure 8.20. Postdistraction, a neocondyle with a new cortical outline was noted on the CT scan (A) as compared to the preoperative image (B).

a patient with bony ankylosis after a gap arthroplasty. This patient had previously undergone costochondral graft reconstruction after condylar tumor resection. She had limited painful mouth opening secondary to bony fusion of the costochondral graft laterally to the temporal bone (Figure 8.22). A gap arthroplasty was preformed followed by a reverse L osteotomy and placement of an external distractor. No intervening tissue was placed into the gap arthroplasty site. The transport disc was advanced 1 mm per day until contact was made with the glenoid fossa. The segment was held in place until a cortical outline was seen radiographically. Postdistraction, the cut edge of the transport disc was noted to have remodeled to become a neocondyle (Figure 8.23). A new cortical outline was noted on

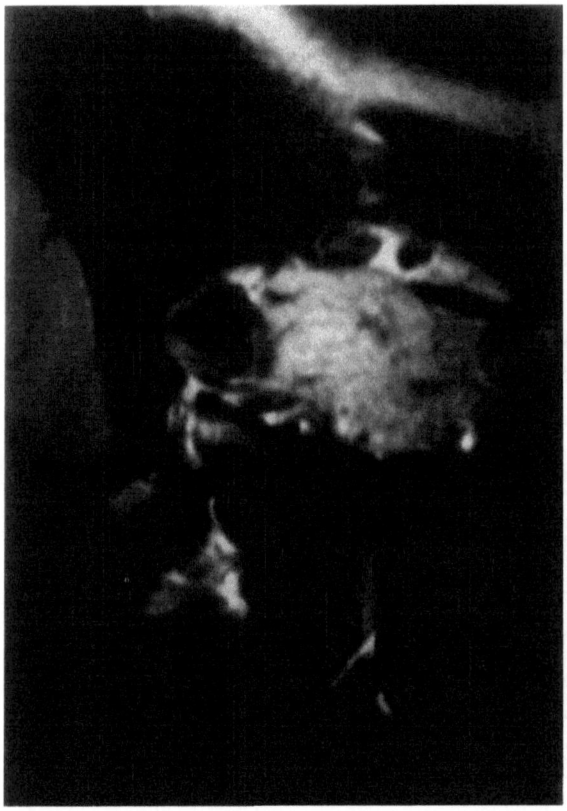

Figure 8.21. An intervening pseuodisc was noted on the postdistraction MRI scan.

the neocondyle, now seated in the glenoid fossa.

The use of transport distraction osteogenesis for the construction of a new temporomandibular articulation has been successful in part because of the formation of a fibrocartilaginous cap in the leading edge of the transport disc during the process of distraction. Active physical therapy is obligatory during the period of distraction and postdistraction fixation. Without encouraged jaw movements (wide mouth opening and lateral and protrusive excursive motions), functional remodeling will not optimally occur. Transport distraction osteogenesis is now being applied to patients with other forms of degenerative temporomandibular joint disease, including idiopathic condylar resorption as observed after orthoganthic surgery, and TMJ proplast-Teflon implant failures.

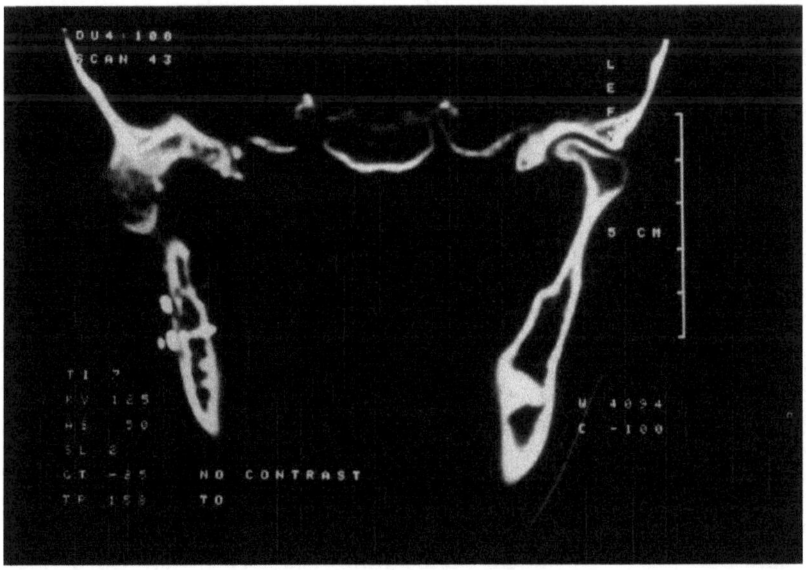

Figure 8.22. CT scan showing lateral bony fusion of a previously placed costochondral graft with an empty glenoid fossa.

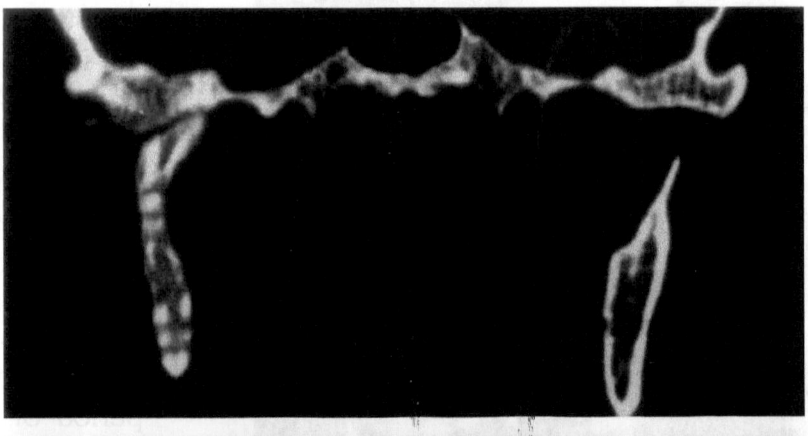
A

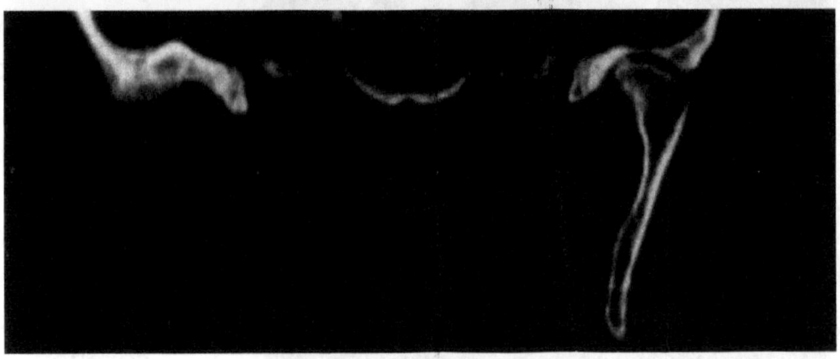
B

Figure 8.23. After distraction, the leading edge of the transport disc was noted on CT scan image to have remodeled to form a neocondyle with a new cortical layer with seating of the articulation in the glenoid fossa. (A) Predistraction CT scan. (B) Postdistraction CT scan.

References

1. Mankin H, Radin E. Structure and function of joints. In: McCarty D, ed. *Arthritis and Allied Conditions*, 10th ed. Philadelphia: Lea & Febiger, 1985.
2. Buchbinder D, Kaplan AS. Biology of the temporomandibular joint. In: Kaplan A, Assail L, eds. *Temporomandibular Disorders. Diagnosis and Treatment*. Philadelphia: WB Saunders, 1991.
3. Mohl N. The temporomandibular joint. In: Mahl N, Zarb G, Carlsson G, Rugh J, eds. *A Textbook of Occlusion*. Chicago: Quintessence, 1988.
4. Perry H, Xu Y, Forbes D. The embryology of the temporomandibular joint. *J Craniomand Pract* 3:126, 1985.
5. Pruzansky S. Not all dwarfed mandibles are alike. In: Begoma D, ed. *Malformation Syndromes*. II. Baltimore: Williams & Wilkins for the National Foundation—March of Dimes, *Birth Defects* 2:120, 1969.
6. Mulliken JB, Kaban LB. Analysis and treatment of hemifacial microsomia in childhood. *Clin Plast Surg* 14:91, 1987.
7. Kaban LB, Moses MH, Mulliken JB. Surgical correction of hemifacial microsomia in the growing child. *Plast Reconstr Surg* 82:9, 1988.
8. McCarthy JG. Craniofacial microsomia. In: Seratin D, Georgiade NG, eds. *Pediatric Plastic Surgery*. St. Louis: CV Mosby, 1984.
9. Kaplan RG. Induced condylar growth in a patient with hemifacial microsomia. *Angle Orthod* 59:85, 1989.
10. Coung PH, Nam IW, Kim KS. Vascularized cranial bone grafts for mandibular and maxillary reconstruction. *J Cranio Maxillofac Surg* 19:235, 1991.
11. Kamiji T, Ohmori K, Takada H. Chinical experience with patients with facial bone deformities associated with hemifacial microsomia. *J Craniofac Surg* 2:181, 1982.
12. Kummoona R. Chondro-osseous iliac crest for stage reconstruction of the ankylosed TMJ in children. *J Maxillofac Surg* 14:215, 1986.
13. Dingman RD. Follow-up clinic: Reconstruction of both mandibular condyles with metatarsal bone grafts. *Plast Reconstr Surg* 47: 594, 1971.

14. Siemssen SO. Temporomandibular arthroplasty by transfer of the sternoclavicular joint on a muscle pedicle. *Br J Plast Surg* 35:225, 1982.
15. Mulliken JB, Ferraro NF, Vento AR. A retrospective analysis of growth of the constructed condyle-ramus on children with hemifacial microsomia. *Cleft Palate J* 26:312, 1989.
16. Munro IR, Phillips JH, Griffin G. Growth after conservation of the temporomanibular joint in children with hemifacial microsomia. *Cleft Palate J* 26:312, 1989.
17. Guyuron B, Lasa CI. Unpredictable growth pattern of costochondral graft. *Plast Reconstr Surg* 90:880, 1992.
18. McCarthy JG, Schrieber J, Karp N, Thorne CH, Grayson BH. Lengthening of the human mandible by gradual distraction. *Plast Reconstr Surg* 89:1, 1992.
19. McCarthy JG. The role of distraction osteogenesis in the reconstruction of the mandible in unilateral craniofacial microsomia. *Clin Plast Surg* 21:625, 1994.
20. McCarthy JG. Mandibular bone lengthening. *Open Tech Plast Reconstr Surg* 1:99, 1994.
21. Molina F, Ortiz-Monasterio F. Mandibular elongation and remodeling by distraction: A farewell to major osteotomies. *Plast Reconstr Surg* 96:825, 1995.
22. Ortiz-Monasterio F, Molina F. Mandibular distraction in hemifacial microsomia. *Oper Tech Plast Reconstr Surg* 1:105, 1994.
23. Havlick RJ, Bartlett SP. Mandibular distraction lengthening in the severely hypoplastic mandible: A problematic case with tongue aplasia. *J Craniofac Surg* 5:305, 1994.
24. Habal MB. New bone formation by biologic rhythmic distraction. *J Craniofac Surg* 5: 344, 1994.
25. Rachmiel A, Levy M, Laufer D. Lengthening of the mandible by distraction osteogenesis: Report of cases. *J Oral Maxillofac Surg* 53:838, 1995.
26. McCormick SU, McCarthy JG, Grayson BH, Staffenberg D, McCormick SA. Effect of mandibular distraction on the temporomandibular joint: Part 1, Canine study. *J Craniofac Surg* 6:358, 1995.
27. McCormick SU, Grayson BH, McCarthy JG, Staffenberg D. Effect of mandibular distraction on the temporomandibular joint: Part 2, Clinical study. *J Craniofac Surg* 6:364,1995.
28. Stucki-McCormick SU, Molina F, Ortiz-Monasterio F. Unpublished data, 1996.
29. Ellis E, III Hinton RJ. Histologic examination of the temporomandibular joint after advancement with and without rigid fixation. *J Oral Maxillofac Surg* 49:1316, 1991.
30. Arnett GW. A redefinition of bilateral sagittal osteotomy (BSO) advancement relapse. *Am J Orthod Dentofac Orthop* 104:506, 1993.
31. Karaharju-Suvanto T, Peltonen J, Ranta R, Laitinen Kahri A. The effect of gradual distraction of the mandible on the sheep temporomandibular joint. *Int J Oral Maxillofac Surg* 25:125, 1996.
32. Ilizarov GA, Ledyaev VI. The replacement of tubular bone defects by lengthening distraction osteotomy of the fragments. *Clin Orthop* 280:7, 1992.
33. Ilizarov GA. The principles of the Ilizarov method. *Bull Hosp J Dis* 48:1, 1988.
34. Ilizarov GA. Clinical application of the tension-stress effect of limb lengthening. *Clin Orthop* 250:8, 1990.
35. Costantino PD, Shybut G, Friedman CD et al. Segmental mandibular regeneration by distraction osteogenesis. *Arch Otolaryngol Head Neck Surg* 116:535, 1990.
36. Costantino PD, Friedman CD. Distraction osteogenesis. Applications for mandibular regrowth. *Otolaryngol Clin North Am* 24: 1433, 1991.
37. Costantino PD, Friedman CD, Shindo ML, Houston G, Sissons GA. Experimental mandibular regrowth by distraction osteogenesis. *Otolaryngol Head Neck Surg* 119:511, 1993.
38. Gantous A, Phillips JH, Cotton P, Holmberg D. Distraction osteogenesis in the irradiated mandible. *Plast Reconstr Surg* 93:164, 1994.
39. Stucki-McCormick SU. Reconstruction of the mandibular condyle using transport distraction osteogenesis. *J Craniofac Surg.* 8:48, 1997.

CHAPTER 9

VOLUMETRIC STUDIES FOLLOWING MANDIBULAR DISTRACTION

Douglas A. Roth, Richard J. Mackool, and Joseph G. McCarthy

The clinical results of distraction of the hypoplastic mandible have been illustrated qualitatively by the improvement in facial symmetry and appearance, improvement in dental occlusion, and improvement in upper airway obstruction (1,2); however, there has been no established method for quantitative assessment of the new bone volume comprising the bony regenerate. Although distraction osteogenesis was originally developed for and applied to reconstruction of long-bone defects in the extremities many years before being applied in the craniofacial skeleton, there has been no demonstrated method for quantitative volume analysis of newly formed bone (3).

Several authors have used computed tomography scans of the craniofacial skeleton with and without image-analysis software programs to determine intraorbital and intracranial volumes (4–7). This method of CT-derived volume determination has also been used to quantitate the changes after cranial vault remodeling in patients with various craniosynostosis syndromes (8–14).

In a series of patients undergoing unilateral and bilateral distraction of the mandible, a method was developed for quantitative volumetric assessment utlizing the pre- and postdistraction computed tomographic scans (15). The CT-derived volume method was validated by scanning three dry cadaver mandible specimens and comparing the volume data

*Reproduced in part from a paper entitled A CT scan technique for quantitative volumetric assessment of the mandible after distraction ostoegenesis. *Plast Reconstr Surg* 99:1237, 1997.

to those derived from a standard water displacement method. The difference between the two methods was less than 5%. A group of five unilateral mandibular distraction patients had a mean mandibular volume increase of 27%, and a group of five bilateral mandibular distraction patients had a mean mandibular volume increase of 25%. Prior to this study there had been no documentation of the volume of the bony regenerate created by distraction.

Computed tomography scans have been used for nonvolumetric analyses of the craniofacial skeleton. Using multiple linear measurements of the cranio-orbital-zygomatic region on the axial and coronal views of CT scans, Posnick and associates were able to assess quantitatively the presenting deformity of several craniofacial syndromes and the results of cranial vault remodeling (11–13,16–18). The method utilized for the linear measurements was compared to dry skull measurements and found to have satisfactory correlation with a mean difference of 0.9% (19).

Volumetric determinations in craniofacial surgery have previously been employed to estimate intracranial and intraorbital volumes. CT-derived volumetric determinations have been validated by comparison to water displacement technques (9,10,20). In 1955 MacKinnon (21) made direct measurement of intracranial volume in 52 dry adult skulls by filling the skulls with lead shot. Although there was a relationship between the measured volume of the dry skulls and the glabella-opisthocranion distances, estimation of intracranial volume by the single dry skull measurement produced an error of up to 17% with respect to the measured dry skull volume. Subsequently MacKinnon and colleagues (22) determined a formula for the optimum estimate of cranial capacity based on a series of linear measurements recorded from the anteroposterior and lateral skull radiographs. This formula was accurate to within 6.2% of the measured intracranial volume. Based on this calculation, numerous authors have made clinical measurments of intracranial volume in normal pediatric populations (23–29). Radiographically derived measurements of intracranial volume have also been made in French, British, American, East Indian, and West Indian children. Of these studies, only Lichtenberg's (23) data provide statistics on the mean and standard deviation of the intracranial volume in children grouped by age and sex. For this reason, statistical analyses of intracranial volume in pediatric populations have relied on Lichtenberg's normative data (4,8,10). Comparisons of the various studies of intracranial volume in normal pediatric populations show considerable variability from one study to another. The variation in the results and volumetric data may also be due to differences in radiographic technique and the resultant error in the measurements used to calculate intracranial volume, which are derived from plain roentgenograms. This error could have been avoided had a ruler been placed on the patient, allowing measurements from the radiographs to be converted to real measurements (22). Another shortcoming of roentgenographic techniques for determinations of intracranial volume is their reliance on skull symmetry. Due to cranial vault asymmetry, the techniques are not valid in determining intracranial volume in patients with craniofacial synostosis (27). CT-derived volumetric calculations are therefore necessary in patients with skull asymmetry due to cranial synostosis (10).

CT-derived soft tissue volumes were first determined by Koehler and associates (30). The technique was further refined by Brieman and colleagues (31) in calculating organ volumes in cadaver specimens to within 5% of the volume measured by water displacement techniques. Keller and associates (32) described a technique for automatic outlining of regions of the CT scan based on CT density. Bite and colleagues (5) utilized a technique of automatic outlining of regions from CT scans using a software package in order to estimate orbital volumes in patients with enopthalmos. Orbital slices (1.5 mm) were obtained, and intraorbital volume was calculated by counting the number of voxels, or measures of a unit of volume, on each slice. However, it was difficult to determine the accuracy of the method, as the paper on the methodology of the technique was unpublished at the time of the report. In addition, there has been technical difficulty in automated outlining of the ventral surface of the orbit, especially that position toward the orbital rim (6). Manson and colleagues (33) avoided these shortcomings by calculating intraorbital volume in enophthalmos from hand traced images obtained from thin CT slices. The intraorbital volumes estimated from CT scans were correlated to volumes determined from direct measurement. By analyzing intraorbital volume of both bone and soft tissue structures in patients with enophthalmos, the above studies concluded that an increase in the bony intraorbital volume is the major etiologic component of post-traumatic enophthalmos.

Dufresne and colleagues (9) used a software package for automatic contour tracing to determine intracranial volume and intraventricular volume following cranial vault remodeling. While an accurate assessment of the relative change in volume following cranial vault remodeling could be obtained in this study, the absolute volumes were not correlated to real skull volumes. Gooskens and colleagues (34) used a hand-tracing technique to determine intracranial volume in 60 children. While they attempted to provide a CT-derived database for intracranial volume in children, the weaknesses of the study included a lack of correlation between obtained volumes and actual skull volumes and an inconsistent technique in obtaining the CT scans among different patients. Gault and colleagues (4,8) traced the intracranial area by hand from actual CT scan slices to determine intracranial volume with accurate correlation to measured dry skull volumes. Posnick and associates (11) showed that automated contour tracing with a software package also had satisfactory correlation to dry skull volumes. A recent study in our laboratory has shown that in normal skulls without significant asymmetry, there is an accurate correlation between the CT-derived volume, the roentgenographically derived volume, and the measured skull volume at autopsy (10).

Using both the axial slices and the three-dimensional osseous reconstructions from pre- and postoperative CT scans, Lo and colleages measured anterior cranial fossa length-to-width ratios, the supraorbital rim lag, and the orbital volumes of a series of patients to assess the stability of the surgically advanced fronto-orbital segment in nonsyndromic bilateral coronal craniosynostosis patients (35). The technique relied on a software program (Analyze, Biomedical Imaging Resources, Mayo Foundation, Minn.) installed directly at the CT console in order to perform both linear and volumetric analyses of the patient data.

TECHNIQUE

Following distraction osteogenesis, the mandible was maintained in fixation (with the external device attached) for an average of 8 weeks to allow complete consolidation of the regenerate. Each patient was evaluated before and after distraction of the mandible with standardized medical quality photographs, conventional posteroanterior, and lateral cephalograms, and dental casts. Each patient was also evaluated using a GE 9800 Computerized Tomographic Scanner (GE Medical Systems, 3000 North Granview, Waukesha WI 53188). Preoperative and post-distraction CT scans were obtained to define the deformity, determine the feasibility of surgery, plan the site of osteotomy, evaluate the outcome of treatment, and plan any secondary treatment, if necessary. Nine patients were scanned an average of 28 days after removal of the distraction device and one was scanned 26 months after device removal.

All CT scans were obtained using a standard protocol consisting of 3 mm contiguous axial images taken from the hyoid bone to the cranial vertex with the patient in a supine position. In the typical scan, the mandible consisted of 22 to 25 slices from menton to condyle. The CT scanner was set up with a 15-cm diameter scan circle with a 512×512 pixel reconstruction matrix yielding a voxel size (volume element) of $0.27\,mm^3$. Three-dimensional surface reconstructions from the CT scans were used for preoperative planning and for qualitative assessment of the mandibular distraction results.

For CT-derived volume determination, hardcopies of the CT scans (bone windows only) were digitized at 1024×1024 pixels to 8 bits of gray scale using a Lumisys laser film digitizer (Advanced Video Products, Westford, MA, 01886) and transferred to a Macintosh Centris 610 computer (Apple Computer Corp., Cupertino, CA). Each slice was analyzed using image analysis software (36). The level and window of each slice was optimally set by the computer in a standard fashion on all studies to allow precise delineation between bony cortex and soft tissue. An optimal threshold for the bone/soft tissue interface was determined and maintained for consistent use throughout each study. Under direction of the operator, the program automatically outlined the bony contours of the mandible on the basis of this threshold (32).

Figure 9.1 illustrates the technique of outlining the specific contours of the mandible in different axial cuts. The area within the contour can be precisely determined by calibrating the image analysis program with the 5-cm scale reproduced on every hard-copy axial image. For the five unilateral distraction cases in group I, the mandible was divided using two landmarks: On the digitized CT scans a line was constructed between the central incisors and the genial tubercle on the alveolar surface (Figure 9.2). Mandibular volume was computed by first applying Green's theorem to each contour on serial contiguous slices to obtain area (cm^2) within the contour, then muliplying by the slice width (0.3 cm) to obtain the volume contribution of each slice, and finally summing over slices pertaining to the mandible for mandibular bone volume:

$$\text{Volume} = \sum_{\text{all } n} \Bigg[\underbrace{\frac{1}{2} \int (x_n dy_n - y_n dx_n)}_{\text{area}} \times \underbrace{\frac{1}{2}(z_{n-1} - z_{n+1})}_{\text{slice width}} \Bigg].$$

In order to validate the accuracy of the CT-derived volume determination

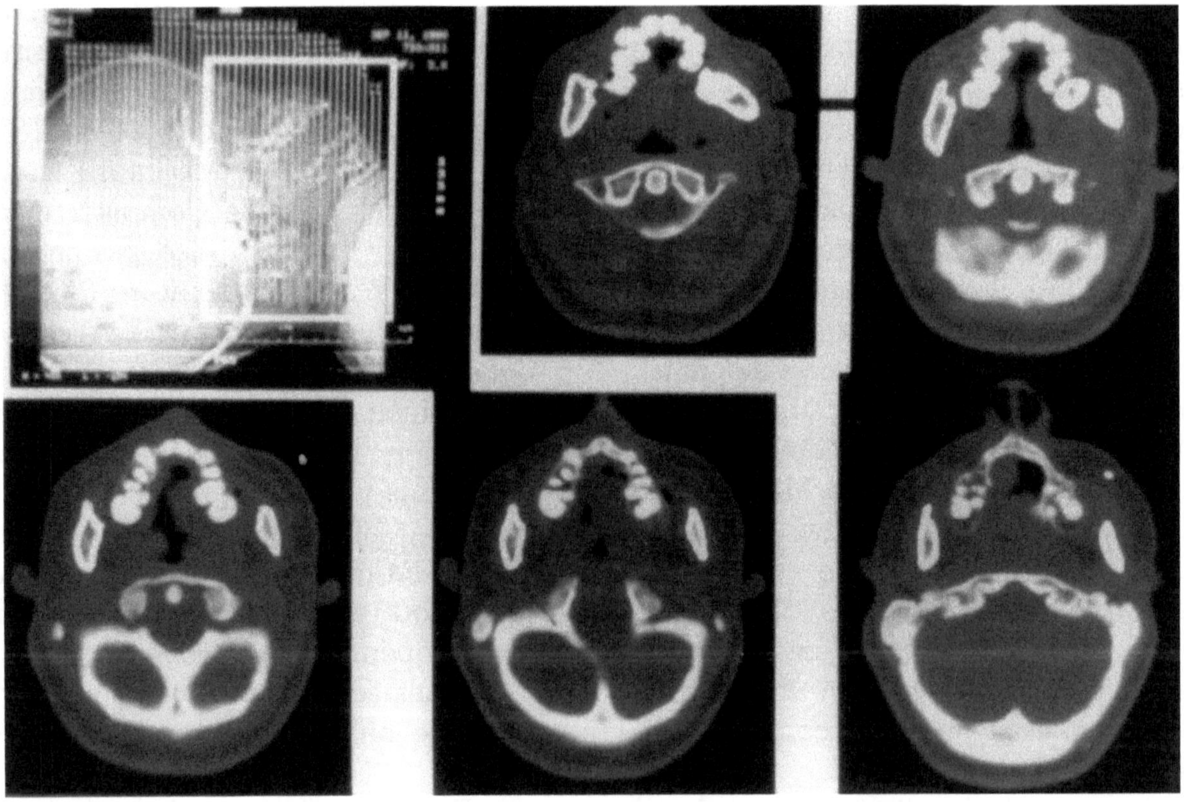

Figure 9.1. Outlining the contour of the mandible on serial axial slices progressing in a cephalad direction along the rami of the mandible. Note the 22–25 slices through the mandible (upper left scout panel).

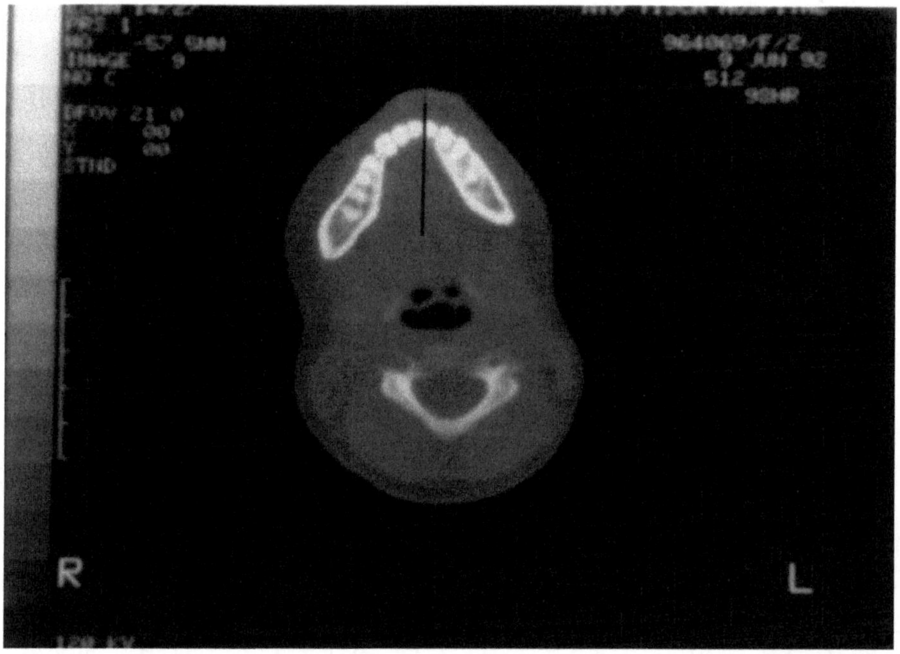

Figure 9.2. For unilateral cases the mandible was arbitrarily divided by a line drawn between the central incisors and the genial tubercle.

technique, several human and canine cadaver mandible specimens were subjected to CT scanning with the identical protocol as the pediatric craniofacial patients. The cadaver specimens underwent standard craniofacial CT scans consisting of 3-mm axial cuts. The same specimens were subjected to volume determination by a water displacement technique. The technique for measuring the volume of the cadaver mandibles by water displacement was as follows: (1) the dry mandibles were first weighed (Mettler Balance Co.); (2) they were covered with a thin layer of heated paraffin wax to occlude all porous surfaces and then reweighed. The difference in weight corresponded to the amount of paraffin wax added. With the known density of the paraffin (Tissue processing medium type 9, Stephen Scientific Co., Riverdale, NJ, 07457-1710) the added volume of paraffin was determined; (3) the paraffin-covered mandibles were placed in graduated cylinders to determine volume by measuring water displacement; (4) the volume of the mandible specimen was determined by subtracting the volume of the extra paraffin wax from the volume of the paraffin-covered mandible. The water displacement volume method was repeated three times for each specimen. The results of both the CT-derived and water-displacement volumes for the cadaver mandible specimens are summarized in Table 9.1. The difference between the two methods was less than 5%.

CLINICAL CASES

The characteristics of five unilateral mandibular distraction patients are summarized in Table 9.2. The results of the

Table 9.1. Correlation of water displacement volume and CT-derived volume of cadaver mandibles. Water displacement and CT-derived volumes are the means of three determinations.

Cadaver mandibles	Water displacement (cc)	CT-derived volume (cc)	Difference (cc)	Difference (%)
#1	59.5	57.3	2.2	3.7
#2	63.4	66.2	2.8	4.4
#3	71.8	68.5	3.3	4.6
				Avg % difference = 4.2

CT-derived volume determinations pre- and postdistraction are summarized in Table 9.3. The average increase in hemimandibular volume was 2.8 cc with an average increase in percentage volume of 27%.

Patient 1 with unilateral craniofacial microsomia underwent 23 mm of distraction osteogenesis on the left side of the mandible. The volumetric analysis showed an increase of 16.4% bone volume following distraction on the left side. Figure 9.3, consisting of the pre- and postdistraction 3D CT scans, illustrates the increased height of the left mandibular ramus with corresponding shift of the pogonion toward the midline. Additional examples of unilateral mandibular distraction are illustrated in Figures 9.4, 9.5, and 9.6.

The characteristics of five bilateral distraction cases are outlined in Table 9.4. The results of the volume analyses for the bilateral distraction group are summarized in Table 9.5. The average increase in total mandibular bone volume was 7.9 cc with an average percentage increase of 25% from the predistraction bone vol-

Table 9.2. Clinical characteristics of the unilateral mandibular distraction patients. The amount of distraction was recorded from the calibration scale on the device at the time of removal.

Unilateral	Age (yrs)	Diagnosis	Length of distraction (mm)
#1	8	UCM	23
#2	10.5	Goldenhaar	28
#3	7.7	UCM	20
#4	2.5	UCM	30
#5	3	UCM	25

UCM = unilateral craniofacial microsomia.

Table 9.3. Results of CT-derived volume measurements for unilateral distraction patients.

Patient (side of distraction)	Pre	Post	ΔV	% ΔV	CT scan interval (mos)
#1	R: 22.6	22.7	0.1	0.3	3
LEFT	**L: 14.2**	**16.5**	**2.3**	**16.4**	
#2	**R: 18.9**	**20.7**	**1.8**	**9.5**	5
RIGHT	L: 23.7	24	0.3	1.2	
#3	R: 18.3	19	0.7	3.8	4
LEFT	**I: 12.0**	**14.4**	**2.4**	**20**	
#4	R: 11.43	11.63	0.2	1.7	3
LEFT	**L: 11.33**	**13.65**	**2.32**	**20.5**	
#5	R: 8.42	13.67	5.25	62.4	31
LEFT	**L: 7.27**	**12.41**	**5.14**	**70.7**	

The distracted side is recorded in bold type. Pre = volume in cc of the right or left hemimandible determined from the predistraction CT scan, Post = postdistraction hemimandibular volume, ΔV = change in volume after distraction osteogenesis, %ΔV = percentage change in volume following unilateral distraction osteogenesis.

ume. Figures 9.7 and 9.8 represent examples of bilateral mandibular distraction and illustrate the improvements in ramus height and pogonion projection in addition to the mandibular volume determinations.

One of the problems encountered in this study was obtaining craniofacial CT scans immediately prior to and following distraction osteogenesis. Patient 5 of the unilateral distraction group underwent predistraction CT scanning 24 months prior to the distraction procedure; the postdistraction CT scan was obtained 30 days after the removal of the device. A similar problem occurred with patient 9 in the bilateral group. For this patient the predistraction CT scan was performed 12 months before distraction, whereas the postdistraction CT scan was performed 35 days after removal of the device. The relatively long interval between CT scans in these two patients adds a potentially large contribution from anticipated growth in the determination of the increase in mandibular bone volume resulting from distraction.

For the unilateral distraction cases the mandible was divided on the axial CT scan slices by a line drawn through the middle of the central incisors and through the genial tubercle on the alveolar surface of the mandible. By dividing the mandible in this fashion, the entire hemimandible on the affected side was analyzed for volume change following distraction. A potential problem with dividing the mandible as described is that there is still a portion of the body of the mandible that was not directly distracted that is included in the bone volume determination.

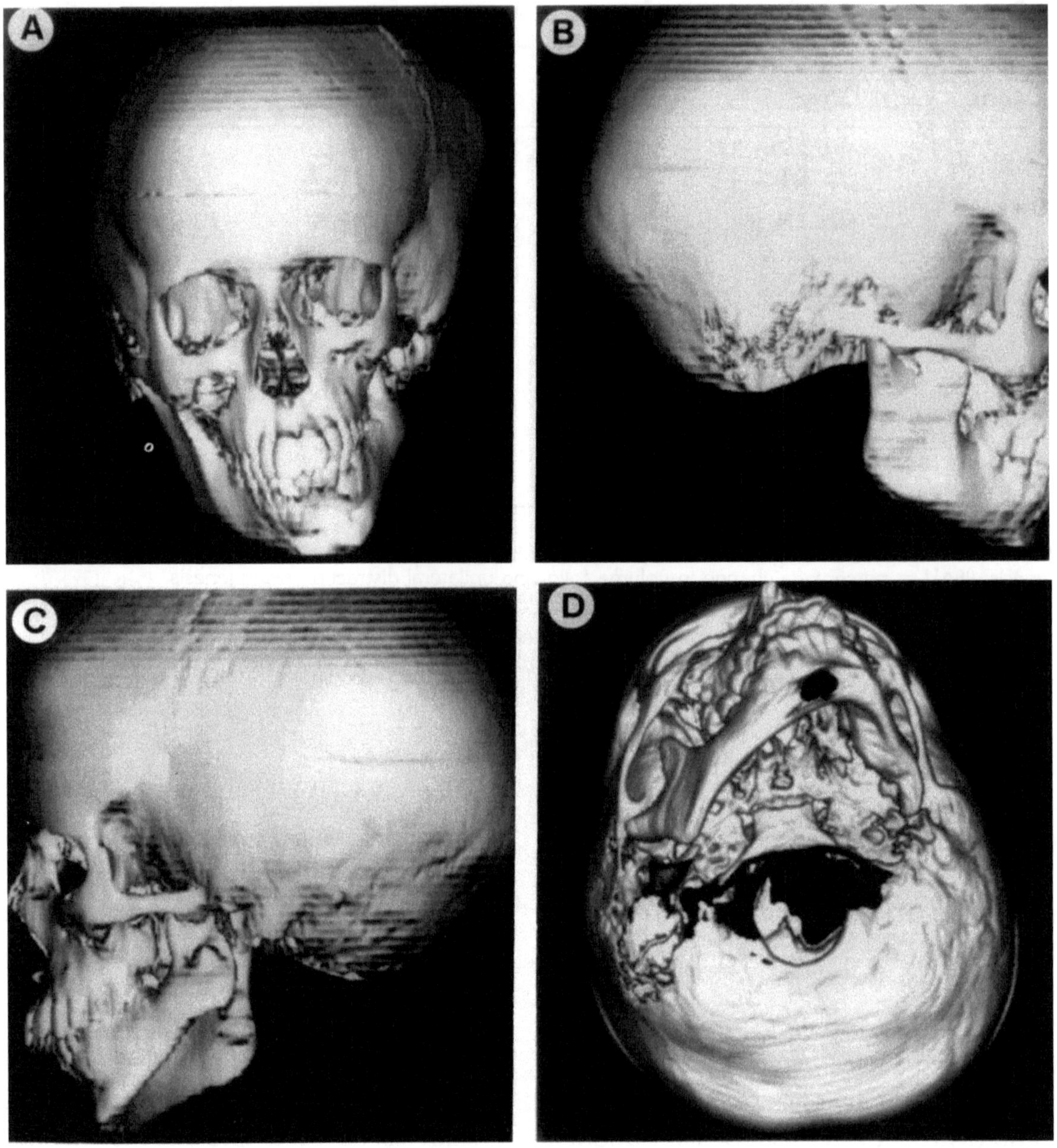

Figure 9.3. (A–D) Predistraction three-dimensional CT scan reconstructions (patient 1). (E–H) Postdistraction three-dimensional CT scan reconstructions. This 8-year-old female with unilateral craniofacial microsomia underwent 23 mm of mandibular distraction on the left side. There was a 16% increase in bone volume. Note that the position of the pogonion postdistraction is closer to the midline. The pinholes are visible on the postdistraction scan as shown in (G). The position, dimensions, and volume of the affected ramus and occlusal plane are improved.

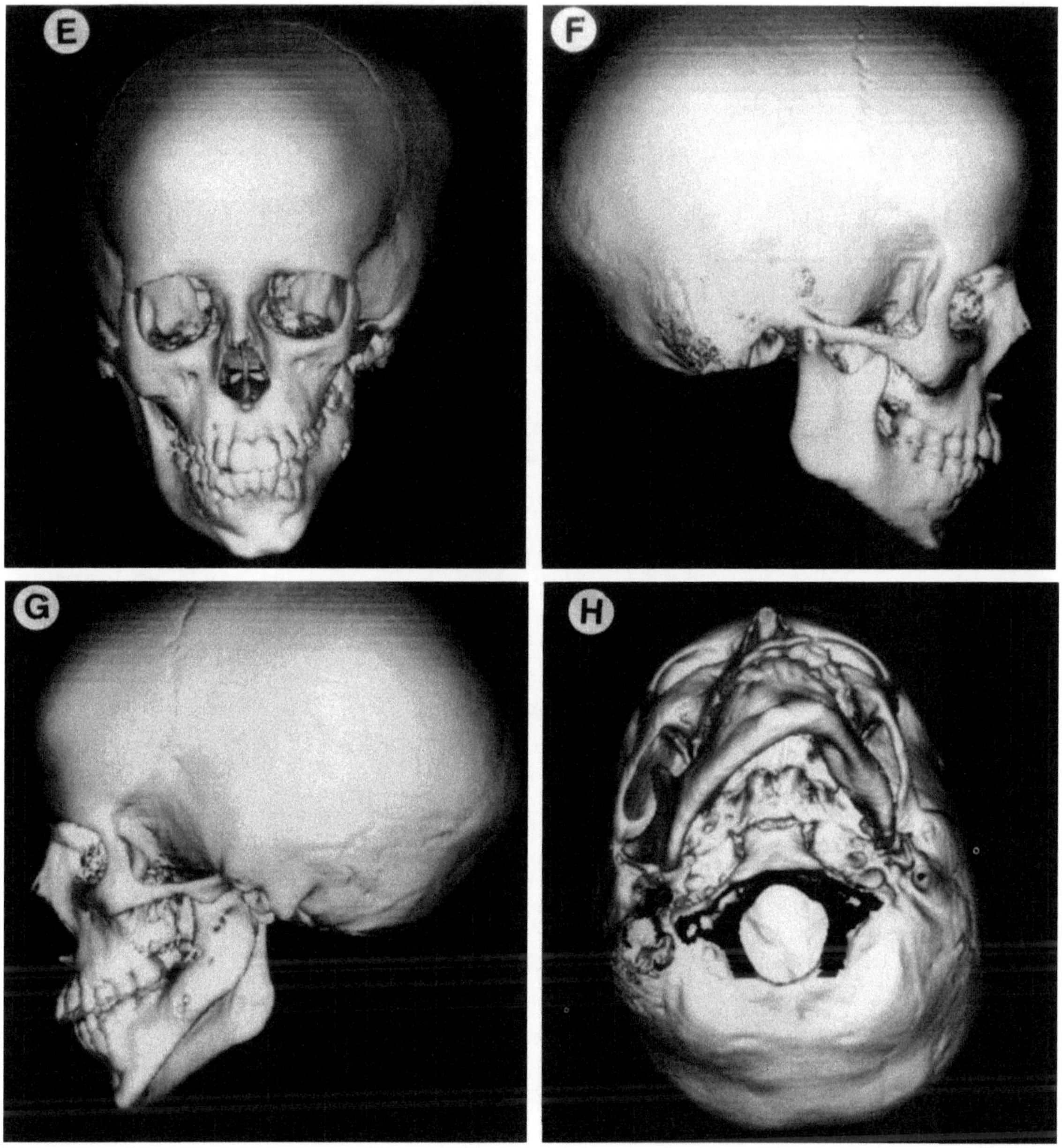

Figure 9.3. *Continued*

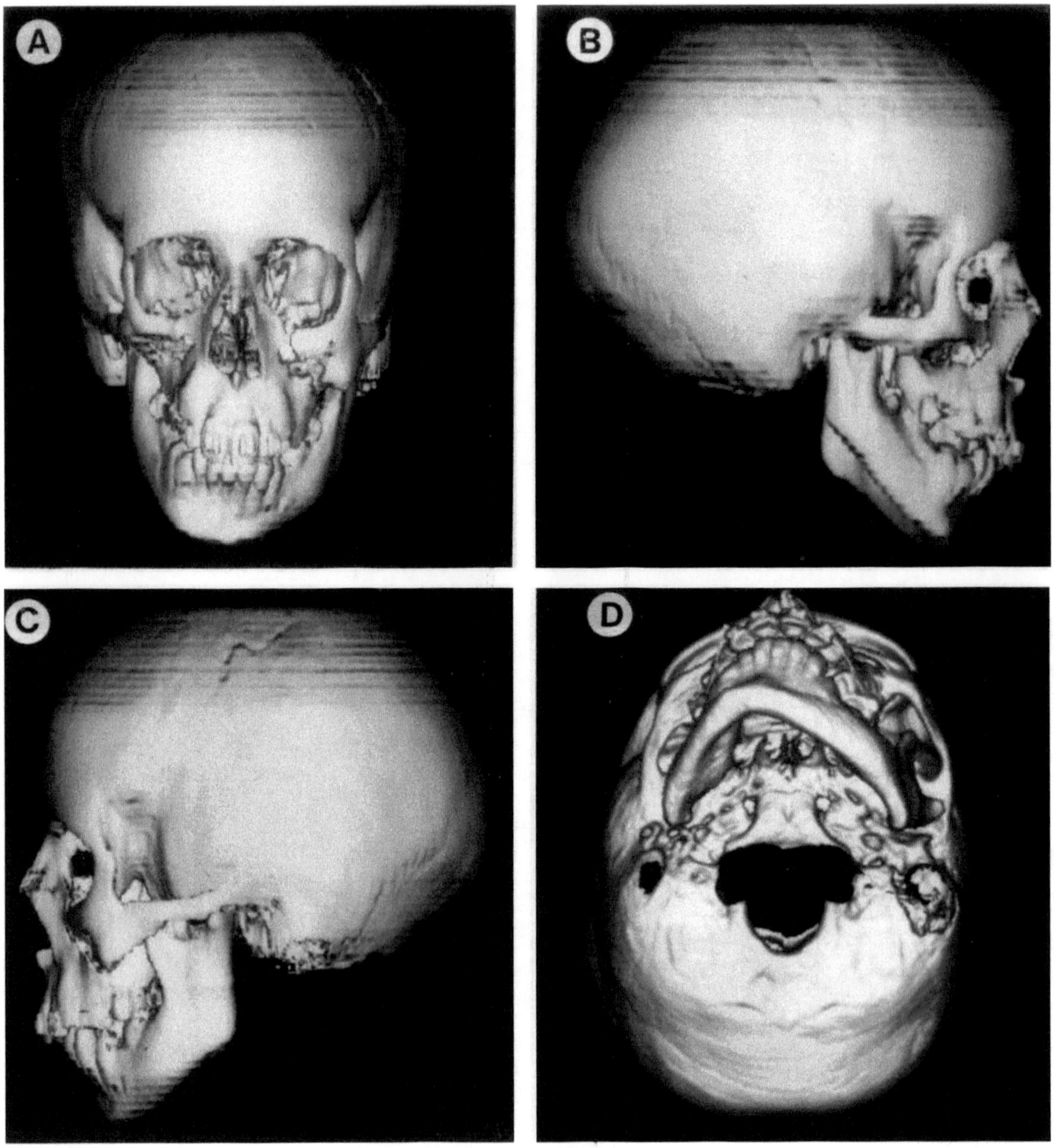

Figure 9.4. (A–D) Predistraction three-dimensional CT scan reconstructions (patient 2). (E–H) Postdistraction three-dimensional CT scan reconstructions. This patient is a 10-year-old female with Goldenhaar syndrome who underwent 28 mm of mandibular distraction on the right side. Note the increased height and more vertical position of the right ramus after distraction. Also note the improved chin position, leveling of the occlusal plane and the increase in the bigonial distance.

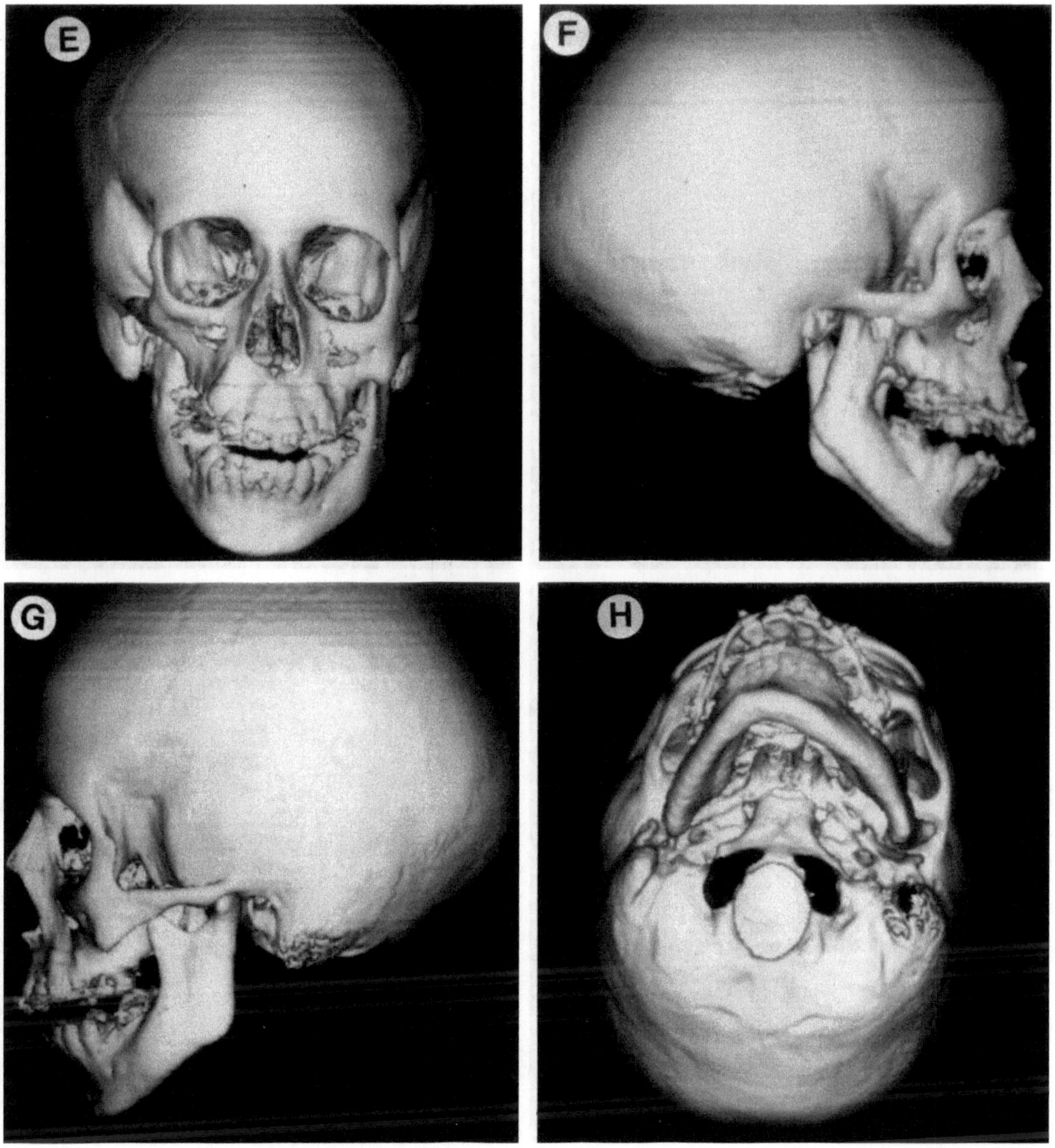

Figure 9.4. Continued

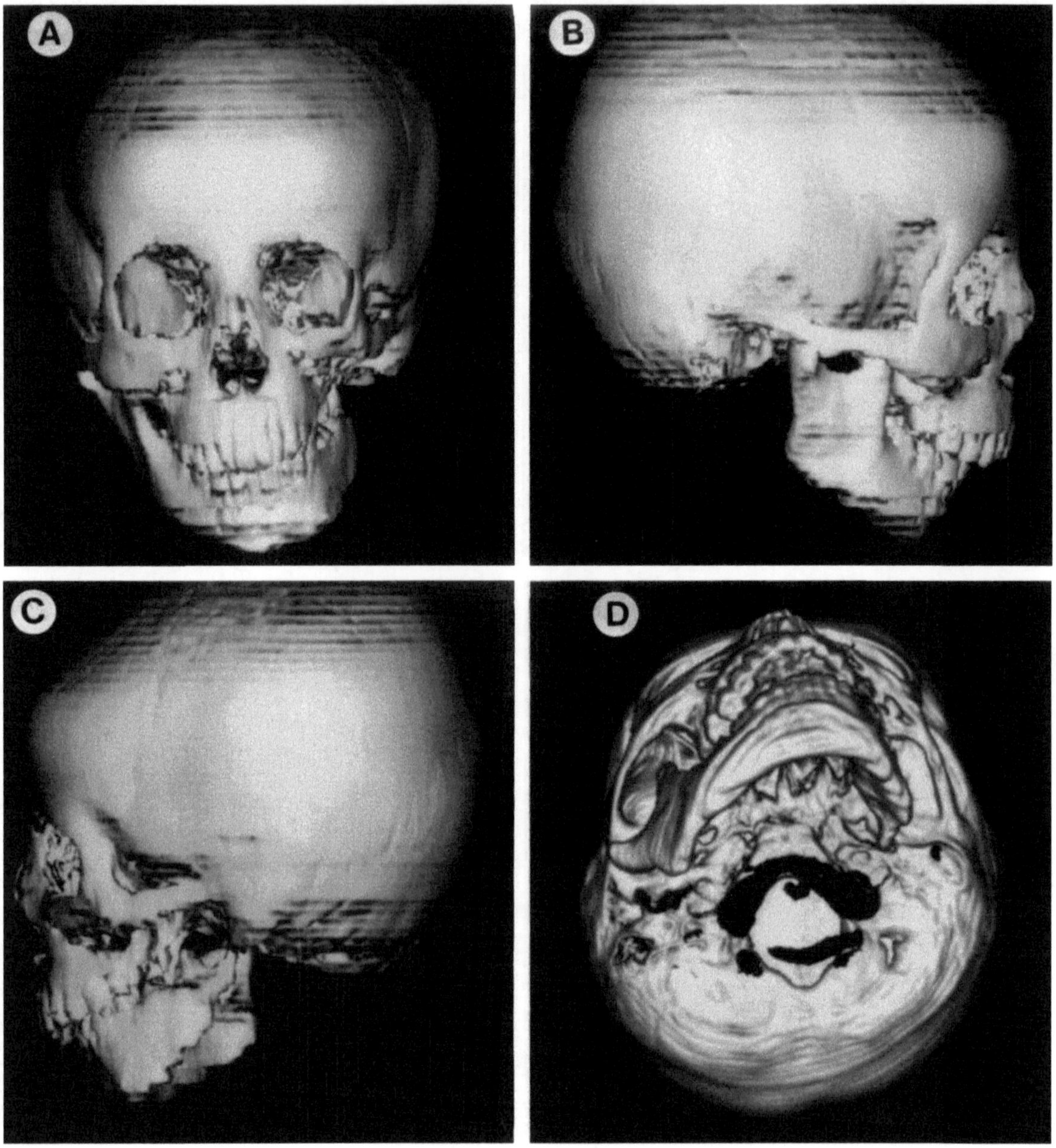

Figure 9.5. (A–D) Predistraction three-dimensional CT scan reconstructions (patient 3). (E–H) Postdistraction three-dimensional CT scan reconstructions. This patient is an 8-year-old with unilateral craniofacial microsomia who underwent 20 mm of mandibular distraction on the left side. Note the improvement in the position of the pogonion, decrease in the occlusal cant, as well as increased bony volume and improved position of the affected (left) ramus.

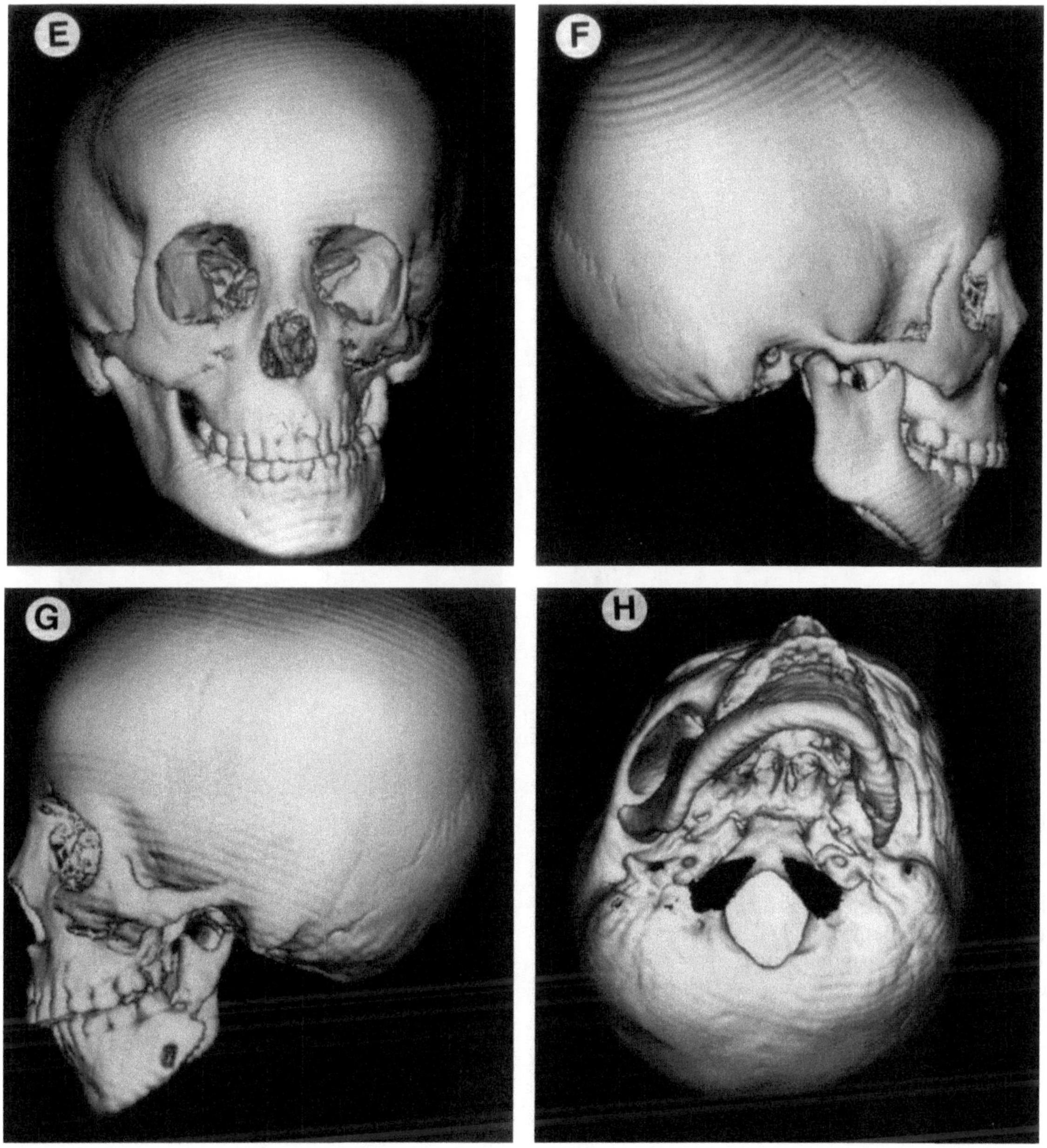

Figure 9.5. Continued

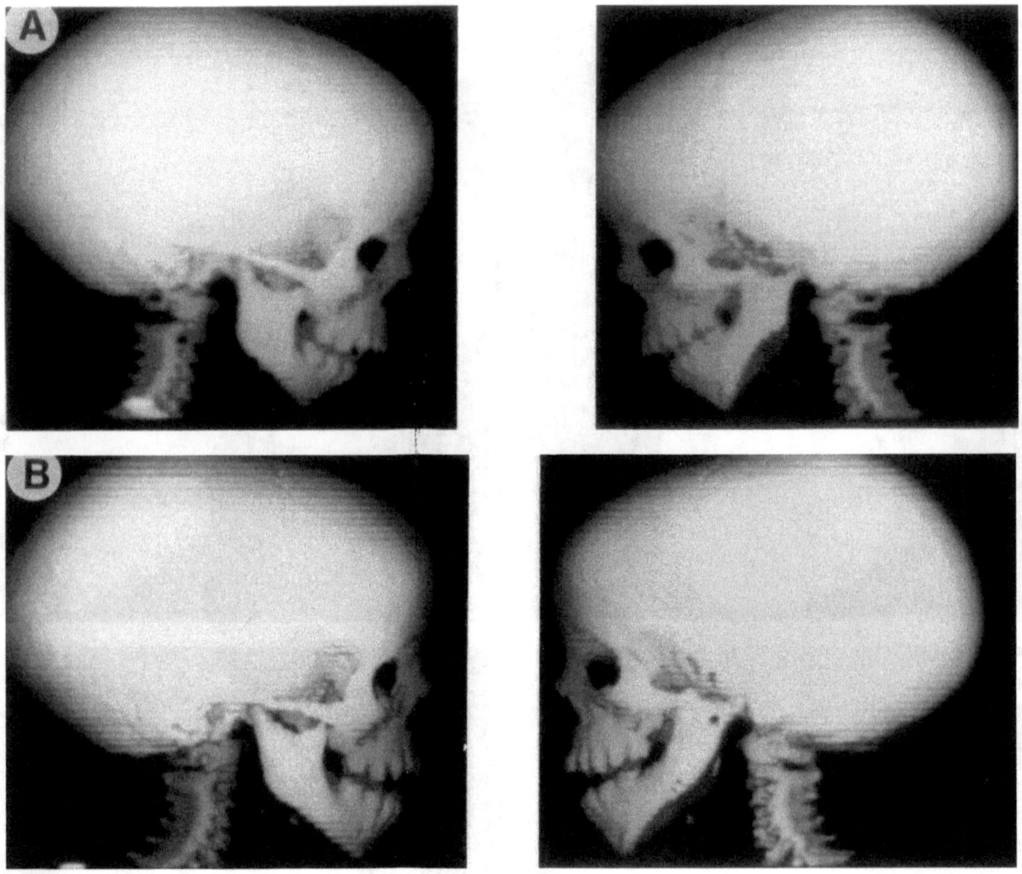

Figure 9.6. (A) Predistraction and (B) postdistraction three-dimensional CT scan reconstructions for patient 4 in Group I. This 30-month-old female patient with left-sided craniofacial microsomia underwent 30 mm of mandibular distraction on the left side. The increase in bone volume was 20.5%. Note the pin holes from the distraction device in the left side of the mandible in the postdistraction CT. Note the increase in the vertical dimension of the affected ramus and the increased projection of the pogonion.

Table 9.4. Clinical characteristics of bilateral mandibular distraction patients. The amount of distraction was recorded from the calibration scale on the device at the time of removal.

Bilateral	Age (yrs)	Diagnosis	Length of distraction (mm)
			Right, Left
#6	4	TC	20, 20
#7	19	BCM	21, 21
#8	3	DM	29, 28
#9	13.7	TC	19, 21
#10	3.3	NAGER	21, 21

BCM = bilateral craniofacial microsomia, TC = Treacher Collins syndrome, DM = developmental micrognathia.

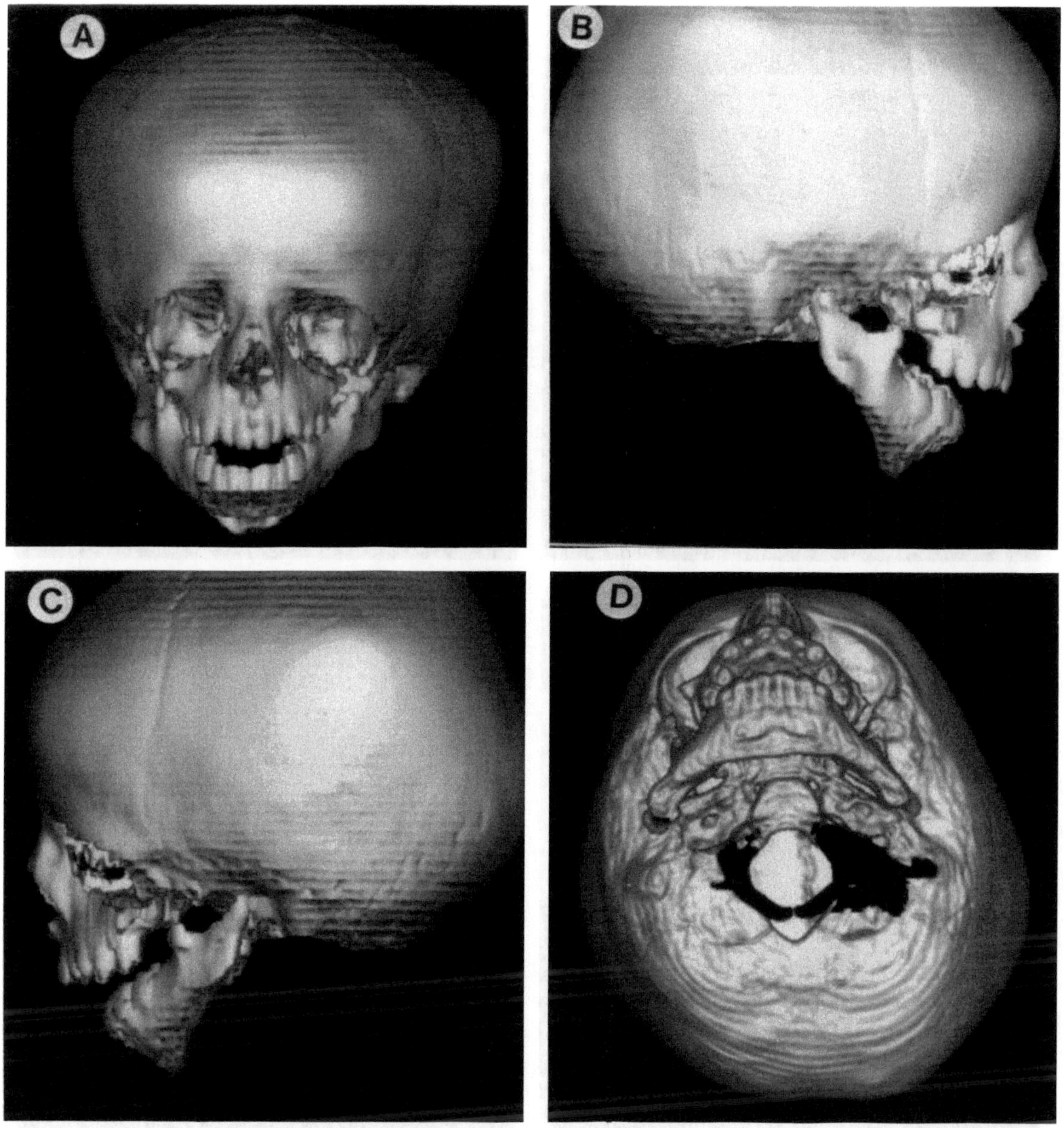

Figure 9.7. (A–D) Predistraction three-dimensional CT scan reconstructions (patient 6). (E–H) Postdistraction three-dimensional CT scan reconstructions. This 4-year-old male patient with severe Treacher Collins syndrome underwent 20 mm of distraction bilaterally. The increase in bone volume was 25%. Note the increase in projection of the pogonion, the increased dimensions of the bodies and the increase in vertical height of the rami. The anterior occlusal relationships are significantly improved but the open bite remains.

(Continued)

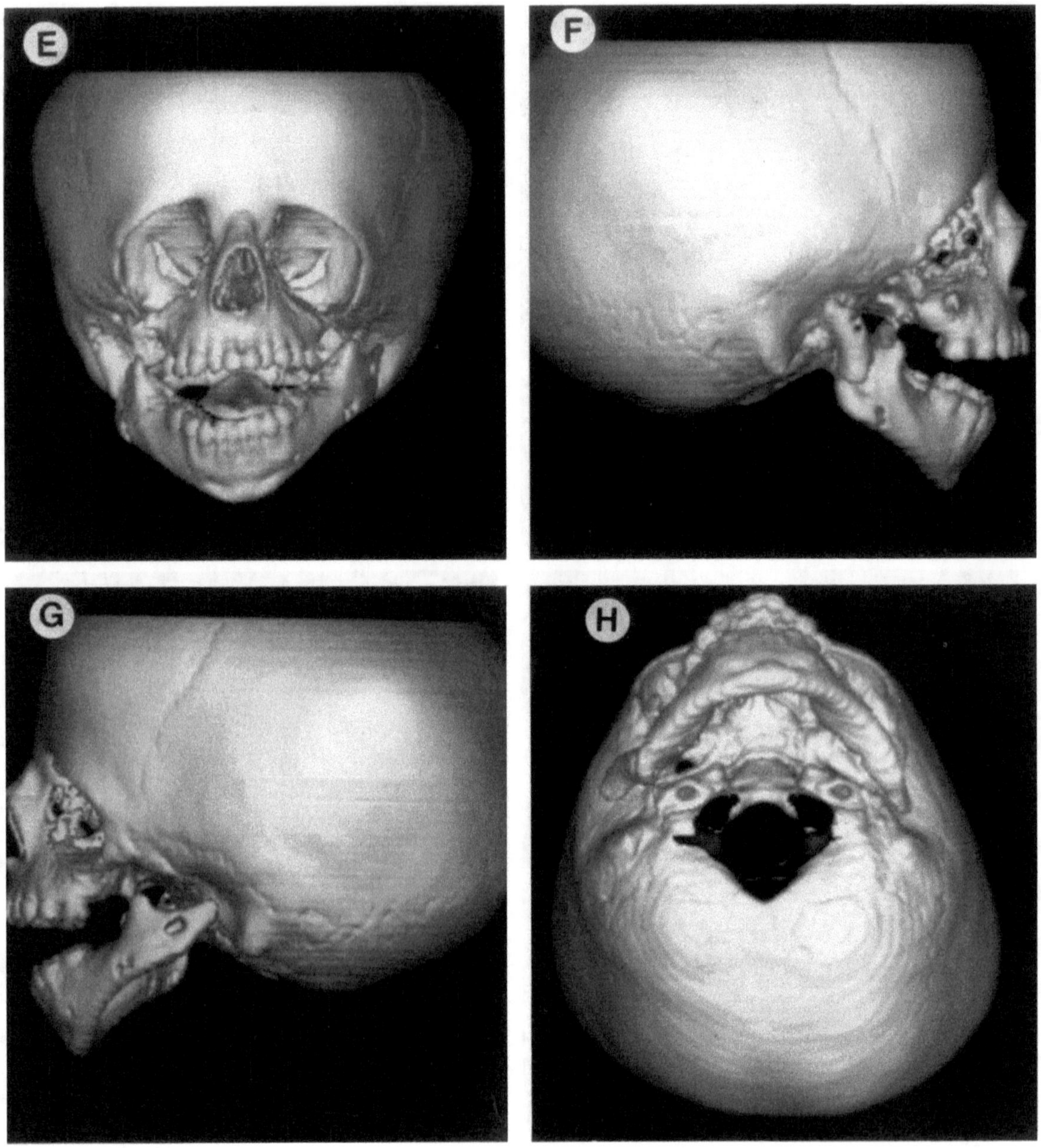

Figure 9.7. *Continued*

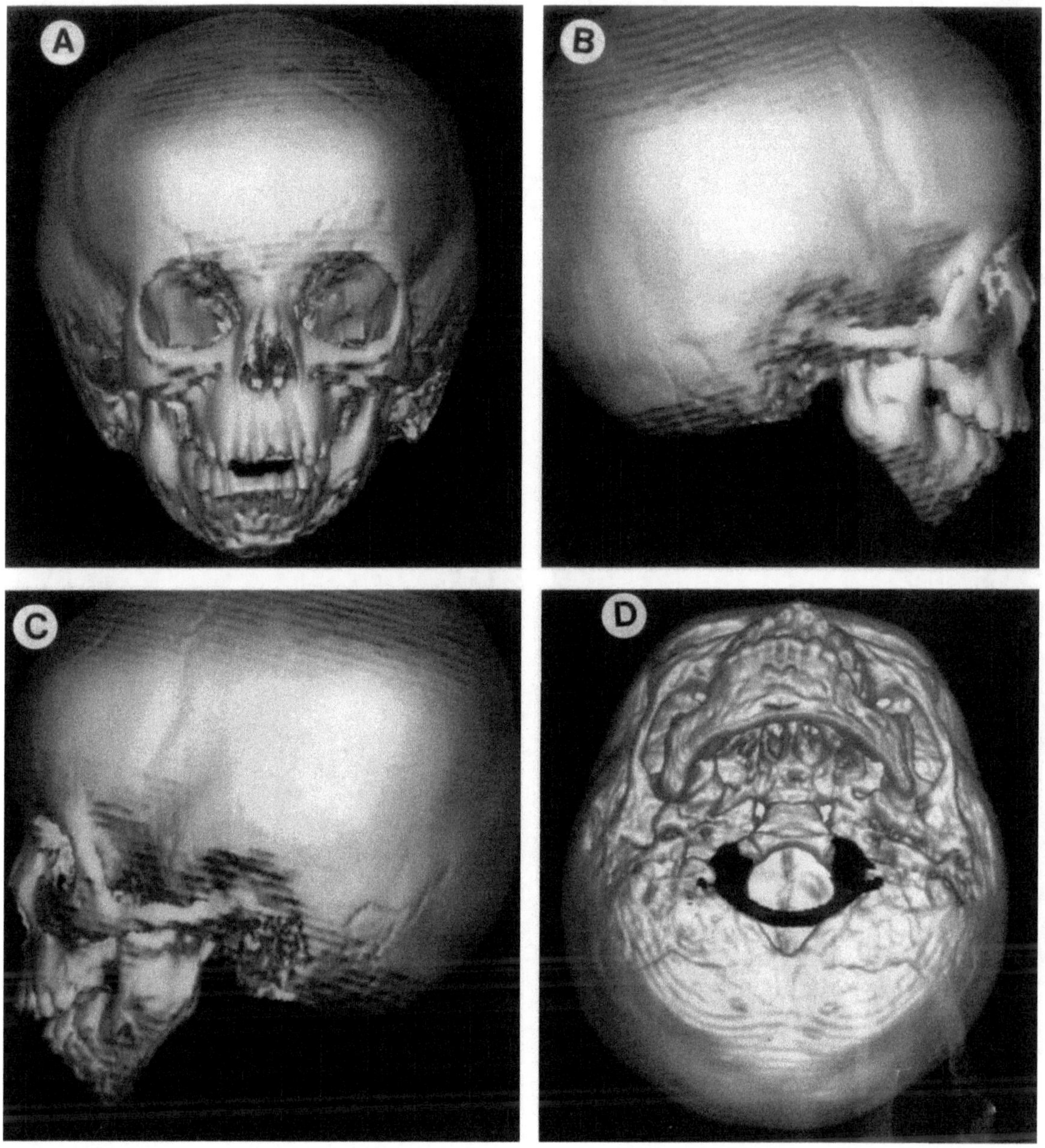

Figure 9.8. (A–D) Predistraction three-dimensional CT scan reconstructions (patient 8). (E–H) Postdistraction three-dimensional CT scan reconstructions. This 3-year-old male with developmental micrognathia underwent bilateral distraction (29 mm on right, 28 mm on left). The increase in bone volume was 30%. Note the increase in the vertical height of the rami, the increased dimensions of the bodies, and the counterclockwise rotation of the mandible with sagittal thrust of the pogonion (right profile views).

(*Continued*)

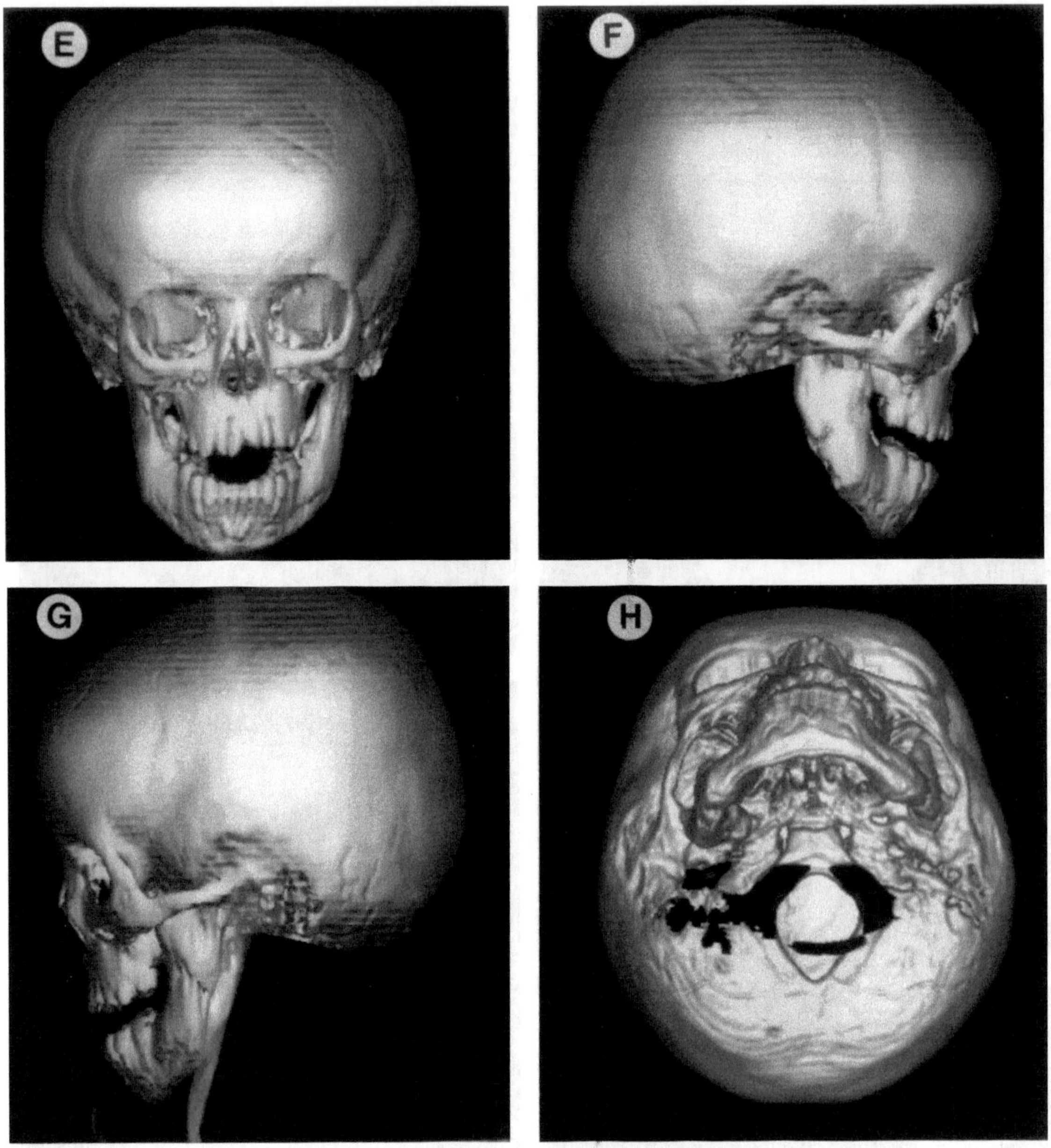

Figure 9.8. *Continued*

Table 9.5. Results of CT-derived volume for bilateral distraction patients.

Patient	Pre	Post	ΔV	% ΔV	CT scan interval (mos)
#6	18.4	23	4.6	25	3.5
#7	47	58.3	11.25	24	7
#8	34	44.3	10.3	30	5
#9	29.3	33.8	4.5	15.4	18*
#10	27.8	36.8	9	32.4	8

Pre = total mandibular volume in cc determined from predistraction CT scan, Post = total mandibular volume determined from postdistraction CT scan, ΔV = change in volume in cc between pre- and postdistraction CT scans, % ΔV = percentage change in total mandibular volume between pre- and postdistraction CT scans.

However, to study the mandibular ramus alone in order to focus specifically on the distraction zone would have required an arbitrary point of division of the mandible approximately where the ramus joins the body and would not have been consistent from one CT scan to another or from one patient to another.

References

1. McCarthy JG, Schreiber J, Karp N, Thorne CH, Grayson BH. Lengthening the human mandible by gradual distraction. *Plast Reconstr Surg* 89:1, 1992.
2. Moore MH, Guzman-Stein G, Proudman TW, Abbott AH, Netherway DJ, David DJ. Mandibular lengthening by distraction for airway obstruction in Treacher–Collins syndrome. *J Craniofac Surg* 5:22, 1994.
3. Garcia-Cembrelo E, Olsen B, Ruiz-Yague M, Fernandez-Baillo N, Munuera-Martinez L. Ilizarov technique. Results and difficulties. *Clin Orthop* 283:116, 1992.
4. Gault D, Brunelle F, Renier D, Marchac D. The calculation of intracranial volume using CT scans. *Childs Nerv Syst* 4:271, 1988.
5. Bite U, Jackson IT, Forbes GS, Gehring DG. Orbital volume measurements in enopthalmos using three-dimensional CT imaging. *Plast Reconstr Surg* 75:502, 1985.
6. Vannier M, March JA. Orbital volume measurments in enopthalmos using three-dimensional CT imaging (Discussion). *Plast Reconstr Surg* 75:508, 1985.
7. Geist CE, Stracher MA, Grove AS. Orbital augmentation by hydroxyapatite based composites: A rabbit study and comparative analysis. *Ophthal Plast Reconstr Surg* 7:8, 1991.
8. Gault DT, Renier D, Marchac D, Ackland FM, Jones BM. Intracranial volume in patients with craniosynostosis. *J Craniofac Surg* 1:1, 1990.
9. Dufresne DR, McCarthy JG, Gutting CB, Epstein FJ, Hoffman WY. Volumetric quantification of intracranial and ventricular volume following cranial vault remodeling: A preliminary report. *Plast Reconstr Surg* 79:24, 1987.
10. Gosain AK, McCarthy JG, Glatt P, Staffenberg D, Hoffman RG. A study of intracranial volume in Apert syndrome. *Plast Reconstr Surg* 95:284, 1995.
11. Posnick JC, Bite U, Nakano P, Davis J, Armstrong D. Indirect intracranial volume measurements using CT scans: Clinical applications for craniosynostosis. *Plast Reconstr Surg* 89:34, 1992.
12. Posnick JC, Armstrong D, Bite U. Metopic and sagittal synostosis: Intracranial volume measurements prior to and after cranio-orbital reshaping in childhood. *Plast Reconstr Surg* 96:299, 1995.
13. Posnick JC, Armstrong D, Bite U. Crouzon and Apert syndromes: Intracranial volume measurements before and after cranio-orbital reshaping in childhood. *Plast Reconstr Surg* 96:539, 1995.
14. Spinelli HM, Irizarry D, McCarthy JG, Cutting CB, Noz ME. An analysis of extradural dead space after fronto-orbital surgery. *Plast Reconstr Surg* 93:1372, 1994.
15. Roth DA, Gosain, AK, McCarthy JG, Stracher MA, Lefton DR, Grayson BH. A CT scan technique for quantitative volumetric assessment of the mandible after distraction osteogenesis. *Plast Reconstr Surg* 99:1237, 1997.
16. Posnick JC, Lin KY, Chen P, Armstrong D. Metopic synostosis: Quantitative assessment of presenting deformity and surgical results based on CT scans. *Plast Reconstr Surg* 92:1015, 1993.
17. Posnick JC, Lin KY, Chen P, Armstrong D. Sagittal synostosis: Quantitative assessment of presenting deformity and surgical results based on CT scans. *Plast Reconstr Surg* 92:1027, 1993.
18. Posnick JC, Lin KY, Chen P, Armstrong D. Apert syndrome: Quantitative assessment of presenting deformity and surgical results based on CT scans. *Plast Reconstr Surg* 93:489, 1994.
19. Waitzman AA, Posnick JC, Armstrong DC, Pron GE. Craniofacial skeletal measurements

based on computed tomography Part I. Accuracy and reproducibility. *Cleft Palate Craniofac J* 29:112, 1992.

20. Disler DG, Mar DS, Rosenthal DI. Accuracy of volume measurements of computed tomography and magnetic resonance imaging phantoms by three-dimensional reconstruction and preliminary clinical applications. *Invest Radiol* 29:739, 1994.
21. MacKinnon II. The relation of the capacity of the human skull to its roentgenological length. *AJR* 74:1026, 1955.
22. MacKinnon II, Kennedy JA, Davies TV. The estimation of skull capacity from roentgenological measurements. *AJR* 76:303, 1956.
23. Lichtenberg R. Radiographie du crane de 226 enfants normauz de la naissance à 8 ans: Impressions digitifomes, capacité, angles et indices. Thesis, University of Paris, 1960.
24. Gordon IRS. Measurement of cranial capacity in children. *Br J Radiol* 39:377, 1966.
25. Bray PF, Shields WD, Wolcott GJ, Madsen JA. Occipitofrontal head circumference: An accurate measure of intracranial volume. *J Pediatr* 75:303, 1969.
26. Walia HK, Sodhi JS, Gupta BB, Gulati DR. Roentgenologic determination of the cranial capacity in the first four years of life. *Indian J Radiol* 26:250, 1972.
27. Buda FB, Reed JC, Rabe EF. Skull volume in infants. *Am J Dis Child* 129:1171, 1975.
28. Fernandez F, Moule N, Singhi S. Roentgenographic skull volume in Jamaican children between the ages of one month and five years. *West Indian Med J* 33:227, 1984.
29. Singhi S, Walia BNS, Singhi P, Walia HK. A simple roentgenographic alternative for skull volume measurements in children. *Indian J Med Res* 82:150, 1985.
30. Koehler PR, Anderson RE, Baxter B. The effect of computed tomography viewer controls an anatomical measurements. *Radiology* 130:189, 1979.
31. Breiman RS, Beck JW, Korobkin M et al. Volume determination using computed tomograph *AJR* 138:329, 1982.
32. Keller JM, Edwards FM, Rundle R. Automatic outlining of regions of CT scans. *J Comput Tomograph* 5:240, 1981.
33. Manson PN, Grivas MA, Rosenbaum A et al. Studies on enopthalmos: II. The measurement of orbital injuries and their treatment by quantitative computed tomography. *Plast Reconstr Surg* 77:203, 1986.
34. Gooskens RH, Gielen CC, Hanto PW et al. Intracranial spaces in childhood macrocephaly: Comparison of length measurements and volume calculations. *Dev Med Child Neurol* 30:509, 1988.
35. Lo L, Marsh JL, Yoon J, Vannier MW. Stability of fronto-orbital advancement in nonsyndromic bilateral coronal synostosis: A quantitative three-dimensional computed tomographic study. *Plast Reconstr Surg* 98: 393, 1996.
36. NIH Image 1.54 is a public domain program written by Wayne Rasband at NIH, Research Services Branch, National Institute of Mental Health, Bethesda, MD, USA.

Part 3
The Midface and the Zygomas

CHAPTER 10

DISTRACTION OF THE MIDFACE AND THE ZYGOMA

EXPERIMENTAL STUDIES

Paul M. Glat and Joseph G. McCarthy

Distraction osteogenesis has been evaluated for eventual clinical use in the reconstruction of the mandible, cranial vault, midface, orbit, and other areas of the craniofacial skeleton. Many studies have been performed in animal models and subsequently applied in humans. The earliest use of distraction osteogenesis in the craniofacial skeleton was described in the orthodontic literature and involved the rapid expansion of the midpalatal suture of the maxilla. The zygoma has not received as much investigative attention as the other anatomic areas, but the technique is now being evaluated in this region as well.

MIDPALATAL SUTURE

One of the first experimental descriptions of distraction was published in 1965 by Cleall and associates (1). The authors expanded the midpalatal suture in the monkey and were able to move not only the teeth and alveolar processes but also the maxilla. Twelve rhesus monkeys were included in the study, comparable in age to a 7- to 9-year-old human. A custom-made acrylic expansion appliance was fabricated from models and attached to the hard palate. An expansion screw was embedded in the midline. The animals were sacrificed sequentially after 2 weeks (4 mm of expansion), 3 months (6 mm of expansion), 6 months (6 mm of expansion, 3 months of fixation), and 9 months (6 mm of expansion, 3 months of fixation, and 3 months without any appliance). The maxilla was then removed and examined histologically and radiographically. The midpalatal suture was found to have opened when strong expansion forces were applied to the maxillary arch and new bone formation was demonstrated on the free surfaces within 3 months. A fibrous, inflammatory reaction was present at 2 weeks. In the animals fixated for 3 months, the sutural bone was more mature and more mineralized. The final group demonstrated evidence of even more mature bone. The amount of new bone formation and the amount of relapse were not discussed.

A follow-up study, published by the same group in 1971, discussed the tissue response to rapid maxillary expansion (2). The authors found that the midpalatal suture split secondary to resorption, and heavy deposition of bone attempted to maintain sutural morphology. Four rhesus monkeys underwent rapid palatal expansion, similar to the technique described above. The bone was expanded at the rate of 0.25 mm/day. The animals were sacrificed at 24 hours, 4 days, 7 days, and 14 days. There was no change in the bone at 24 hours. After 4 days, there was evidence of disruption of the midpalatal suture with an increase in the density and cellularity of the connective tissue as well as increased vascularity. In addition, the bone edges were scalloped, showing osteoclastic activity. After 7 days, the connective tissue became organized in a linear configuration and was less dense. There was evidence of new bone deposition at the free edges of the suture. Finally, after 14 days, heavy bone deposition was observed. The dental changes were also discussed in the paper.

In 1971, Ekstrom and associates described the mineralization in the suture after expansion in a 10-year-old human child (3). Using radiographic techniques, the authors determined that the greatest amount of mineralization occurred in the first month. The suture was stable after retention for 3 months with a fixed appliance and mineralization remained stable in the patient.

In 1980, Haas described a 20-year clinical experience of using palatal expansion in humans (4). The author advocated the use of the technique and recommended a minimum of 10 mm of expansion. The expansion was stable, and relapse did not occur during a follow-up period approaching 20 years.

MIDFACE

After the mandible, the next most common site of investigation for the application of the techniques of distraction osteogenesis has been the midface (maxilla). Midface hypoplasia has been traditionally corrected by using various types of Le Fort advancement osteotomies associated with wide surgical exposure. The procedures suffer the disadvantages of hemorrhage (and transfusion), airway management, and the need for bone grafts with requisite retained hardware and donor site problems. The application of distraction osteogenesis to this clinical problem offers the potential of eliminating the above-mentioned problems associated with traditional Le Fort osteotomies and midface advancements.

The first such study was undertaken by Rachmiel and colleagues in 1993 (5). Midface osteotomies were performed on five mature sheep (Figure 10.1). A single external device was used to perform midface distraction at the rate of 2 mm/day for 21 days. Fixation was maintained for 6 weeks. New bone formation was evident radiographically, clinically, and histologically. Class II malocclusion developed with distraction, and there was subsequent difficulty in mastication (Figure 10.2). A one-year follow-up of this study

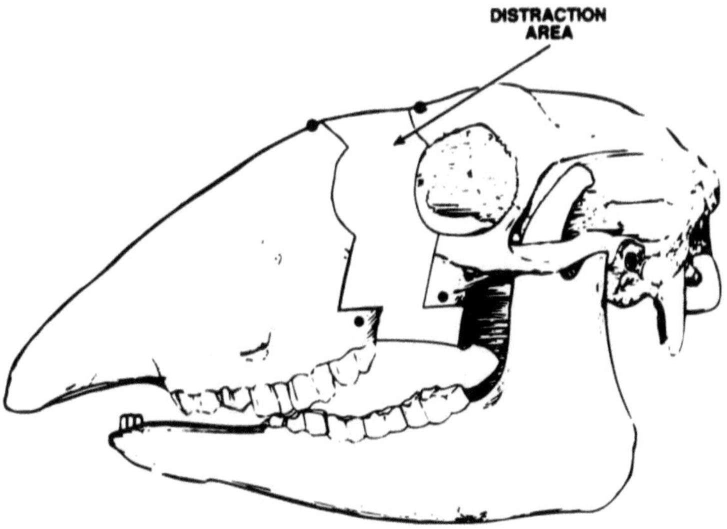

Figure 10.1. Diagram showing the area of midface distraction after removal of a bone-lengthening appliance. Note the increased distance between the bone markers (solid circles). Reproduced with permission from Rachmiel A, Potparic Z, Jackson IT et al. Midface advancement by gradual distraction. *Br J Plast Surg* 46:202, 1993.

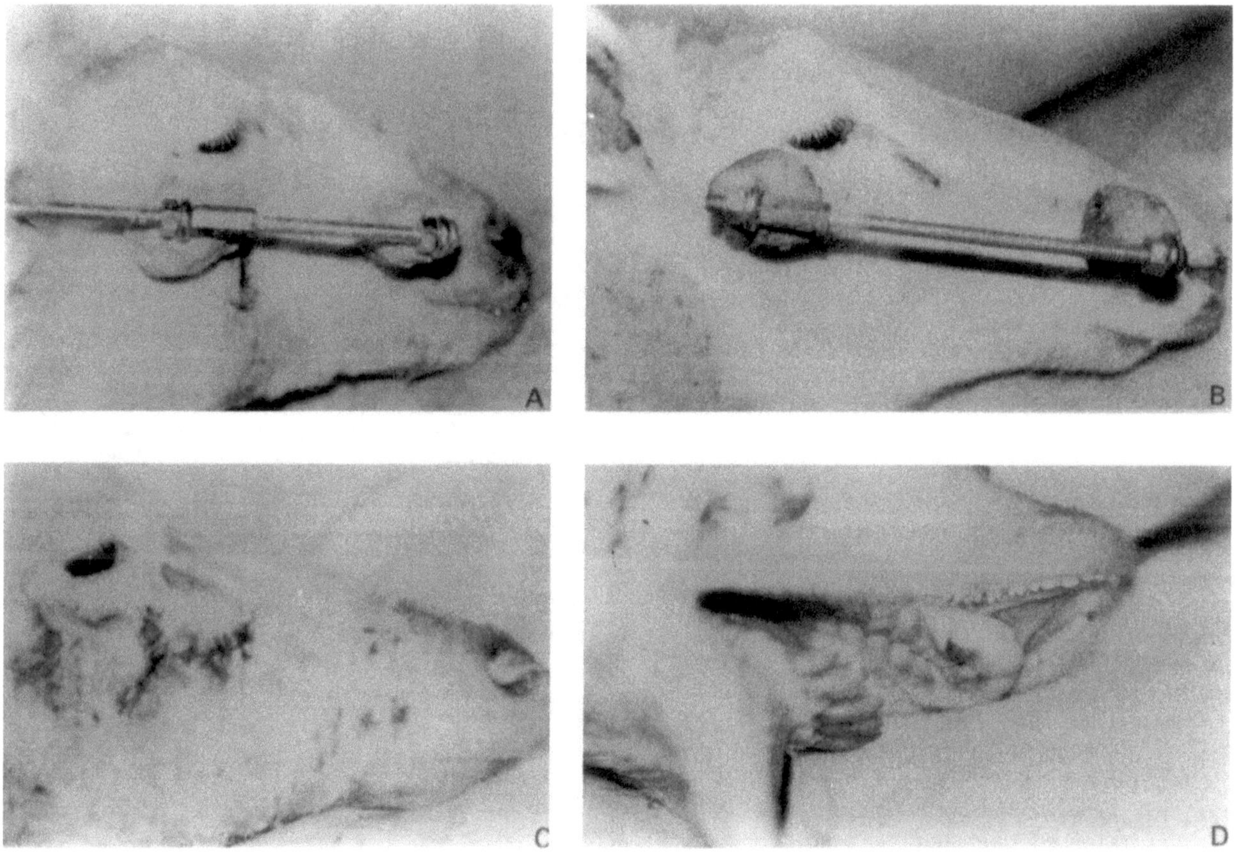

Figure 10.2. (A) Immediately after surgery showing an expansion device before the commencement of distraction. (B) Midface protrusion after distraction. (C) After removal of the distraction device. (D) Note the Class II malocclusion after distraction. There are no teeth on the anterior portion of the maxillary arch in sheep. Reproduced with permission from Rachmiel A, Potparic Z, Jackson IT et al. Midface advancement by gradual distraction. *Br J Plast Surg* 46:203, 1993.

was published by the same group in 1995 (6). The same animals were assessed one year after cessation of distraction. Through the use of radio-opaque markers, 2 to 3mm of relapse of the advanced segment was documented. This occurred within the first 3 months after removal of the fixation device. The documented minimal amount of relapse supports the hypothesis that distraction osteogenesis can be used for major maxillary advancement or inferior repositioning without the need for bone grafting.

Block and associates reported the use of an intraoral device to achieve an anterior maxillary advancement by distraction after performing an osteotomy in dogs (7,8). The distance between the tooth cusps on either side of the distracted segment was found to be greater than the length of distraction accomplished in the maxilla itself. On histologic examination, the gap was bridged by new bone within 12 weeks after distraction. When skeletal movement was compared to dental movement, there was significantly greater amount of dental movement. Because of this finding, fixation of the maxilla itself is necessary, and the teeth probably cannot provide an adequate means of

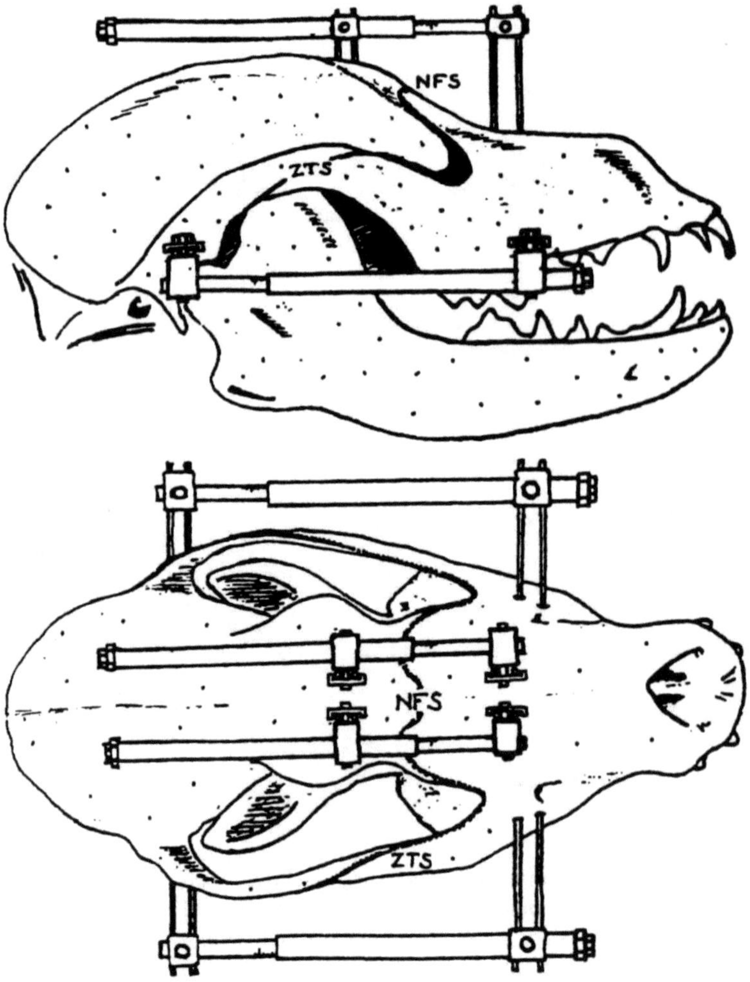

A

B

Figure 10.3. Drawing illustrating the placement of the distraction devices across the nasofrontal (NFS) and zygomaticotemporal (ZTS) sutures. (A) Lateral view prior to midface expansion. (B) Dorsal view prior to midface expansion. (C) Lateral view after midface expansion (distraction area shown in black). (D) Dorsoventral view after midface expansion (distraction area shown in black). Reproduced with permission from Staffenberg DA, Wood RJ, McCarthy JG, Grayson BH, Glasberg SB. Midface distraction in the canine without osteotomies. *Ann Plast Surg* 34:513, 1995.

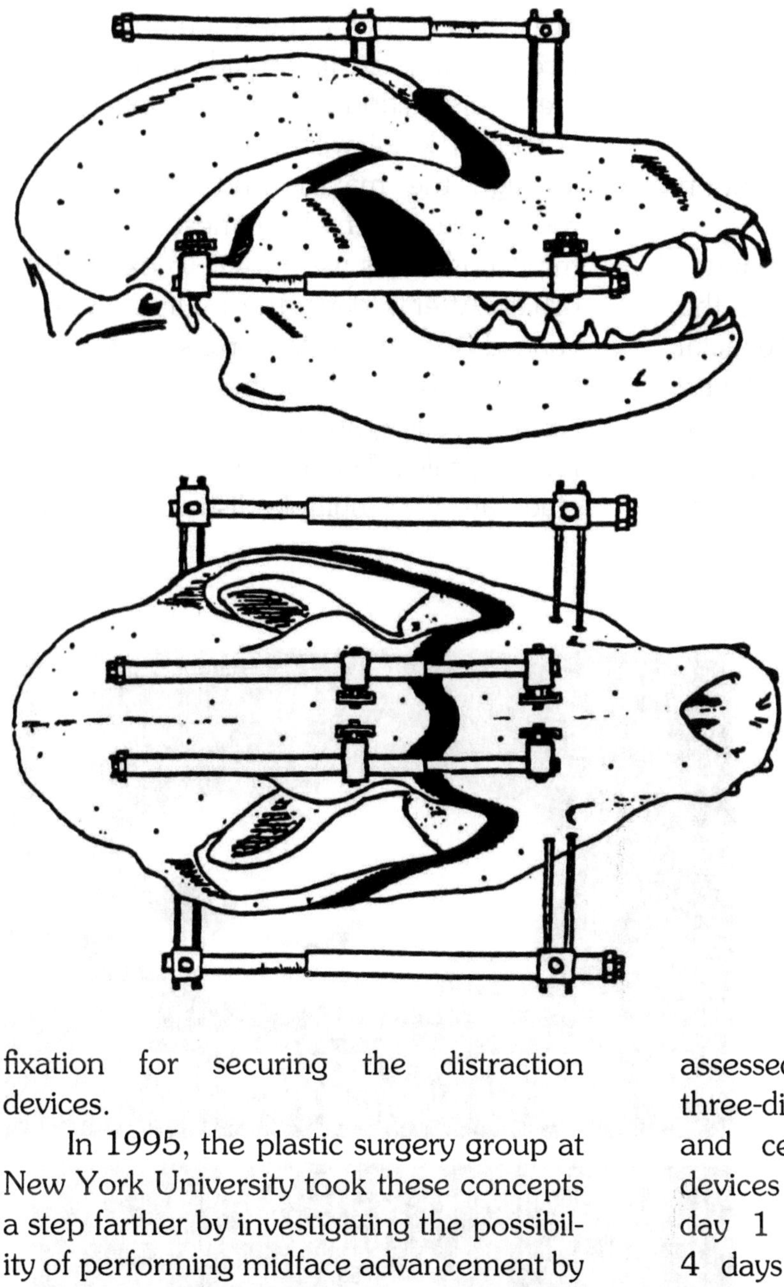

C

D

Figure 10.3. *Continued*

fixation for securing the distraction devices.

In 1995, the plastic surgery group at New York University took these concepts a step farther by investigating the possibility of performing midface advancement by distraction *without* osteotomy (9). Three immature 10-week-old canine pups were compared to two 5-year-old (mature) animals. Craniofacial maturity is attained in the canine by 9 months of age. All animals underwent the placement of four external distraction devices across the nasofrontal and zygomaticotemporal sutures (bilateral) (Figure 10.3). The periosteum was preserved. The results were assessed by pre- and postoperative three-dimensional CT scans (Figure 10.4) and cephalograms. Distraction of all devices was commenced on postoperative day 1 at the rate of 0.5mm/day for 4 days and 1.0mm/day for 28 days. In the immature animals, physical examination revealed the development of bilateral enophthalmos (Figure 10.5), dolichocephaly, and Class II malocclusion. None of these findings was observed in the mature animals. Cephalograms revealed a 28-mm overjet in the immature animals while the mature animals showed only 2mm of overjet and no evidence of distraction effects. The authors hypothesized that this technique may be applicable to human infants and would significantly reduce the length of hospitalization and operating times, while also lowering the relapse and complication rates.

In 1996, Rachmiel and colleagues further expanded the indications for the use of distraction osteogenesis in the facial skeleton (10). The authors performed a Le Fort II osteotomy combined with circumferential orbital osteotomies in young adult sheep. Titanium bone screws were placed as markers and a lengthening device was applied to provide multiple segment distraction. Two transfixing pins (175-mm long) were placed transversely through the maxilla and two threaded rods were attached to these rods. Two minilengtheners were used to expand the orbits. After 7 days, the midface was advanced 30 mm and the orbits were moved forward 20 mm. New bone was demonstrated radiographically, clinically, and histologically. The implications from this study are that multiple distraction devices

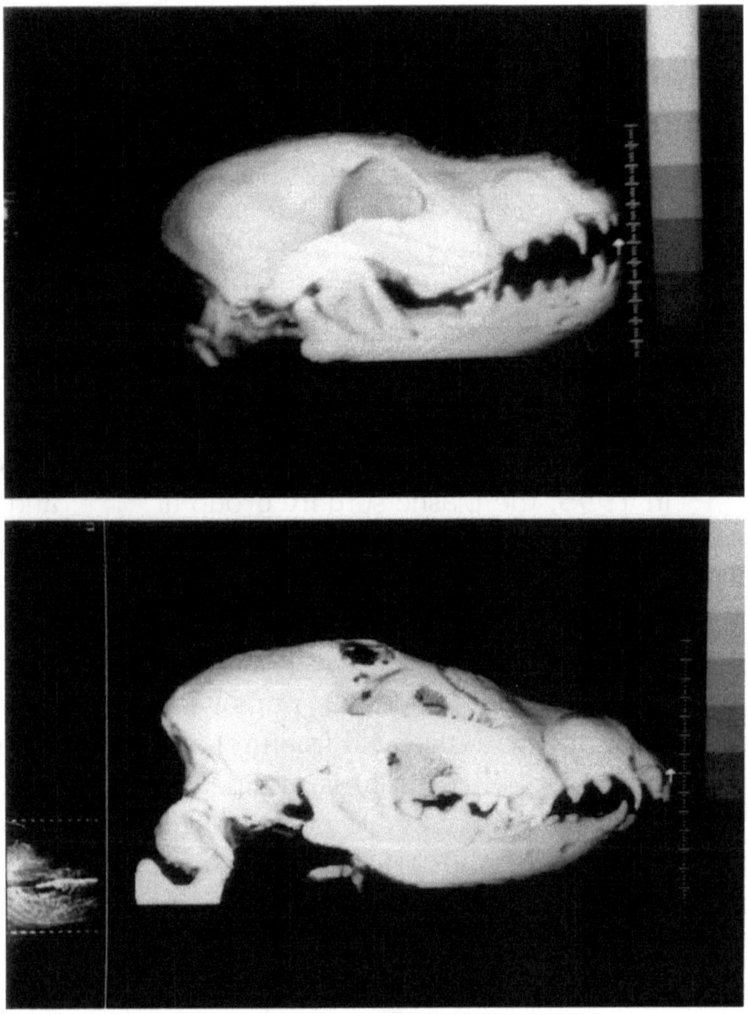

A

B

Figure 10.4. (A) Preoperative craniofacial three-dimensional CT scan in an immature animal. The arrow designates anterior teeth relationships. (B) Craniofacial three-dimensional CT scan in the same animal after midface distraction. Note the widening of the nasofrontal and zygomaticotemporal sutures (see Figures 10.3C and 10.3D), as well as thinning of the ethmoid complex and the development of a Class II malocclusion-overjet (arrow). Reproduced with permission from Staffenberg DA, Wood RJ, McCarthy JG, Grayson BH, Glasberg SB. Midface distraction advancement in the canine without osteotomies. *Ann Plast Surg* 34:516, 1995.

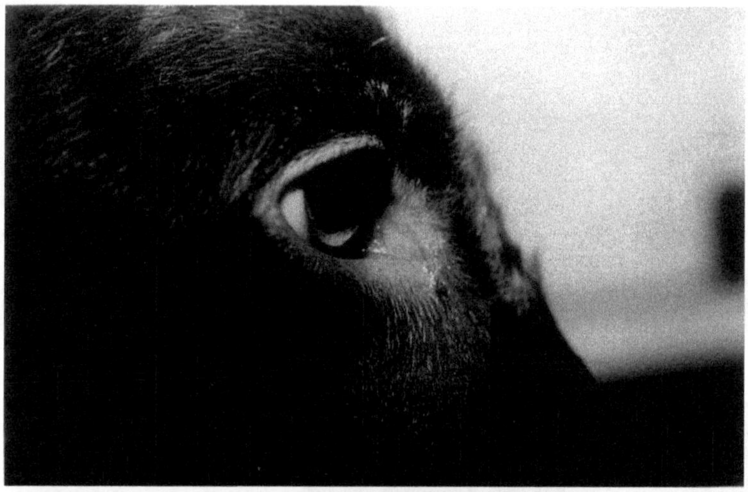

A

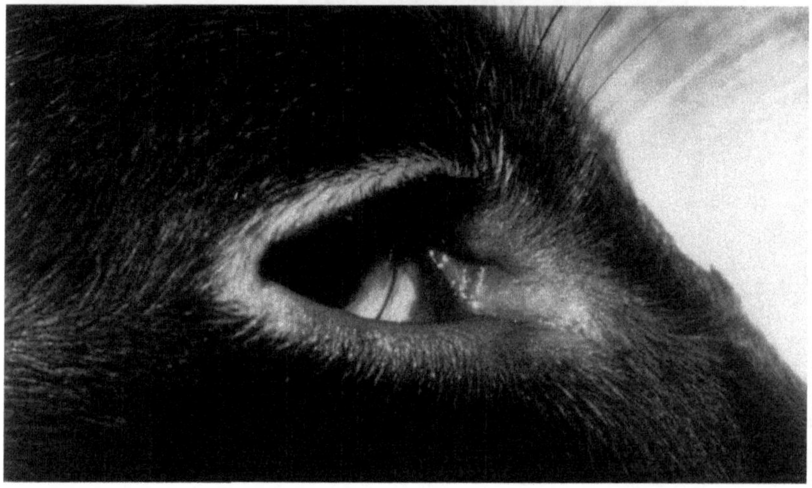

B

Figure 10.5. (A) Immature animal: orbital appearance before midface distraction. (B) Same animal: orbital appearance after a completed course of distraction, illustrating the presence of enophthalmos. Reproduced with permission from Staffenberg DA, Wood RJ, McCarthy JG, Grayson BH, Glasberg SB. Midface distraction advancement in the canine without osteotomies. *Ann Plast Surg* 34:514, 1995.

can be designed to offer three-dimensional, multisegment, controlled correction of facial deformities.

ZYGOMA

Two animal studies have been reported in which the zygoma alone was subjected to distraction osteogenesis. In 1992, Phillips, Forrest, and Gruss described using an osteotomy of the zygoma through the orbital rim and zygomatic arch in three adult dogs to lengthen the zygoma (11). Percutaneous threaded K-wires were placed into the zygoma on both sides of the osteotomy. The distraction device was applied unilaterally (Figure 10.6). Lengthening was performed at the rate of 0.7 mm/day for a total gap of 2.1 cm (Figure 10.7). New bone formation with a fibrous inner zone and subsequent total ossification were observed. Histologic studies indicated direct bone formation,

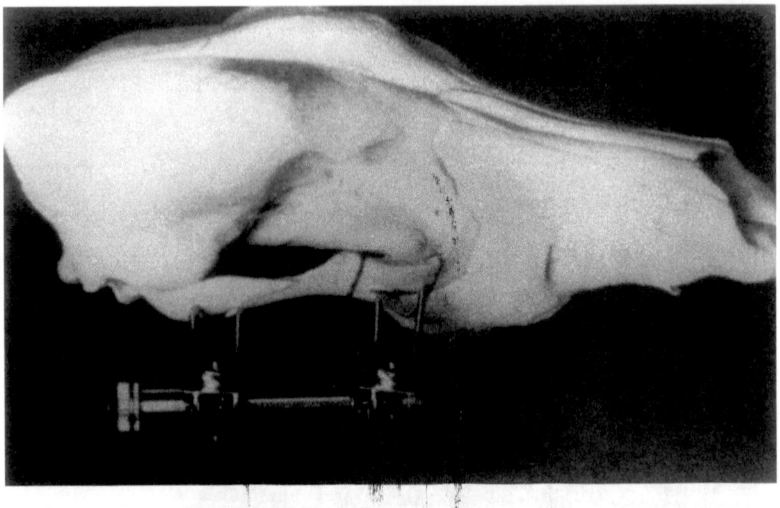

Figure 10.6. Dry skull model of the osteotomized zygoma of an adult mastiff dog with localization of the percutaneous threaded K-wires. Reproduced with permission from Phillips JH, Forest CR, Gruss JS. Current concepts in the use of bone grafts in facial fractures: Basic science considerations. *Clin Plast Surg* 19:53, 1992.

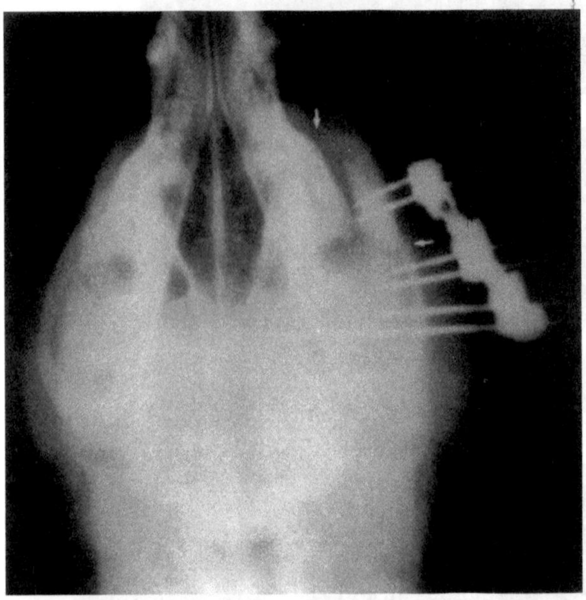

A

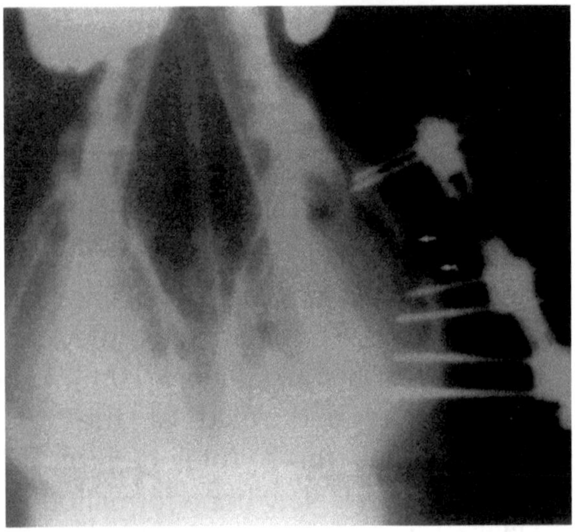

B

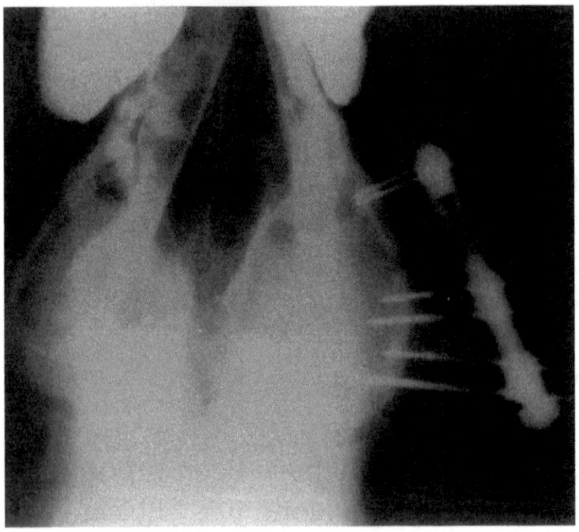

C

Figure 10.7. (A) Radiographic demonstration of the osteotomized zygomatic segment in the adult mastiff dog. Arrows indicate the osteotomy sites. (B) Total lengthening of 2.1 cm in the adult dog zygoma. Arrows indicate a distraction gap of 2.1 cm. (C) New bone formation in the 2.1 cm distraction gap. Reproduced with permission from Phillips JH, Forest CR, Gruss JS. Current concepts in the use of bone grafts in facial fractures: Basic science considerations. *Clin Plast Surg* 19:54–55, 1992.

and physical exam demonstrated an obvious asymmetry.

The second animal study was reported by Glat and the plastic surgery group at New York University in 1994. The authors employed a distraction device to move the zygoma out of the plane of the long axis of the zygoma in a canine model (12). In this study, four mongrel dogs were used. Two osteotomies were made in the zygomatic arch after which a custom-made distraction device was fixed to the zygoma (Figure 10.8). The device consisted of percutaneous K-wires placed in the zygoma, two anterior and two posterior to the two osteotomies and parallel to the long axis of the bone. The lengthener was attached perpendicular to the bone and fixated by passing two unthreaded, right-angle pins through holes drilled through the central portion of the osteotomized segment. After 7 days of fixation, the osteotomized segment was lengthened 1 mm/day at a right angle to the long axis of the zygoma for an interval of 15 days. External fixation was maintained for an additional 4 weeks. CT scans with three-dimensional reconstruction and dorsoventral skull radiographs documented multidimensional bone lengthening with marked increase in the thickness of the zygoma as well as its lateral projection when compared with the control zygoma (Figures 10.9 and 10.10). Histologic analysis confirmed the presence of new cortical bone in the expanded areas. Physical examination on the expanded side revealed marked enlargement of the zygomatic complex with the illusion of enophthalmos.

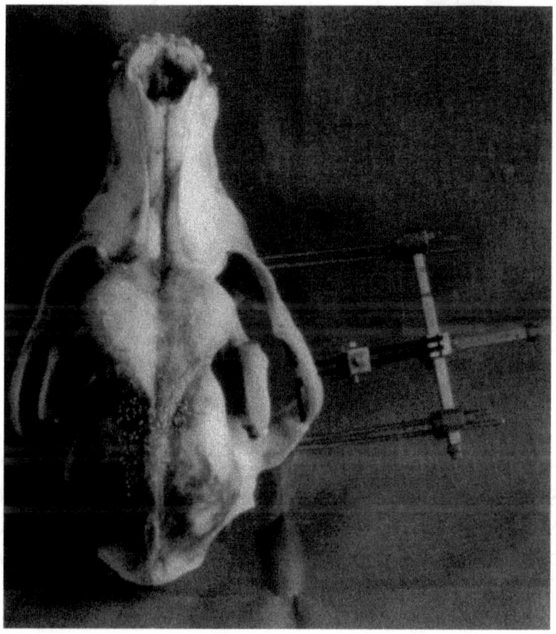

Figure 10.8. Bone distraction device in place on the canine skull. Note the adjustable brace (parallel to the long axis of the zygoma) and the lengthener that is perpendicular to the brace and attached to the osteotomized segment. The brace is secured by two pairs of half-pins. Reproduced with permission from Glat PM, Staffenberg DA, Karp NS, Holliday RA, Steiner G, McCarthy JG. Multidimensional distraction osteogenesis: The canine zygoma. *Plast Reconstr Surg* 94:754, 1994.

One study in the literature demonstrated distraction of the zygoma in conjunction with lengthening of the cranial vault (13). The authors utilized an expandable craniotactic appliance to distract continuously the disarticulated frontofacial complex from the posterior cranium in a rabbit model (Figure 10.11). In order to do this, the temporozygomatic sutures had to be released and distraction had to be performed longitudinally across the suture, in a manner similar to the technique used by Phillips and his group (11). In addition to lengthening of the entire skull length, the findings demonstrated marked elongation of the zygoma itself. Histology revealed the formation of new bone within the distraction zone.

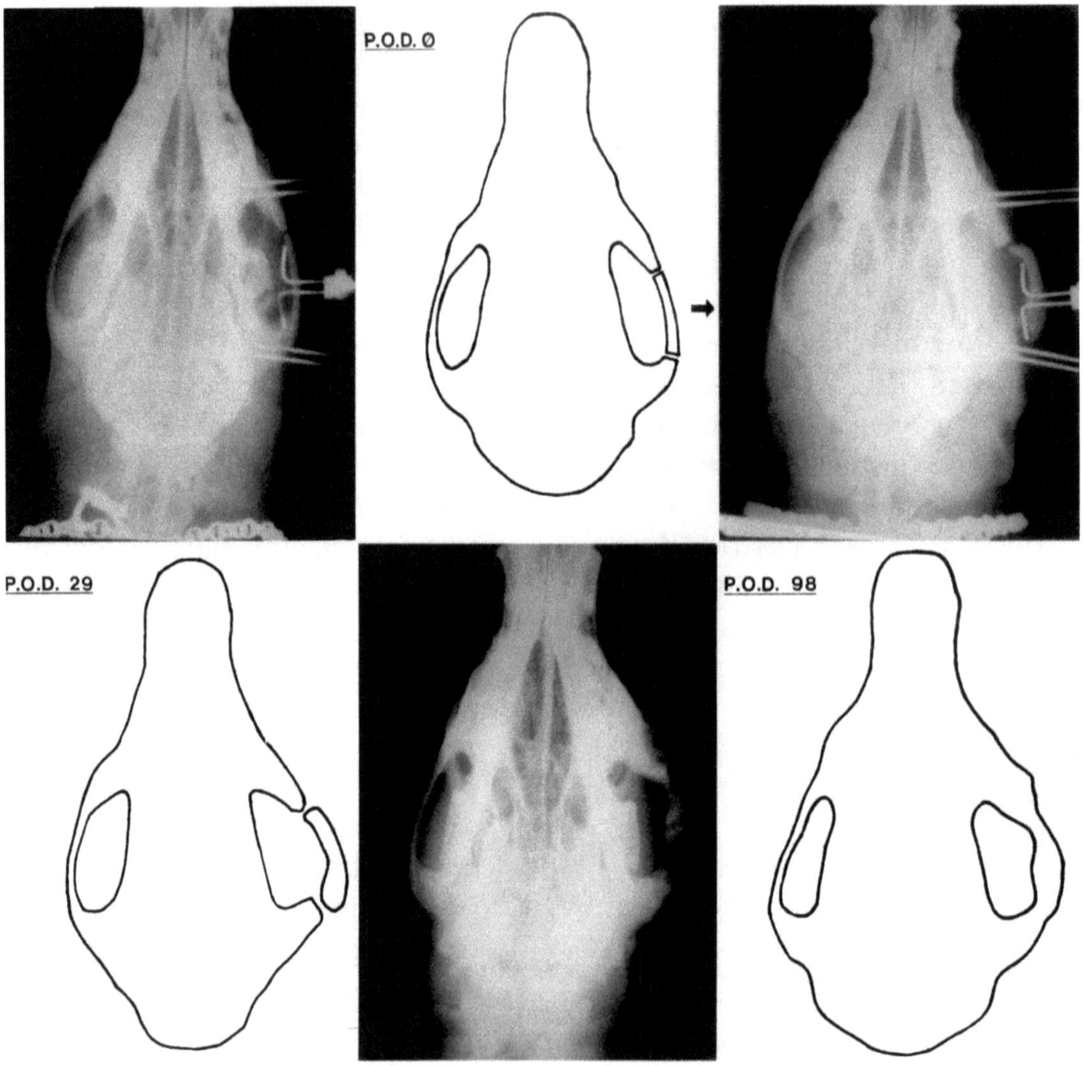

Figure 10.9. (Top, left) Dorsoventral skull radiograph on postoperative day 0. (Top, center) Tracing of skull radiograph on postoperative day 0. (Top, right) Dorsoventral skull radiograph on postoperative day 29. (Bottom, left) Tracing of skull radiograph on postoperative day 29. (Bottom, center) Dorsoventral skull radiograph on postoperative day 98. (Bottom, right) Tracing of skull radiograph on postoperative day 98. Reproduced with permission from Glat PM, Staffenberg DA, Karp NS, Holliday RA, Steiner G, McCarthy JG. Multidimensional distraction osteogenesis: The canine zygoma. *Plast Reconstr Surg* 94:755, 1994.

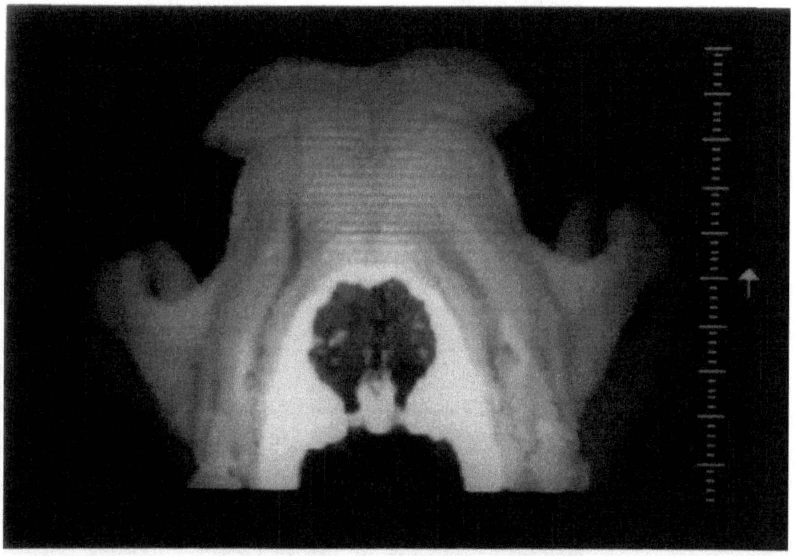

A

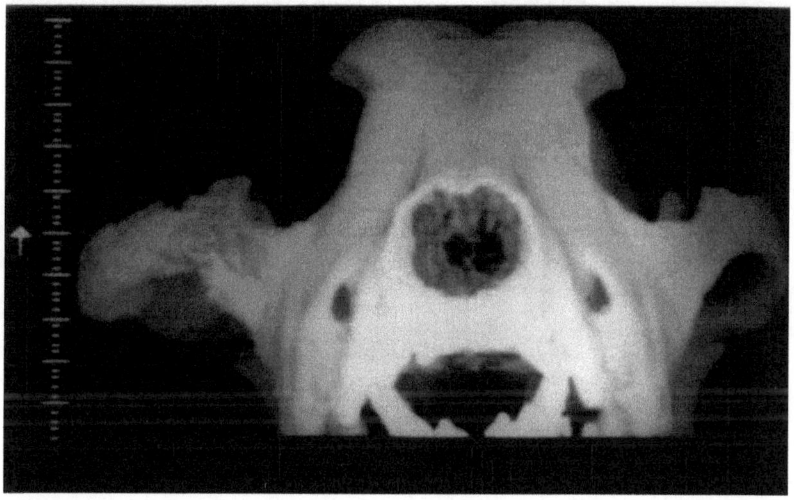

B

Figure 10.10. (A) Three-dimensional CT scan, anterior view, preoperative. (B) Three-dimensional CT scan, anterior view, postoperative after unilateral zygomatic distraction. Note the increase in bone volume and projection (C) Three-dimensional CT scan, ventral view, preoperative. (D) Three-dimensional CT scan, ventral view, postoperative after unilateral zygomatic distraction. Note the increased zygomatic projection. Reproduced with permission from Glat PM, Staffenberg DA, Karp NS, Holliday RA, Steiner G, McCarthy JG. Multidimensional distraction osteogenesis: The canine zygoma. *Plast Reconst Surg* 94:756, 1994.

(*Continued*)

Figure 10.10. *Continued*

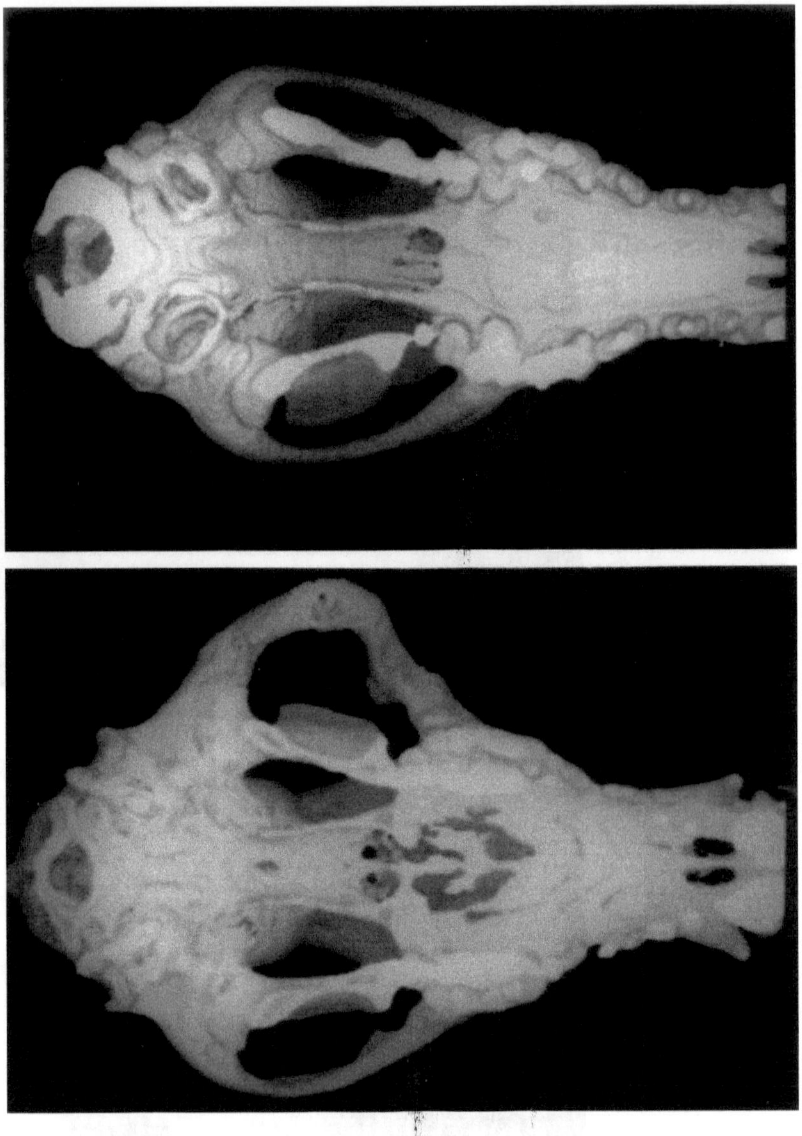

C

D

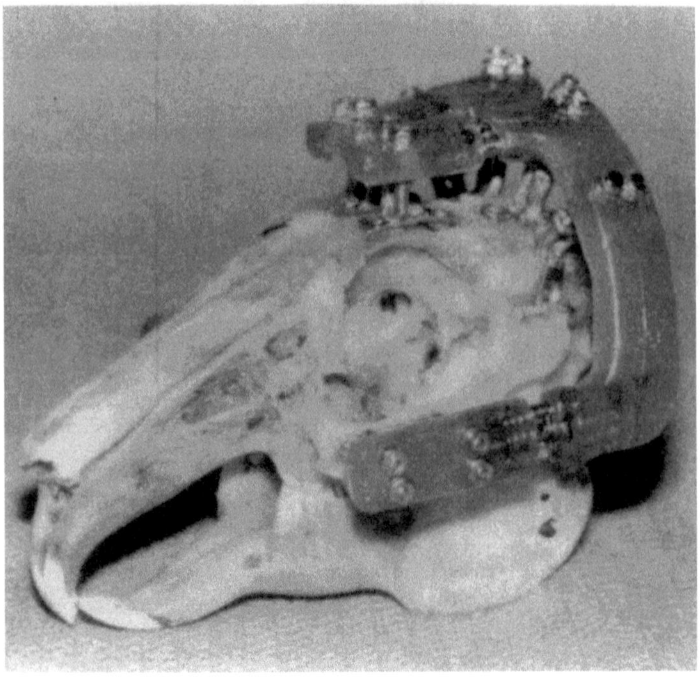

Figure 10.11. Craniotactic appliance on a dry skull specimen. Reproduced with permission from Remmler D, McCoy FJ, O'Neil D et al. Osseous expansion of the cranial vault by craniotasis. *Plast Reconstr Surg* 89:788, 1992.

The zygoma has been used infrequently as a site for distraction osteogenesis within the craniofacial skeleton. Animal studies, however, have shown the feasibility of performing distraction both parallel and perpendicular to the long axis of the zygoma, even without an osteotomy. Further refinement of the technique may make distraction of the zygoma more widely applicable for use in the human craniofacial skeleton (eg, Treacher Collins syndrome). The technique allows for an increase in bone stock without the need for bone grafts or donor site morbidity.

REFERENCES

1. Cleall JF, Bayne DI, Posen JM, Subtelny JD. Expansion of the midpalatal suture in the monkey. *Angle Orthod* 35:23, 1965.
2. Murray JM, Cleall, JP. Early tissue response to rapid maxillary expansion in the midpalatal suture of the rhesus monkey. *J Dent Res* 50:1654, 1971.
3. Ekstrom C, Henrikson CO, Jensen R: Mineralization in the midpalatal suture after orthodontic expansion. *Am J Orthod* 71:449, 1971.
4. Haas AJ. Long-term posttreatment evaluation of rapid palatal expansion. *Angle Orthod* 50:189, 1980.
5. Rachmiel A, Potparic Z, Jackson IT et al. Midface advancement by gradual distraction. *Br J Plast Surg* 46:201, 1993.
6. Rachmiel A, Jackson IT, Potparic Z, Laufer D. Midface advancement in sheep by gradual distraction: A 1-year follow-up study. *J Oral Maillofac Surg* 53:525, 1995.
7. Block MS, Brister GD. Use of distraction osteogenesis for maxillary advancement: Preliminary results. *J Oral Maxillofac Surg* 52:282, 1994.
8. Block MS, Cervini D, Chang A, Gottsegen GB. Anterior maxillary advancement using tooth-supported distraction osteogenesis. *J Oral Maxillofac Surg* 53:561, 1995.
9. Staffenberg DA, Wood RJ, McCarthy JG, Grayson BH, Glasberg SB. Midface distraction advancement in the canine without osteotomies. *Ann Plast Surg* 34:512, 1995.
10. Rachmiel A, Levy M, Laufer D, Clayman L, Jackson IT. Multiple segmental gradual distraction of the facial skeleton: An experimental study. *Ann Plast Surg* 36:52, 1996.
11. Phillips JH, Forrest CR, Gruss JS. Current concepts in the use of bone grafts in facial fractures: Basic science considerations. *Clin Plast Surg* 19:41, 1992.
12. Glat PM, Staffenberg DA, Karp NS, Holliday RA, Steiner G, McCarthy JG. Multidimensional distraction osteogenesis: The canine zygoma. *Plast Reconstr Surg* 94:753, 1994.
13. Remmler D, McCoy FJ, O'Neil D et al. Osseous expansion of the cranial vault by craniotasis. *Plast Reconstr Surg* 89:787, 1992.

CHAPTER 11A

DISTRACTION OF THE MAXILLA

Fernando Molina

Distraction osteogenesis has become an accepted, and often preferred, technique for the reconstruction of deficient mandibles and has simplified the treatment of congenital mandibular hypoplasia (1–8). Laboratory studies have also demonstrated the feasibility and efficacy of midface distraction (9, 10).

The absence of maxillary hypoplasia and Class III malocclusion in unrepaired cleft palate patients suggests that the surgical procedures employed to correct cleft lip and palate may be related to the development of this condition (11). The resulting midface deficiency may be manifest at the nasal, paranasal, infraorbital, and zygomatic regions as well as at the occlusal level.

The results of maxillary advancement using the principles of distraction osteogenesis are presented as an alternative treatment technique in patients with cleft lip and palate and associated maxillary hypoplasia during the period of mixed dentition.

Maxillary distraction was performed in 36 patients between the ages of 6 and 12 years (mean: 8 years): 18 unilateral cleft lip and palate (UCLP), 9 bilateral cleft lip and palate (BCLP), 5 unilateral cleft palate (UCP), 2 mandibular prognathism, and 2 nasomaxillary hypoplasia. All of the patients demonstrated moderate to severe underdevelopment of the maxilla and Class III malocclusion, with partial or total anterior and posterior crossbite.

According to the study protocol, photographs, cephalograms (posteroanterior and lateral), and dental models were obtained preoperatively, in the immediate postdistraction period and at 6-month intervals thereafter. Lateral and posteroanterior cephalometric studies were done to determine basal, sagittal, vertical, and transverse dimensions of the maxilla, as well as their relationships to the cranial base. A preoperative panoramic roentgenogram (panorex) was used to locate the position of the tooth buds. The dental occlusion was documented with dental casts.

Orthodontic requirements were satisfied prior to maxillary distraction: transverse skeletal and/or dentoalveolar expansion of the upper jaw, alignment of the permanent incisors in the cleft area in some patients, and bone grafting at age 8 to 10 years in patients with significant alveolar clefts.

SURGICAL TECHNIQUE

The day before surgery, a modified quadhelix fixed applicance, prepared by the orthodontist, is placed across the palate (Figure 11A.1).

Under general anesthesia bilateral maxillary vestibular incisions (3–4cm in length) are made, leaving a 2-cm central mucosal bridge between the incisions. Subperiosteal dissection is performed on the anterior aspect of the maxilla, and dissection on the nasal floor is limited to the lateral aspect. The septal base (vomer) is left intact. With a side-cutting burr, an incomplete osteotomy is performed above the roots of the canines and molar tooth buds (Figure 11A.2). The osteotomy must preserve the integrity of the maxillary antral mucoperiosteum in order to maintain vascularity. Dissection in the nasal floor/septal base and pterygomaxillary disjunction with Rowe forceps is not performed. The mucosal incision is approximated and closed with absorbable sutures.

On the fifth postoperative day, the application of the distraction forces is initiated by using the fixed applicance system as an anchorage for a modified "Petit" facial mask resting on the skin of the forehead and chin (see Figure 11.4B). The initial mechanical force used for distraction is approximately 900g. The face mask is used mainly at night and at some periods during the day for a total of 16 to 18 hours every day.

A combination of forward and downward distraction forces can be used in patients with a decreased vertical dimension of the maxilla.

At approximately 8 to 10 weeks postdistraction, there is radiographic evidence of new cortical bone at the site of the corticotomy. The bone step formed by the horizontal distraction technique is replaced with mature cortical bone. There is evidence of increase in the size of the tuberosity at the pterygomaxillary junction with new tissue that has the radiographic appearance of bone (Figure 11A.3).

RESULTS

The projected advancement (range 4–12mm) was achieved in all of the patients. The esthetic results were excellent (Figure 11A.4). The soft-tissue profile changed from a prognathic to a well-proportioned orthognathic face.

Dental occlusion was changed to a distal sagittal molar relationship with moderate overjet. On cephalometric examination a counterclockwise rotation of 2 to 7° was achieved as well as a mean increase of 2.7 to 7.4° at the ANB angle.

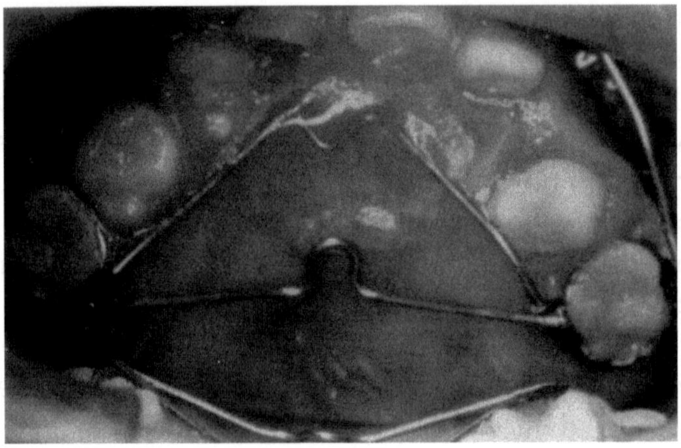

Figure 11A.1. Intraoral device in place. The horizontal bar is designed to maintain transverse maxillary expansion during distraction. Note the acrylic button behind the incisors and the vestibular hooks.

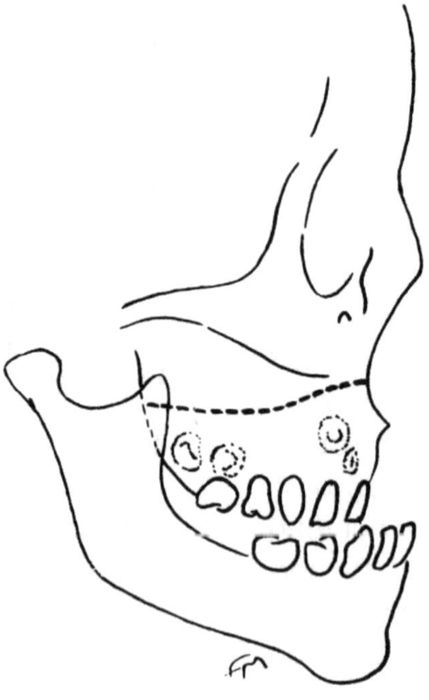

Figure 11A.2. Line of osteotomy. The septum and pterygomaxillary junctions are spared.

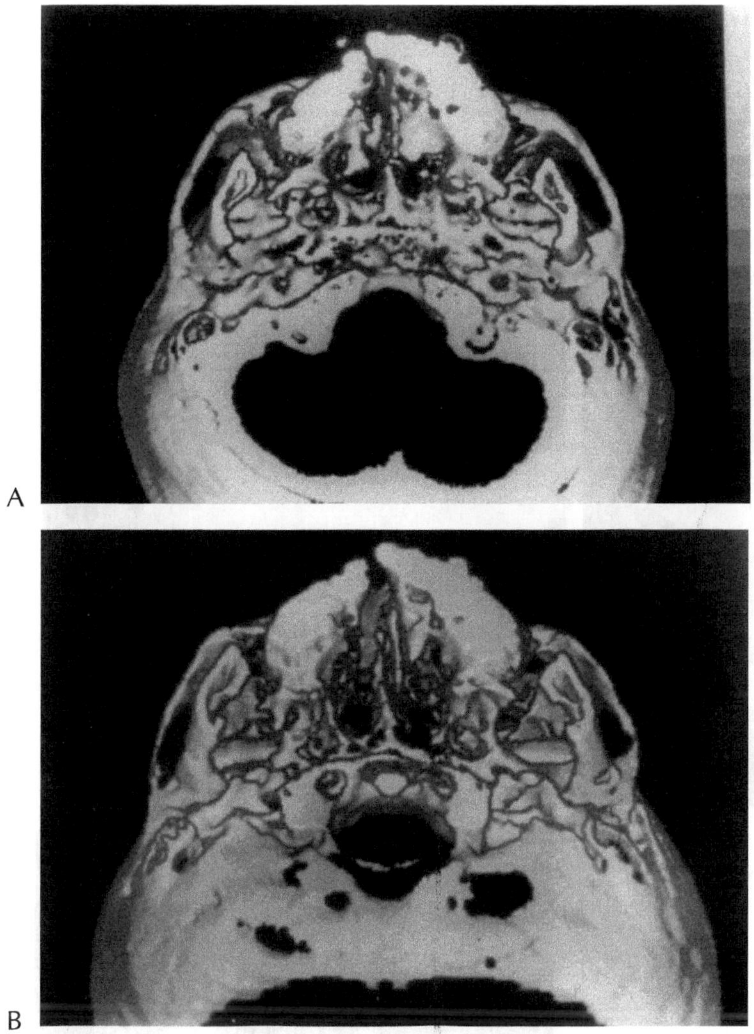

Figure 11A.3. Evidence of new bone formation along the osteotomy line. (A) Predistraction CT scan. (B) Postdistraction CT scan. Note the new bone formation in the pterygomaxillary junction.

In five patients the simultaneous horizontal and vertical maxillary dimensional increases varied from 3 to 5mm. The esthetic improvement in and restoration of the facial appearance have also been impressive (Figures 11A.5–11A.7). It was considered essential to stabilize the postdistraction maxilla with a fixed palatal arch in order to proceed with orthodontic treatment such as alignment of the permanent incisors in the cleft area.

No significant relapse has been observed in the patients in these series during the 3 years of maximum follow-up. However, in cases with an unfavorable growth pattern, a functional orthodontic device (Frankel III) may be considered as an active retainer treatment option.

The main patient complaint has been the discomfort of wearing a facial mask. The procedure is essentially painless and there was no evidence of infection, bone necrosis, loss of teeth, mucosal fistulae, or delayed healing.

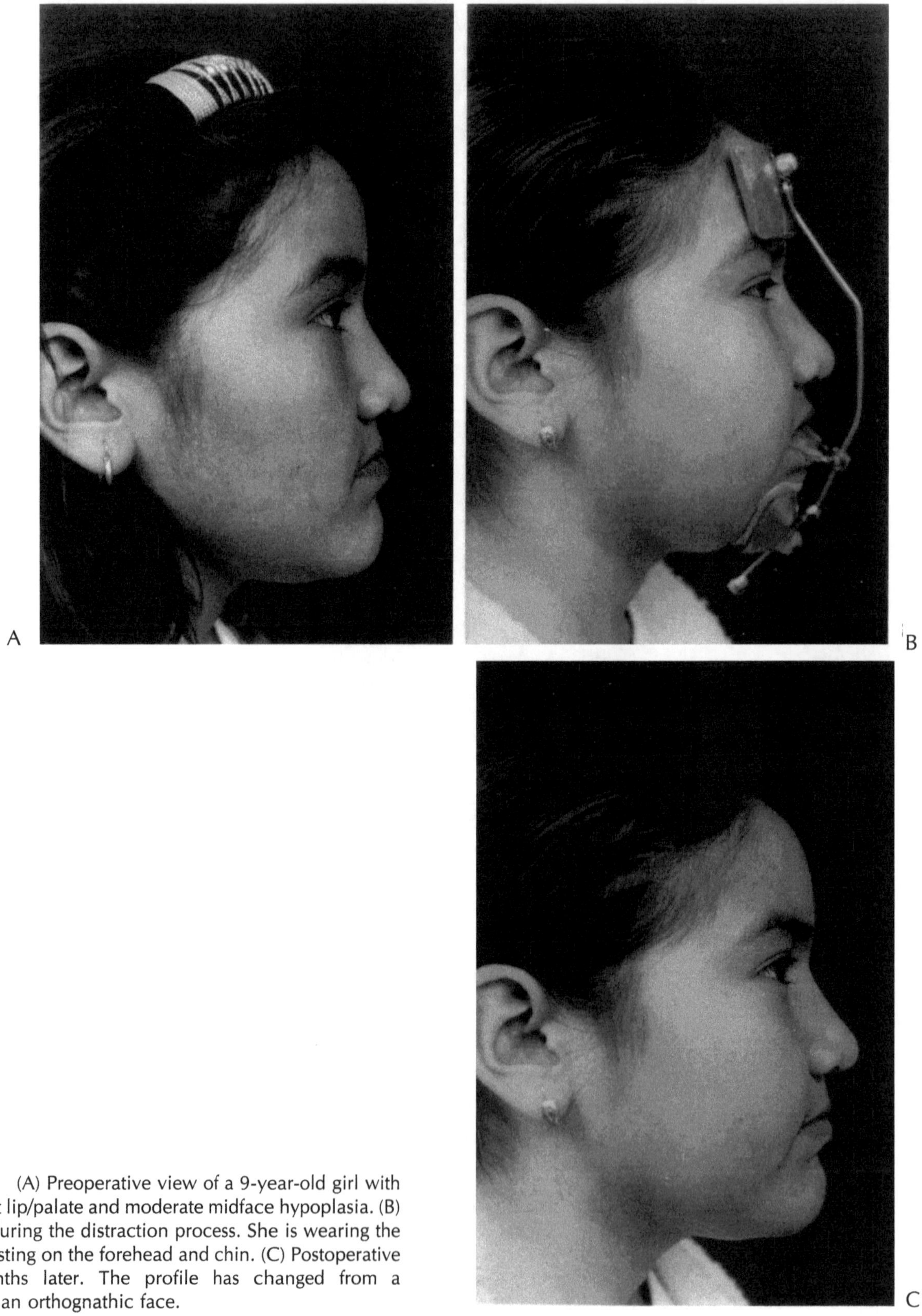

Figure 11A.4. (A) Preoperative view of a 9-year-old girl with unilateral cleft lip/palate and moderate midface hypoplasia. (B) Appearance during the distraction process. She is wearing the facial mask resting on the forehead and chin. (C) Postoperative result 6 months later. The profile has changed from a prognathic to an orthognathic face.

DISCUSSION

Early esthetic and functional rehabilitation of children with cleft lip/palate has been considered a major treatment goal. The maxillary distraction technique offers exciting treatment possibilities by eliminating the need for bone grafts, rigid skeletal fixation, blood transfusion, prolonged hospitalization, or intermaxillary fixation. The treatment can also be initiated as early as the period of mixed dentition.

A source of concern at the initiation of the study was the quality and density of the new regenerate tissue formed at the pterygomaxillary junction. Cephalograms and computed tomographic scans present an image similar to that of new bone at the site of the osteotomy on the anterior maxillary surface (see Figure 11A.3).

The preoperative planning of the distraction vectors is fundamental to achieving optimal results. The most commonly used vector is a sagittal one in which the vector must be parallel to the occlusal plane following the projected molar and incisor relationship, thus avoiding the development of an anterior open bite.

A
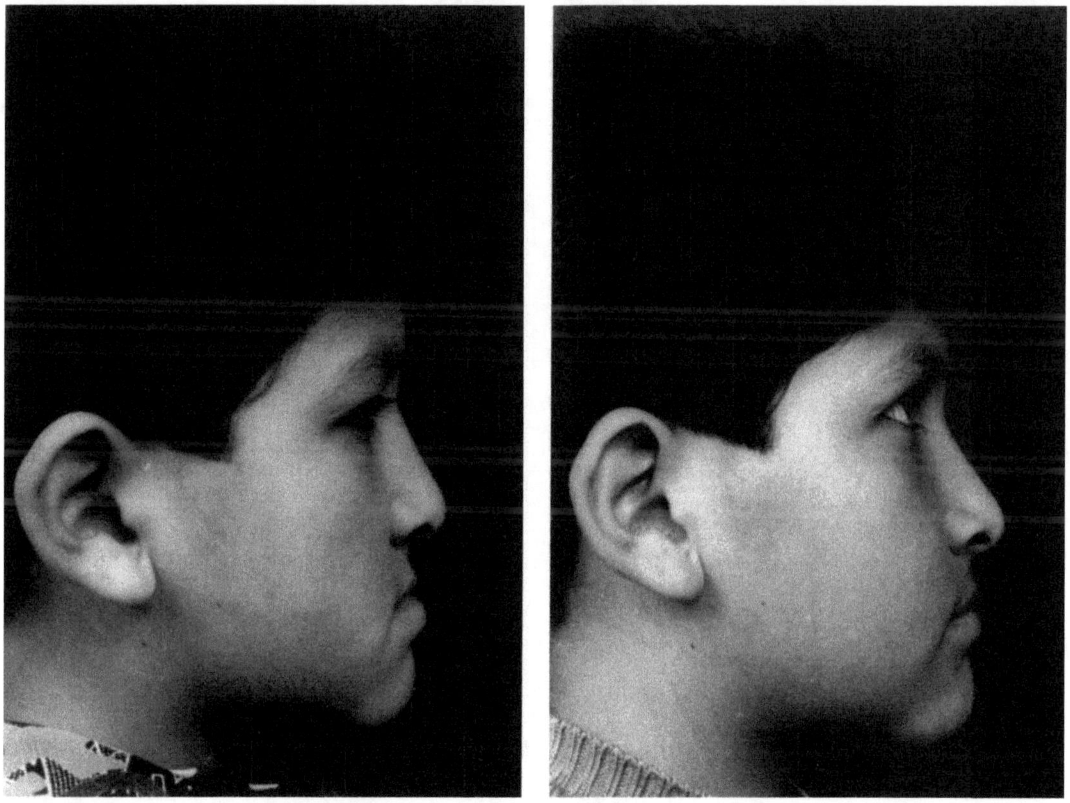
B

Figure 11A.5. (A) Preoperative view of an 8-year-old boy with repaired unilateral cleft palate and severe midfacial retrusion. (B) Postoperative view 6 months after correction by maxillary distraction (6 mm) and anterior advancement. Note the improved relationship between the soft tissues and the skeletal framework around the mouth and nose.

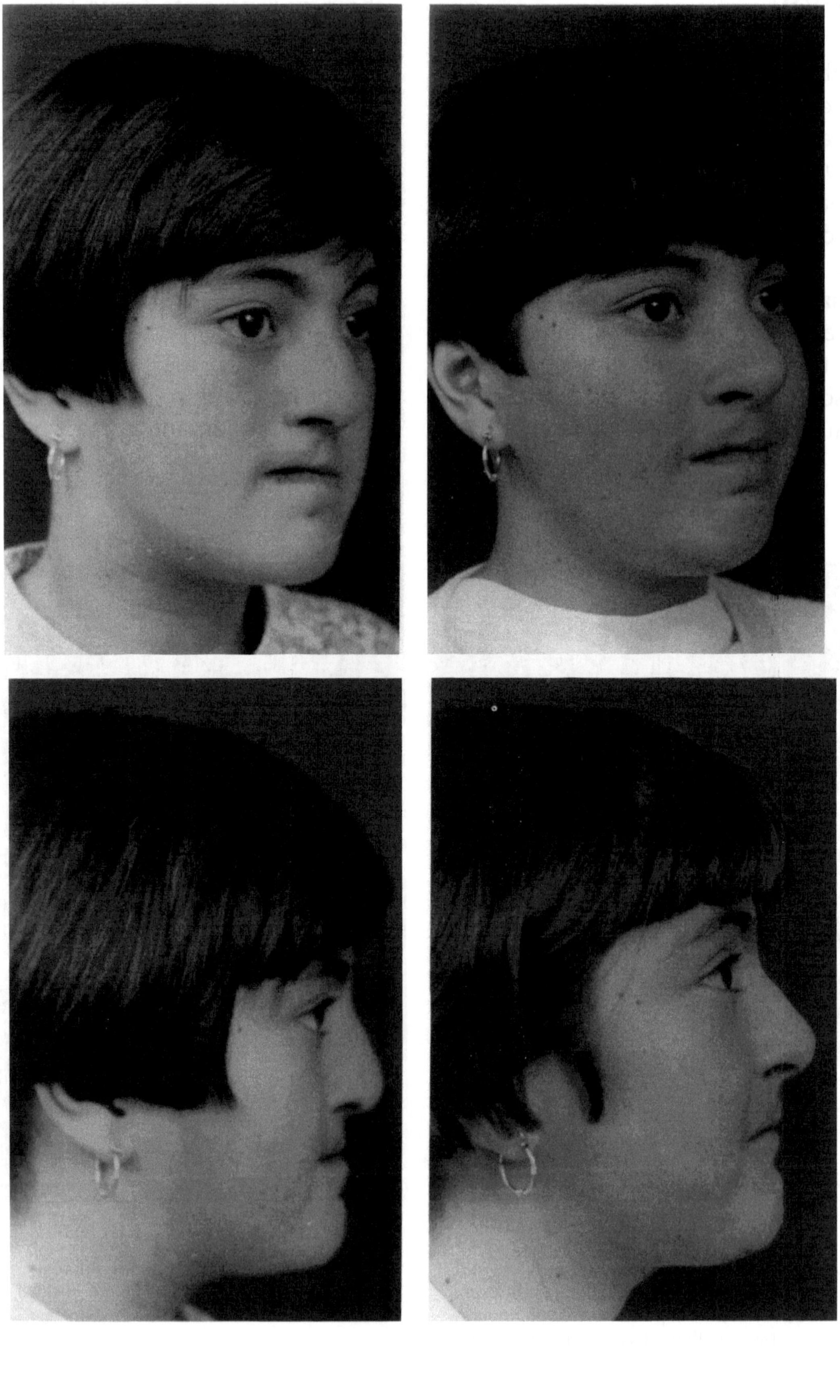

A B C D

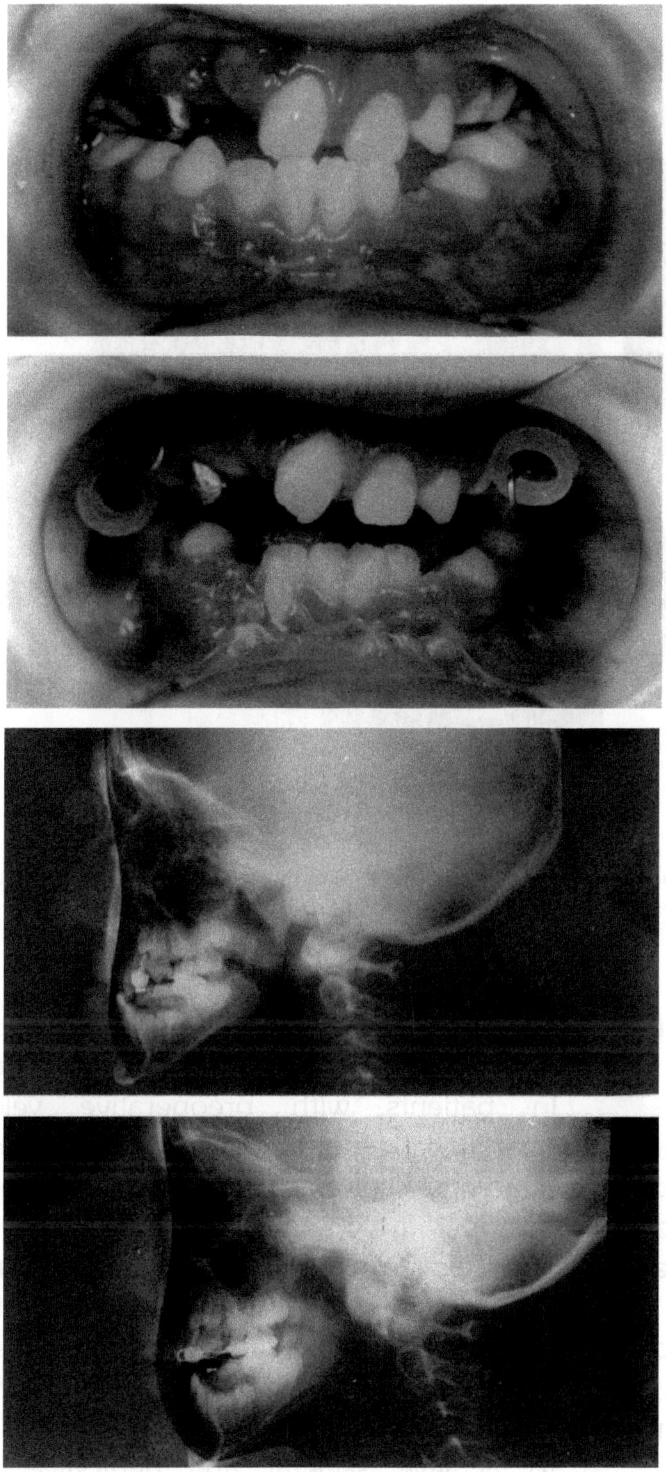

E

F

G

H

Figure 11A.6. (A) Preoperative oblique view of a 10-year-old girl with the sequelae of unilateral cleft lip and palate and midfacial retrusion. (B) Postoperative view showing correction with anterior maxillary advancement by distraction (7 mm). Note the improved relationship of the soft tissues around the mouth and nose. (C) Preoperative lateral view showing the midfacial retrusion. (D) Postoperative view 6 months later. Note the changes in the nasolabial angle with the maxilla in the advanced position. (E) Preoperative occlusion. Note the anterior crossbite. (F) Postoperative occlusion at the end of the distraction period. Note the bands that are used for maxillary distraction in a lateral direction. (G) Preoperative lateral cephalogram. Note the hypoplastic maxilla and the disturbed molar relationships. (H) Postoperative lateral cephalogram. The maxilla has been advanced 7 mm by distraction and the molar relationship is class II.

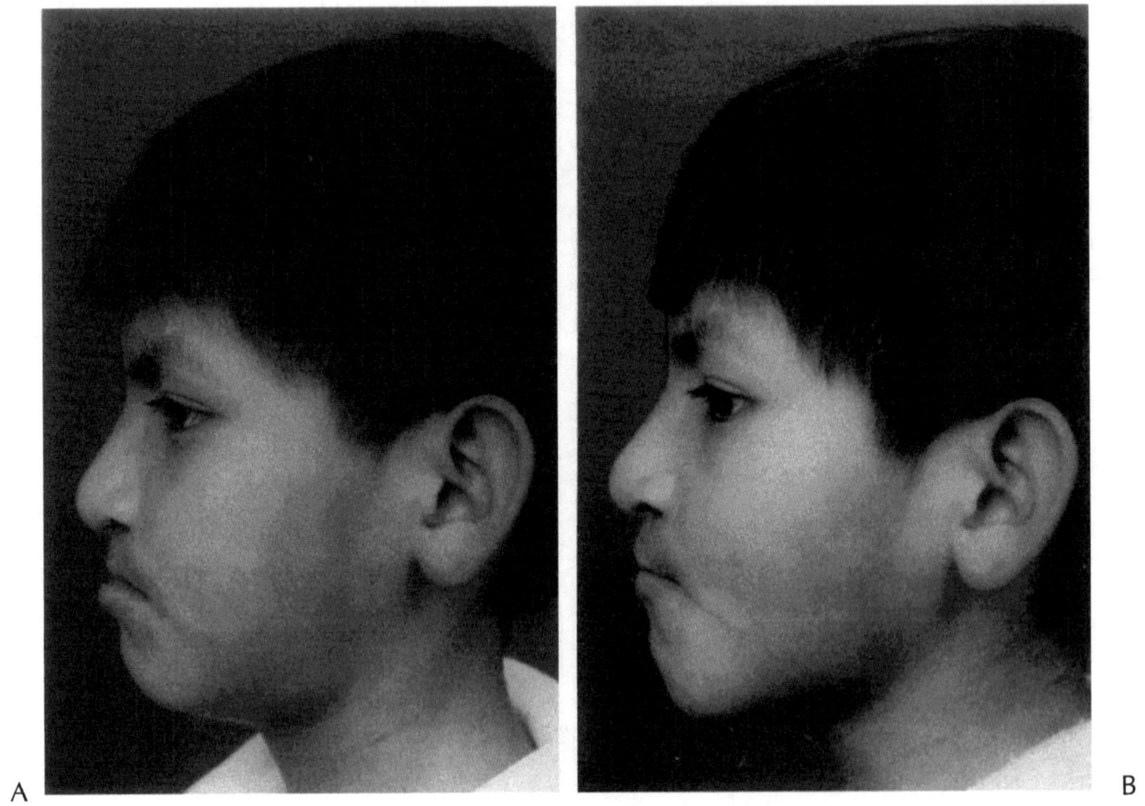

Figure 11A.7. (A) Preoperative view of a 7-year-old boy with midfacial retrusion due to the sequelae of cleft lip/palate. (B) Appearance 6 months later following 6 mm of maxillary advancement by distraction.

Overcorrection with a Class II molar relationship is always sought. This surgical goal is critical because during the remaining postoperative growth phase the individual midface growth pattern tends to revert to the original tendency of reduced maxillary growth and an anterior crossbite may come reestablished.

Gradual maxillary distraction also produced functional changes affecting respiration. Nasal breathing, as well as air flow and patency of the nasal airway, was improved. In this clinical series, six patients presented with documented obstructive sleep apnea; however, after an anterior distraction of 4 to 5 mm, the airway compromise was resolved.

Another concern was the potential deterioration of velopharyngeal function. In patients with preoperative velopharyngeal competence, the velopharyngeal sphincter remained functional postoperatively.

Two relevant points must be considered to predict the difficulties with the midfacial distraction technique: first, the quality of the palatal soft tissue including scarring, and second, the need to achieve skeletal and dentoalveolar transverse maxillary expansion by orthodontic means prior to distraction. These factors determine the stability of any maxillary advancement after distraction.

With maxillary distraction, a simultaneous soft-tissue expansion is observed, and the skin, fat, and muscles have a more favorable distribution around the mouth. The nasal base remains unchanged and the position of the lips, teeth, and tongue is in better relationship.

The technique can also be performed before the permanent dentition has erupted as the tooth-buds remain intact since the dental follicles are not injured by the corticotomy.

SIMULTANEOUS MANDIBULAR AND MAXILLARY DISTRACTION IN ADULTS

In the older patient in whom maxillary growth is completed, the dental occlusion is severely altered after mandibular distraction and an unacceptably prolonged orthodontic treatment program or secondary orthognathic surgery is required. This group of older patients with untreated unilateral craniofacial microsomia has slanted occlusal planes, but the dental occlusion is efficient and stable. Thus, simultaneous maxillo-mandibular distraction is indicated to correct the facial-dental deformity.

The surgical technique consist of a vestibular incision and subperiosteal dissection of the anterior and lateral aspects of the maxilla with exposure extended to the level of the pterygomaxillary junction. The nasal spine is dissected and the subperiosteal undermining is extended along the lateral walls and floor of the nose freeing the nasal septum from its caudal insertion. A full thickness osteotomy is made on the maxilla at the level of the pyriform aperture on both sides. The pterygomaxillary junction is liberated with a curved osteotome and Rowe forceps applied only on the affected side. The pterygomaxillary junction on the unaffected side remains intact and will serve as a pivot point for the midface elongation-rotation of that side.

A second incision is made in the inferior buccal sulcus of the hypoplasic mandible. The periosteum is elevated and, after the lateral and extended corticotomy is made, a unidirectional distraction device is applied. A vertical distraction vector is usually indicated for the adult patients. Both incisions are closed and five days later mandibular distraction is initiated at the rate of 1 mm/day and on the same day intermaxillary fixation is initiated with elastic bands. In general, the distraction period is completed in 3 to 4 weeks and a consolidation period of 8 to 10 weeks is necessary prior to removing the device.

The clinical results have demonstrated that, with the mandibular elongation, the maxilla follows the mandible changes and achieves simultaneous elongation, medial rotation and advancement. With a mean of 18 mm of new bone formation in the ascending ramus facial asymmetry was corrected with associated descent of the buccal commissure (Figure 11A.8). Preoperatively the deviation of the occlusal plane from the horizontal was a mean of 14 degrees. After the combined distraction procedure there was a minimal remaining deviation of 1 degree (Figure 11A.8C). Before distraction the vertical dimension of the maxilla was reduced, and the most posterior mandibular molar was in an exceedingly close relationship with the malar bone. Postdistraction the verti-

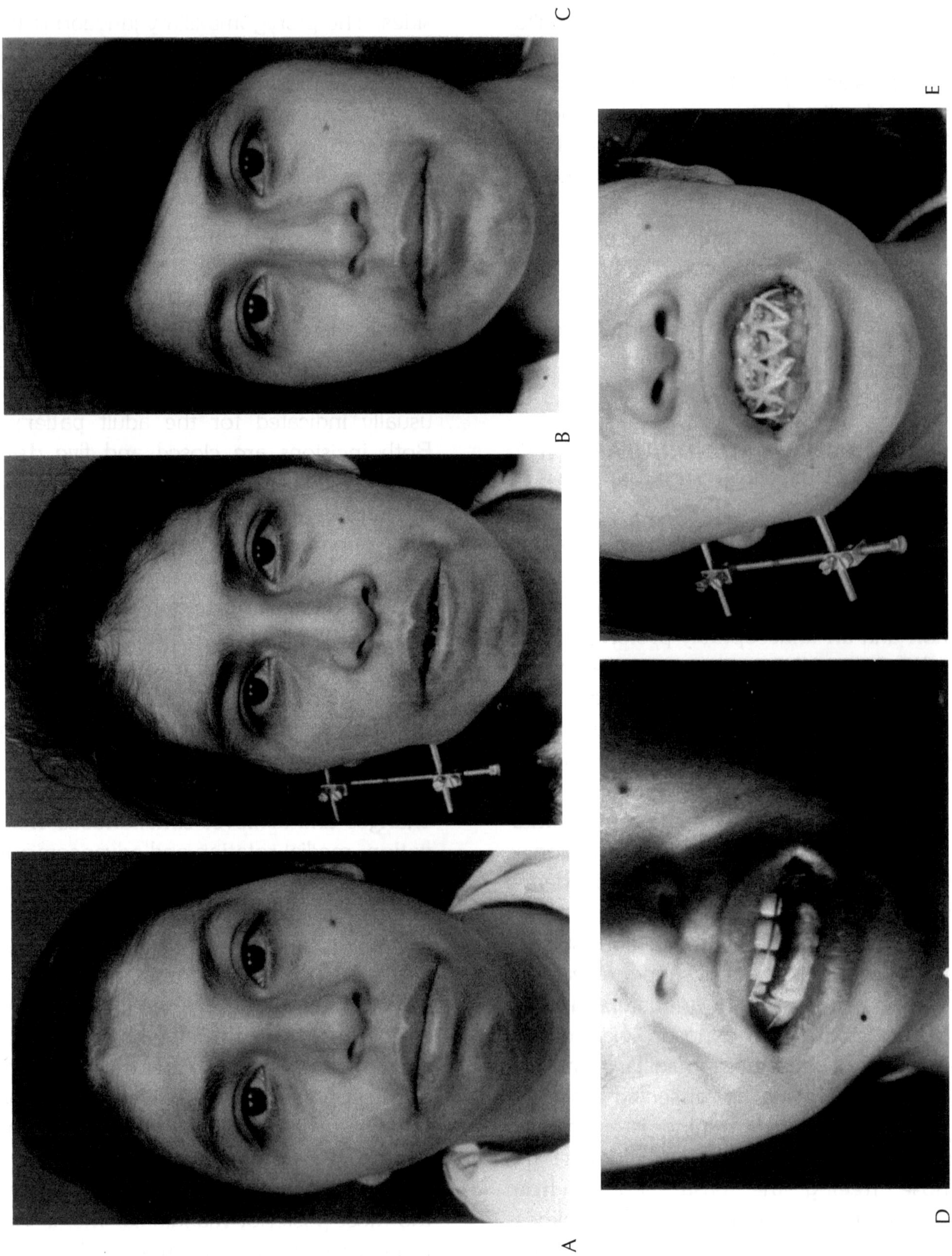

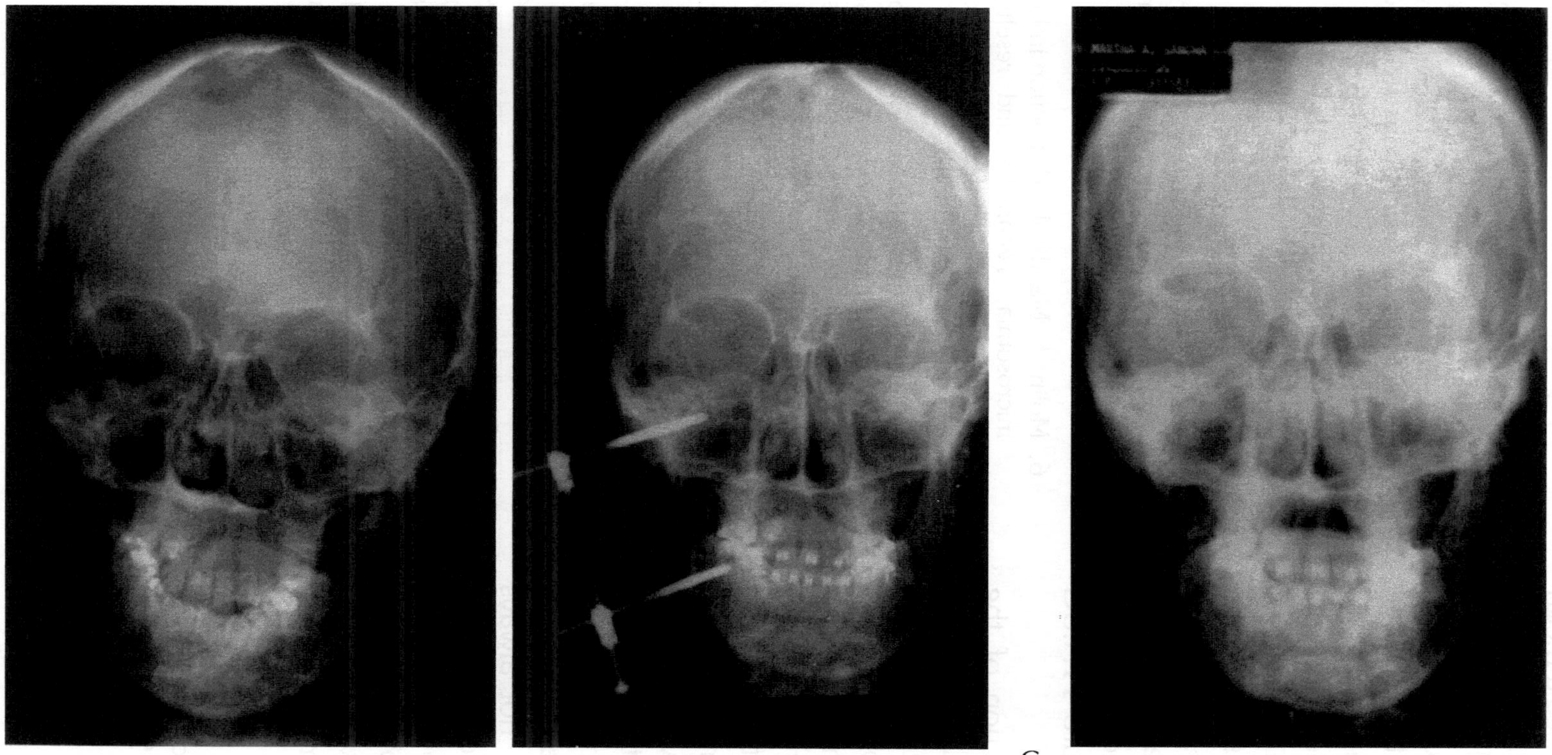

Figure 11A.8. (A) A 28-year-old female with untreated right craniofacial microsomia. (B) Appearance during the consolidation period (after 18 mm of mandibular elongation combined with 9 mm of maxillary elongation). (C) Appearance one year later. (D) Preoperative occlusal view showing the slanted occlusal plane. (E) The occlusal plane has been corrected after the combined maxillo-mandibular distraction (consolidation period). (F) Preoperative posteroanterior cephalogram showing the hypoplasic mandibular angle and ascending ramus with the diminished vertical dimension of the maxilla. (G) Posteroanterior cephalogram during the consolidation period. (H) The final posteroanterior cephalogram showing the following skeletal changes: a new dimension of the right ascending ramus with improvement in the size and volume of the condyle in the temporomandibular joint; a longer vertical dimension of the right maxillary buttress approximating that on the left side; correction of the dimensions of the nasal septum and nasal floor. The menton still remains undercorrected.

cal maxillary dimensions increased a mean of 10 mm, representing a 98% correction compared with the unaffected side. All of the new bone formation resulted in the simultaneous correction of the oblique nasal floor, as well as the movement of the nasal septum into a more normal position, thus increasing the volume of the nasal cavity. The preexisting dental occlusion has been preserved, after elongation of the superior and inferior midline incisors with positioning in the midline of the craniofacial skeleton (Figure 11A.8G and H).

The simultaneous distraction of the mandible and the maxilla is a logical treatment for older patients with unilateral craniofacial microsomia and produces satisfactory esthetic and functional results. It also eliminates the need for costly and prolonged orthodontic treatment. The maxilla, attached to the mandible by intermaxillary fixation, follows the rotational mandibular movements produced by the unidirectional distraction device.

The chin is always medialized by the distraction but in adults it is not always possible to achieve a normal central position. For this reason, the procedure does not eliminate the need for a sliding genioplasty at the time of device removal to improve the final esthetic result.

References

1. Ilizarov GA. The principles of the Ilizarov method. *Bull Hosp Joint Dis* 48:1, 1988.
2. Karp NS, Thorne CH, McCarthy JG, Sissons HA. Bone lengthening in the craniofacial skeleton. *Ann Plast Surg* 24:231, 1990.
3. McCarthy JG, Coccaro PJ, Schartz MD. Velopharyngeal function following maxillary advancement. *Plast Reconstr Surg* 64:180, 1979.
4. McCarthy JG, Schreiberg J, Karp N, Thorne CH, Grayson BH. Lengthening the human mandible by gradual distraction. *Plast Reconstr Surg* 89:1, 1992.
5. Molina F, Ortiz Monasterio F. Extended indications for mandibular distraction: Unilateral, bilateral and bidirectional. *Int Craniofacial Cong* 5:79, 1993.
6. Molina F. Mandibular distraction in hemifacial microsomia. Technique and results in 56 patients. The Craniofacial Society of Great Britain, 1994 (abstract).
7. Molina F, Ortiz-Monasterio F. Mandibular elongation and remodeling by distraction: A farewell to major osteotomies. *Plast Reconstr Surg* 96:825, 1995.
8. Snyder CC, Levine GA, Swanson HM, Brone EZ Jr. Mandibular lengthening by gradual distraction. *Plast Reconstr Surg* 51:506, 1973.
9. Staffenbery DA, Wood RJ, McCarthy JG, Grayson BH, Glasberg SB. Midface distraction advancement in the canine without osteotomies. *Ann Plast Surg* 34:512, 1995.
10. Rachmiel A, Potparic Z, Jackson IT, Sugihara T, Clayman L, Topf JS. Midface avancement by gradual distraction. *Br J Plast Surg* 46:201, 1993.
11. Ortiz Monasterio F, Rebeil AS, Valderrama M, Cruz R. Cephalometric measurements on adult patients with non-operated cleft palates. *Plast Reconstr Surg* 24:53, 1959.

CHAPTER 11B

Rigid External Maxillary Distraction

John W. Polley and Alvaro A. Figueroa

In 1992 McCarthy opened new hori zons in craniofacial surgery with the publication of the first application of distraction osteogenesis in the human craniofacial skeleton (1). Since the introduction of this pioneering work, distraction osteogenesis has rapidly become the keystone for the reconstruction of many craniomaxillofacial anomalies. For the management of severe maxillary hypoplasia, maxillary distraction osteogenesis is becoming one of the most important aspects of treatment planning. In this chapter, we present our technique for the reconstruction of severe maxillary hypoplasia utilizing rigid external distraction (RED).

The traditional orthodontic–surgical approach for the treatment of patients with severe maxillary hypoplasia, commonly associated with orofacial clefts, has several limitations. A major disadvantage is that long-term facial esthetics are often compromised in order to obtain skeletal and occlusal stability. In fact, bimaxillary surgery has often been advocated for many of these patients with setback of the mandible, which is usually normal in morphology and position. With this treatment the mandible is retrodisplaced from its ideal esthetic position, and the maxilla is not advanced sufficiently to obtain ideal upper face projection and convexity. As a result, facial esthetics are compromised.

Another major disadvantage with traditional orthognathic approaches in the treatment of maxillary hypoplasia is that surgical correction must be delayed until the teenage years when skeletal maturity has been reached. This treatment philosophy means that a young child with a significant maxillary hypoplasia must endure facial disfigurement and its functional and psychosocial consequences throughout the important developmental and formative years.

The application of maxillary distraction techniques has eliminated many of the significant disadvantages associated with traditional surgical approaches for the management of patients with severe maxillary hypoplasia. Through properly performed maxillary distraction, one can now achieve esthetic and occlusal correction of the deformities. Another advantage of maxillary distraction is that it can also be applied in children. It is no longer necessary to wait years before an affected child undergoes reconstruction. With maxillary distraction one can successfully treat severe maxillary hypoplasia, with minimal morbidity, as early as 5 or 6 years of age.

We initially attempted maxillary distraction utilizing an orthodontic face mask with elastic traction. With this technique, it was impossible to obtain the required amount of maxillary advancement. In addition, some patients suffered skin ulceration of the chin with wearing of the mask. Based on these early unsatisfactory results with elastic maxillary distraction, we modified the distraction technique to incorporate a rigid external system based on cranial fixation (2). Rigid external distraction employs a head frame stabilized to the cranium with scalp screws (Figure 11B.1). The head frame supports an adjustable vertical bar to which is attached an adjustable horizontal bar with adjustable distraction screws. The distraction screws are linked to an intraoral orthodontic appliance with a surgical wire (Figure 11B.2). The distraction process is performed at home by turning the distraction screws. With the use of rigid external distraction, changes can be made in the vertical and horizontal vectors of distraction, without discomfort to the patient, throughout the period of active distraction. The flexibility of the system allows customization of the distraction process based on each patient's esthetic and occlusal requirements.

The technique of rigid external distraction of the maxilla has been utilized in 30 patients with excellent results and minimal morbidity. In patients in whom the occlusal relationships and dental arches are well coordinated, maxillary distraction has been a definitive procedure. In patients whose arches are not well coordinated and in very young patients, maxillary distraction is an essential intermediate procedure that allows the surgeon to obtain substantial maxillary advancement with satisfactory alignment of the basal skeleton between the upper and lower jaws. In such patients, a definitive LeFort I osteotomy may be indicated at a later date to obtain the final ideal occlusal relationships. However, the amount of horizontal and vertical change of the maxilla required at the time of this final surgery should be minimal.

Maxillary distraction with the use of rigid external distraction offers several unique advantages. The most important of these include the following:

1. Freedom of Osteotomy Design. When utilizing external distraction the sole determinant in the design of the LeFort I osteotomy is the esthetic requirement of the patient. A complete zygomatico–maxillary osteotomy with mobilization of all segments is required, including

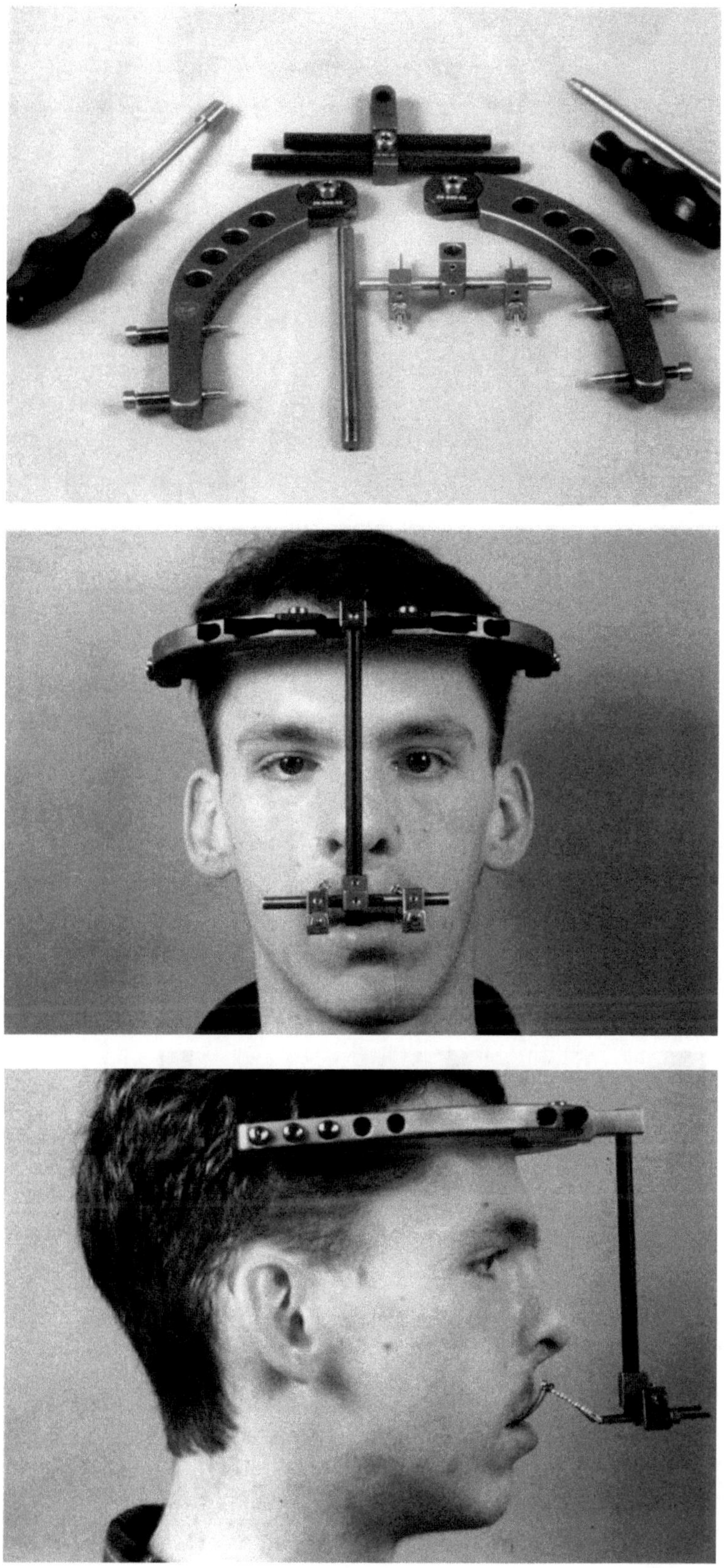

A

B

C

Figure 11B.1. Disassembled rigid external distraction (RED) device (A). Frontal (B) and profile (C) views of a patient undergoing maxillary distraction. Note the cranially fixated halo with vertical bar from which a movable horizontal bar containing the distraction screws is attached.

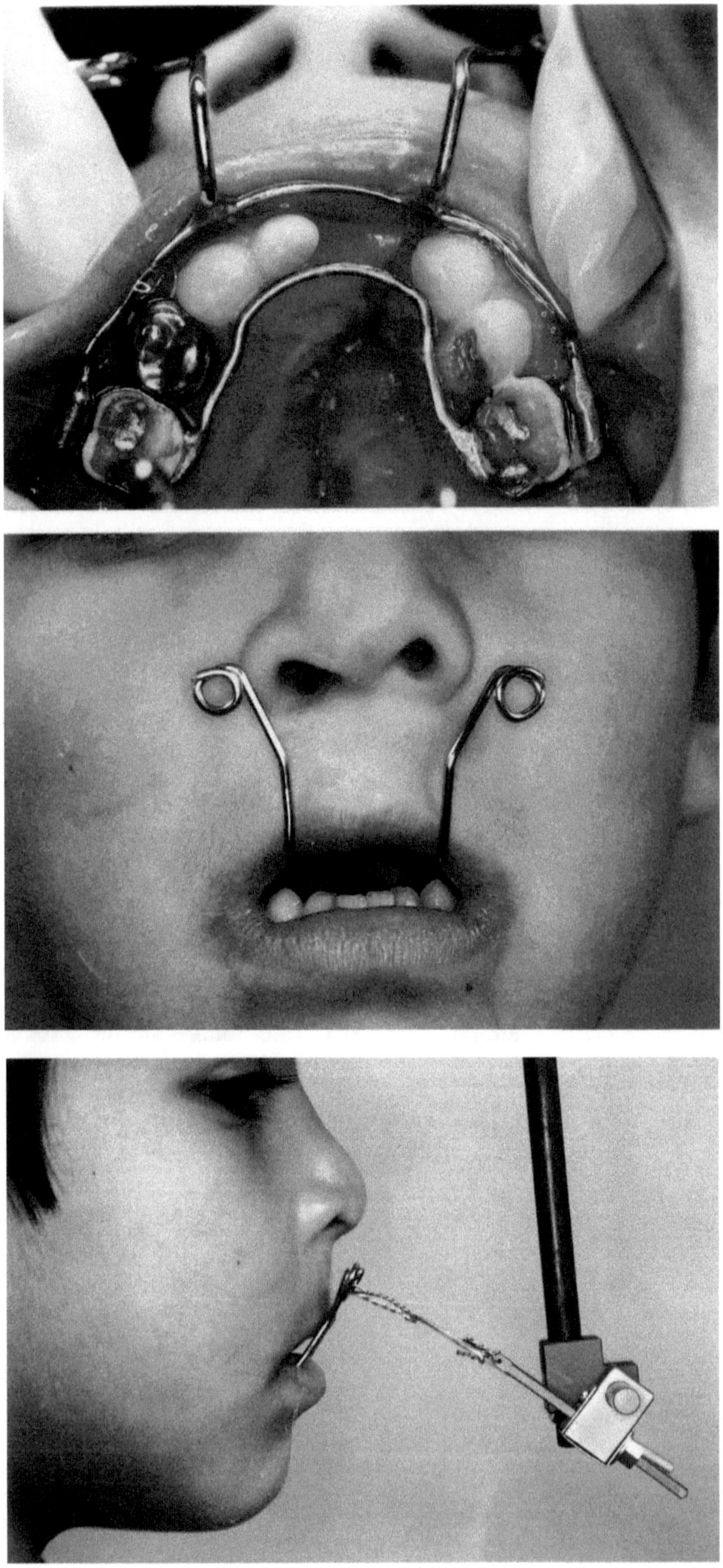

Figure 11B.2. Intraoral view (A) of the custom built intraoral splint. Extraoral traction hooks soldered to the intraoral splint positioned at the level of the palatal plane (B). Extraoral traction hook connected with a surgical wire to the adjustable distraction screw (C). Note the direction of pull or vector in a downward and forward fashion. The vector can be modified at any time during the distraction process by moving the horizontal bar. The intraoral splint is further secured by circumdental wiring to as many teeth as possible.

A

B

C

pterygomaxillary and septal dysjunction. The height of the transverse maxillary osteotomy is determined by the preoperative esthetic evaluation of the patient. Most patients will require a high transverse osteotomy, which includes most or all of the anterior projection of the zygoma. The level of the osteotomy is determined by the amount of malar and perinasal advancement required. In addition, in young children the osteotomy must avoid the developing dentition. The osteotomy design is not limited by the placement of internal devices which requires stable bone above and below the osteotomy for fixation.

2. Distraction Control. Rigid external distraction allows for complete control over the distraction process. The force vectors can be changed at any time during the distraction process. These adjustments are simply performed without discomfort to the patients, titrating the distraction to meet the specific esthetic and occlusal requirements.

3. Placement, Compliance, Removal. At surgery, after completion of the LeFort osteotomy, the external distraction device is easily placed. There is no discomfort wearing the head frame and no pin site care is required. As the head frame is not removable, compliance is assured. The external distraction device is quickly removed in an outpatient setting with infiltration of a minimal amount of local anesthetic at the pin sites. No secondary operative procedure is required for removal of the device.

4. Age of Treatment. An important advantage of rigid external distraction is that it can be utilized from the age of 5 or 6 years through adulthood. The only limitations to external distraction are behavioral constraints of young age, dental requirements for fitting of the intraoral appliance (full deciduous dentition or older), and the surgeon's confidence in performing the LeFort osteotomy without damaging the permanent tooth follicles.

The distraction protocol with rigid external distraction (RED) is as follows:

1. Latency period: 4 to 6 days following osteotomy and application of the device.
2. Active distraction: 1 to 1.5 mm per day
3. Rigid retention: distraction device in place without active distraction 2 to 3 weeks
4. Final retention: Elastic retention with face mask for 4 to 6 weeks at nighttime only (two 6-oz elastics)

The following are representative cases illustrating the use of rigid external distraction for the treatment of severe maxillary hypoplasia.

Case Studies

Case 1. A 5-year-10-month-old female presented with a repaired left cleft lip and palate with associated midfacial hypoplasia, Class III skeletal and dental relations, and anterior and posterior crossbite (Figure 11B.3). The patient had severe overclosure because of horizontal and vertical maxillary hypoplasia. The patient underwent maxillary distraction utilizing rigid external distraction. After insertion of the intraoral splint with external hooks, a high two-piece LeFort I maxillary osteotomy with pterygomaxillary and septal dysjunction was performed. Care was taken to avoid all developing tooth buds. At the time of surgery the external distraction device was anchored through scalp pins to the cranium. The patient was discharged from the hospital the following morning and maxillary distraction was commenced on the fifth postoperative day at a rate of 1mm/day. She underwent a maxillary advancement of 10mm utilizing rigid external distraction. At the completion of active distraction the patient was retained with the external device for 3 weeks. This was followed by a period of 6 weeks with a removable face mask worn at night only.

After distraction, the midfacial concavity was corrected from the infraorbital region to the upper lip. The convexity of the face and the vertical relationships were restored. The nose-lip relationships were greatly improved and the posterior and anterior crossbites were also corrected. The postoperative cephalometric radiographs demonstrated improvement of the skeletal convexity as well as the maxillomandibular and dental relationships. The velopharyngeal mechanism of the patient was not affected and the speech demonstrated an improvement in articulation. The changes on this patient have remained stable 12 months after distraction.

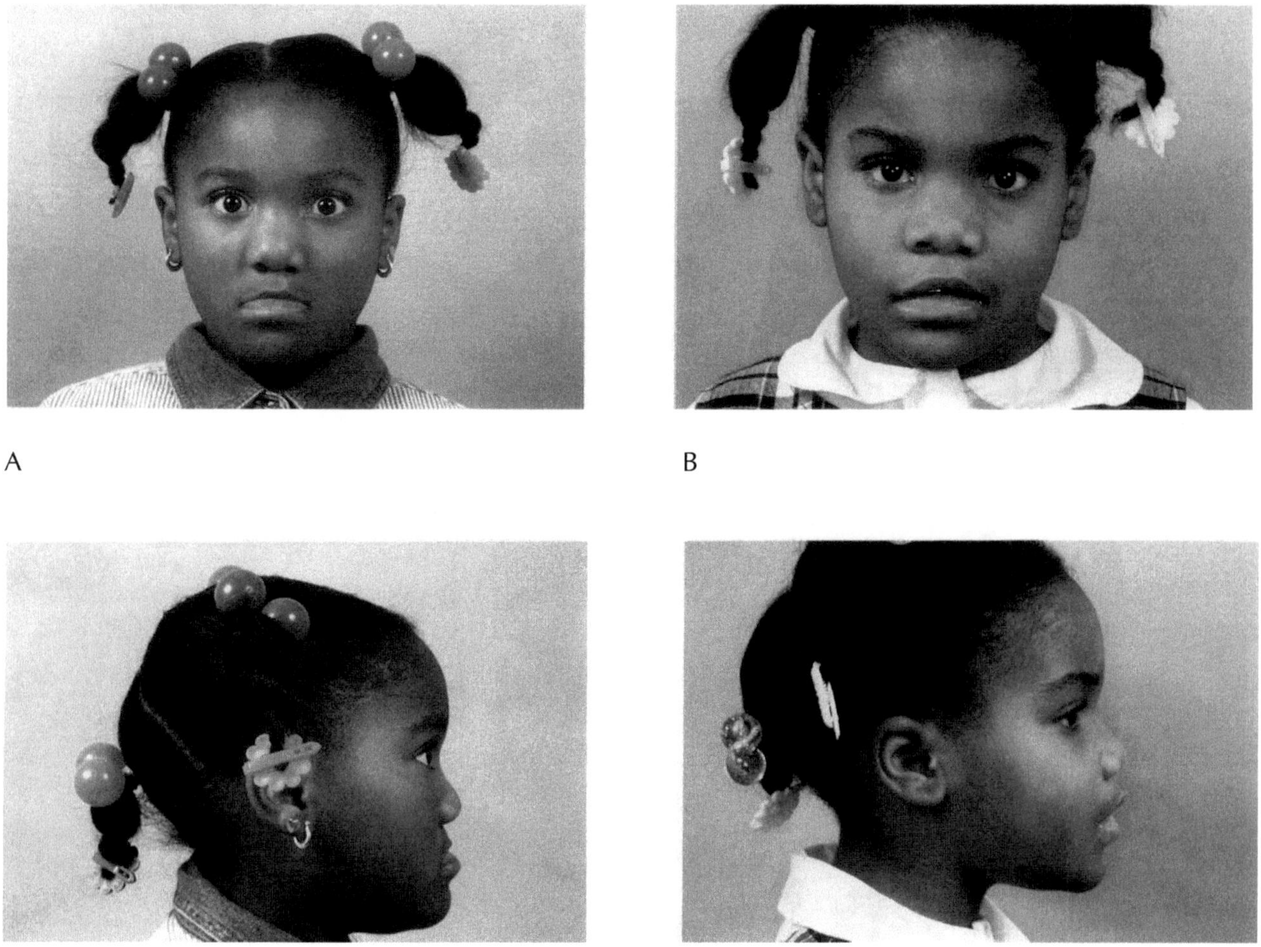

A B C D

Figure 11B.3. Case 1. A 5-year-10-month-old female with left cleft lip and palate who underwent maxillary distraction with the rigid external distraction device. Note the improvement in facial convexity including malar prominences, nasal tip and upper lip. The dental relations are also improved.

(A) Predistraction frontal view.

(B) Postdistraction frontal view.

(C) Predistraction right profile.

(D) Postdistraction right profile.

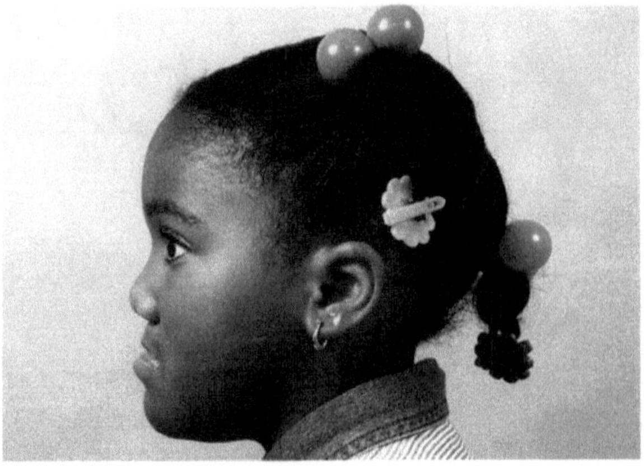

E

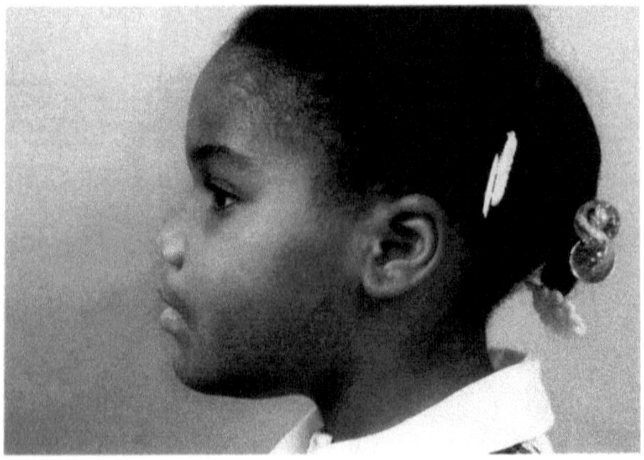

F

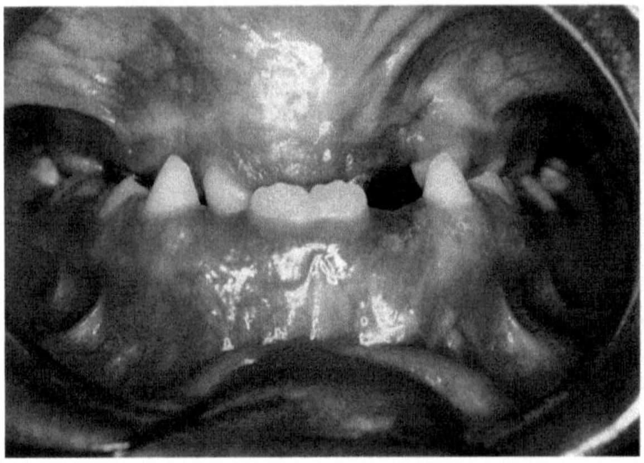

G

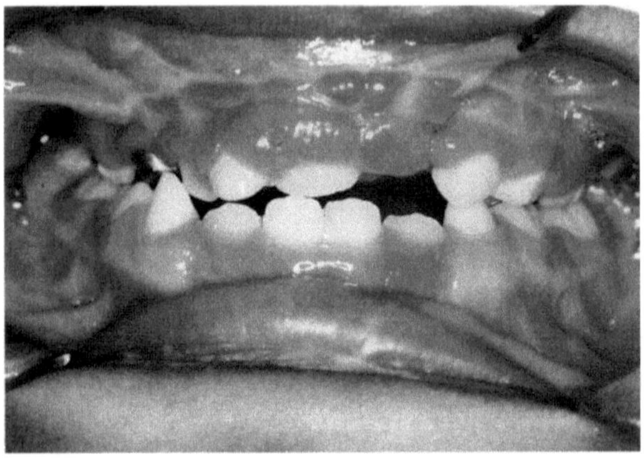

H

Figure 11B.3. Case 1. *Continued*

(E) Predistraction left profile.

(F) Postdistraction left profile.

(G) Predistraction frontal intraoral view.

(H) Postdistraction frontal intraoral view.

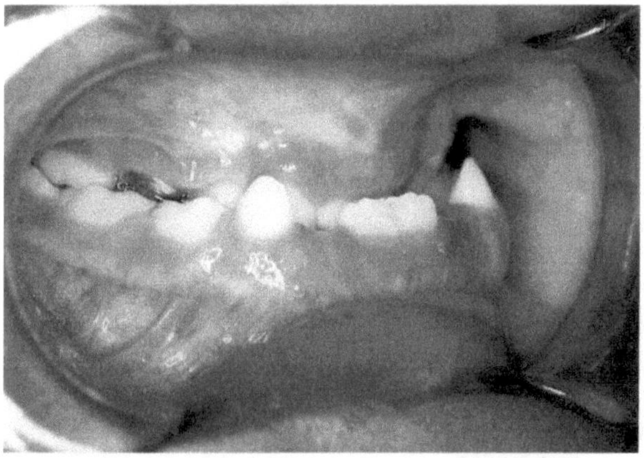

I

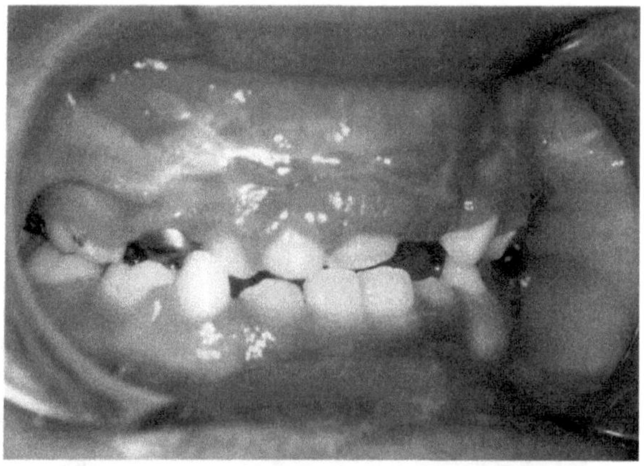

J

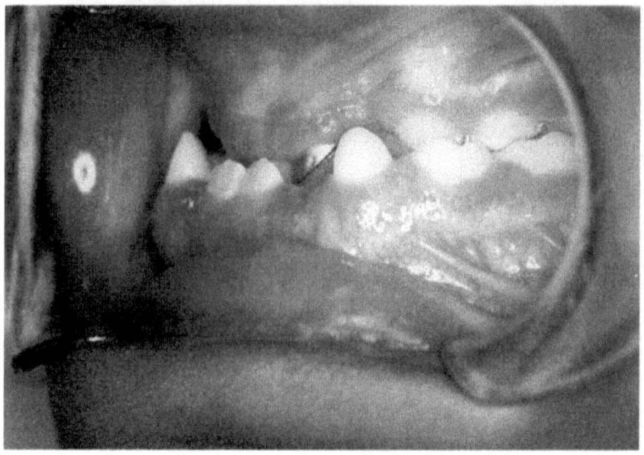

K

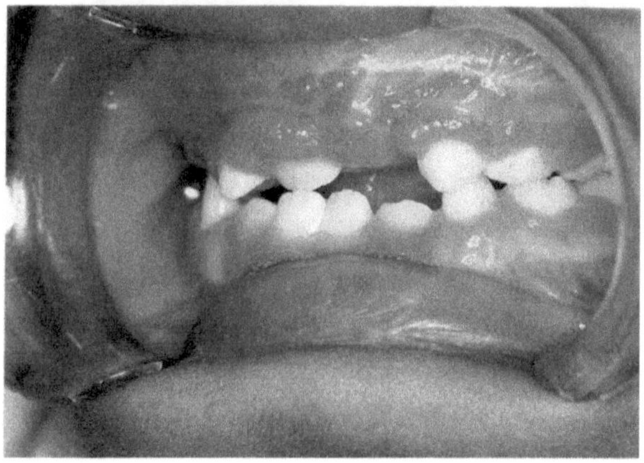

L

Figure 11B.3. ***Case 1.*** *Continued*

(I) Predistraction oblique intraoral view.

(J) Postdistraction oblique intraoral view.

(K) Predistraction oblique intraoral view.

(L) Postdistraction oblique intraoral view.

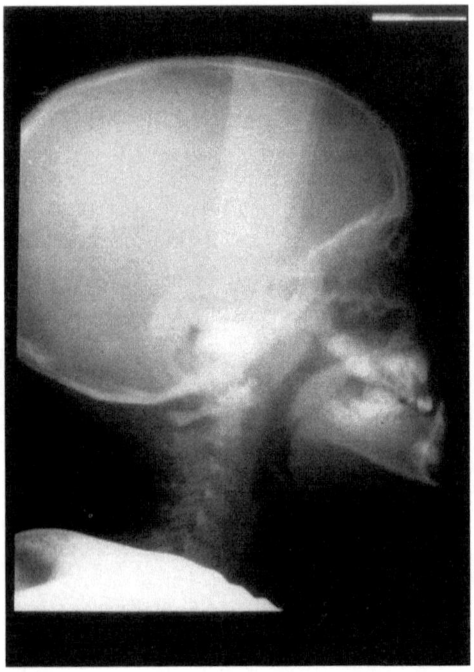

M

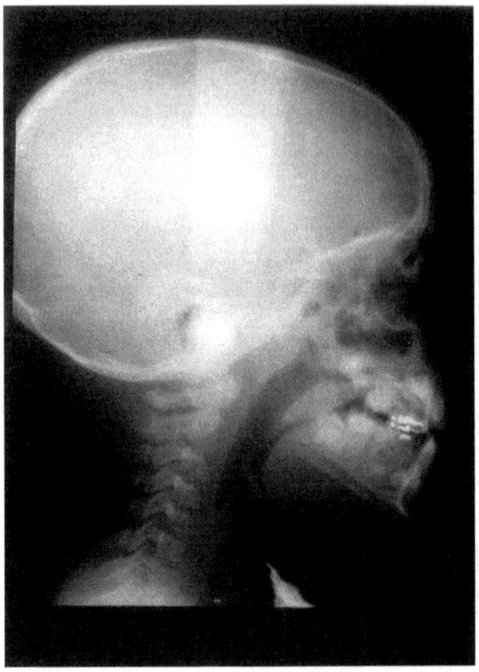

N

Figure 11B.3. ***Case 1.*** *Continued*

(M) Predistraction lateral cephalogram.

(N) Postdistraction lateral cephalogram.

Case 2. A 5 year-2-month-old male presented with a repaired right cleft lip and palate with maxillary deficiency, vertical overclosure as well as Class III skeletal and dental relations hips with anterior and posterior crossbites (Figure 11B.4). After insertion of the intraoral splint with external traction hooks, the patient was scheduled for maxillary distraction. The patient underwent a high two-piece LeFort I osteotomy with pterygomaxillary and septal dysjunction and avoidance of all permanent tooth buds. After completion of the osteotomy, the external device was secured to the cranium. The patient was discharged from the hospital the following morning. Maxillary distraction was commenced on the fifth postoperative day at the rate of 1mm/day. After active distraction the external device was left in place for 3 weeks for consolidation, followed by 6 weeks of retention with an orthodontic face mask and elastics at night only. As demonstrated by the cephalometric radiographs (Figures 11B.4M and 11B.4N) and tracings, the maxilla was advanced 11mm with minimal changes in the vertical position of the mandible. The concave skeletal and facial deformity was corrected to normal facial relations and proportions. The anterior and posterior crossbites were also corrected after distraction. The facial contour, position of the nasal tip and lip and nose relationships were improved after maxillary distraction without the need for nasal reconstructive procedures. The skeletal and dental changes have remained stable 18 months after distraction.

Distraction osteogenesis has revolutionized the treatment of patients with severe craniofacial deficiencies (1). Maxillary distraction osteogenesis utilizing rigid external distraction permits successful and predictable treatment of patients with severe maxillary hypoplasia at almost any age. Long term follow-up studies of these patients will answer specific questions concerning stability, growth, and dental development.

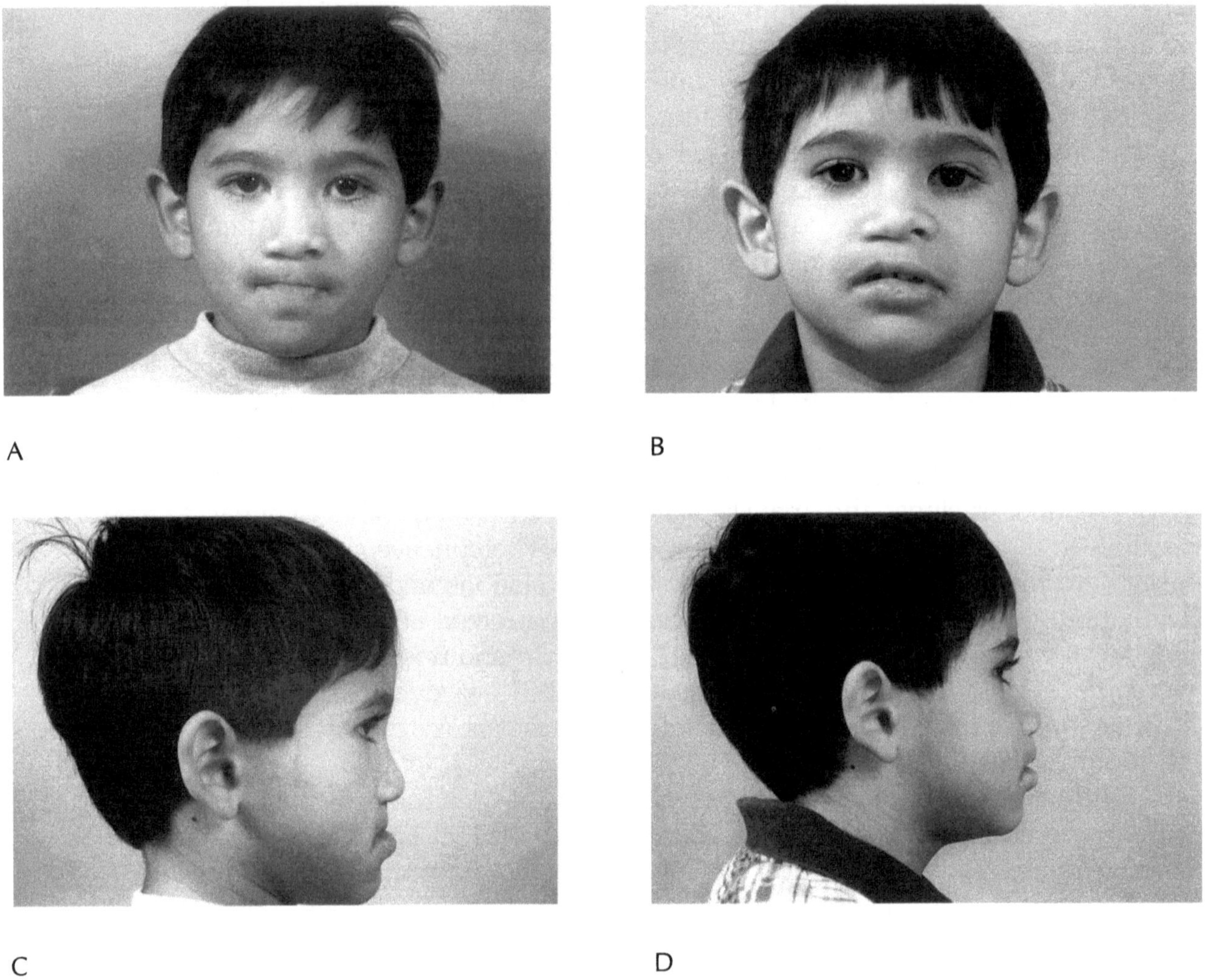

Figure 11B.4. **Case 2.** A five-year-two-month-old male with right cleft lip and palate who underwent maxillary distraction. Note the correction of the concave skeletal profile with restoration of normal horizontal and vertical maxillomandibular and dental relationships.

(A) Predistraction frontal view.

(B) Postdistraction frontal view.

(C) Predistraction right profile.

(D) Postdistraction right profile.

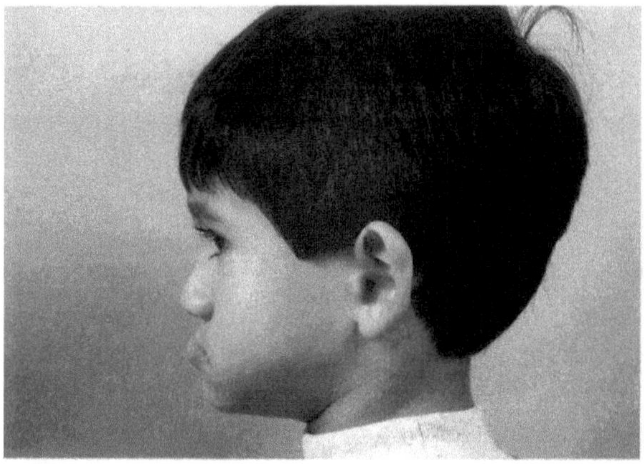

E

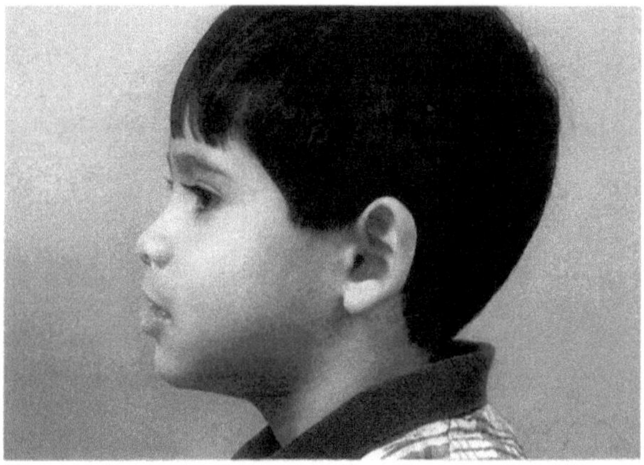

F

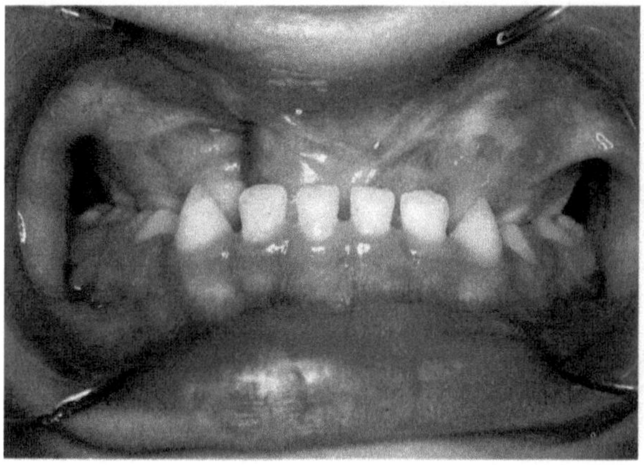

G

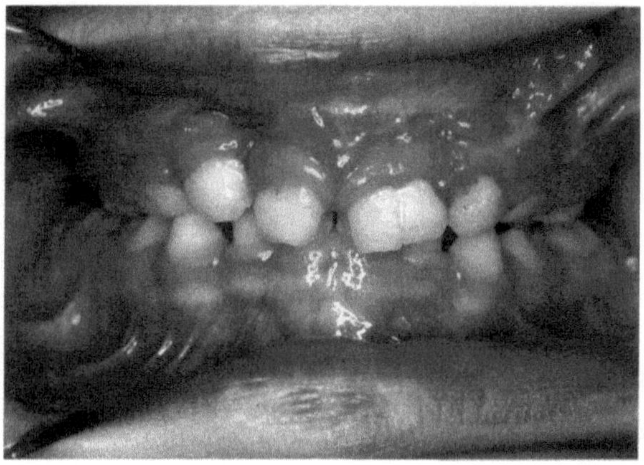

H

Figure 11B.4. Case 2. *Continued*

(E) Predistraction left profile.

(F) Postdistraction left profile.

(G) Predistraction frontal intraoral view.

(H) Postdistraction frontal intraoral view.

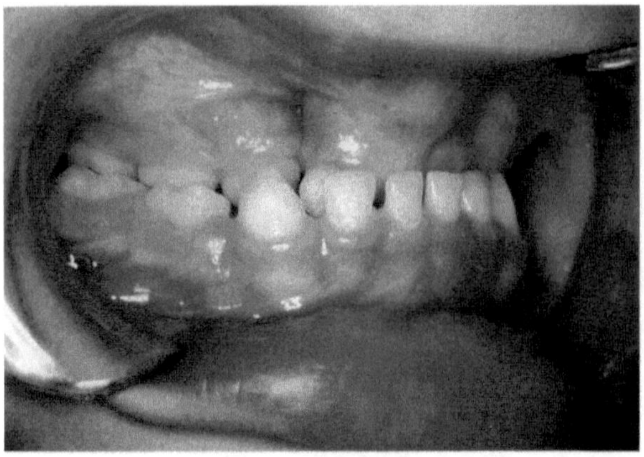

I

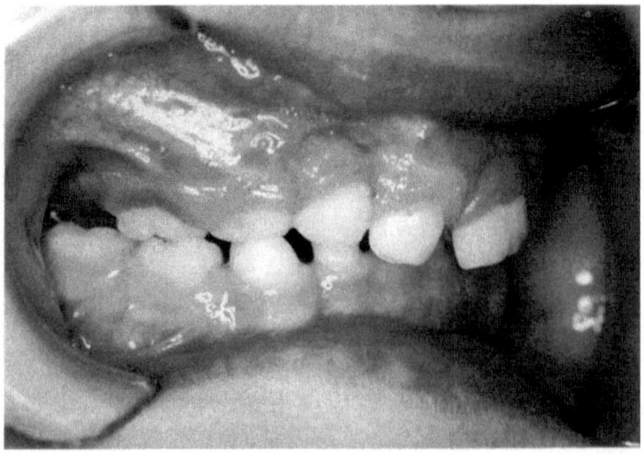

J

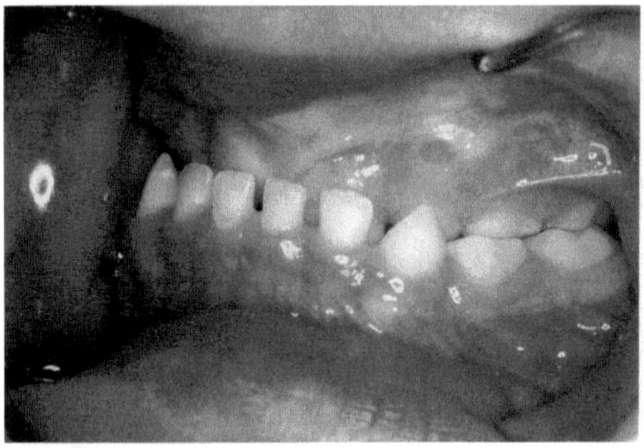

K

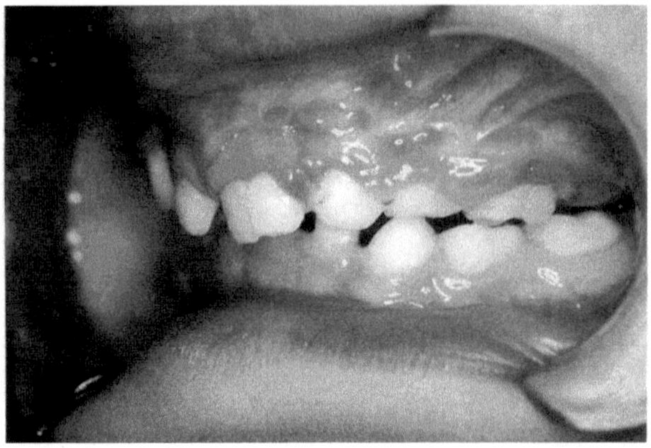

L

Figure 11B.4. ***Case 2.*** *Continued*

(I) Predistraction oblique intraoral view.

(J) Postdistraction oblique intraoral view.

(K) Predistroction oblique intraoral view.

(L) Postdistraction oblique interval view.

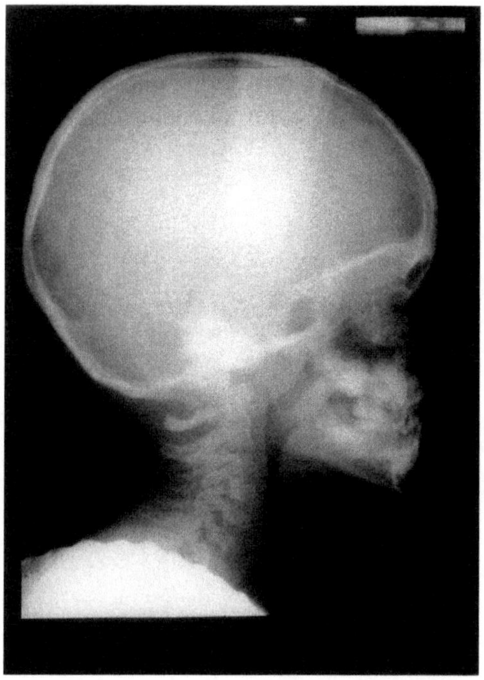

M

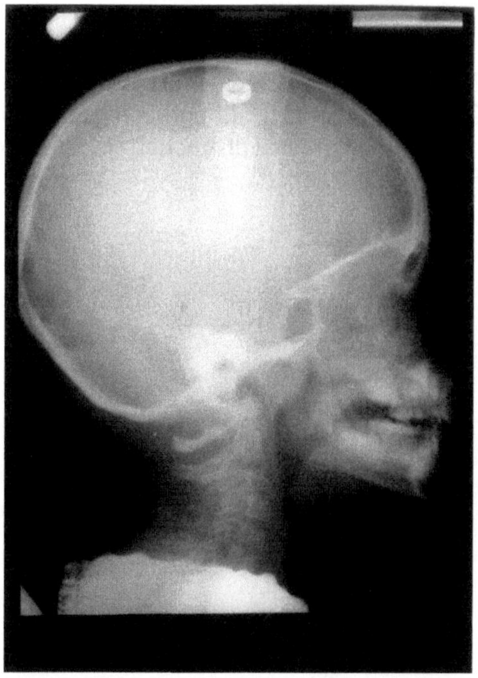

N

Figure 11B.4. ***Case 2.*** *Continued*

(M) Predistraction lateral cephalogram.

(N) Postdistraction lateral cephalogram.

References

1. McCarthy JG, Schreiber J, Karp N, Thorne CH, Greyson BH. Lengthening the human mandible by gradual distraction. *Plast Reconstr Surg* 89:1, 1992.

2. Polley JW, Figueroa AA. Management of severe maxillary deficiency in childhood and adolescence through distraction osteogenesis with an external, adjustable, rigid distraction device. *J Craniofac Surg* 8:181, 1997.

CHAPTER 12

DISTRACTION OF THE MIDFACE AND THE ZYGOMA

CLINICAL STUDIES

Jeffrey D. Fairley, Wolfgang Muhlbauer, and Hans Anderl

Distraction osteogenesis, a technique initially used and described in the correction of lower limb deficiencies and discrepancies (1–4), has recently been adapted, at first in animal models and later in the human, to the craniofacial skeleton and has gained popularity as the devices have become more sophisticated and the techniques more refined (5–13).

Distraction lengthening, a technique first described by Codivilla in 1905, delineated a method for generating new bone by the stretching or lengthening of callus (1). This concept was popularized by Ilizarov who recognized that there exists in the "organic regeneration" (bone, muscle, nerve, blood vessels, and skin) the inherent capacity for living tissue that is mechanically stressed to respond by growing in the direction of that stress (2,3). Bone lengthening by gradual distraction is a well-known and standard procedure for the lengthening of enchondral bones of the extremities (4). In 1973 Synder and associates (5) applied this principle to the membranous bones of the canine mandible and additional experimental studies on membranous bone lengthening have been subsequently reported (6,7,14,15). More recently Karp and associates at New York University described an adaption of this technique to the canine mandible (7), and in 1992 McCarthy and colleagues reported the first clinical cases of mandibular lengthening by gradual distraction using an extraoral device in Nagers syndrome and unilateral craniofacial microsomia (11).

Despite early operative midface disjunction, mobilization, and advancement (LeFort III or Monobloc) in infancy or early childhood, the continued intrinsic growth deficiency in syndromic craniofacial synostosis usually results in midface imbalance and maxillomandibular dysharmony (16–18). This is reflected in the myriad of surgical procedures described to correct combined midface and maxillary deficiencies (19). The results are often unsatisfactory and not therapeutically as comprehensive, especially with regard to occlusal correction and restoration of the contour of the hypoplastic midface. The need for a surgical alternative to well-established craniofacial advancement procedures consequently became apparent. A dynamic distraction device was developed that not only fulfilled the criteria of mechanical distraction but allowed growth during the most explosive growth phase to take place. In addition, the device was esthetically acceptable for young patients and their parents.

CLINICAL SERIES

Since May 1993, 10 infants with Apert syndrome underwent midface distraction at a mean age of 6.8 months (Table 12.1). The diagnosis of Apert syndrome was established on the basis of bilateral coronal suture synostosis on radiographic examination and the associated extremity syndactyly. The first four cases were subjected to a fronto-orbito-facial advancement (monobloc procedure) followed after an interval of one month by midface distraction; the last six patients underwent a fronto-orbital surgical advancement combined with midface distraction alone and without a delay interval.

The clinical series can be analyzed as follows:

Case 1: Distraction was initiated one month after monobloc advancement and the device was turned five times in the remaining 4 months (Table 12.2).

Case 2: Distraction was begun 1 month after monobloc advancement and the device was turned eight times in the remaining 7 months.

Case 3: Distraction was initiated 1 month after monobloc advancement and the device was turned seven times in the remaining 8 months.

The remaining patients (cases 5–10, excluding case 4 of monobloc advancement)

Table 12.1. Midface distraction in patients with Apert syndrome.

Case	Intraoperative fronto-orbital advancement (mm)	Postoperative midface distraction (mm)	
		Right	Left
1	20	10	8
2	20	14	14
3	20	14	14
4	15	20	20
5	20	16	14
6	25	14	17
7	25	22	12
8	20	7	13
10	20	16	16
x	21.0	14.8	14.3

Note the amount (mm) of fronto-orbital advancement and midface distraction.

Table 12.2. Midface distraction (months).

	1	2	3	4	5	6	7	Removal (postoperative months)
1		5x						8
2		8x						7
3		7x						11

Distraction in the first three patients was initiated one month after Monobloc advancement. The number of times that the device was turned is also designated.

were subjected to a different regimen from the initial surgical procedure (ie, fronto-orbital advancement alone followed one week later by the initiation of midface distraction, which continued for an additional 3 weeks). The miniplate fixation device used for stabilization was removed at 4 weeks following the initial procedure, and the distraction devices were removed 3 months after their insertion.

TECHNIQUE OF MONOBLOC (FRONTO-ORBITAL-FACIAL) ADVANCEMENT

Following orotracheal intubation, a bilateral coronal incision with elevation of the anterior scalp flap was performed. Dissection was extended in a subperiosteal plane over the midforehead region and in a superior, lateral, and medial direction around the orbits, and continued deep to the superficial layer of the deep temporal fascia, exposing the zygomatic arches laterally and the anterior maxilla. Through a subcilliary incision of the lower lids, exposure was obtained of the inferior orbital rim and the medial orbital wall. Subperiosteal mobilization of the orbital contents was completed.

A bifrontal craniotomy was performed with separation of the cranial bones from the dura; the zygomatic arches were divided and a circular orbitotomy ensued. Separation of the bony nasal septum from the anterior cranial base, separation of the pterygomaxillary junction and midfacial advancement were performed (20,21).

TECHNIQUE OF FRONTO-ORBITAL ADVANCEMENT

This technique is essentially the same as that described for the fronto-orbital-facial advancement except that the following surgical maneuvers were omitted: pterygomaxillary disjunction and osteotomy of the lower half of the orbit or zygomatic arch.

The distraction device (Figure 12.1), applied bilaterally, is made of a gold and vitallium alloy and composed of two parts: an anterior segment, which is screwed into the posterior surface of the zygomatic arch, and a posterior segment (attached to a universal joint allowing movement in a horizontal plane) connected to the temporal bone (Figures 12.2 and 12.3). The anterior and posterior segments are con-

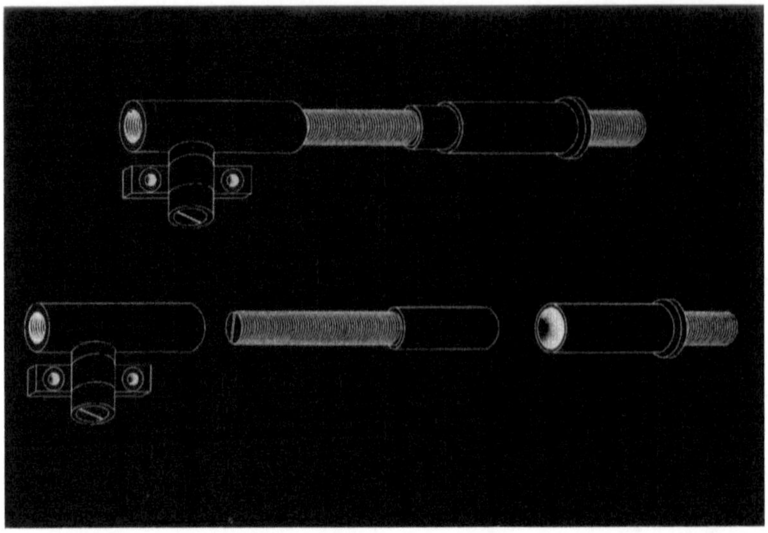

Figure 12.1. Distraction device. The distraction device is composed of an anterior and posterior segment connected to each other via a spindle, which is threaded in the posterior portion. The anterior portion of the spindle is unthreaded, as is the anterior segment of the distraction device. The anterior segment of the distraction device is held in place by the spindle, "floating" on the latter. Distraction is initiated with the use of a screwdriver that activates the posterior end of the spindle through an opening in the posterior segment. One turn of the screwdriver moves the spindle 1 mm forward, and the anterior end of the spindle thus abuts on the anterior segment of the device. The anterior segment, which is flared at its furthermost end, is screwed into the posterior surface of the zygoma.

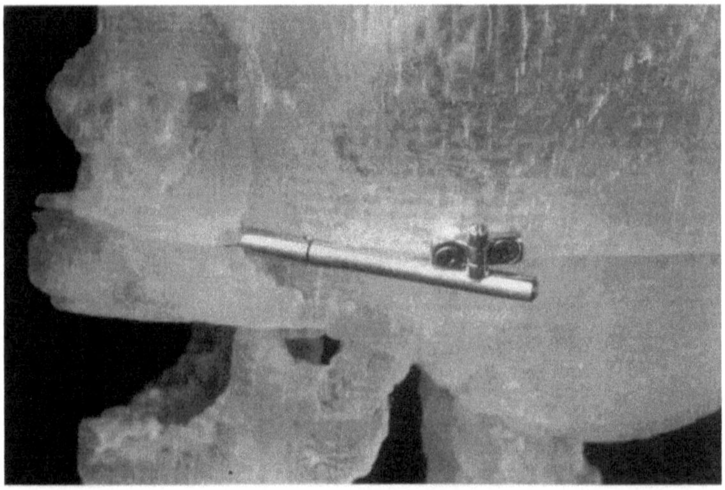

Figure 12.2. The distraction device attached to a stereolithographic model of a neonatal skull. The anterior segment is screwed into the posterior surface of the zygoma; the posterior surface is attached to the temporal bone. A device is placed on each side of the craniofacial skeleton (not illustrated).

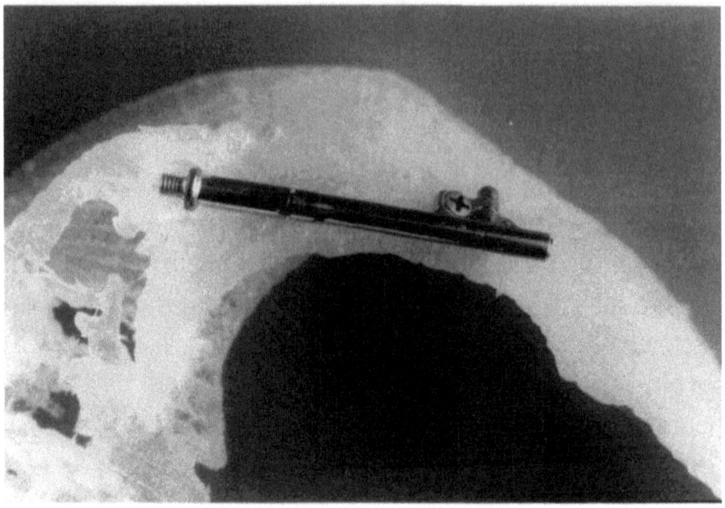

Figure 12.3. Caudal view of the distraction device attached to a stereolithographic model of a neonatal skull. The device is screwed into the zygoma anteriorly and attached to the temporal bone posteriorly.

nected via a threaded spindle, which is activated through a dorsal opening in the device. One complete rotation of the device moves it forward one millimeter allowing controlled mechanical distraction and advancement of the midface. The anterior segment has no thread and holds the spindle in place, while at the same time allowing for spontaneous growth in the region of the midface. Activation of the spindle pushes it against the interface of the anterior segment, thus causing mechanical distraction. The device is exteriorized through a stab wound in the skin at the dorsal end to facilitate activation, which is performed on an ambulatory basis (Figures 12.4–12.6). As in cases 5 to 10, active distraction begins one week following surgery and is continued on a daily basis for 14 to 21 days at the rate of 1mm/day. After this interval the device is left in situ for an additional 3 months, after which time it is removed (Table 12.3).

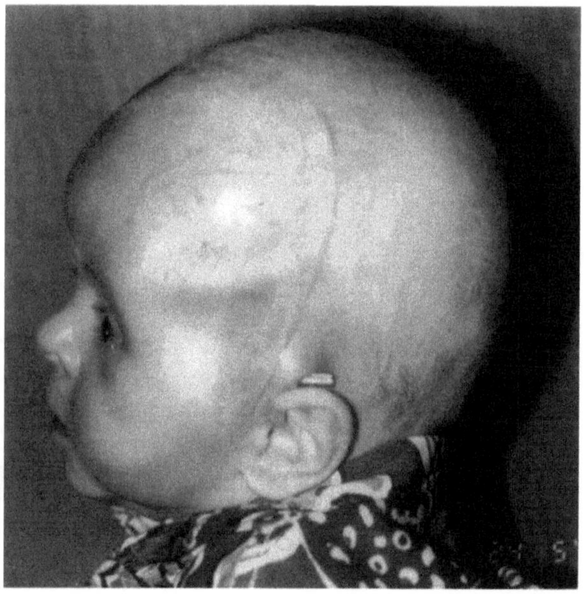

Figure 12.4. The device is exteriorized behind the ear, thus facilitating activation on an ambulatory basis.

RESULTS

Cephalometeric studies were carried out to determine the SNA angle in the 10 patients with Apert syndrome preoperatively (Table 12.4) and one year postoperatively (Figures 12.7–12.9). The control group was represented by a group of 10 Apert cases following monobloc advancement alone without distraction (Table 12.5), and in this group the same cephalometric evaluation was performed preoperatively and one year postoperatively.

In the group with midface distraction the mean intraoperative fronto-orbital advancement at the time of surgery was 21mm, and an additional postoperative

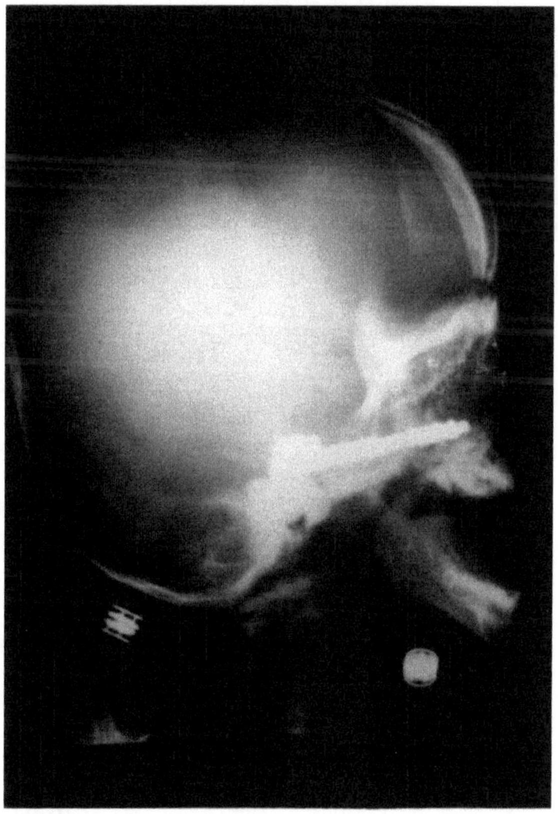

Figure 12.5. A lateral radiographic view showing the distraction device in place.

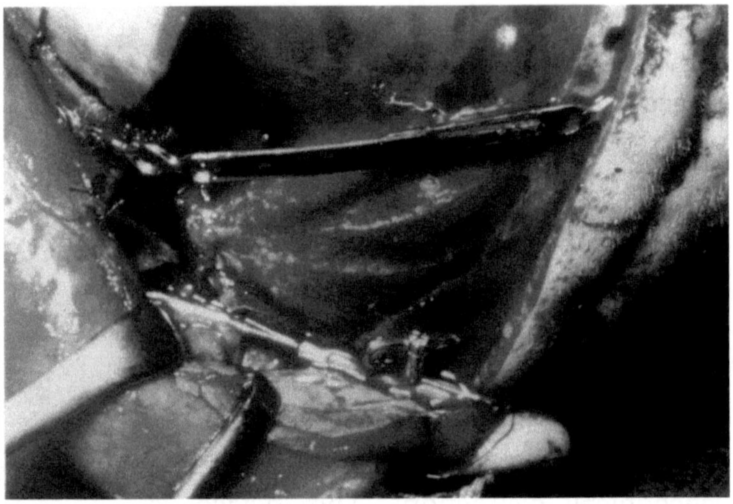

Figure 12.6. An intraoperative view demonstrating the position of the distraction device (lower) with a dynamic miniplate (upper) for temporary stabilization following fronto-orbital advancement.

Table 12.3. Midface distraction (weeks).

	1	2	3	4	5	6	7	8	9	10	11	12	13	14	Removal (post-operative weeks)
1		■	■	■											12
2		■	■	■	■										14
3		■	■	■											13
4				■	■	■									14
5					■	■	■								12
6		■	■	■											12
7		■	■	■											12

The shaded areas designate the time periods of distraction in the seven patients who underwent fronto-orbital advancement and midface distraction, the latter initiated one week postoperatively.

Table 12.4. SNA angle following distraction.

Case	Preoperative	1 year postoperative
1	70	80
2	72	80
3	72	80
4	65	78
5	74	85
6	70	82
7	66	82
8	72	80
9	68	80
10	74	82
x	70.3	80.9

Cephalometric evaluation (SNA) after Monobloc surgical advancement and midface distraction.

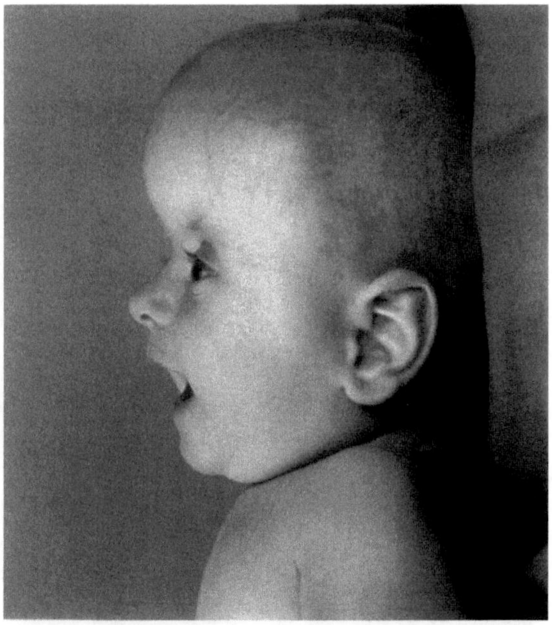
A

Figure 12.7. (A) Lateral view of a 6-month-old patient with Apert syndrome. (B) Frontal view one-year postoperatively following midface/zygoma distraction. (C) Lateral view one-year postoperatively following midface/zygoma distraction. Note the improvement in zygomatic and nasal projection.

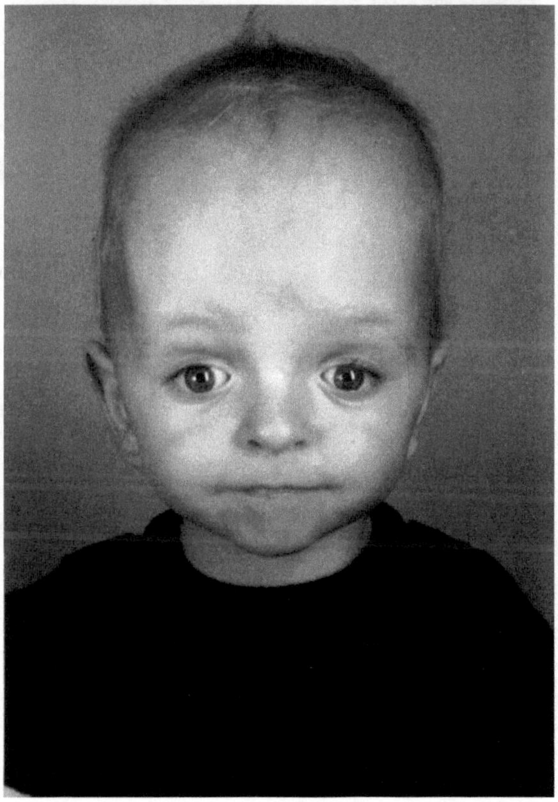
B

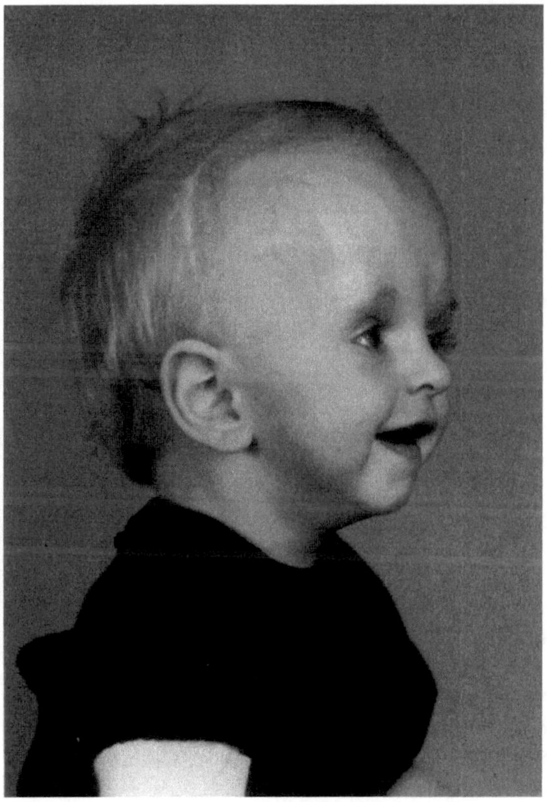
C

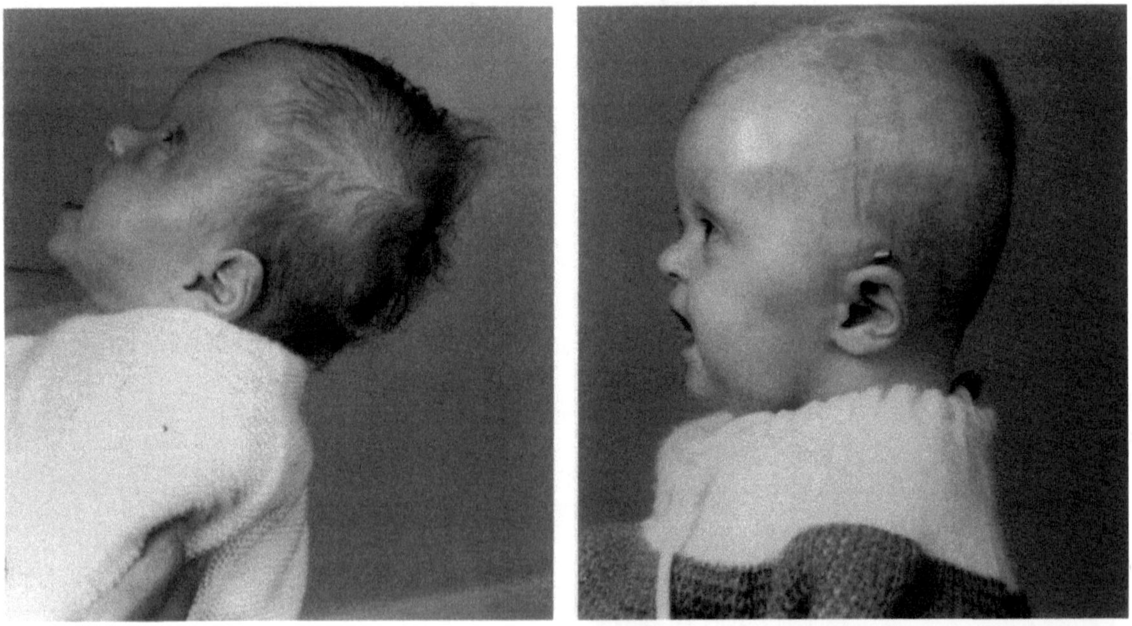

A B

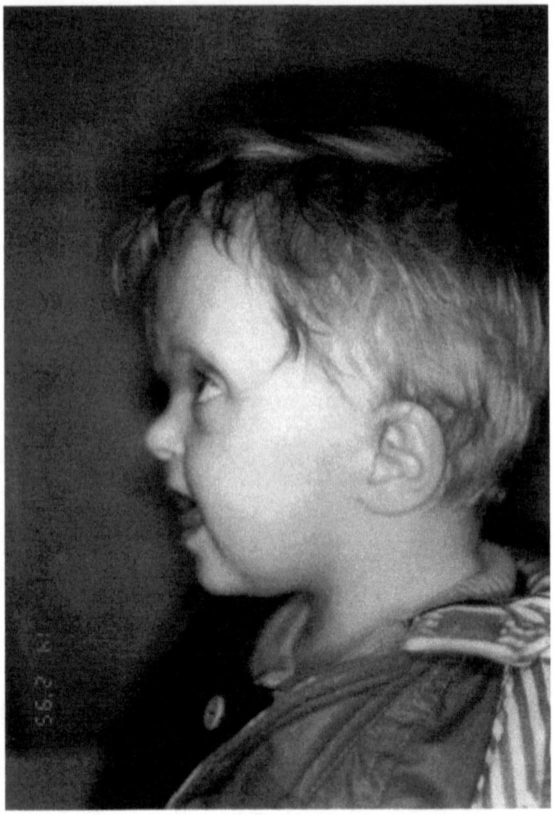

C

Figure 12.8. (A) Lateral view of a 7-week-old infant with Apert syndrome. (B) Lateral view one-month postoperatively during midface/zygoma distraction. (C) Lateral view 6-months postoperatively following midface/zygoma distraction. Note the improved projection of the zygomas, nose, and inferior orbital rims.

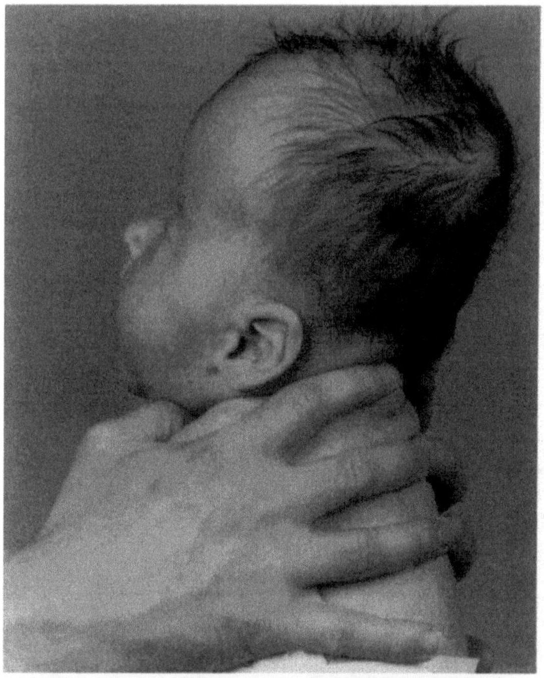

A

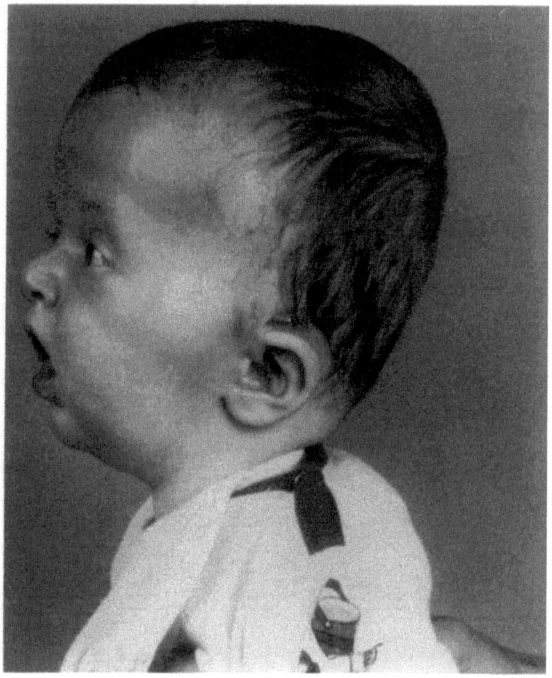

B

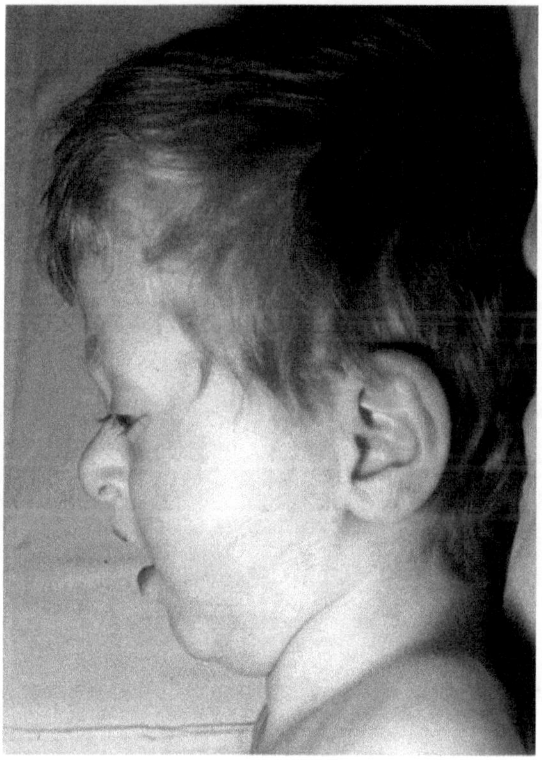

C

Figure 12.9. (A) Lateral view of a 10-week-old infant with Apert synrome. (B) Lateral view one-month postoperatively during midface/zygoma distraction. (C) Lateral view 21-months postoperatively following midface/zygoma distraction. Note the improvement in zygomatic projection.

Table 12.5. SNA angle without distraction.

Case	Preop	1 year postop
1	76	76
2	70	70
3	78	76
4	68	72
5	72	65
6	74	70
7	80	78
8	76	74
9	72	76
10	68	74
x	73.4	73.1

Cephalometric evaluation (SNA) in the control group (Monobloc procedure alone without distraction).

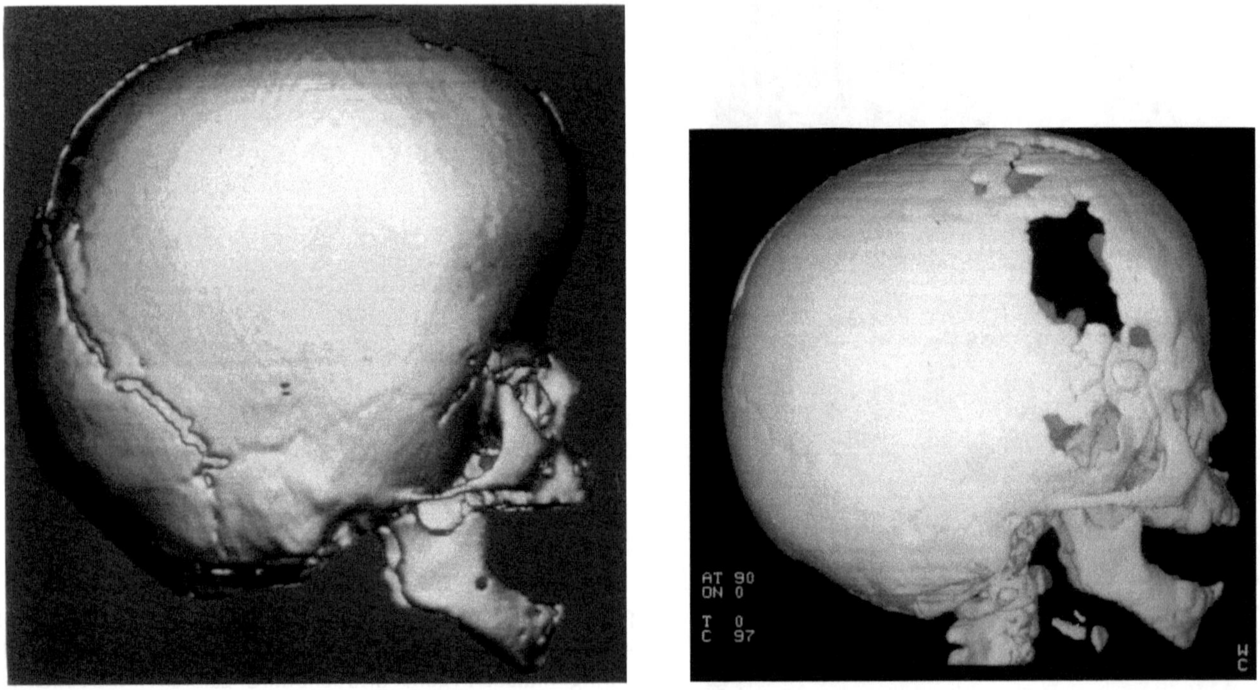

A B

Figure 12.10. Demonstration of lengthening and augmentation of the zygomatic complex after distraction and fronto-orbital advancement *without* ostesotomy of the lower half of the orbit or zygomatic arch. (A) Preoperative lateral radiograph. (B) Postoperative and postdistraction lateral radiograph.

distraction of 14.8mm on the right and 14.3mm on the left side was achieved. The results show that the SNA angle, one of nature's constants at 82°, (Table12.4) improved in the distracted group from 70.3 preoperatively to 80.9 postoperatively, whereas the group in which no distraction took place remained stationary at 73.4° preoperatively and 73.1° postoperatively (see Table 12.5).

The zygomatic region (without osteotomy) demonstrated increased lengthening and an overall augmentation of the zygomatic complex (Figure 12.10). This area could serve as an additional aid in providing support and stability after the desired effect of distraction has been achieved.

It has been shown that an infant fronto-orbital advancement, a standardized operation associated with low morbidity rates, fails to promote midface development and that midfacial development remains retarded in most syndromic craniosynostosis patients and that these patients require some type of Le Fort III advancement procedure with increasing age (16,17,22).

The current surgical treatment of midface hypoplasia is to perform multiple osteotomies, fill the defects with autogenous bone grafts and, to ensure stability of the advanced segments, apply rigid fixation with miniplates and screws. The complications of such procedures can be significant and include donor site morbidity, bone graft infection, resorption of the bone graft, and a skeletal relapse rate of between 50% and 60% with the development of a malocclusion (19,23–25). In infants, passive intracranial translocation of the fixation devices has also been noted (26). This finding would imply that miniplate fixation and even a distraction device in the neonate and infant should be a temporary measure.

Based on our clinical findings, there is reason to believe that midface advancement without osteotomies can be achieved in the infant patient with syndromic craniosynostosis and midface hypoplasia. Lengthening of the human zygoma in infants following distraction without osteotomy was achieved (Figure 12.10). It should also be noted that midface distraction without osteotomies has also been demonstrated in the immature canine model (10).

References

1. Codivilla A. On the means of lengthening in the lower limbs, muscles and tissues which are shortened through deformity. *Am J Orthop Surg* 2:353, 1905.
2. Ilizarov GA. The tension-stress effect on the genesis and growth of tissues: Part I. The influence of stability of fixation and soft tissue preservation. *Clin Orthop* 238:249, 1989.
3. Ilizarov GA. The tension-stress effect on the genesis and growth of tissues: Part II. The influence of the rate and frequency of distraction. *Clin Othop* 239:263, 1989.
4. De Bastiani G, Aldegheri R, Renizi-Brivio L, Trivella G. Limb lengthening by callus distraction (callotasis). *J Pediatr Orthop* 7:129, 1987.
5. Snyder CC, Levine GA, Swanson HM, Brown EZ Jr. Mandibular lengthening by gradual distraction. *Plast Reconstr Surg* 51:506, 1973.
6. Michaeli S, Miotti B. Lengthening of mandibular body by gradual surgical-orthodontic distraction. *J Oral Surg* 35:187, 1977.
7. Karp NS, Thorne CHM, McCarthy JG, Sissons HA. Bone lengthening in the craniofacial skeleton. *Ann Plast Surg* 24:231, 1990.

8. Rachmiel A, Potparic A, Jackson IT et al. Midface advancement by gradual distraction. *Br J Plast Surg* 46:201, 1993.
9. Glat PM, Staffenberg DA, Karp NS et al. Multidimensional distraction osteogenesis: The canine zygoma. *Plast Reconstr Surg* 94:753, 1994.
10. Staffenberg DA, Wood RJ, McCarthy JG et al. Midface distraction advancement in the canine without osteotomies. *Ann Plast Surg* 34:512, 1995.
11. McCarthy JG, Schreiber J, Karp N et al. Lengthening of the mandible by gradual distraction. *Plast Reconstr Surg* 89:1, 1992.
12. Cohen SR, Rutrick RE, Burstein FD. Distraction osteogenesis of the human craniofacial skeleton: Initial experience with a new distraction system. *J Craniofac Surg* 6:368, 1995.
13. Sugihara T, Kawashima K, Igawa H, Ohura T, Yamamura M, Ohata N. Mandibular lengthening by gradual distraction in humans. *Eur J Plast Surg* 18:7, 1995.
14. Komuro Y, Tsuyoshi T, Kiyonori H, Yoshiyuki Y. The histologic analysis of distraction osteogenesis of the mandible in rabbits. *Plast Reconstr Surg* 94:152, 1994.
15. Karaharju-Suvanto T, Karaharju EO, Ranta R. Mandibular distraction. An experimental study on sheep. *J Craniomaxillofac Surg* 18:280, 1990.
16. McCarthy JG, Epstein F, Sadove M, Grayson B, Zide B. Early surgery for craniofacial stenosis: An eight year experience. *Plast Reconstr Surg* 73:521, 1984.
17. Whitaker LA, Bartlett SP, Schut L, Bruce D. Craniosynostosis: An analysis of the timing, treatment, and complications in 164 consecutive patients. *Plast Reconstr Surg* 80:195, 1987.
18. Wolfe SA, Morrison G, Page LK, Berkowitz S. The monobloc frontofacial advancement: Do the pluses outweigh the minuses: *Plast Reconstr Surg* 91:977, 1993.
19. Schmitz JP, Tiner BD, Van Sickels JE. Stability of simultaneous modified Le Fort III/Lefort I osteotomies. *J Craniomaxillofac Surg* 23:287, 1995.
20. Muhlbauer W, Anderl H, Heeckt P et al. Early facial advancement in craniofacial stenosis *Craniofacial Surgery*. Springer-Verlag. Heidelberg, 1987.
21. Muhlbauer W, Anderl H et al. Radical treatment of craniofacial anomalies in infancy and the use of miniplates in craniofacial surgery. *Clin Plast Surg* 74:707, 1987.
22. Marchac D, Renier D. Craniofacial surgery for craniosynostosis improves facial growth: A personal case review. *Ann Plast Surg* 14:43, 1985.
23. Laurie SW, Kaban LB, Mulliken JB, Murra JE. Donor site morbidity after harvesting rib and iliac bone. *Plast Reconstr Surg* 73:933, 1984.
24. Jackson IT. Maxillary hypoplasia. *Clin Plast Surg* 16:757, 1989.
25. Bell WH, Scheiderman CB. Correction of vertical maxillary deficiency: Stability and soft tissue changes. *J Oral Surg* 39:666, 1981.
26. Goldberg DS, Bartlett SP, Yu JC, Hunter JV, Whitaker LA. Critical review of microfixation in pediatric craniofacial surgery. *J Craniofac Surg* 6:301, 1995.

CHAPTER 13

DISTRACTION OF THE MIDFACE

Bryant A. Toth and Martin Chin

Distraction osteogenesis has emerged as an important surgical modality in the management of complex problems of the craniomaxillofacial skeleton. In combination with the standard LeFort III osteotomy it offers the potential of significantly improved results in the treatment of severe midface hypoplasia. Moreover, it has become common for the authors to double the amount of advancement (distance), when compared to the classical LeFort III surgical procedures.

The orthopedic surgical experience has demonstrated the principles of skeletal distraction to regenerate bone in the management of a variety of limb deficiencies (1). Ilizarov defined the specific biological basis of the these techniques and established firm guidelines for its practical clinical use (2). The early clinical application of these techniques for the correction of mandibular deformities relied on the application of similar orthopedic devices to achieve the transport and fixation of bone (3–5).

Distraction of the midface in animals was first reported in animals with (6) and without osteotomies (7), the latter in immature canines. In 1995 the authors reported their experience using a completely internal device for the distraction of the maxillofacial skeleton. Included in these case examples was the distraction of the midface at the time of LeFort III osteotomy (8). It is in this setting at the midface level that a combination of surgery and distraction gives some of its most satisfactory results.

The authors are indebted to McCarthy and his colleagues who have reported their experience in using a miniature Hoffman-type device to distract the mandible in canines (3) and humans (4). It is an extrapolation of this device and technology that led the authors to develop an entirely implantable device. The practical application of distraction technology to the midface required not only a modification of the existent hardware but also changes in both the surgical technique and distraction protocol as originally described.

The pediatric craniofacial skeleton is a unique anatomical site. Many of the problems observed in long-bone distraction are almost never found in the growing pediatric midface. Nonunion, for example, has been a rare if ever present occurrence. Therefore, the authors have abandoned the traditional distraction (Ilizarov) protocol. Corticotomy has been replaced by full-thickness osteotomy. There is no latent period observed prior to the initiation of distraction. The previous distraction rate of 1 millimeter/day has been replaced by continuous midface distraction beginning intraoperatively and continuing for approximately 5 to 7 days postoperatively, or until the ideal or close to ideal goal of midface distraction has been achieved.

THE RATIONALE OF MIDFACE DISTRACTION

The severe midface hypoplasia that accompanies many craniofacial syndromes, most commonly syndromic craniofacial synostosis, has challenged craniofacial surgeons for decades. The experience of delaying midfacial surgery until adolescence has often left a severely undercorrected midface, one that is also associated with psychosocial problems and commonly requires secondary or tertiary surgery. Because of associated airway and corneal exposure problems manifest in early childhood, the authors initiated a program of distracting the midface in the 4- to 6-year age group. Having in the past been frustrated by surgical relapse, the authors have avoided fixating the LeFort III segment and have distracted the midface in the operative and immediate postoperative period. This type of distraction, in most instances, has doubled the amount of skeletal advancement usually achieved in a traditional midfacial osteotomy in a similar age group.

Baumrind (9) has made available data revealing typical dimensions of normal adult orbits relative to the anterior cranial base. The data are expressed in mean measurements from porion to orbitale (PO-ORB). When compared to the dimensions recorded in the patient with midface hypoplasia, an estimate of the magnitude of deficiency can be made. For example, the midface deficiency as reflected by infraorbital rim retrusion in a syndromic child is typically 25 mm. Therefore, the surgical objective of midfacial distraction in childhood is to advance the orbital rim into the anticipated adult position. The distraction devices are fabricated to accommodate the calculated transport distance.

Baumrind (9) has also made available longitudinal data projecting the effective normal growth observed at the orbital rim position. From these data it is anticipated that in the normal individual orbitale grows forward less than 2 mm between the ages of 8.5 and 18.5 years. It is, therefore, reasonable to advance the midface in children to adult orbital dimensions. However, because this degree of deficiency exceeds the capability of correction by conventional midface osteotomy surgical techniques, the authors have combined intraoperative surgery with distraction techniques. Conventional osteotomy surgery is limited by the resistance of the soft tissue envelope which, in the authors' opinion, can be managed only by gradual distraction or multiple surgical procedures. The results of midface osteotomy advancement with rigid fixation typically fall short of the desired goal. The role of distraction in midface advancement is thus to increase the amount of correction that can be achieved in a single procedure, enabling a more complete anatomic correction and possibly sparing the patient multiple staged procedures.

DEVICE DESIGN

For each child undergoing midfacial advancement, two distraction devices are designed and fabricated for placement at the zygoma osteotomy site. Measurements recorded from axial and three-dimensional (CT) images are used in the design of the devices. Computer aided design (CAD) allows manipulation of the distractor dimensions and contours to satisfy the particular requirements of each patient. The design of each device is unique and determined by: (1) the dysmorphology of the osteotomy site, (2) the magnitude of the desired skeletal transport, (3) the axis of the skeletal transport, (4) the strength of the implant material, (5) the anticipated load, and (6) the mode of access for placement and removal of the device. The CAD design process derives a virtual image defined within a three-dimensional coordinate system. The CAD data are transferred to a vertical milling machine, which is used to form the distractors from medical-grade titanium. The lead screw components are formed on a lathe.

In the design of a midface distractor multiple assumptions were made. Any device must be not only internal but also completely submergible and potentially permanently implantable. The device must be self-retaining since one cannot rely upon screw fixation in the pediatric facial skeleton either to hold the device in place or to bear the forces that are transmitted with distraction. The screws serve merely as a point of stabilization for avoiding rotation. In addition, the distraction device must be able to bear 10 kilograms or 22 pounds of force in addition to transporting the skeletal segments from 10 to 20 mm. The force transmitted was determined by force as measured by a torque wrench. A final but extremely important assumption was that the device could be easily removable. Any distraction device needs to be removed either transorally or transconjunctivally, allowing any secondary procedure to be executed on an outpatient basis and avoiding reopening of the coronal incision.

To accomplish these distraction device features, a system was developed involving customized bone plates that are joined by a screw component (Figure 13.1). The latter is percutaneously activated, and when the desired amount of distraction is achieved, the activating component can be removed allowing the device to remain submerged as a rigid

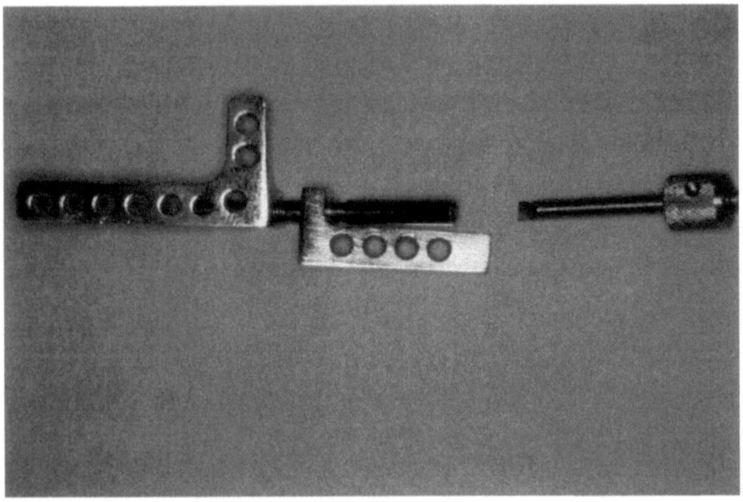

Figure 13.1. Midface distraction device showing customized bone plates joined by a screw component. The activation component is separate.

fixation unit. The design of the device is such that the primary distraction force is transmitted from the bone directly to the bone-plate component. The cortex screws stabilize the device to assure that the axis of distraction remains stable (Figure 13.2). The screws, however, do not bear the primary force of distraction. Given the forces required to achieve distraction and the friable nature of the bones in the pediatric craniofacial skeleton, cortex screws cannot be relied upon to bear the primary stabilizing force for distraction. To date, all distraction devices have been left in place for a minimum of 6 months. The devices have been designed so that the implant can be left in place permanently if one desires (Figure 13.3).

TECHNIQUE

Prior to embarking on midface surgery with distraction, it is imperative that a preoperative two-dimensional CT scan, preferably in the coronal plane, be ob-

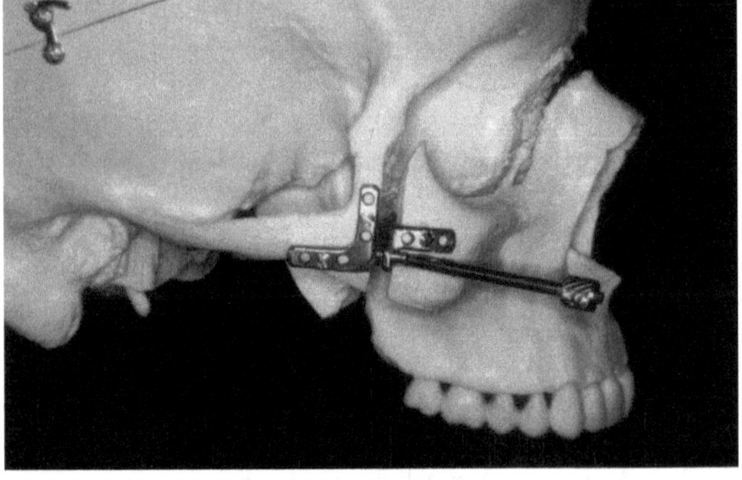

Figure 13.2. Midface distraction device in position. Note the activation component which is removed percutaneously.

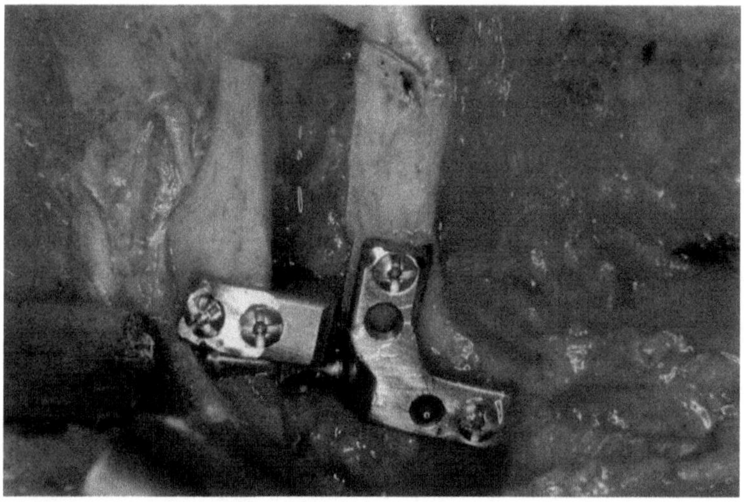

Figure 13.3. Intraoperative view of distraction device in place at time of LeFort III osteotomy. Note intraoperative distraction of approximately 10 mm.

tained to allow the surgeon to determine the location of the cribriform plate. It is not uncommon that the cribriform plate is inferiorly displaced in syndromic children, thereby necessitating a low osteotomy across the nasion. Exposure of the midface and orbits is obtained through a standard coronal incision. In most patients there is a coronal scar from a previous cranial vault remodeling procedure. In reoperative cranial surgery, particularly in children with a history of cranial vault remodeling, one must pay careful attention to the elevation of the coronal flap. Not uncommonly there are areas where there is no bone protection of the dura, and if one is careless, dural penetration can result. In additional, it is often easiest in reoperative surgery to proceed at a plane just above the neoperiosteum since much of the bleeding from the calvarial bone that has been generated can be avoided. It has not been necessary to perform a transpalpebral incision to provide orbital access and distraction placement. Not uncommonly the coronal incision needs to be extended slightly in front of the upper portion of the ear to allow for adequate exposure in the temporozygomatic area. At the temporal level the dissection extends deep to the deep temporal fascia so that the soft-tissue envelope can be reflected off the lateral orbital rim and zygoma. The dissection is carried anteriorly over the maxilla with gentle stretching of the midfacial soft tissue envelope to minimize the forces restricting the midfacial advancement. The dissection is also carried down to the distal point of the nasal bones. The dissection is extended on top of the septum and upper lateral cartilages as far as the nasal tip. This maneuver allows for easy access when a bone graft is necessary for nasal recorstruction. The dissection is carried medially within the orbit down to the nasolacrimal groove without disruption of the medial canthal ligament. In the lateral orbit the dissection is extended so that the inferior orbital fissure is clearly visualized. A tunnel connecting the medial and lateral subperiosteal dissection is created.

The LeFort III osteotomy is initiated (Figure 13.4). The first osteotomy is the

Figure 13.4. LeFort III osteotomy as intended in a patient undergoing advancement osteotomy and distraction. Note the posterior location of the osteotomy across the base of the nose and medial wall of the orbit which includes the nasolacrimal apparatus in the mobilized segment.

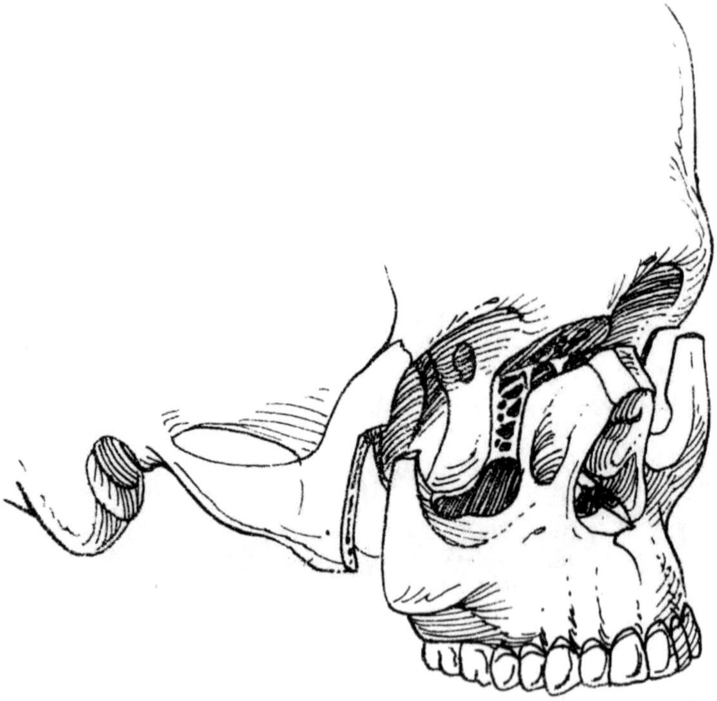

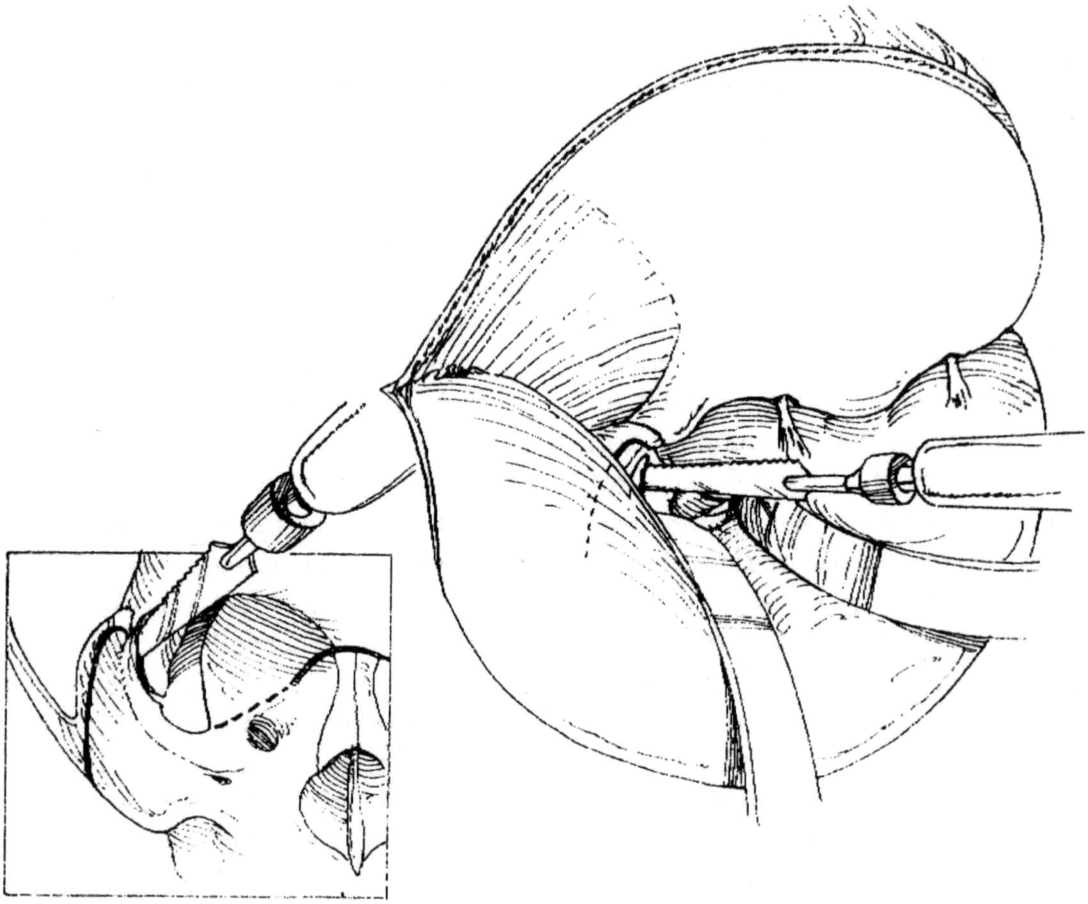

Figure 13.5. Osteotomy extending from the inferior orbital fissure along the lateral wall to the frontozygomatic suture. Note that the zygomatic osteotomy has already been made on the zygoma, as noted in the inset.

lateral osteotomy designed so that it extends from the bottom of the zygoma splitting the lateral orbital rim in half (Figure 13.5). It is extended in a cephalic direction to end at approximately the level of the zygomaticofrontal suture. The osteotomy is extended intraorbitally with a retractor protecting the orbital contents. The intraorbital osteotomy is angled down from the lateral rim to the inferior orbital fissure. Both osteotomies are ideally done with a reciprocating saw. After both lateral osteotomies are completed, attention is directed to the medial osteotomies. The CT scan is again reviewed to verify the position of the cribriform plate. After this has been done, the horizontal osteotomy extending over the nasal base is undertaken (Figure 13.6). The medial orbital osteotomy is extended posterior to the nasolacrimal apparatus and the insertion of the medial canthal ligaments (Figure 13.7). This maneuver allows for a thicker segment of facial bone and the advancement of the nasolacrimal apparatus and medial canthal tendons anteriorly with the midface fragment. The connection between the medial orbital and lateral orbital osteotomy is often made with a 6-mm osteotome that can be manually pushed through the thin bone of the orbital floor.

The surgical exposure is extended intraorally. An incision is made at the base

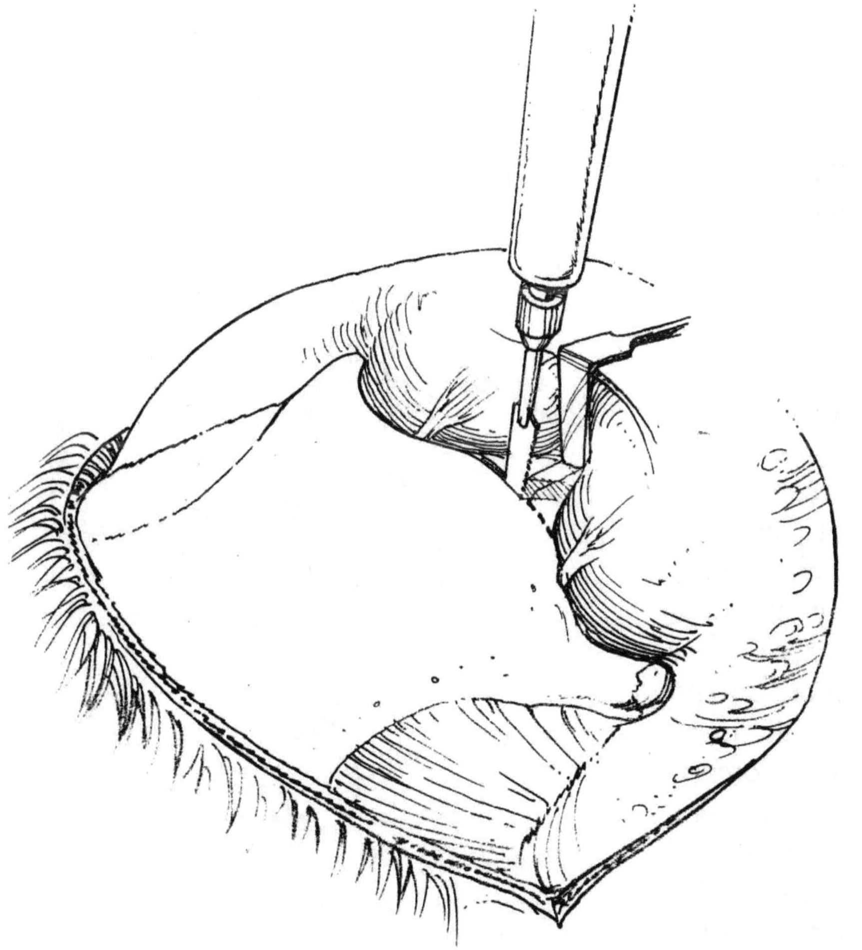

Figure 13.6. The osteotomy across the base of the nose. It is imperative that one check a preoperative coronal CT scan to verify the location of the cribriform plate.

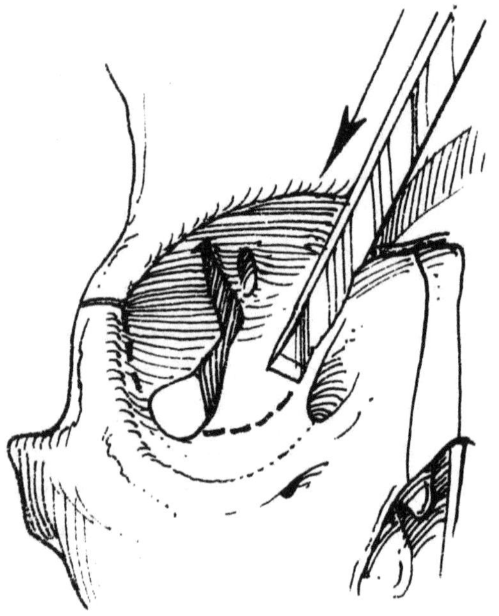

Figure 13.7. A 6.0-mm osteotome is used to extend the osteotomy across the medial wall and orbital floor.

of the zygomatic buttress, and a subperiosteal tunnel is created leading back to the junction of the maxilla and the pterygoid plate. This allows placement of a curved osteotome to separate the junction of the pterygoid plate and the posterior maxilla (Figure 13.8). The actual craniofacial disfunction is achieved by using Rowe Kiley forceps (Figure 13.9). This is best done using the forceps along with a previously made dental plate that fits over the maxillary and mandibular teeth and minimizes the amount of trauma on the teeth and the palatal mucosa. After the plate is placed into position on the maxillary segment, as well as on the mandibular segment, the Rowe Kiley forceps are placed intranasally and intraorally. The midface disfunction is accomplished with gentle rocking and traction done with the Rowe Kiley forceps. Gentle movement is initially done to ensure that the midface is moving in one piece. Downward and anterior forces are directed with stretching of the overlying soft tissue envelope. If necessary, Tessier maxillary disimpaction forceps can be used in an effort to facilitate anterior midface distraction. At all points in the procedure, one must carefully avoid excess or unnecessary traction on the orbital neurovascular structures.

The distraction devices are placed on the midface distraction fragment and the proximal zygomatic segment. Grooves allowing for the placement of the hardware are carved into the zygomatic segment on both the distraction fragment and the

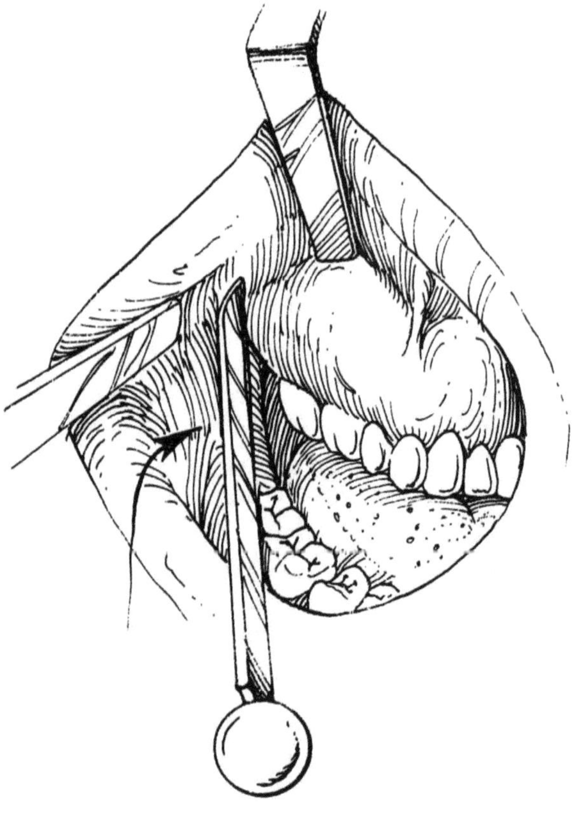

Figure 13.8. Pterygomaxillary separation with a curved osteotome.

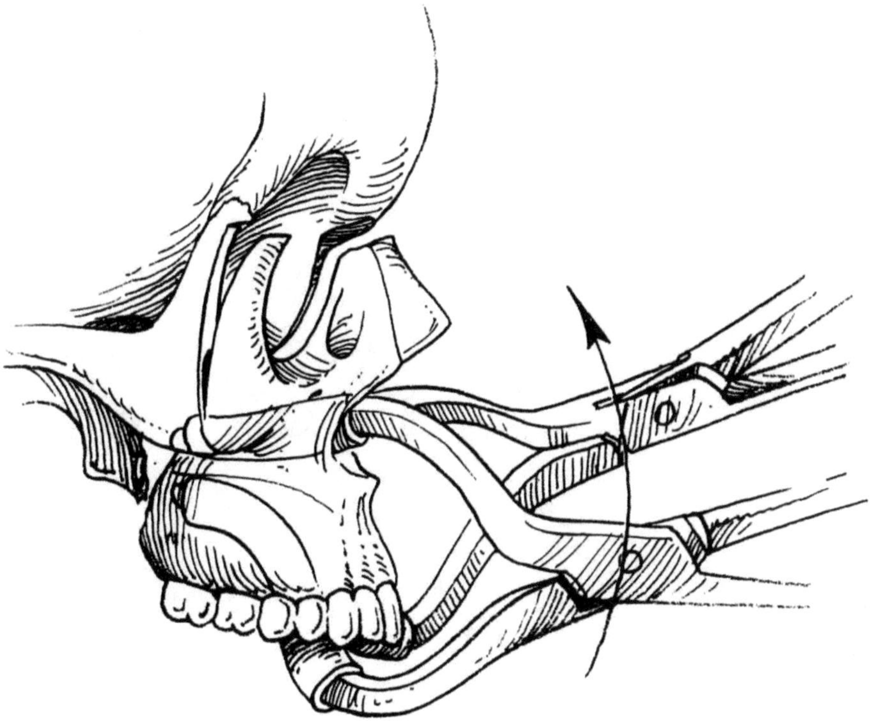

Figure 13.9. Midface separation with gentle traction after careful placement of the Rowe Kiley forceps. A dental splint has previously been made, which prevents the oral limb of the forceps from lacerating the palatal mucosa.

proximal segment (Figure 13.10). This is done generally with an up-biting Lempert rongeur. The fixation plates are placed in position in a self-retaining fashion with the screws providing only device orientation, not the bearing of the torque generated by the distraction device. After both segments are attached to the distraction device, a percutaneous hole allowing for the passage of the activation component is made. This is done by using a no. 11 blade and the activation device is passed from the outside to the inside over an introducing trochar. The trochar is removed and the activating pin is passed through the cannula and engaged in the screw mechanism of the distraction device (Figure 13.11). The interlock is retained by a friction fit of the tapered components. With the activating pin in place, the devices are activated to verify that the access of distraction is secure, that the bony segments are stabilized, and that the distraction devices will withstand distraction forces.

In the initial clinical experience, autogenous bone grafts were harvested to place in the defects resulting from immediate distraction. At the present time the only bone grafts used are onlay nasal bone grafts. Distraction of the midface is done for a minimum of 10mm or to a point where the surgeon would ordinarily leave the patient following a standard LeFort III osteotomy (ie, 10 to 24mm).

The wounds are irrigated with antibiotic-containing solution and the coronal flap is redraped over the skeleton. A no. 15 round Jackson-Pratt drain is placed under the scalp flap. Bilateral lateral canthopexies are done in an effort to elevate the lateral aspect of the palpebral aperture. The coronal flap is closed in a standard two-layer technique.

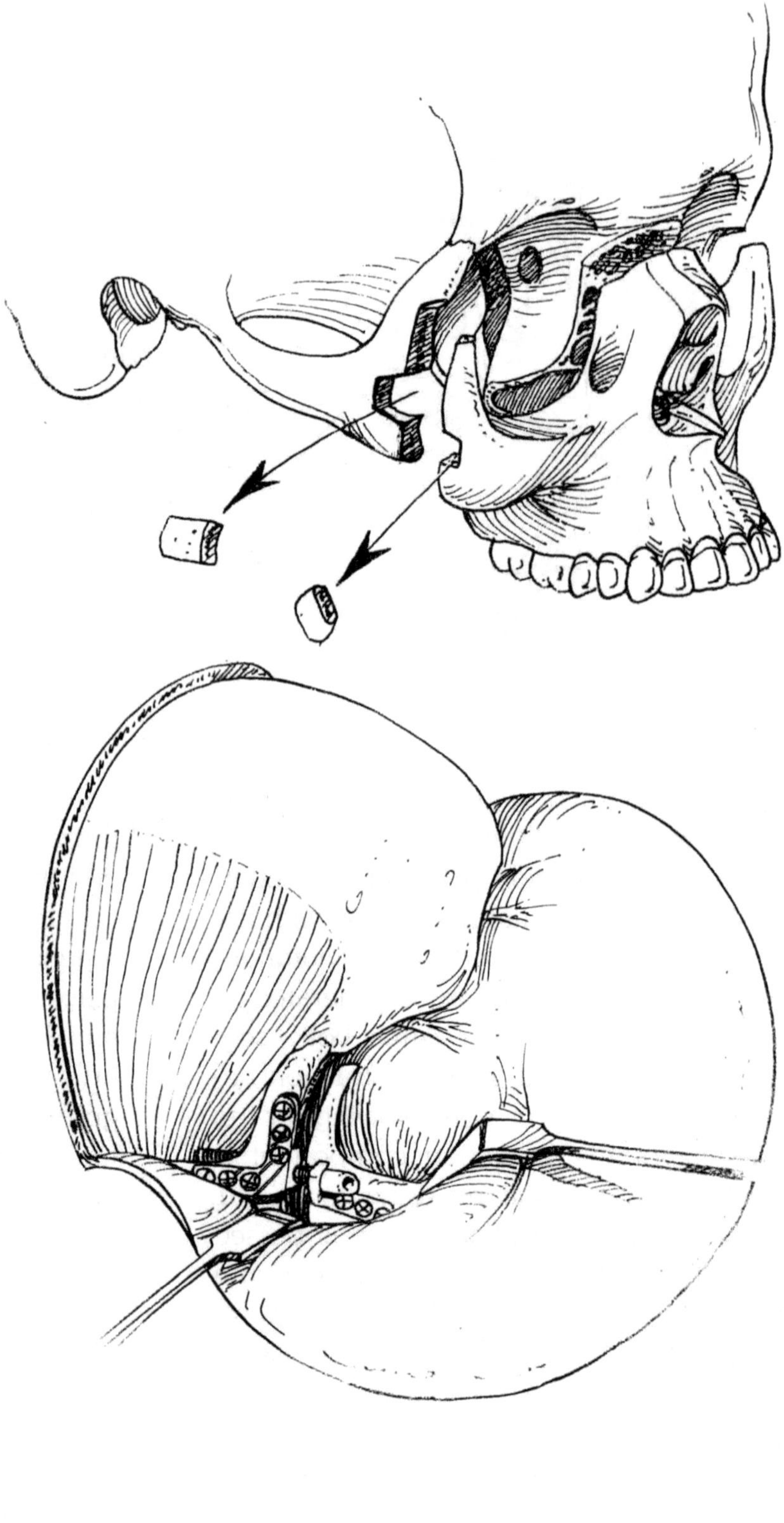

Figure 13.10. Preparation of the proximal and midface segments for application of the midface distraction device. Note in the inset that the distraction device is self-retaining, thereby avoiding traction and tension. The midface distraction device is in place with advancement having been initiated.

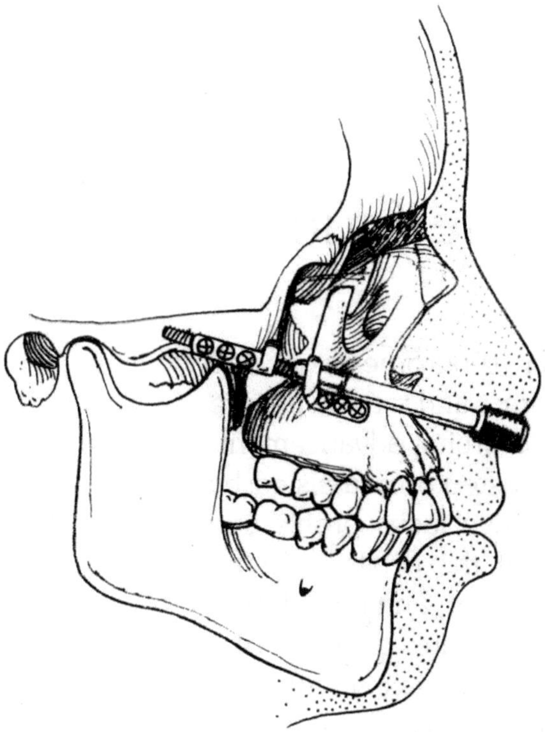

Figure 13.11. Postoperative result with midface distraction device in position. Also note the percutaneous activation pin.

The distraction is continued over the next 3 to 6 days postoperatively. There is no limit to the amount of distraction that takes place per day, although the amount of force generated is controlled by a torque wrench. No torque is allowed that exceeds what has been achieved in the operating room. When adequate distraction has been obtained and this approximates the predicted value as determined by Baumrind (9), the percutaneous fixation is removed. This always takes place prior to the patient's discharge from the hospital (between postoperative days 5 and 7).

CLINICAL RESULTS

The clinical experience will be illustrated by five patients who underwent continuous midfacial distraction at the time of and subsequent to the LeFort III osteotomy.

Case Studies

Case 1. RS is a 12-year-old boy with Pfeiffer syndrome who had severe midface hypoplasia involving the orbits, zygoma, and maxilla (Figure 13.12). At the age of 7 years, he underwent fronto-orbital advancement. The procedure involved a LeFort III advancement osteotomy assisted by distraction. Figures 12.2A,B illustrate the preoperative facial profile and lateral cephalogram. The zygoma, inferior asfect of the orbits, and the nasomaxillary complex were osteotomized as a single unit, and the midface was advanced 10 mm during surgery. Distractors were fixed to the osteotomy sites in the zygomatic regions using 2-mm cortex screws. For activation, each distractor incorporated a transcutaneous pin that emerged in the infraorbital region. In the immediate postoperative period, the distractors were activated 0.5 millimeters 4 to 6 times per day; no latency period was observed. After 5 days, the right distractor had moved 9 mm and the left 11 mm. The difference in right versus left distraction allowed correction of an asymmetry in the maxillary dental midline. The postoperative view and lateral cephalogram demonstrate the improved relationship between the midface, mandible, and cranium (Figure 13.12C,D). The combination of intraoperative movement and postoperative distraction advanced the midface 19 mm and 21 mm on the right and left, respectively. On the fifth postoperative day, the transcutaneous pins were disengaged, and the patient was discharged from the hospital.

Figure 13.12. Case 1. Twelve-year-old boy with Pfeiffer syndrome.

(A) Preoperative lateral view.

(B) Preoperative lateral cephalogram.

(C) Postoperative lateral view (after LeFort III osteotomy-distraction).

(D) Postoperative lateral cephalogram. Note the change from Class III to Class II occlusion and the improvement in the overlying soft-tissue envelope.

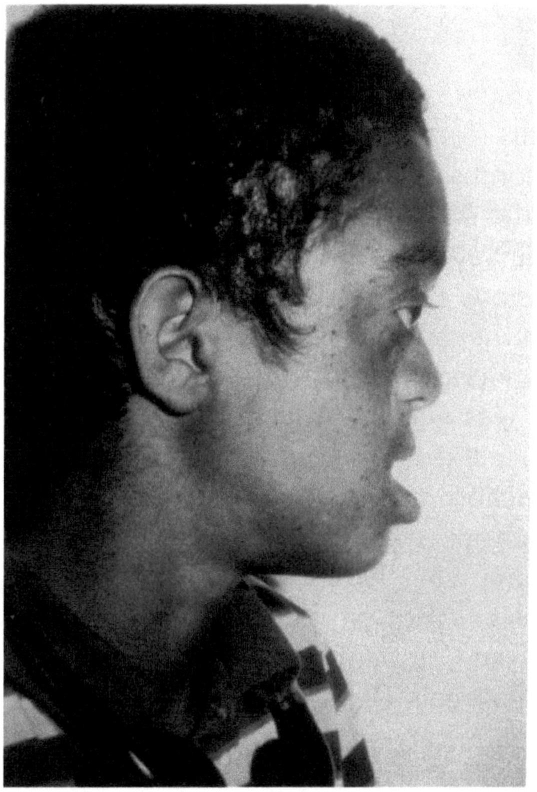

A

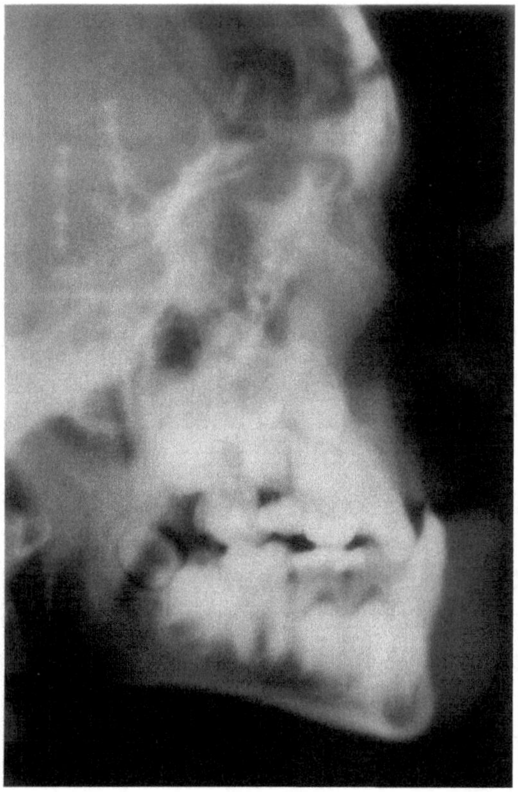

B

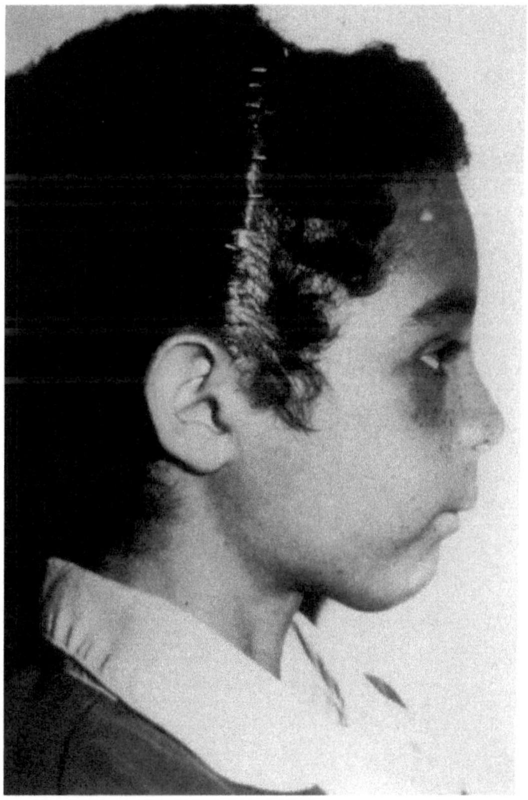

C

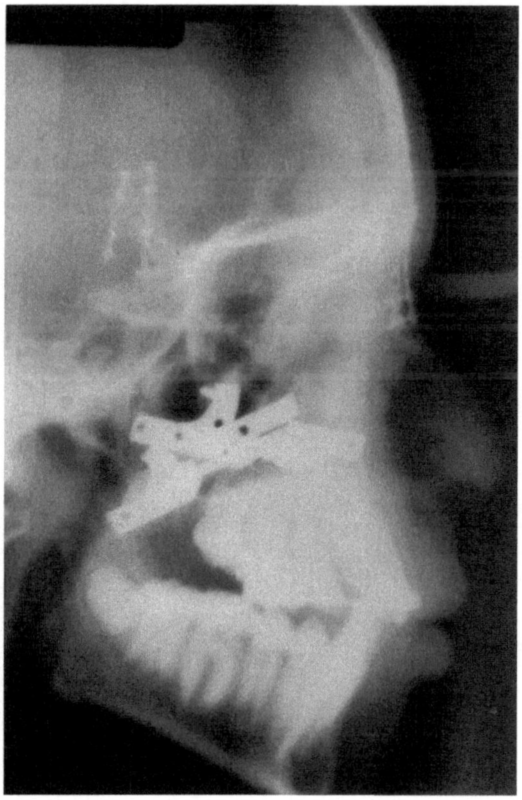

D

Case 2. ALH underwent LeFort III osteotomy with continuous midface distraction at age four-and-one-half years for severe midface retrusion secondary to Crouzon syndrome. At six months of age the patient had undergone fronto-orbital advancement. Over the subsequent interval, the patient required continuous noctural positive airway (C-PAP) pressure because of severe sleep apnea. On multiple occasions prior to definitive midface surgery a discussion was entertained for permanent tracheostomy. At the time of surgery a LeFort III osteotomy was undertaken and 8 mm of advancement was obtained intraoperatively. This was achieved on both sides since the orbits were spatially symmetric. Over the immediate post-operative period, an additional 11 mm of distraction was able to be obtained for a total of approximately 20 mm of advancement bilaterally. Autogenous bone grafts were used at the osteotomy site. Figure 13.13 illustrates patient ALH on the left with her twin sister ARH on the right. Preoperative frontal and lateral photographs reveal the amount of severe midface hypoplasia. A postoperative cephalogram reveals Class II occlusion. Note the improved skeletal and soft-tissue relationships in the frontal and lateral views. The patient no longer requires C-PAP therapy and on repeat sleep study at one year postoperative there was no evidence of sleep apnea.

Figure 13.13. Case 2.

(A) Pediatric sisters with Crouzon syndrome (ALH and ARH).

(B) Frontal preoperative view of patient (ALH).

(C) Preoperative lateral new.

(D) Postoperative frontal view.

(E) Postoperative lateral view.

(F) Preoperative lateral cephalogram.

(G) Postoperative lateral cephalogram.

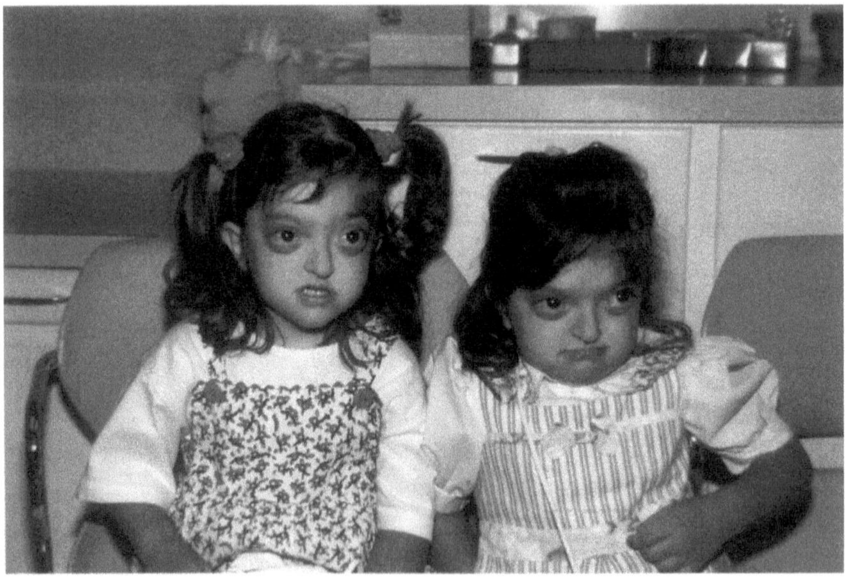

A

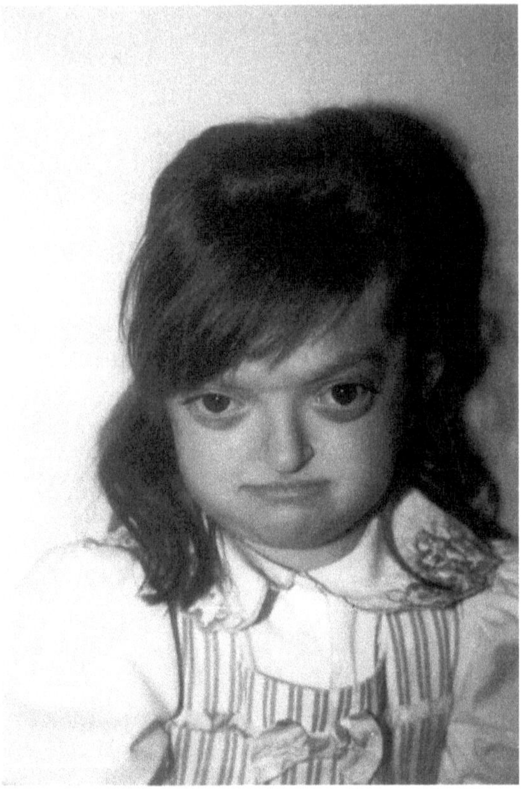

B

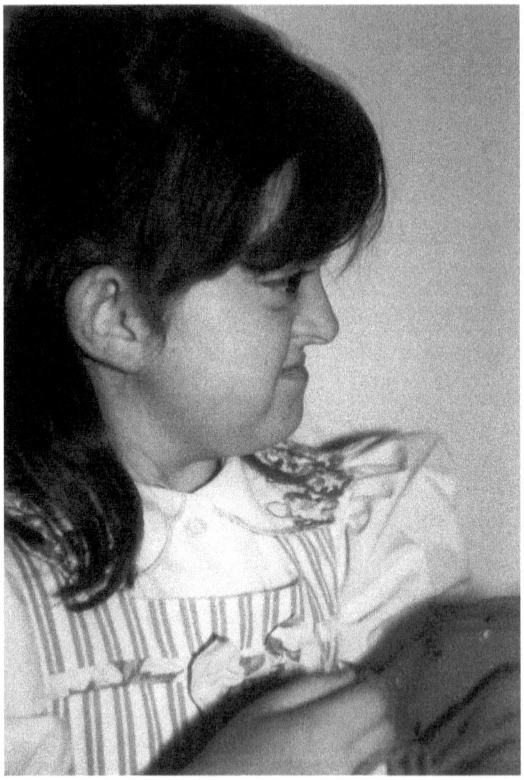

C

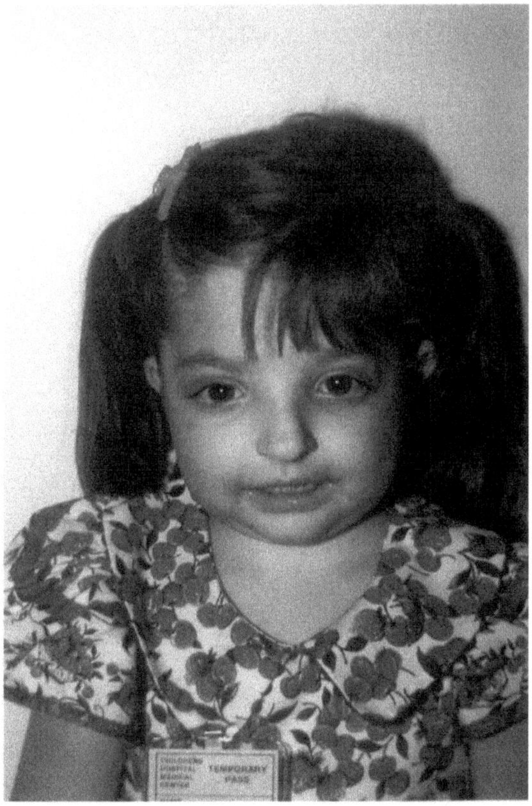

D

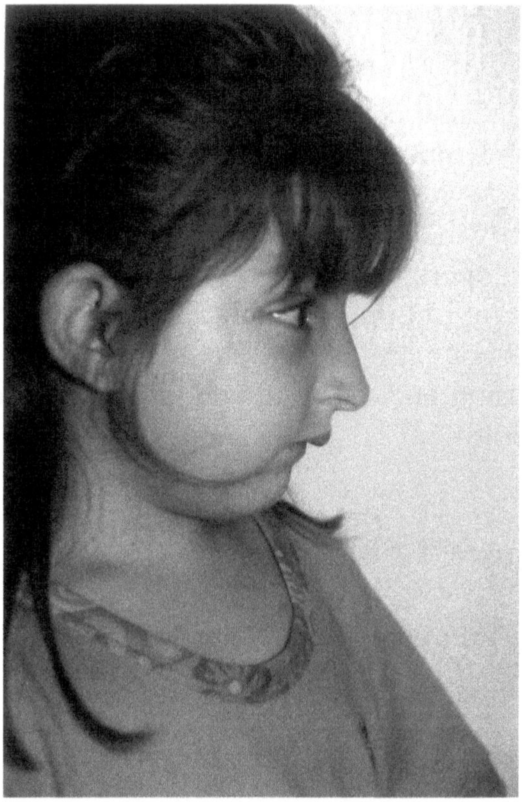

E

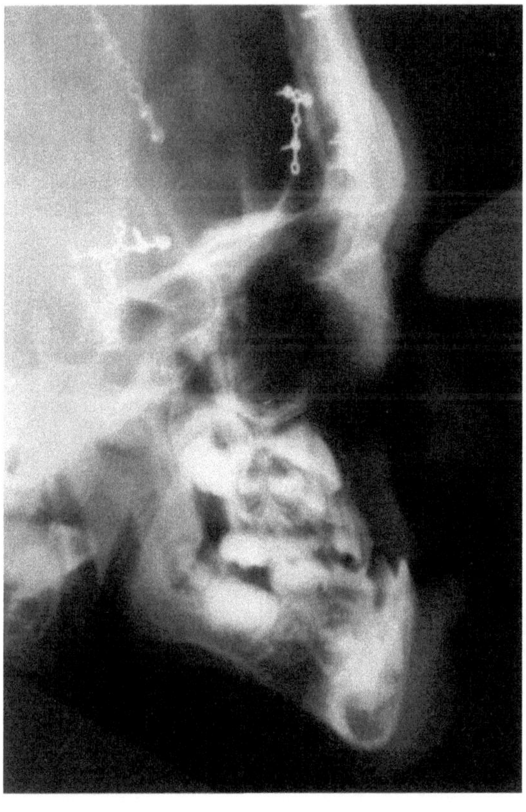

F

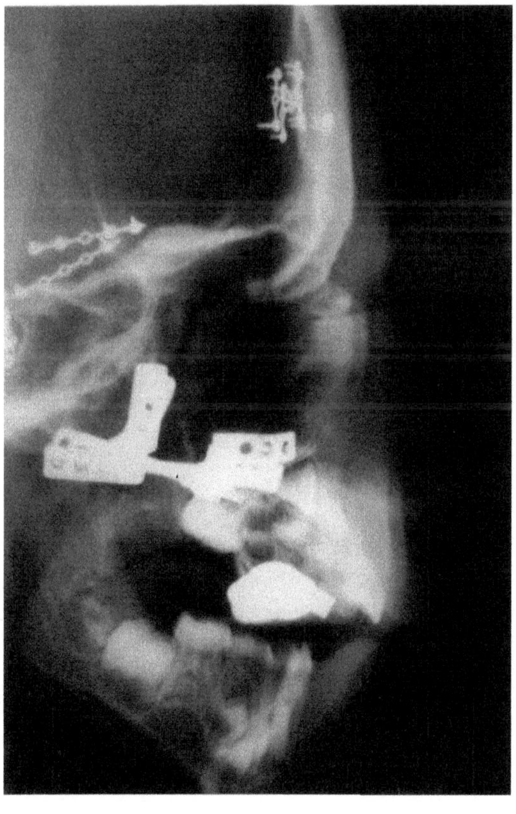

G

Case 3. ARH is the twin sister of ALH (Case 2) and was also born with Crouzon syndrome (Figure 13.14). Surgery at four-and-one-half years of age was performed in an effort to do the exact procedure as executed on her twin. A midfacial advancement of 8mm was obtained on each side intraoperatively, followed postoperatively by 11-mm bilateral distraction for a total of approximately 20mm advancement. The postoperative course was complicated by a pin-tract infection on the right side that necessitated incision and drainage and ultimate removal of the distraction device at 6 months.

Figure 13.14. Case 3. Twin sister (see Figure 13.13) at age 4.

(A) Preoperative frontal view.

(B) Preoperative lateral view.

(C) Postoperative frontal view.

(D) Postoperative lateral view.

(E) Preoperative lateral cephalogram.

(F) Postoperative lateral cephalogram.

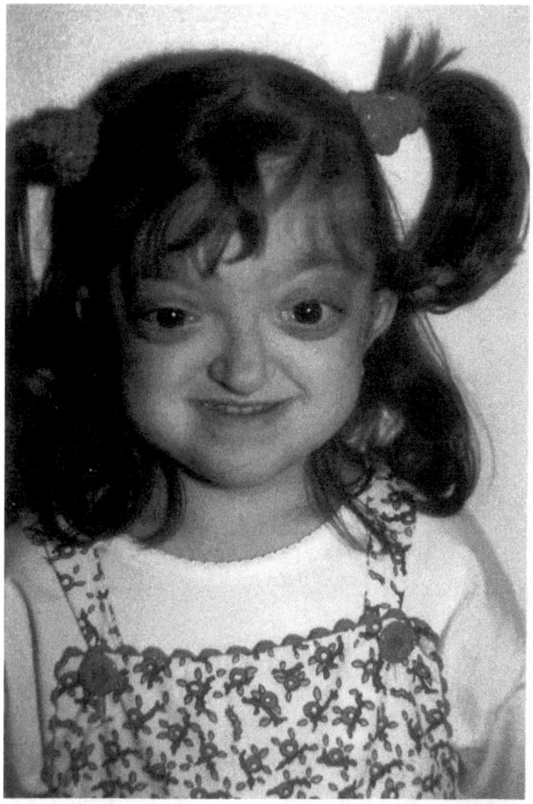

A

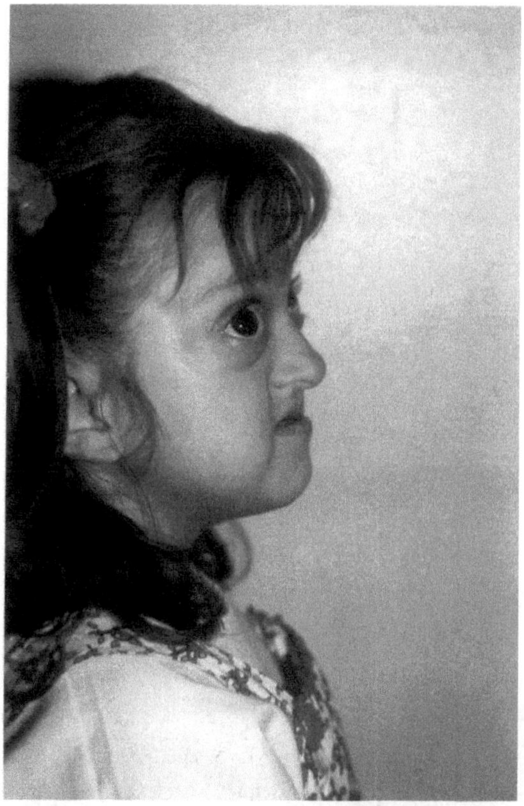

B

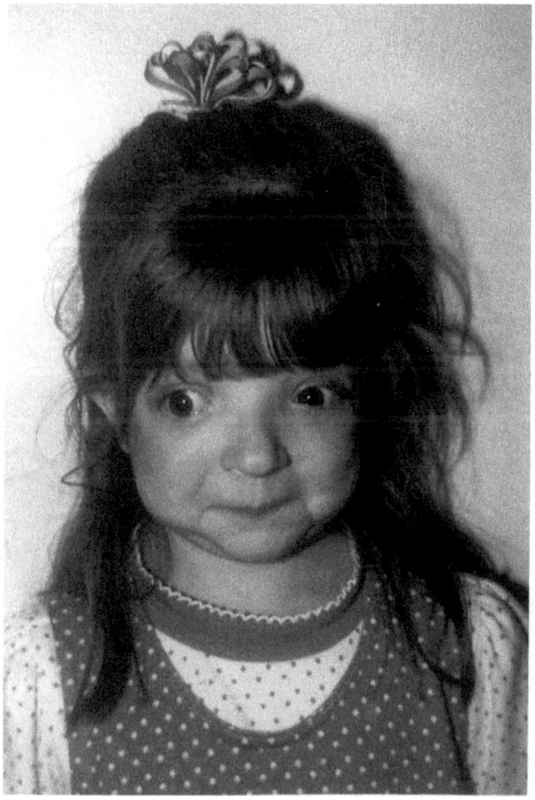

C

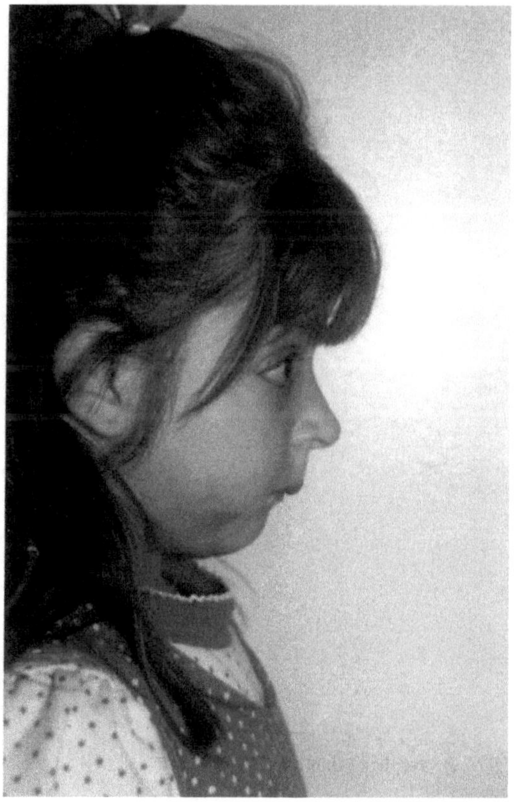

D

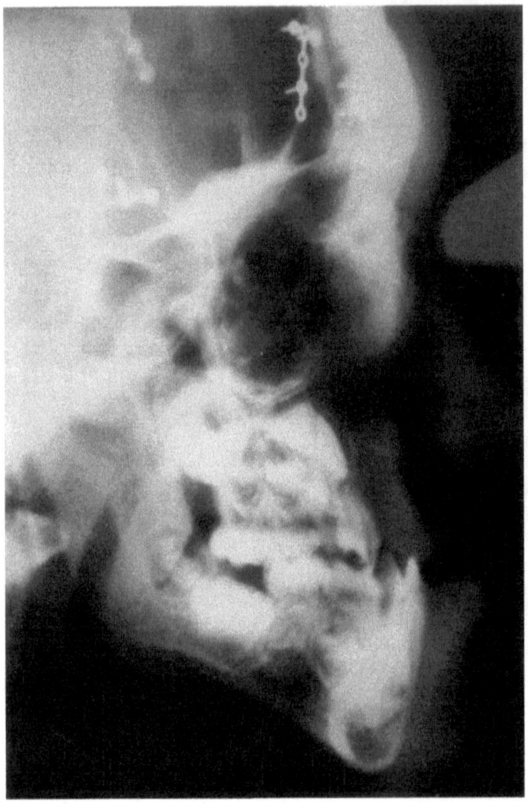

E

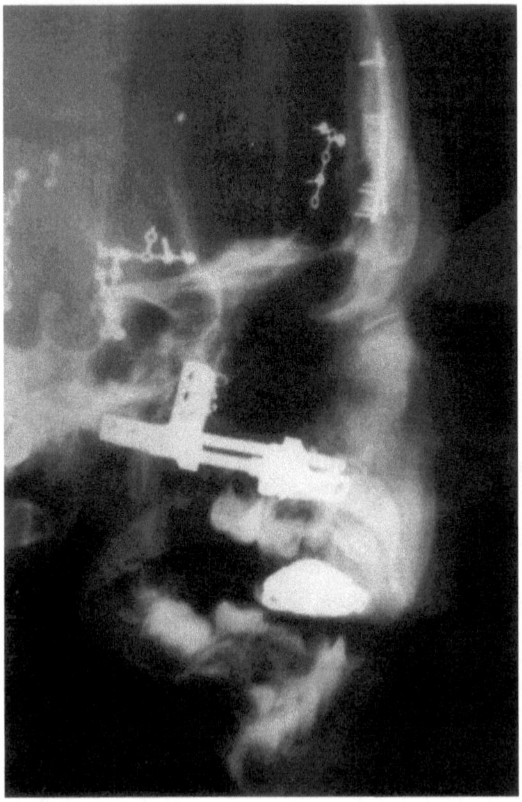

F

Case 4. ST is a ten-and-a-half-year-old girl with Crouzon syndrome (Figure 13.15). She underwent fronto-orbital advancement at 6 months of age for the correction of an asymmetric calvarial deformity consistent more with plagiocephaly than brachiocephaly. Over the ensuing 10 years, the patient developed a progressive Class III malocclusion, and she was extremely concerned about the dysmorphic appearance of her face. The patient was distracted a total of 15mm intraoperatively to place her in a Class II occlusion. Postoperatively she had an uncomplicated course. The mother reported significant psychological improvement in the child's behavior. It is anticipated that no future midface manipulation, other than orthodontic therapy, will be required.

Figure 13.15. Case 4. Ten-year-old girl with Crouzon syndrome.

(A) Preoperative frontal view.

(B) Preoperative lateral view.

(C) Postoperative frontal view.

(D) Postoperative lateral view.

(E) Preoperative occlusal relationships.

(F) Postoperative occlusal relationships.

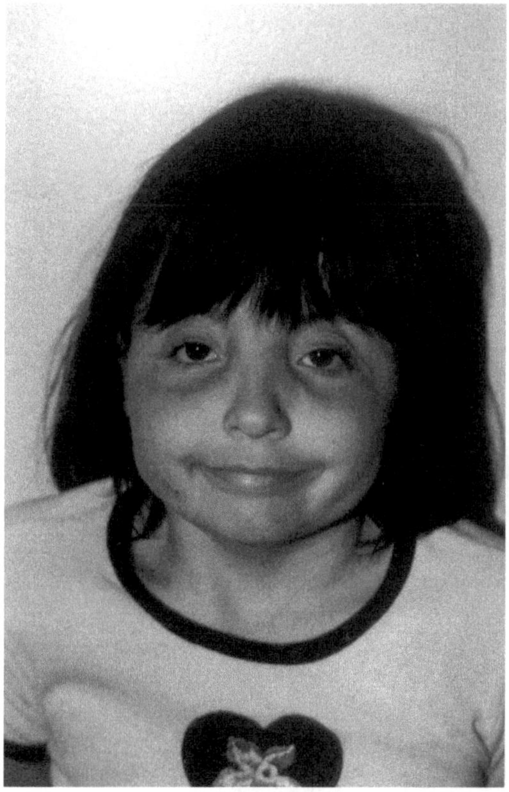

A

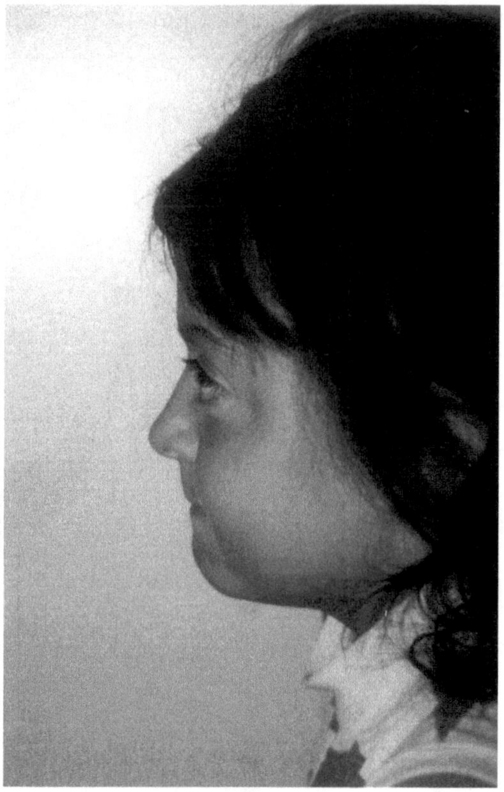

B

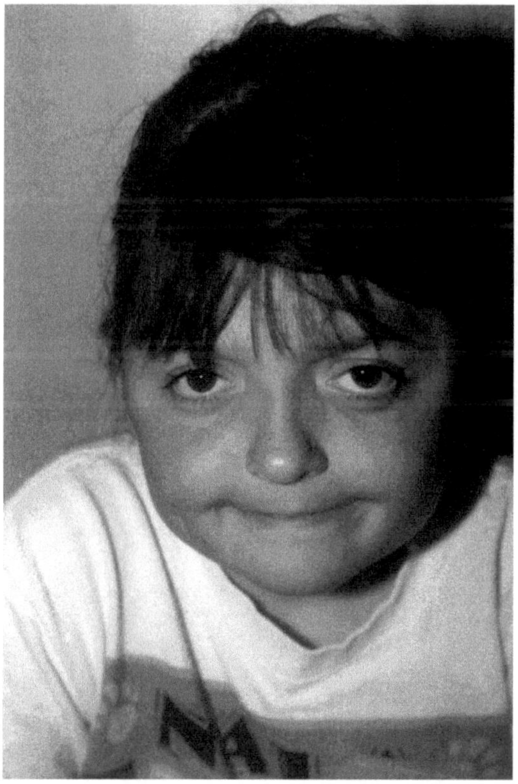

C

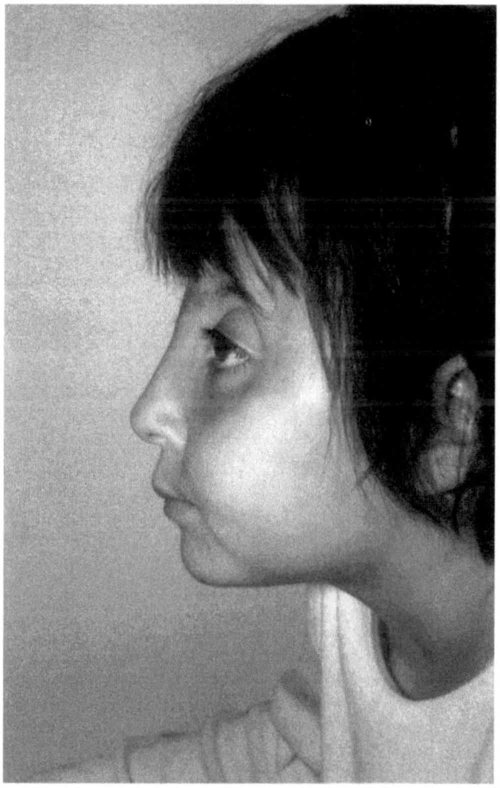

D

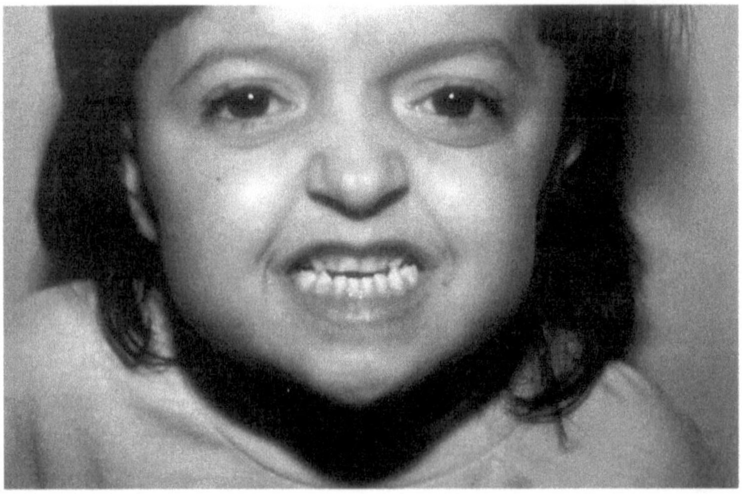

E

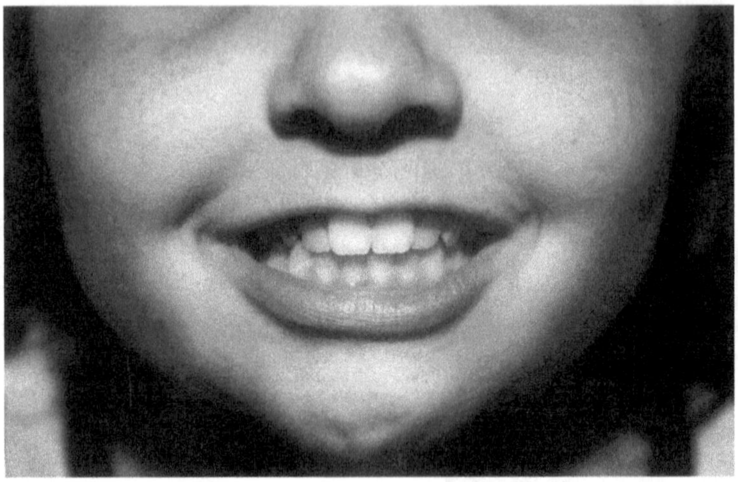

F

Case 5. DC is a five-and-a-half-year-old boy with Apert syndrome (Figure 13.16). At 3 months of age he underwent bicoronal strip craniectomy with remodeling of the orbits, frontal bone, and calvarium. Because of severe towering of the skull (turricephaly) he underwent total cranial vault remodeling at 8 months of age. Over the subsequent interval the patient developed asymmetric bilateral exorbitism in addition to progressive towering of the calvarium. The midface hypoplasia, likewise, progressed considerably with respiratory compromise consisting of snoring and sleep apnea, which worsened over the same interval. The patient underwent 9.5 mm of bilateral distraction intraoperatively. An additional 8.3 mm of distraction was accomplished in the immediate postoperative period for a total of 17.8 mm of distraction.

Figure 13.16. Case 5. A five-year-old boy with Apert syndrome.

(A) Preoperative frontal view.

(B) Preoperative lateral view.

(C) Postoperative frontal view.

(D) Postoperative lateral view.

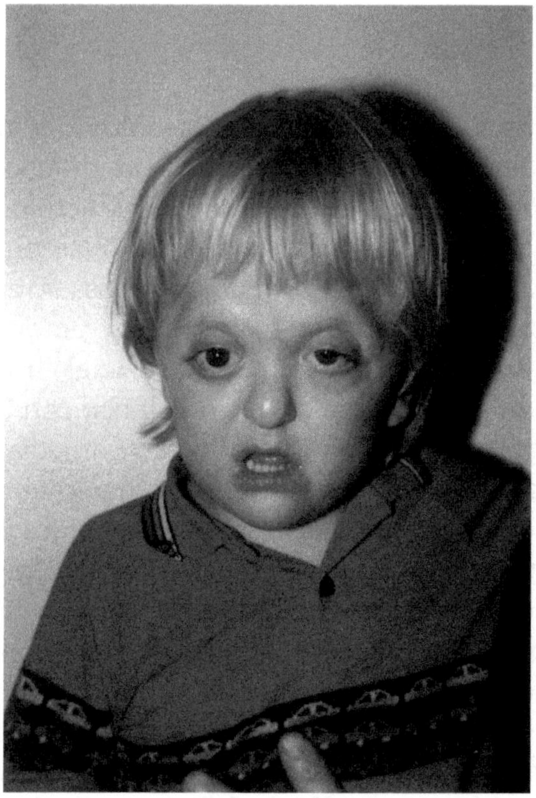

A

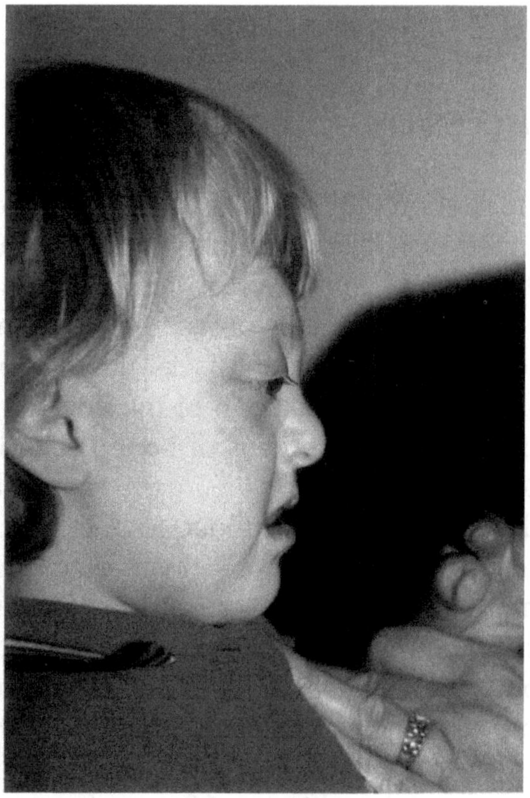

B

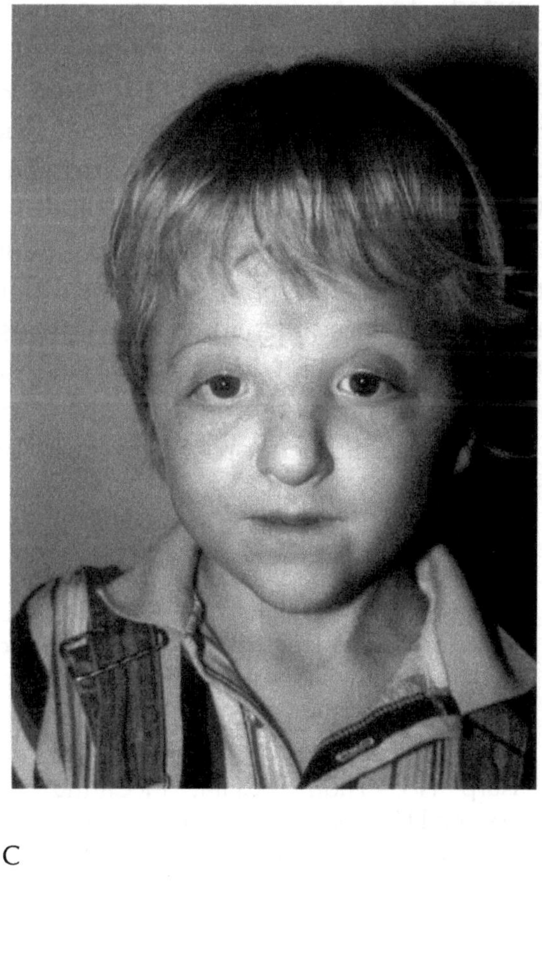

C

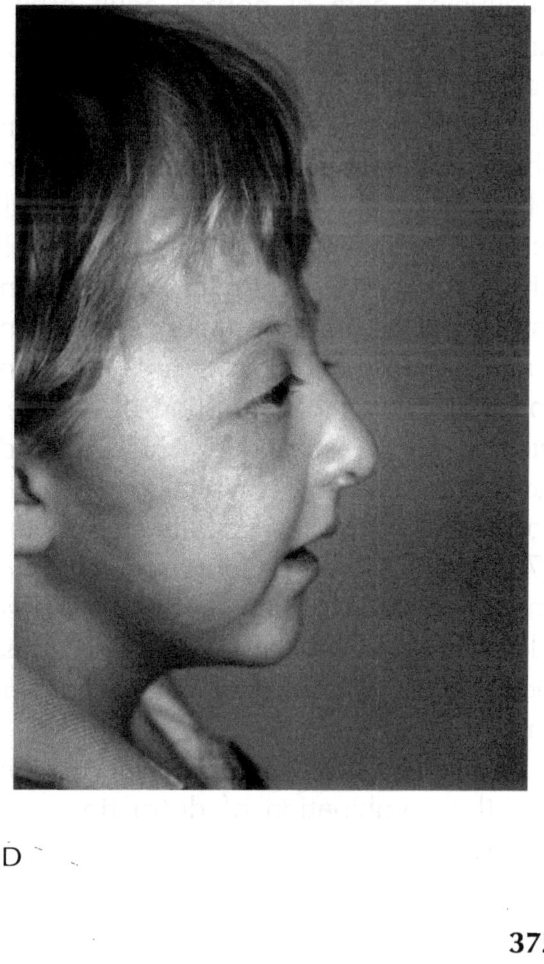

D

DISCUSSION

The LeFort III osteotomy, as first described by Gillies and Harrison (10), but later refined and popularized by Tessier (11), is an extensive procedure involving the creation of a craniofacial dysjunction followed by rigid fixation of the advanced midface and placement of bone grafts in the resultant defects. Surgery not only advances the midface but also expands the orbital volume by increasing the anteroposterior and vertical dimensions. The range of advancement possible with conventional LeFort III osteotomy and rigid fixation techniques has been reported to be between 8 and 20 mm, with most patients achieving 10 mm of correction (12–14).

Direct comparisons can be made with longitudinal data of normal adult orbital dimensions (9). The projected orbital deficiency of a child with syndromic craniofacial synostosis is approximately 24 mm. The deficit, as measured by the amount of retrusion at the infraorbital rim, usually exceeds the amount of correction possible with a traditional LeFort III advancement osteotomy. Clinical studies have confirmed that undercorrection is frequent and that a significant portion of children will require a secondary midfacial advancement (13,15). Whitaker (15) reported that in the severely affected group, 67 percent of the patients required secondary midface surgery as they reached adolescence, even after the child had monobloc advancement surgery performed at an early age.

Based on this background it is evident that the combination of distraction with midface advancement surgery may offer advantages over midface osteotomy/rigid fixation techniques currently in practice. The major benefit of gradual distraction is that it allows the surgeon to overcome resistance of the overlying soft-tissue envelope, which is the main limiting factor in the mobilization of large skeletal fragments. The force of this resistance can be significant when performing an immediate LeFort III advancement. Incremental movement using distraction mechanics allows the displacement of skeletal fragments over greater distances because the soft-tissue envelope is allowed to accommodate gradually. By using the described methods an average correction of 18.7 mm was achieved in the authors' series of patients. While falling short of the preoperative goal of 24 mm, this magnitude of lengthening is almost twice that reported for traditional advancement procedures. These results suggest that combining osteotomies with gradual distraction can significantly increase the amount of correction possible, thereby allowing mobilization of the infraorbital rim in these children to near the normal adult dimension and changing the occlusal pattern from a Class III to, in most instances, a Class II relationship. Moreover, relapse should be decreased and the need for a secondary midface procedure may be obviated.

References

1. DeBastiani G, Oldegheri R, Renzi-Brivo L, Trivella G. Limb lengthening by callus distraction. *J Pediatr Orthop* 7:129, 1987.
2. Ilizarov GA. The principles of the Ilizarov method. *Bull Hosp Joint Dis* 48:1, 1988.
3. Karp NS, Thorne CHM, McCarthy JG, Sissons HA. Bone lengthening in the craniofacial skeleton. *Ann Plast Surg* 24:231, 1990.

4. McCarthy JG, Schreiber J, Karp N, Thorne CH, Grayson BH. Lengthening the human mandible by gradual distraction. *Plast Reconstr Surg* 89:1, 1992.
5. Takato T, Harii K, Hirabayashi S, Komuro Y, Yonehara Y, Susami T. Mandibular lengthening by gradual distraction: Analysis using accurate skull replicas. *Br J Plast Surg* 46:686, 1993.
6. Rachmiel A, Potparic Z, Jackson IT, Sugihara T, Clayman L, Topf JS, Forte RA. Midface advancement by gradual distraction. *Br J Plast Reconstr Surg* 46:201, 1993.
7. Stafferberg DA, Wood RJ, McCarthy JG, Grayson BH, Glasberg SB. Midface distraction or advancement in the canine without osteotomies. *Ann Plast Surg* 34:512, 1995
8. Chin M, Toth BA. Distraction osteogenesis in maxillofacial surgery using internal devices: Review of five cases. *J Oral Maxillofac Surg* 54:45, 1996.
9. Baumrind S. Personal communication, 1996.
10. Gillies H, Harrison SH. Operative correction by osteotomy of recessed malar maxillary compound in a case of oxycephaly. *Br J Plast Surg* 3:123, 1950.
11. Tessier P. The definitive plastic surgical treatment of the severe facial depormities of craniofacial dysostosis, Crouzon's and Apert's disease. *Plast Reconstr Surg* 48:419, 1971.
12. McCarthy JG, Grayson B, Bookstein F, Vickery C, Zide B. LeFort III advancement osteotomy in the growing child. *Plast Reconstr Surg* 74:343, 1984.
13. McCarthy JG, LaTrenta GS, Breitbart AS, Grayson BH, Bookstein FL. LeFort III advancement osteotomy in the child under 7 years of age. *Plast Reconstr Surg* 86:633, 1990.
14. Ousterhout DK, Vargervik K, Clark S. Stability of the maxilla after LeFort III advancement in craniosynostosis syndromes. *Cleft Palate J* 23(suppl):91, 1986.
15. Whitaker LA, Barlett SP, Schut L, Bruce D. Craniosynostosis: An analysis of the timing, treatment, and complications in 164 consecutive patients. *Plast Reconstr Surg* 80:195, 1987.

Part 4
THE CRANIUM AND THE ORBITS

CHAPTER 14

DISTRACTION OF THE CRANIAL VAULT

John A. Persing and Constance M. Barone

In an effort to improve skull shape deformities induced by craniosynostosis, various surgical techniques have been developed. Initially, the linear craniectomy procedure was described; it consisted of removal of the prematurely fused suture and a minimal amount of adjacent cranial bones (1,2). Although this was effective to some degree, dissatisfaction with the lack of complete correction of the deformity stimulated others to modify the procedure. Because it was presumed that the reason for the incomplete correction of the skull deformity following linear craniectomy was the "refusion" of the craniectomy site, surgeons devised alternative methods to prevent it. Polyethylene film was applied to the cut edges of the bone to serve as a barrier to new bone formation across the craniectomy site. However, the polyethylene film neither prevented the "refusion" nor significantly improved skull shape, particularly when there was a severe degree of skull deformity or advanced patient age.

The era of direct reshaping or remodeling of the skull followed, initially localized to the pathologic areas of stenosis and morphologic change, proceeding ultimately to the areas of secondary compensation throughout the cranial vault (3–9). Although the more recent measures are more successful in improving skull form, they are also more time consuming, require greater use of physical resources, and still are not uniformly successful in returning skull shape to normal. This is particularly true for patients with the craniosynostosis syndromes like Apert and Crouzon, in whom the skull base deformity is more resistant to change following cranial vault remodeling. One persistent abnormality is oftentimes a shortened anterior cranial base. The cranial base is the "template" or foundation for both the cranial vault and the facial skeleton. Its shape influences the morphology of these regions, and different approaches to alter cranial base shape need to be undertaken in order to achieve a truly normal shape of the cranial vault.

LABORATORY STUDIES

A laboratory model of craniosynostosis was developed in which immobilization of the coronal suture in 9-day-old New Zealand white rabbits was achieved by the topical application of methylcyanoacrylate adhesive over a growing cranial vault suture. (Figure 14.1). The adhesive resulted in restriction of growth at the coronal suture leading to a brachycephalic skull shape, a phenocopy consistent with the clinical observation of brachycephaly in bilateral coronal synostosis in humans. In addition, with restriction of growth at the coronal suture, the cranial base became secondarily deformed and foreshortened due solely to the cranial vault suture growth restriction (10). Subsequently, a linear craniectomy of the immobilized coronal suture was performed on these animals at different time periods in development demonstrating the potential for, at least, a partial recovery to normal skull shape by this surgical approach. Early surgery (ie, at a time when significant brain and bone growth remained) resulted in the greatest improvement. However, later in skull development, this surgical approach only ameliorated the deformity and failed to return the skull shape to normal (11). This laboratory finding is similar to the clinical situation that clinicians now face: surgical procedures improve but frequently do not fully correct the established cranial deformities.

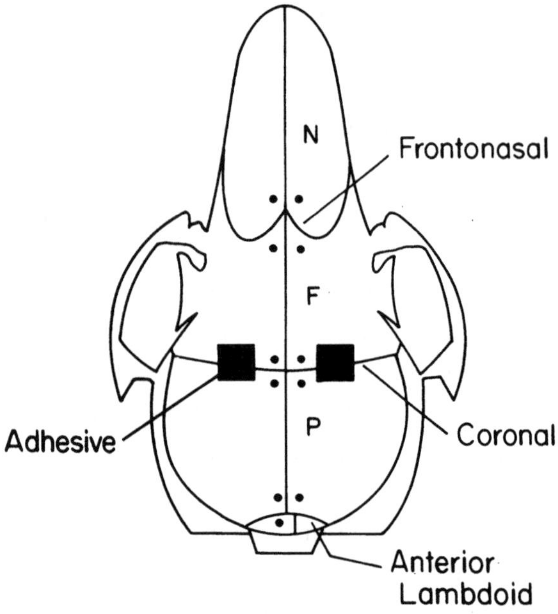

Figure 14.1. Diagram of rabbit's skull viewed from above with radiopaque markers (dots) placed adjacent to the frontonasal, coronal, and anterior lambdoid sutures. Adhesive (solid squares) is applied to the coronal suture bilaterally. N = nosal bone, F = frontal bone, P = parietal bone.

With this observation, a device was constructed that was designed to offer a positive growth influence at the area of previous growth restriction (fused suture) on a continual basis postoperatively. In these animals, following linear craniectomy, a "spring expander" or distraction device was inserted in the region of the suture to enhance further the separation of the bones at the cranial base suture (12). Two significant observations were made. First, the placement of the spring at the cranial vault suture resulted in greater expansion of the frontal and parietal bones adjacent to the coronal suture (Figure 14.2). This allowed an expansion to a

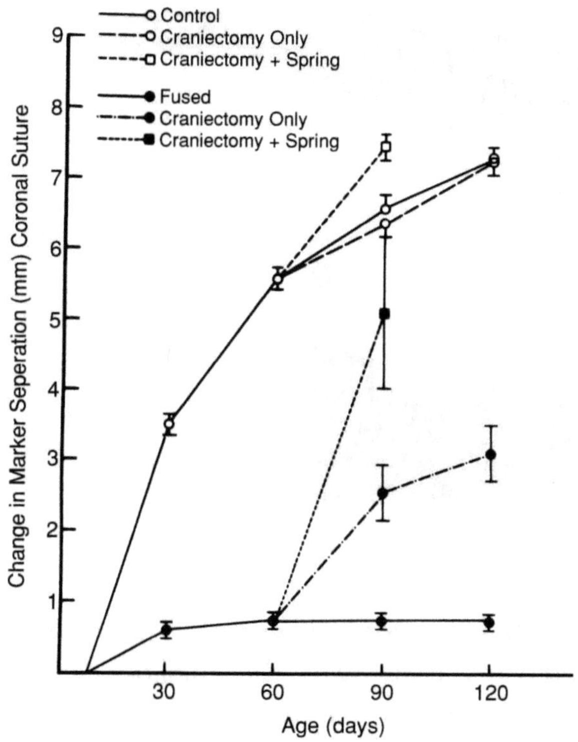

Figure 14.2. Coronal suture marker separation (solid circles) following coronal suture fusion, linear craniectomy, and craniectomy plus spring distraction. Note return to normal marker separation at the coronal suture following supplemental use of the implanted distraction device. Control animals are depicted with open circles. Reproduced with permission from Persing JA, Babler WJ, Nagorsky MJ, Edgerton MT, Jane JA. Skull expansion in experimental craniosynostosis. *Plast Reconstr Surg* 78:594, 1986.

point where local skull morphology recovered to normal dimensions. The mechanism by which this occurred, as Ten Cate and associates (13) had described, was stretching and probable disruption of the transosseous binding fibrous tissue at the craniectomy site. The second finding is more significant. The influence of the vault suture expander was more generalized and not just localized to the immediate environ of the previously fused suture. The contralateral coronal suture showed a temporary increase in growth (or distraction) as well, but this was not sustained over the longer course of the study. On the other hand, more remote sites in the cranial base, specifically, the cribriform plate (corresponding to the anterior portion of the anterior cranial base) demonstrated a persistent and significant increase in length (following the placement of the spring at the craniectomy site in the cranial vault). This observation suggests the possibility that not only could the expander exert a local effect at the suture, but it also might have a positive "remote" effect in the cranial base. This latter finding has particular significance, because as stated earlier, it has been the cranial base deformities that persist following many cranial vault remodeling procedures for craniosynostosis, and these residual deformities may account for the incomplete shape corrections in the skull observed postoperatively.

A second study was performed in order to address the concept of residual cranial base deformity as being the cause of persistent skull deformity (14). Immature New Zealand white rabbits received a cranial base expansion device inserted at the basal extension of the coronal suture (ie, the frontosphenoidal suture) (Figure 14.3). In this study, it was elected to define the consequences of placement of the expansion device in a previously *normal* animal as an initial step to determine how effective it would be in an animal model of craniosynostosis. Thirty-day-old rabbits received a mechanical spring that served to develop distraction forces across the frontosphenoidal suture.

It was observed that the mechanical spring device was effective in altering the ipsilateral coronal suture growth to a de-

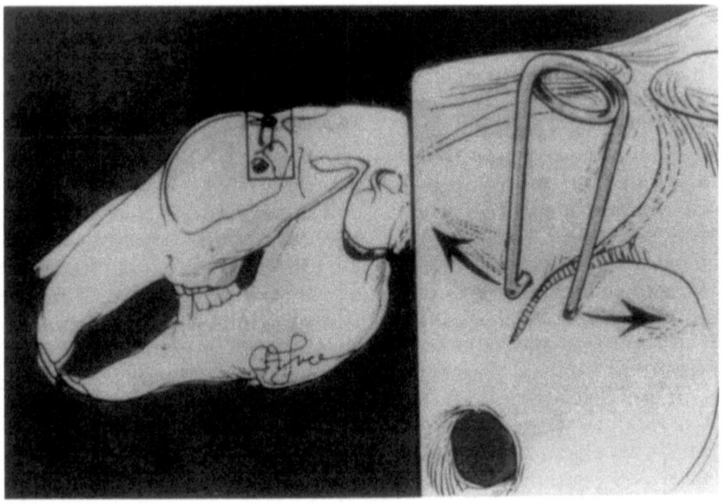

Figure 14.3. Drawing of placement of the spring distraction device across the frontosphenoidal suture in the left orbit (rabbit). Reproduced with permission from Persing JA, Morgan EP, Cronin AJ, Wolcott WP. Skull base expansion: Craniofacial effects. *Plast Reconstr Surg* 87:1028, 1991.

gree greater than normal "control" levels (Figure 14.4). The remainder of the cranial vault, cranial base, and facial skeleton, however, remained unaffected. That the growth expansion effect was regionalized solely to the side ipsilateral to the vault suture and spring placement is significant. The midline portion of the cranial base was unaltered by this relatively lateral cranial base spring placement. This finding indicates that, with the midline cranial base structure remaining unaltered, the midface structures and the remainder of the cranial vault skeleton, likewise, were unaffected. It may mean that in order for the anteroposterior dimension of the face to change, the sagittal dimensions of the cranial base must also change. These stud-

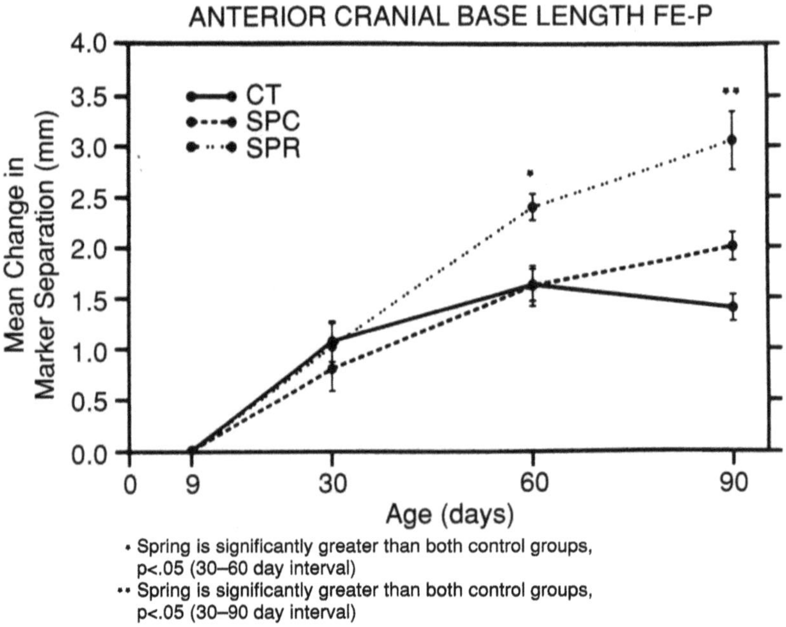

Figure 14.4. Anterior cranial base (FE-P) growth (marker separation) following spring distraction. Note statistically significant increase in growth of the skull at the coronal suture after spring expansion compared with both control groups. Reproduced with permission from Persing JA, Morgan EP, Cronin AJ, Wolcott WP. Skull base expansion: Craniofacial effects. *Plast Reconstr Surg* 87:1028, 1991.

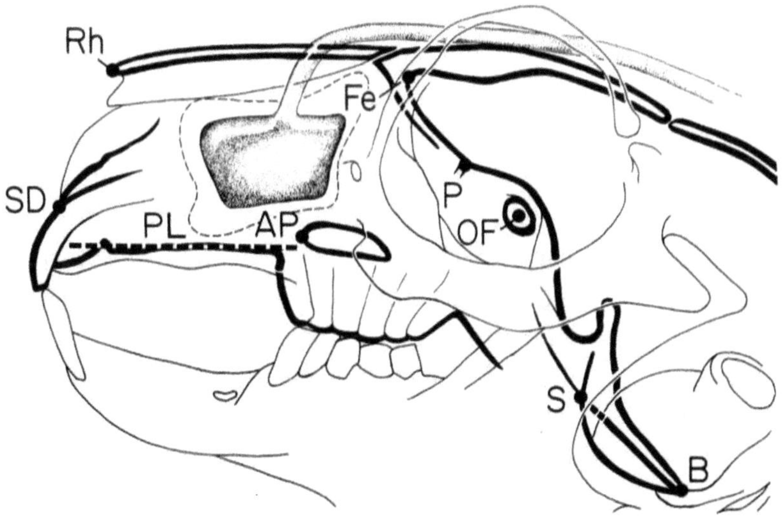

Figure 14.5. Drawing of lateral cephalogram with defined points and superimposed tissue expander in the maxillary sinus. Reproduced with permission from Persing JA, Gampper TJ, Morgan EP, Wolcott WP. Experimental expansion of the maxillary sinus. *J Craniofac Surg* 5:11, 1994.

ies further support the concept that there is a relationship between cranial vault and cranial base suture growth and that the pathway of influence is reciprocal.

As a feature of this search for an alternate site to influence midline cranial base growth, a third study was performed (15). An inflatable expander device was placed in the maxilla of the growing rabbit (Figure 14.5). At 30 days of age, immature or growing rabbits underwent placement of a tissue expander in the maxillary sinus that, when inflated, was intended to increase the size of the maxilla and alter the cranial base structure secondarily. This goal was achieved as evidenced by elongation of the anterior cranial base in a vertical dimension. There was, however, a deleterious effect on midface anteroposterior (sagittal) growth. Skeletal growth in this dimension was reduced compared to normal, but the height of the midface was elongated (Figure 14.6) commensurate with the lengthening of the

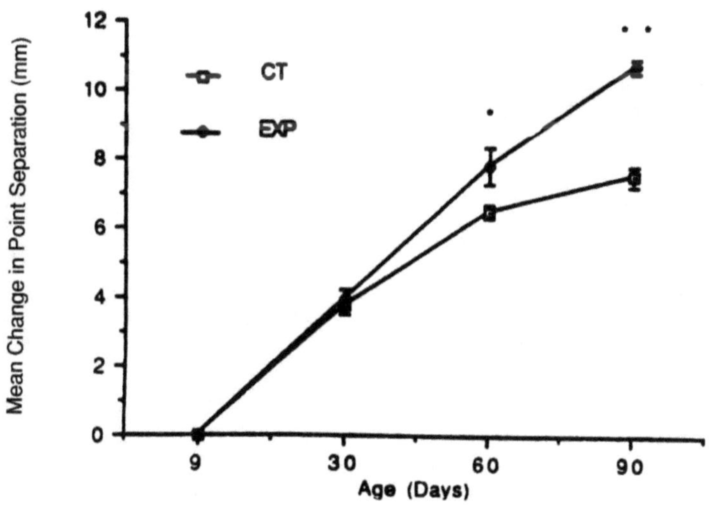

* EXP had growth greater than CT, p<.0.5, 30–60 day interval.

** EXP had growth greater than CT, p<.0.5, 60–90 and 30–90 day interval.

Figure 14.6. Posterior midface (FE–PL) growth following inflation of the maxillary sinus expander. Note the statistically significant increase in midface height (FE–PL) with expansion or distraction when compared with the control group (CT = control group, EXP = expander or distraction group). Reproduced with permission from Persing JA, Gampper TJ, Morgan EP, Wolcott WP. Experimental expansion of the maxillary sinus. *J Craniofac Surg* 5:11, 1994.

anterior cranial base. It was surprising that this had no significant effect on cranial vault dimensions. This finding heightened the perception that in order for a cranial expander to be effective in reversing established cranial deformities, the site for the distraction device and the degree of expansion must be well defined and controllable. The opposite effect of the intended expansion may result with "improper" placement of the expanding influence. Remmler and colleagues (16) developed a device that could provide a calculated amount of distraction to a potentially hypoplastic region of the skull on a gradual basis. Like earlier reports, this has been effective in "expanding" the cranial skeleton but has the important and additional advantage of being adjustable.

A similar approach to fronto-orbital advancement has been undertaken by Barone and colleagues (17). In this study, 22-week-old rabbits were divided into three groups: control, where frontal craniotomy alone was performed; a second group, sham control, where frontal craniotomy was performed and a distraction device was applied but not expanded, and an experimental group, in which a frontal craniotomy was performed. The distraction device was applied and expanded at a rate of one millimeter every other day for a period of 8 weeks. The direction of expansion however was not in the plane of the skull as in earlier studies (12,14,15,16). Rather, it was perpendicular to the plane of the surface of the skull. It was demonstrated that this distraction approach was also effective in translocating the bone outside the normal plane of the skull (Figure 14.7). Therefore, the bones of the skull may be expanded multidirectionally, depending on the orientation of the distraction device and the rate at which it is expanded.

In summary, it has been demonstrated in animals that it is technically feasible to increase the growth at cranial vault and cranial base sutures with the placement of distraction devices. What is needed at this point is to define which sites in the skull are capable of the greatest degree of expansion, in which

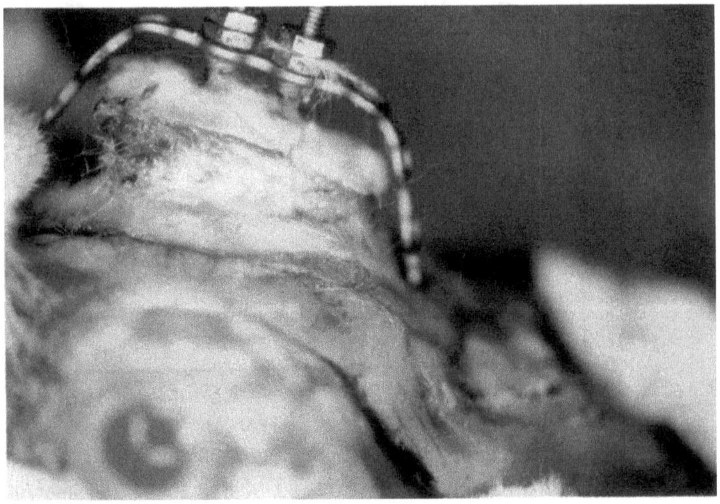

Figure 14.7. Distraction of the frontal bone perpendicular to the plane of the cranial vault in the rabbit. Note the two-pin distraction device and the bone regenerate.

direction expansion will occur, and which method is associated with the least morbidity. The clinical implications of this methodology are many.

References

1. Lane LC. Linear craniectomy for relief of mental imbecility due to premature sutural close and microcephalus. *JAMA* 18:49, 1892.
2. Lannelongue OM. De la craniectomie dans la microcephalie. *Compt Rend Acad Sci* 110:1382, 1890.
3. Ingraham FD, Matson DD, Alexander E. Experimental observations in the treatment of craniosynostosis. *Surgery* 23:252, 1948.
4. Hoffman HJ, Mohr JP. Lateral canthal advancement of the supraorbital margin. A new corrective technique in the treatment of coronal synostosis. *J Neurosurg* 45:376, 1976.
5. Persing JA, Jane JA, Delashaw JB. Treatment of bilateral coronal synostosis in infancy: A holistic approach. *J Neurosurg* 72:171, 1990.
6. Marchac D, Renier D. *Craniofacial Surgery for Craniosynostosis*. Boston: Little, Brown, 1982: p. 1–195.
7. McCarthy J, Epstein FJ, Wood-Smith D. Craniosynostosis. In McCarthy JG, ed. *Plastic Surgery*. 1990: Vol. 4, pp. 3013–3053.
8. Persing JA, Edgerton MT, Park TS, Jane JA. Barrel stave osteotomy for correction of turribrachycephaly craniosynostosis deformity. *Ann Plast Surg* 18:488, 1987.
9. Persson KM, Roy WA, Persing JA, Rodeheaver GT, Winn HR. Craniofacial growth following experimental craniosynostosis and craniectomy in rabbits. *J Neurosurg* 50:187, 1979.
10. Babler WJ, Persing JA. Experimental alteration of cranial suture growth: Effects on the neurocranium, basicranium, and midface. In: Dixon AP, Sarnat BG, eds. *Factors and Mechanisms Influencing Bone Growth*, New York: Alan R. Liss, 1982: pp. 333–345.
11. Persing JA, Babler WJ, Winn HR, Jane JA, Rodeheaver GT. Age as a clinical factor in the success of surgical correction of craniosynostosis. *J Neurosurg* 54:601, 1981.
12. Persing JA, Babler WJ, Nagorsky MJ, Edgerton MT, Jane JA. Skull expansion in experimental craniosynostosis. *Plast Reconstr Surg* 78:594, 1986.
13. Ten Cate AR, Freeman E, Dickinson JB. Sutural development: Structure and its response to rapid expansion. *Am J Orthod* 71:622, 1977.
14. Persing JA, Morgan EP, Cronin AJ, Wolcott WP. Skull base expansion: Craniofacial effects. *Plast Reconstr Surg* 87:1028, 1991.
15. Persing JA, Gampper TJ, Morgan EP, Wolcott WP. Experimental expansion of the maxillary sinus. *J Craniofac Surg* 5:11, 1994.
16. Remmler D, McCoy FJ, O'Neil D. Osseous expansion of the cranial vault by craniotasis. *Plast Reconstr Surg* 89:787, 1992.
17. Barone CM, Ferder M, Jimenez DF. Distraction of the frontal bone outside the cranial plane: A rabbit model. *J Craniofac Surg* 4:177, 1993.

CHAPTER 15A

DISTRACTION OF THE ORBIT

Barry L. Eppley and A. Michael Sadove

Congenital anophthalmos/microphthalmos or early enucleation in the infant child removes the stimulation for subsequent development of the surrounding bones of the orbit (1–4). This has adverse growth effects with resultant decrease in all orbital dimensions. In addition, the growth disturbances may be transferred to the development of the zygomaticomaxillary complex and mandible depending on how early the eye is absent from the orbit during development (Figures 15A.1 and 15A.2) (1).

Orbital growth results from an interplay of several regulatory mechanisms, not all of which are fully understood. Craniofacial growth results primarily from its enveloping soft tissue and functional matrix (eg, muscle pull and tension, neurovascular flow, pressure) (5,6). The internal forces of the expanding globe, combined with external soft tissue tension provided by the downward growth of the nasomaxillary complex and the anterolateral movement of the zygomas, collectively work toward creating the final orbital position and shape, thus supporting the functional matrix theory (Figure 15A.3) (5,6). Other theories speculate that craniofacial growth is regulated by internal osseous cellular mechanisms (ie, a genetic blueprint) (7). However, the dramatic skeletal changes manifest after early orbital evisceration question the significance of these mechanisms.

Conventional treatment of the microphthalmos or enucleated orbit involves the early intraorbital placement of spherical silicone implants. These are serially replaced with ones of enlarging size as the child develops (8,9). While the implants have some effect on enlarging the bony orbit, their use is often complicated by extrusion and diffic-

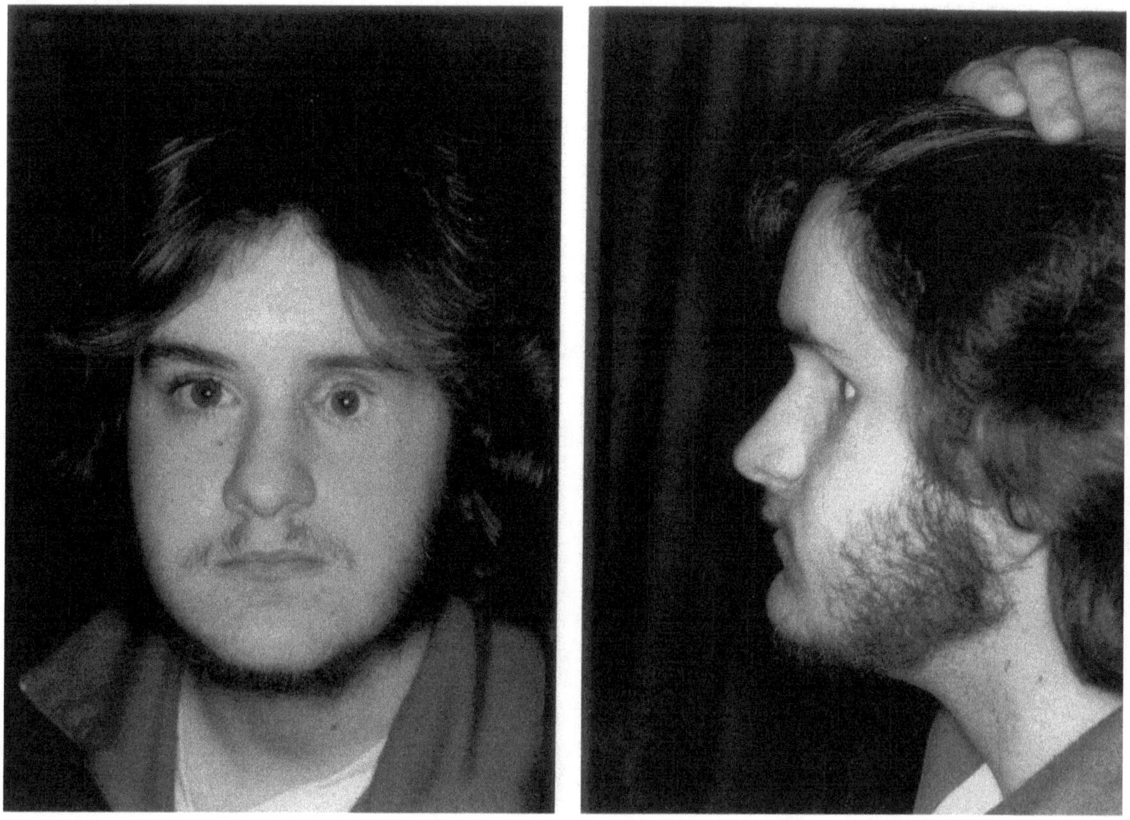

A B

Figure 15A.1. Male patient following removal of the left eye at age 7 with evidence of mild orbital hypoplasia but without underlying facial hypoplasia. A, Frontal view. B, Lateral view.

ulties in maintaining their intraorbital position.

Another method of orbital enlargement is the application of three-dimensional expansion osteotomies (10,11). Surgical repositioning of the orbital rims and walls effectively enlarges orbital volume and improves symmetry with the contralateral normal orbit. However, the technique does not promote growth of the expanded orbit postoperatively unless aided by the subsequent use of serial spherical implants. Therefore, surgical orbital expansion may need to be repeated when craniofacial skeletal growth has finished. Furthermore, the procedure does not improve the overlying soft-tissue envelope (eyelids) which, like the underlying skeleton, is also deficient.

An alternative approach, employing the biology of the functional matrix theory and the biomechanical influences of distraction osteogenesis, is to expand the anophthalmic orbit during growth and development through the use of an internal expandable implant.

EXPERIMENTAL STUDY

Twenty-one kittens were randomized equally into three experimental groups: unoperated controls (Group A), unilateral enucleations (Group B), and unilateral enucleations with postoperative intraorb-

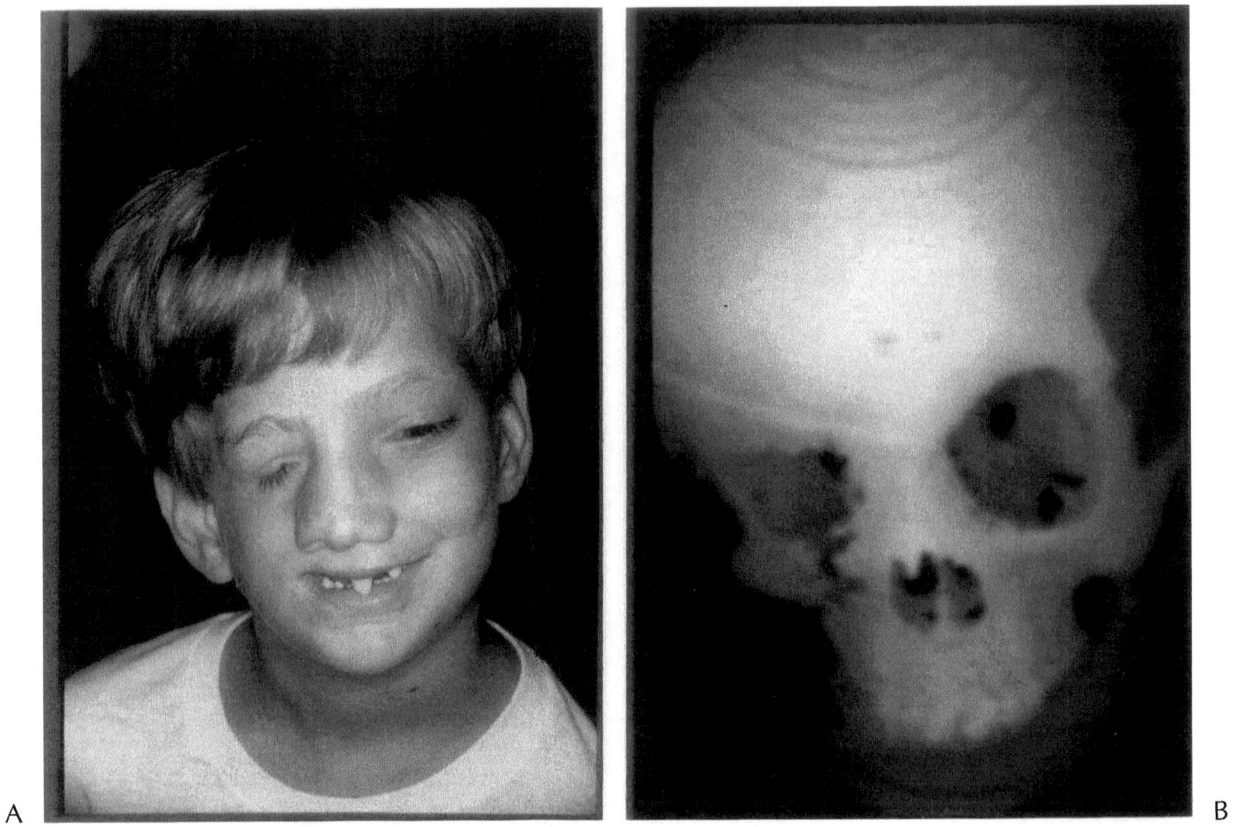

Figure 15A.2. Congenital microphthalmos in a young patient with marked facial shortening. A, Frontal view. B, 3D CT scan demonstrating a contracted orbit, hypoplastic zygoma and maxilla, rotated mandible, and canted occlusal plane on the affected side.

ital expansion or distraction (Group C). The enucleations were performed at the third postnatal week and the animals allowed to grow until 20 weeks of age.

A custom-designed expander (Mentor, Goleta, CA) was developed that consisted of a spherical design to simulate the shape of the globe and a peripheral injection port (Figure 15A.4). The maximal inflation volume was 5 ml which was serially achieved with 0.25 ml weekly saline installations over a 3-month interval after an initial 2-ml fill at the time of placement.

Under intraperitoneal sedation and periorbital infiltration anesthesia, Group B and Group C animals underwent a right-sided enucleation. Through a lateral canthotomy and conjunctival incision, the dissection was extended posteriorly along the lateral orbital wall as far as the optic neurovascular bundle. The latter was transected after being initially ligated. Additional release of the conjunctiva along the superior and inferior fornices, as well as further dissection posteriorly in an extraconal plane, permitted delivery of the globe. The conjunctival incision was reapproximated anteriorly with interrupted 5-0 resorbable suture. In Group C animals an expander was introduced through the superolateral (cleft) portion of the orbit with the aid of a skin incision. The injection port was placed in a subcutaneous tunnel extended from the skin incision over the occiput and into the neck. The expander was stabilized within the orbit by a 4-0 monofilament suture placed between the orbital rim and wrapped around the injection tubing at a position distal to the expander. The expander was instilled with 2 ml of saline and the skin incision and eyelids (tarsorrhaphy) closed with interrupted 5-0 monofilament sutures.

After a final saline installation at the beginning of the 20th week of age (17th postoperative week), the animals were sacrificed and the expanders removed to permit nondistorted radiographic images. CT scans with 3D reconstruction employing 1-mm thick sections (GE 9800 Quick, M level software, GE Medical Systems, Milwaukee, WI) were printed in life-size dimensions for assessment. The scans were used to make bilateral linear (height and width) measurements of the orbits as well as the zygomaticomaxillary complex in a frontal orientation. The orbital heights were measured along a straight line drawn from the midpoint of the supraorbital rim (at a point medial to the superolateral orbital cleft) to the midpoint of the infraorbital rim (superior to the infraorbital foramen). The orbital widths were measured on a straight line drawn from the most centric point along the medial orbital rim (anterior to the lacrimal fossa) to the point of greatest convexity along the lateral orbital rim (inferior to the superolateral orbital rim cleft). The zygomaticomaxillary height was measured between the inferior orbital rim at a point superior to the infraorbital foramen to the highest point of the alveolus inferiorly on a straight line. The zygomaticomaxillary width was measured from the nasomaxillary junction medially to the most lateral prominence of the zygomatic body.

The animal skulls were also used to make direct orbital volume measurements. This was done by lining the orbits with metallic foil and filling them with water and measuring the volume to the nearest 0.1 ml.

All values for both linear and volume measurements were averaged and the group means compared by a test.

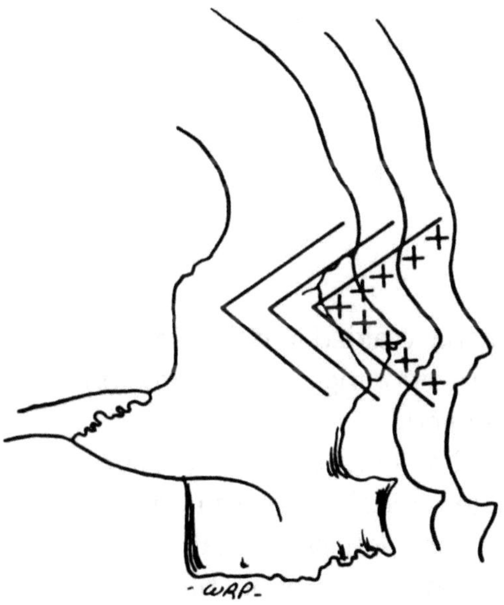

Figure 15A.3. Orbital growth is explained by the V-principle (a cone that moves in the direction of its opening) in which intraorbital bone deposition enlarges, rather than reduces, internal or intraorbital volume. Reproduced with permission from *Facial Growth*, 3rd ed., Enlow DH (ed), WB Saunders, 1990, p. 127.

RESULTS

All animals survived enucleation and tissue-expander implantation without complications. There was one incident of

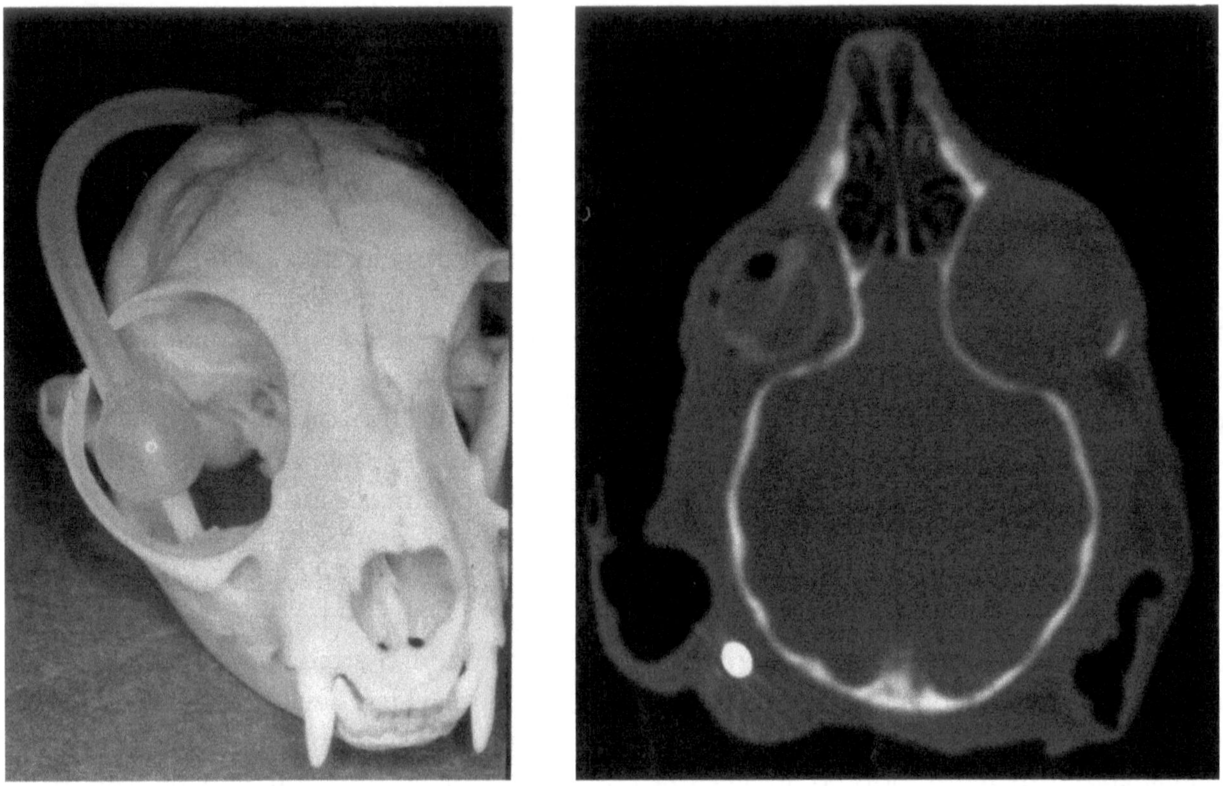

A B

Figure 15A.4. Spherical intraorbital tissue expander. (A) In place (noninflated) in the adult cat orbit. Inflation to 5 ml approximates the globe size of the adult cat. (B) Axial CT section with the intraorbital expander undergoing serial inflation.

implant extrusion in a Group C animal because the implant could not be adequately contained within the orbit by the tarsorrhaphy. This animal was excluded from the study, reducing Group C animals to six and the total number of study animals to twenty. All tissue expanders in the Group C animals functioned without failure during inflation over the study period without apparent loss of saline volume at the time of removal. A capsule around the implants consistently appeared and it may have aided in either implant retention or positioning. Body erosion was not observed.

The control orbits (Group A) had average orbital measurements between the right and left sides that were not grossly different in orbital height and width, orbitomaxillary height, zygomaticomaxillary width, or orbital volume (Table 15A.1).

The enucleated animals in Group B, however, had marked differences in orbital configurations between the two sides. The enucleated orbit exhibited underdevelopment of the zygomaticoorbital complex with displacement of this skeletal segment medially with reduction of inferolateral orbital rim length. This anomalous development, combined with expansion of the ethmoid air cells, resulted in a loss of orbital volume (Figure 15A.5). The vertical maxillary dimension on the enucleated side was reduced as evidenced by a maxillary cant. The following were also observed: A discrepancy between the maxillary and mandibular dental midlines, an ipsilateral open bite at the molars, and a more impressive discrepancy between the position of the inferior orbital rims as seen from a cephalic view. The overlying eyelids were shrunken inward; they lacked a supratarsal fold, and they appeared to have reduced overall dimensions than those of the contralateral side.

The enucleated-expanded (distracted) animals (Group C) displayed symmetry between the orientation of the inferior orbital rim, malar eminence, and distal end of the zygomatic arch (Figure 15A.6). The nasomaxillary relationship to the mandible had coinciding midlines between the nasal bones and maxillomandibular dental midlines. The eyelids had a more protrusive appearance, conforming to the anterior surface of the tissue expander.

The differences in the radiographic and clinical appearance of the skulls was further manifest with the Group B orbits (treated side only) being significantly different in orbital height ($p < 0.01$), orbital width ($p < 0.008$), orbito-maxillary height ($p < 0.03$), zygomatico-maxillary width ($p < 0.001$), and orbital volume ($p < 0.02$) from their contralateral orbits. Conversely, the differences between the orbits of the Group A and C animals were not significantly different ($p > 0.05$) in any of the measured values.

DISCUSSION

The developing eye has a profound postnatal growth influence on the size and

Table 15A.1. Orbitomaxillary measurements.

	Controls (A)		Enucleated (B)		Expanded (C)	
	R	L	R	L	R	L
Orbital height (mm)	21.5	20.5	13.5	20.0	19.5	21.0
Orbital width (mm)	21.0	23.5	9.5	22.5	21.5	22.0
Orbito-maxillary height (mm)	31.0	30.5	23.5	31.0	29.5	30.5
Zygomatico-maxillary width (mm)	24.5	25.0	15.0	23.0	24.0	24.5
Orbital volume (cc)	5.1	5.0	1.9	5.4	5.2	5.3

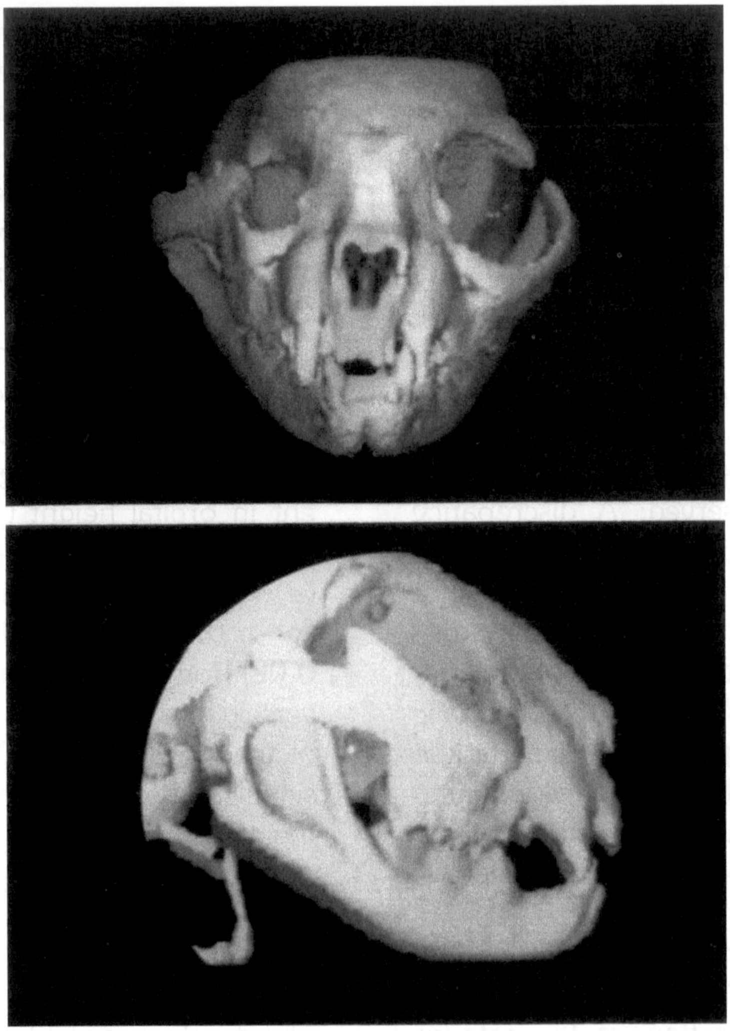

A

B

Figure 15A.5. Three-dimensional CT images of enucleated cat orbit (right). Note the difference in shape and in volume. (A) Frontal view. (B) Lateral view.

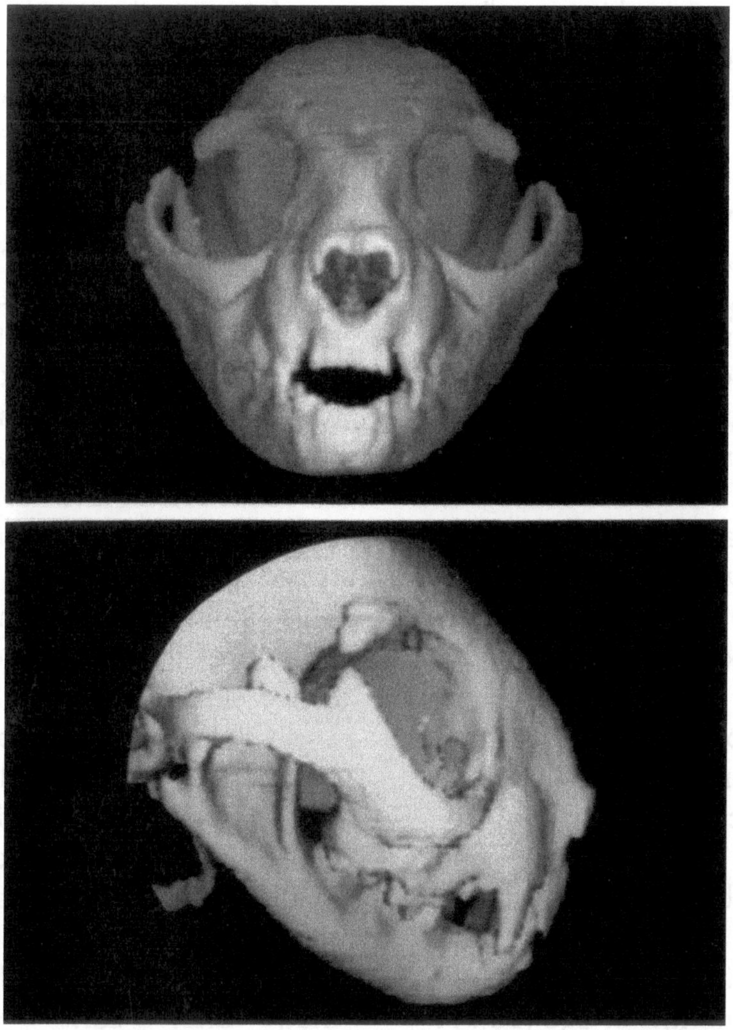

A

B

Figure 15A.6. Three-dimensional CT images of the expanded orbit (right). (A) Frontal view. (B) Lateral view.

morphology of the bony orbit as well as on the surrounding skeletal structures. This phenomenon is due to the rapid increase in volume of the globe during the first few years of life, increasing threefold by adolescence, of which 70% of the increase is attained by age 4 and 90% by age 7 (12). As such, the simplistic law of functional adaptation, Wolff's law, and the functional matrix theory may all be viewed as applicable, with the size of the orbital skeleton increasing in response to the expanding forces of the internal soft-tissue structures. By virtue of orbital position, therefore, the growing globe also indirectly influences the size and orientation of the adjoining maxilla, zygomatic body, and arch.

Numerous experimental investigations have documented the deleterious developmental effects of congenital absence or early loss of the globe. Early enucleations in rabbits at 21 postnatal days decreased the anteroposterior and vertical measurements of the orbit an average of 11% by 9 months of age (13). A direct correlation between the lack of intraorbital tissue mass and reduction in orbital skeletal growth has also been shown in the rabbit enucleation model (14,15).

The definitive animal model, however, was developed in cats by Kennedy and has become the standard reference when referring to the poorly developed anophthalmic orbit (1,3). The cat was chosen as a model in this study because its cranial vault shape more closely simulates that of the human and its orbital rim is nearly intact or circumferential. In addition, compared to other laboratory animals, the visual and orbital axes of the cat are fairly similar to those of man. The experimental findings indicated that the walls of the enucleated orbit were irregular, making true size determination difficult. The adjoining maxillary and ethmoid air cells were enlarged and encroached into the anophthalmic orbit. Shortening of the ipsilateral temporalis muscle was noted with collapse of the lateral orbital wall. The level of the roofs of the orbits was similar; however, an ipsilateral vertical shortening of the maxillary bone was associated with the anophthalmic orbit. The maxilla expanded into the orbit and raised the orbital floor by almost 1 cm. This finding was accompanied by an elevation of the zygomatic arch on the affected side.

Clinical studies also confirm the experimental bony effects and overlying soft tissue sequelae of loss of orbital globe drive. Taylor noted that enucleation in infancy resulted in a deficiency of orbital size and a decrease in medial-lateral canthal distance (16). Pfeiffer determined that, after early enucleation, the anophthalmic orbit is associated with less fullness of the forehead and cheek and a decreased distance from the outer orbital margin to the bridge of the nose (17). Osborne found a significant decrease in the growth of the orbit in children when enucleation was performed before the age of 13 (18).

To date, a completely satisfactory clinical replacement of the globe during the period of rapid orbitofacial growth has not been obtained. The sequential placement of enlarging spherical implants with overlying scleral conformers has had some success at promoting orbital volume change (6). However,the small amount of local orbital enlargement that results is not representative of progressive and expansive growth, and much of the overlying soft-tissue deformity remains, even though the intraorbital implant may be retained. Therefore, the use of a dynamic implant that would internally distract (expand) the orbit appears to be a more desirable biologic globe substitute.

In a previous study, subperiosteal tissue expansion emanating from the orbital roof has proven effective at maintaining normal orbital bone growth in the anophthalmic cat model (19). While the mechanism remains speculative, it was felt that actual orbital bone growth was promoted rather than simple rotation (displacement) or existing skeletal structures. There remains some question as to whether the position of the expander in this study simulated the clinical condition in humans and whether an actual globe placement would be equally, if not more, effective (20). Our results replicate those of the previous expansion study and demonstrate that its effects are dynamic to the surrounding skeleton with normalization of other craniofacial measurements as well as apparent soft tissue (eyelid) adaptation to the underlying enlarging expander. The eyelid development, which is promoted, is of particular importance as often the accompanying soft-tissue deformities are as severe as those of the orbital skeleton in early globe loss or anophthalmos.

The mechanism by which an intraorbital tissue expander supports orbital growth and development would appear to act by simulating that of the epigenetic influence of the actual growing globe. This would cause skeletal changes through a complex relationship between primary remodeling activity along the roof, floor, and walls of the orbit, combined with secondary displacement of the zygoma and maxilla in an inferolateral direction. The expanding intraorbital soft tissue (globe and muscle cone) or expander induces a low-grade force on the surrounding intraorbital bones. This is countered by expansile growth from the cerebrum, periorbital air cells (maxillary and ethmoid), and nasal cavity as well as lateral distraction from the attachment of the temporalis muscle at the zygomatic arch. The entire orbit thus develops with the roof, medial wall, and floor acting as primary bone depository sites and the lateral wall as a resorptive site. This bone development pattern, combined with the generalized forward growth of the orbit through the V-principle, results in an increase in orbital skeletal dimensions that accommodate increasing globe size (See Figure 15A.3). In addition, the divergent growth that results from the skeletal activity between the medial and lateral walls of the orbit serves to add increasing depth to the maturing face. Fluorochrome bone labels in a similar animal study, however, indicated that the type of orbital bone growth seen with expansion is translational in nature with the presence of labeling on both the inner and outer aspects of the orbital rim (21). This finding would suggest that the phenomenon of bone drift may be of greater significance in craniofacial growth than previously appreciated.

An intraorbital expander works effectively in the young cat model presumably because of the thin structure of the lateral

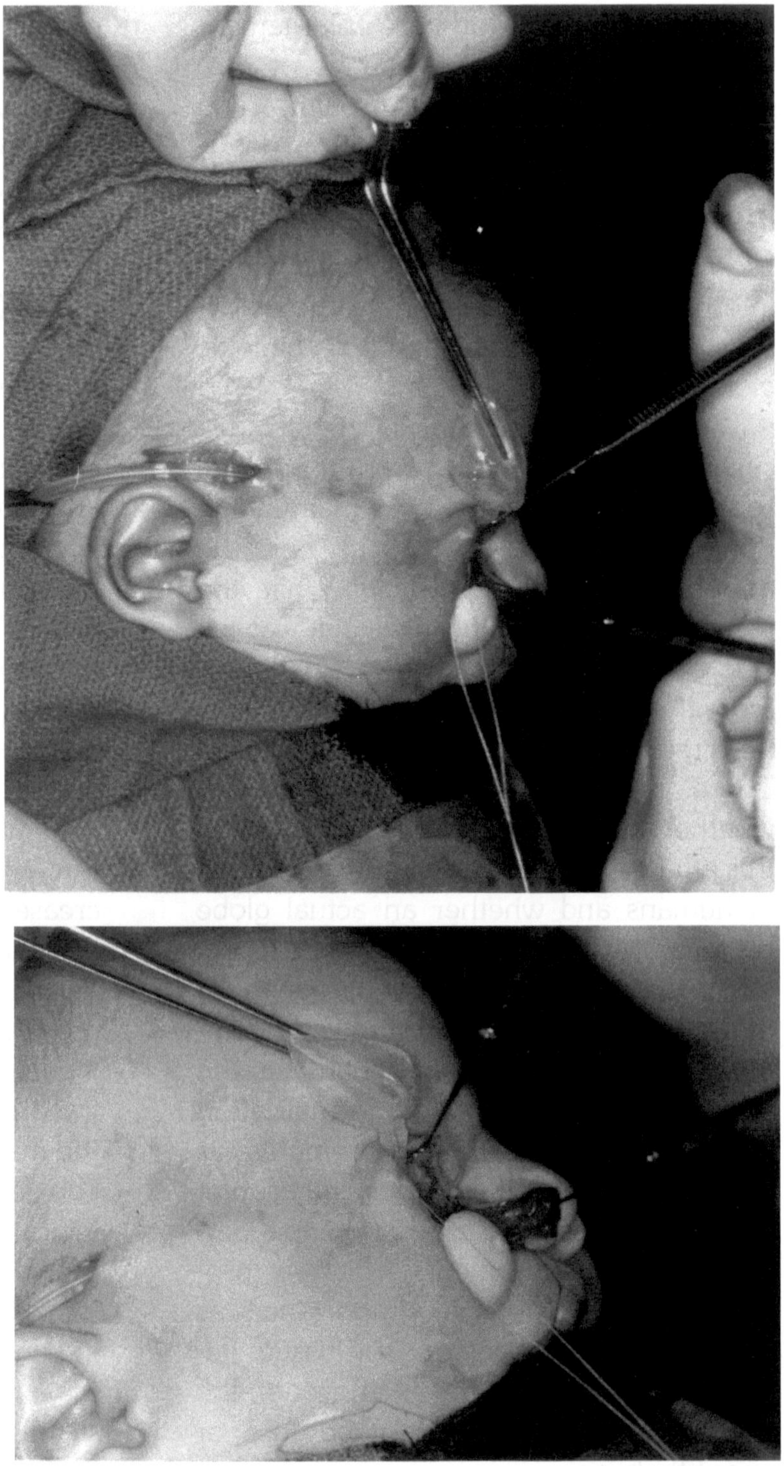

A

B

Figure 15A.7. (A) Intraorbital expander placement in a patient with a remote port exiting the temporal region. Note the accompanying plastic shell. (B) A plastic shell is sutured over the expander to prevent displacement of the expander through the lids with inflation.

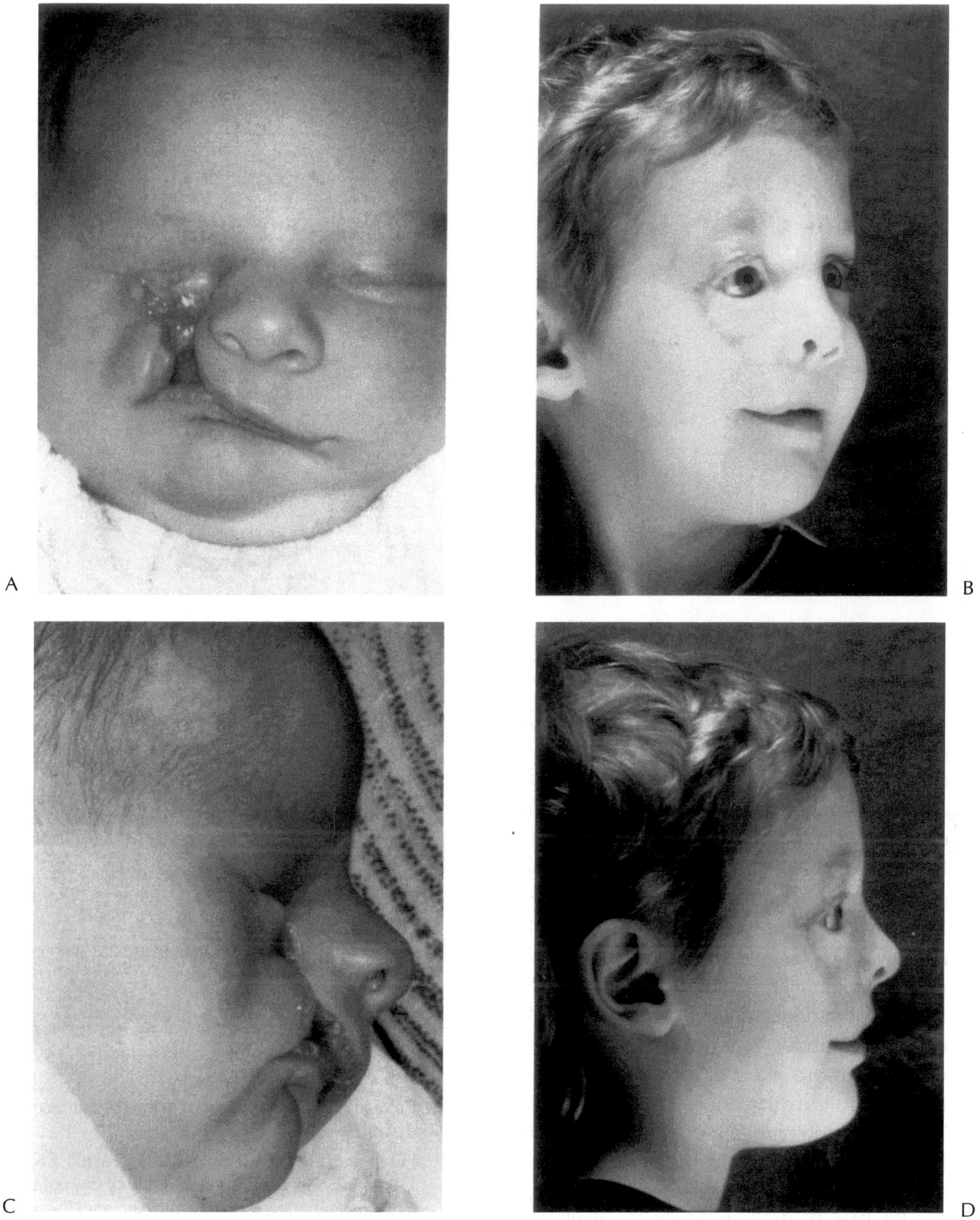

Figure 15A.8. (A) One-month-old infant with a unilateral Tessier IV facial cleft with absence of the globe. (B) Postoperative (5-year) oblique view after early orbital expansion and lower lid reconstruction with a forehead flap (Flap courtesy of S. Anthony Wolfe, MD, Miami, FL). C, Preoperative lateral view. D, postoperative lateral view. E, Preoperative submental view. F, Postoperative submental view.

(Continued)

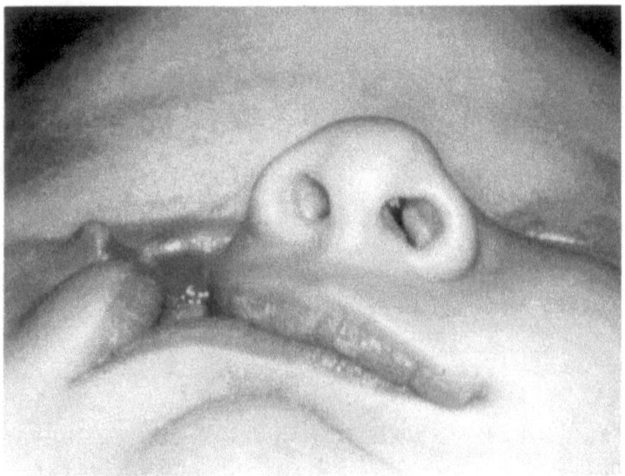
E

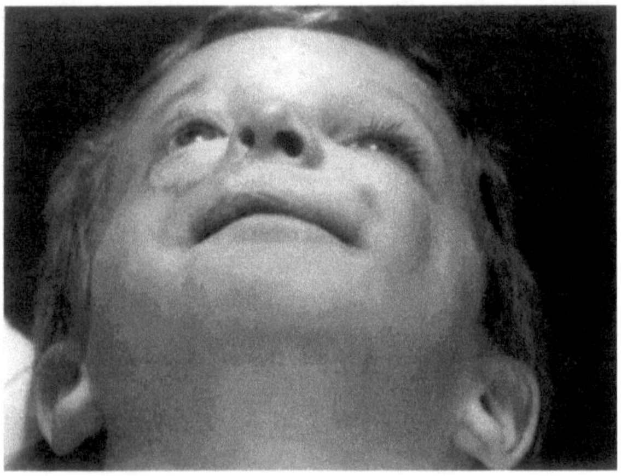
F

Figure 15A.8. *Continued*

orbital wall and the zygomaticomaxillary complex, as well as the lack of bony continuity around the orbital rim. As such, normalization of anatomical position and integrity of bone quality may be relatively easy to achieve. Whether the thicker and circumferentially intact bone of the human orbit may similarly be affected is speculative. It is likely that substantial orbital growth of the human infant can be effected as the expansile forces (pressure) of a growing globe and tissue expander appear quite similar. Unlike the experience in the cat model, however, displacement of the expander anteriorly through the eyelids is more likely to occur in the human due to the differences in bone quality. Therefore, intraorbital expander plans for human application will need to be designed so that they incorporate the ability for fixation to the orbital rim or walls to ensure the location and the direction of the expansile forces (Figures 15A.7 and 15A.8).

References

1. Kennedy RE. Growth retardation and volume determinations of the anophthalmic orbit. *Trans Am Ophthalmol Soc* 70:277, 1972.
2. Van Limborgh J, Tonneyck-Muller I. Orbital growth pattern in experimental microphthalmia. *Mod Probl Ophthalmol* 14:1, 1975.
3. Kennedy RE. The effect of early enucleation on the orbit in animals and humans. *Trans Am Ophthalmol Soc* 62:459, 1964.
4. Apt L, Isenberg S. Changes in orbital dimensions following enucleation. *Arch Ophthalmol* 90:393, 1973.
5. Moss ML. Growth of the calvaria in the rat; the determination of osseous morphology. *Am J Anat* 94:333, 1954.
6. Enlow D. Growth and architecture of the face. *J Am Dent Assoc* 82:763, 1971.
7. Hirabayashi S, Harii K, Sakuria, Takaki EK, Fukuda O. An experimental study of craniofacial growth in a heterotopic rat head transplant. *Plast Reconstr Surg* 82:236, 1988.
8. Price E, Simon JW, Calhoun JH. Prosthetic treatment of severe microphthalmos in in-

fancy. *J Pediatr Ophthalmol Strabismus* 23:22, 1986.

9. Soll DB. Evolution and current concepts in the surgical treatment of the anophthalmic orbit. *Ophthal Plast Reconstr Surg* 2:163, 1986.
10. Marchac D, Cophignon, J, Achard E, Dufourmentel C. Orbital expansion for anophthalmia and micro-orbitism. *Plast Reconstr Surg* 59:486, 1977.
11. Tessier P, Rougier J, Hervouet F, Woillez M, Lekieffre M, Derome P. Microphthalmias and congenital anophthalmias. In: *Plastic Surgery of the Orbit and Eyelids. Report of the French Society of Ophthalmology.* New York: Masson Publishing; 1977: pp. 184–190.
12. Todd TW, Beecher H, Williams et al. The weight and growth of the human eyelball. *Human Biol* 12:1, 1940.
13. Thomson WE. The determination of the influence of the eyeball on the growth of the orbit by experimental enucleation of one eye in young animals. *Trans Opthalmol Soc (UK)* 21:258, 1901.
14. Sarnat BG, Shanedling PD. Orbital volume following evisceration, enucleation, and exenteration in rabbits. *Am J Ophthalmol* 70: 787, 1970.
15. Sarnat BG, Shanedling PD. Orbital growth after evisceration or enucleation without or with implants. *Acta Anat* 82:497, 1972.
16. Taylor WOG. The effect of enucleation of one eye in childhood upon the subsequent development of the face. *Trans Ophthalmol Soc (UK)* 59:361, 1939.
17. Pfeiffer RL. The effect of enucleation on the orbit. *Trans Am Acad Ophthalmol* 49:236, 1945.
18. Osborne D, Harden OB, Deeming LW. Orbital growth after childhood enucleation. *Am J Ophthalmol* 77:756, 1974.
19. Lo AKM, Colcleugh RG, Allen L, Van Wyck LV, Bite U. The role of tissue expanders in an anophthalmic animals model. *Plast Reconstr Surg* 86:399, 1990.
20. Vistnes LM. The role of tissue expanders in an anophthalmic animal model (Discussion). *Plast Reconstr Surg* 86:409, 1990.
21. Buchman SR, Bartlett SP, Wormon III IL, Whitaker LA. The role of pressure on regulation of craniofacial bone growth. *J Craniofac Surg* 5:2, 1994.

CHAPTER 15B

Distraction of the Orbit

Robert G. Colcleugh

Microphthalmos may be either congenital or acquired and results in a small orbit and deformity of the associated skeletal and soft tissues (1,2). Absence of the eye eliminates the stimulus for orbital skeletal growth (1,3–5). In addition, enucleation and irradiation of the orbit have become standard treatment for retinoblastoma. The irradiated orbit fails to grow and often presents with hypoplasia of the associated facial skeletal parts (6,7). Treatment of the affected children using custom-fitted orbital conformers frequently results in extrusion of the prosthesis due to poor retention and the conformers do little to improve facial skeletal/soft tissue anatomy (8–10). Research at our laboratory led to the first reported study of an expander or distraction device in an anophthalmic orbit (11).

LABORATORY STUDIES

Two groups of 6-week-old kittens were studied. One group underwent enucleation of the right orbit while the other group had enucleation and insertion of a custom-made silastic expander in the right orbit (Figure 15B.1). In both groups, the unaffected left orbit served as a control. Every 14 days, 0.5 cc saline was injected into the device to a maximum volume of 5 cc. External horizontal and vertical orbital measurements were obtained weekly and plotted to document bony orbital growth (Figures 15B.2, 15B.3). The average difference in vertical and horizontal orbital measurements between the enucleated and the contralateral control orbit was −27 percent and −13 percent; the greatest change was observed in the vertical orbital dimension. The average differences in vertical and horizontal orbital

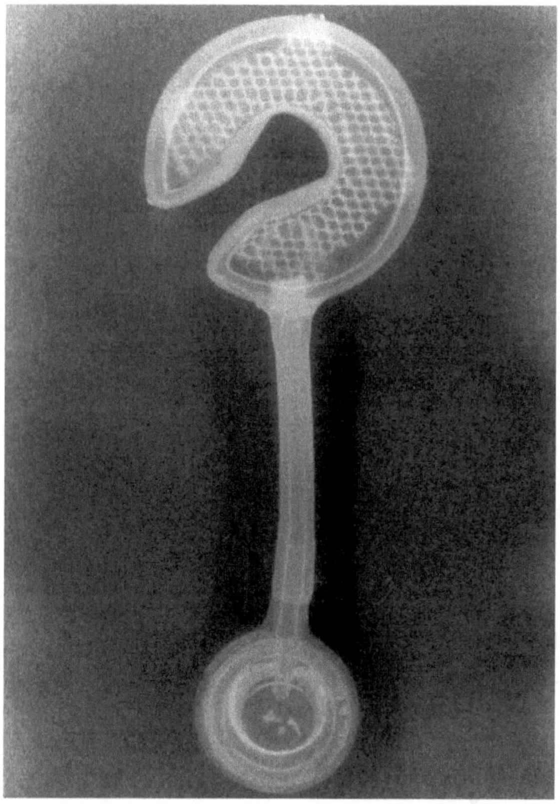

Figure 15B.1. Orbital expander.

measurement between the right expanded orbit and the contralateral control orbit were +4 percent and +2 percent.

Head CT scans were obtained preoperatively and at sacrifice (24 weeks of age) (Figures 15B.4, 15B.5). Dry-skull preparations demonstrated the effects of enucleation as well as distraction (Figure 15B.6). Orbital volumes were calculated from the head CT scans using "CT pac," a software program developed at the University of Western Ontario. Preoperative right and left orbital volumes were equal in both groups. In the enucleation-only group, the operated orbit showed an average decrease of 41 percent in volume when compared with the control orbit (significant at $p < 0.05$). In the enucleation and distracted group, the addition of the device resulted in equal volumes between the expanded and control orbits (−8% not significant at $p < 0.05$).

The dry-skull preparations showed orbital hypoplasia due to delay in lateral wall growth and lowering of the superior rim position as compared to the contralateral side. This study demonstrated that an expander was successful in maintaining normal orbital bony growth in the kitten enucleated orbital model.

The difficulties in dealing with radiation-induced orbital hypoplasia led to additional studies using the kitten-orbit model. The author studied the effects of a standardized dose of irradiation to a growing kitten-orbit model. The animals were anesthetized while head CT scans were obtained. Single beam radiotherapy of the right orbit was begun at 8 weeks of age delivering 500 cGy per treatment through a custom made gantry three times per week for a total of nine treatments (4500 cGy). This dose was calculated to be equivalent to that given a child with retinoblastoma. At 24 weeks the animals were sacrificed and repeat head CT scans obtained. Dry-skull preparations demonstrated that all orbital dimensions were adversely affected (Figure 15B.7). Analysis of orbital volumes in pretreatment and postirradiation animals showed an average difference of 25.3%. In the previous study with enucleation alone, there was an almost complete cessation of orbital growth, whereas in the irradiation model the globe continues to grow more slowly and this is reflected in orbital growth.

The use of an expander device in an irradiated-enucleated orbit was studied us-

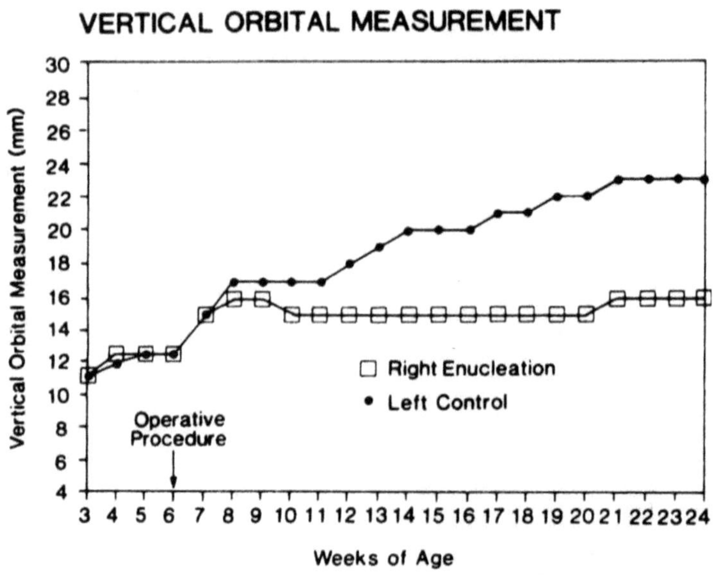

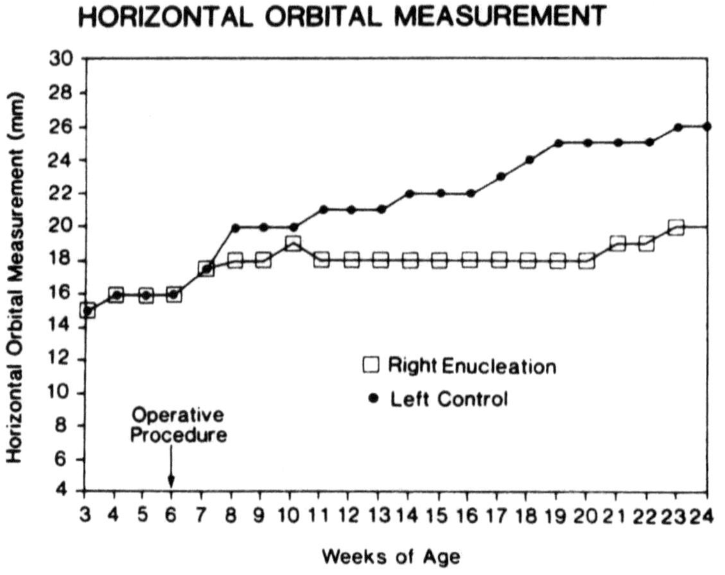

Figure 15B.2. Representative growth curves for Group 1 (enucleation only). (Top) vertical orbital measurement. (Bottom) horizontal orbital movement.

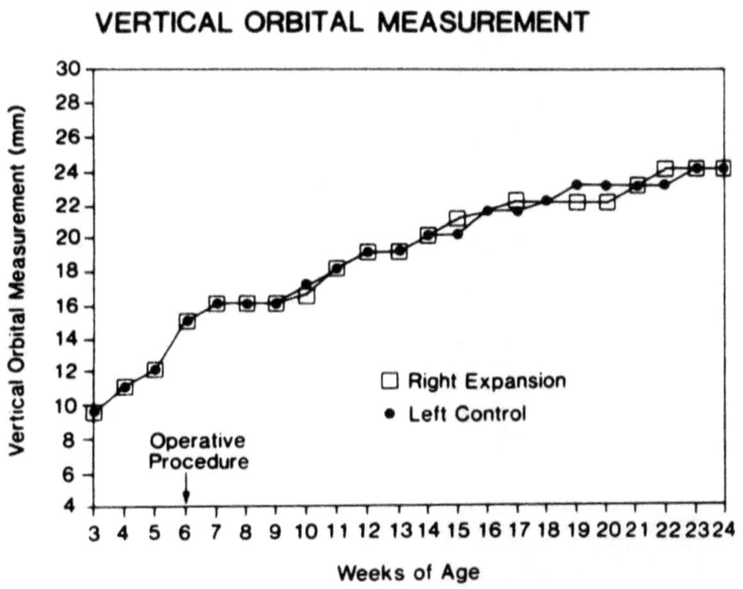

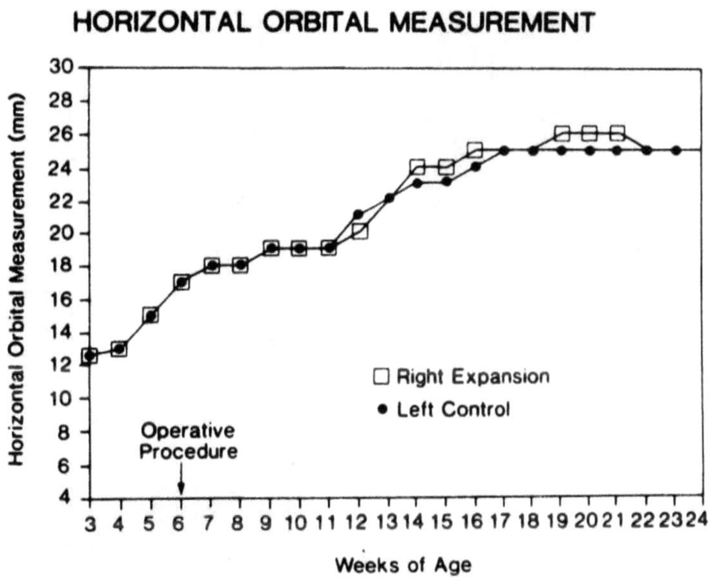

Figure 15B.3. Representative growth curves for Group 2 (enucleation and expansion). (Top) vertical orbital measurement. (Bottom) horizontal orbital measurement.

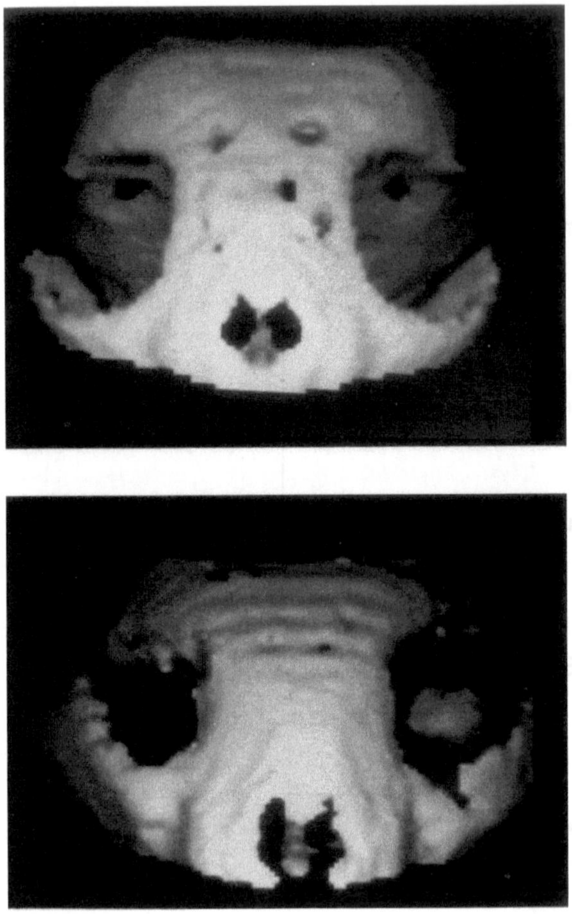

Figure 15B.4. Frontal CT scan (three-dimensional). (Top) preoperative. (Bottom) 24 weeks postenucleation on right side.

ing the kitten-orbit model in six animals. At 6 weeks of age the right orbit was enucleated and an expander placed subperiosteally within the orbit. Under sedation, 500 cGy of external beam radiation was delivered to the right orbit concomitant with expansion of 0.5 cc saline into the expander. Treatments resulted in a total of 4500 cGy over 18 days and an expansion to 5.0 cc over 16 weeks. Horizontal and vertical orbital measurements were obtained and the orbital volume calculated from pretreatment and posttreatment head CT scans. Averaged orbital volumes, comparing expanded-irradiated orbits before and after treatment to controls, showed no difference at the beginning and only a 7.9% difference at the time of sacrifice at 30 weeks (Figure 15B.8). This difference was not statistically significant. The orbital expander therefore appeared as a useful device in the treatment of the irradiated-enucleated orbit.

The mechanism of orbital tissue expansion was also studied in the kitten-orbit

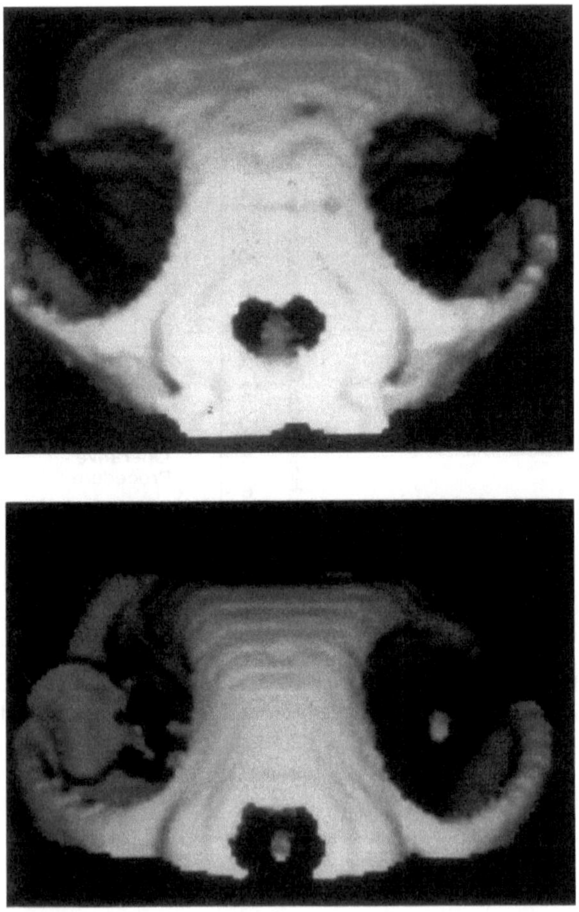

Figure 15B.5. Frontal CT scan (three-dimensional). (Top) preoperative. (Bottom) 24 weeks postexpansion on right side.

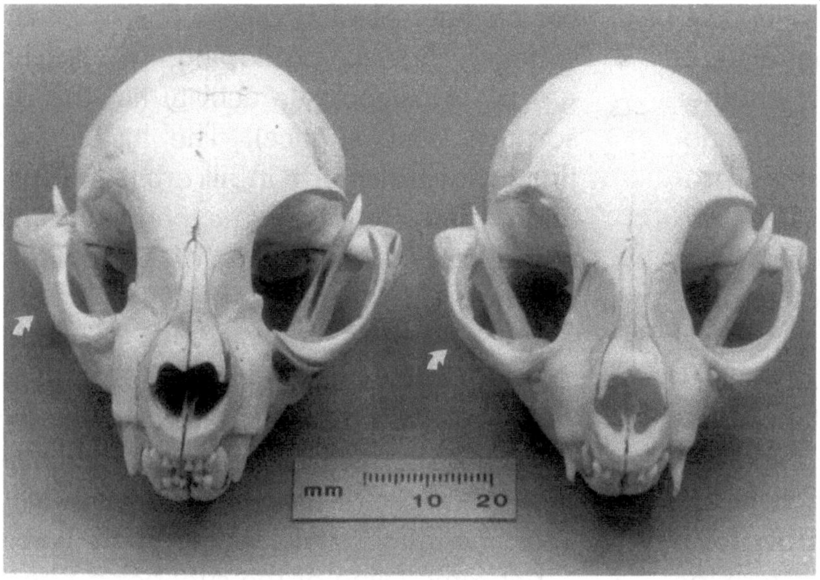

Figure 15B.6. Dry-skull preparations. (Left) effect of enucleation on right side. (Right) effect of enucleation on right side followed by expansion for 24 weeks.

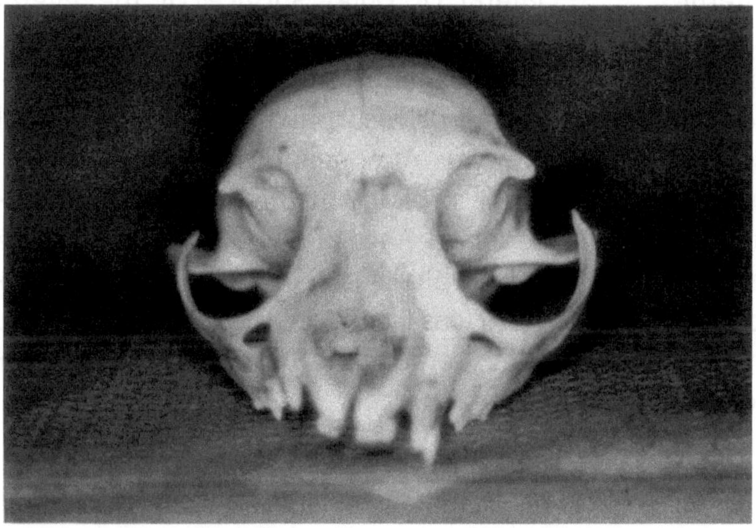

Figure 15B.7. Dry-skull preparation. Note the effect of enucleation and irradiation (generalized hypoplasia) on right side.

Averaged CT scan Orbital Volumes

	Enucleation - Irradiation	Control
At 6 wks	2.11 cc	2.11 cc
At 30 wks	*6.64 cc	7.21 cc

*7.9% difference between radiated expanded orbit and control orbit at 30 wks

Figure 15B.8. Averaged CT scan volumes of the control and manipulated orbits.

model. Groups of animals were enucleated on one side, with the contralateral orbit serving as a control, while another group underwent enucleation and subperiosteal placement. Expansion proceeded as in the original study (11). Two weeks prior to sacrifice, the animals were given two separate injections of tetracycline 6 days apart. At sacrifice, the orbital volumes were calculated and bone biopsies obtained from all four orbital rims.

As in previous studies, the expander was successful in maintaining normal orbital volumes, compared to control orbits. Bone histology was studied to determine the mechanism of orbital growth in the expanded and control orbits. Bone specimens from the superior, inferior, lateral, and medial orbital rim of each orbit were examined under high power magnification. Tetracycline was incorporated in areas of osteoblastic activity and its presence indicated a depository bone surface. This was seen as separate lines in the bone caused by the labeling of the tetracycline. The distance between the two lines represented the amount of new bone laid down between the two periods of injection (ie, an interval of 6 days). The opposite surface showed scalloping, a finding typical of osteoclastic activity (ie, the resorptive bone surface). The histological findings were similar in all orbits (enucleation and enucleation-expanded) and differed only in the rate of osteoblastic activity.

Superior orbital rim (Figure 15B.9): The superior rim demonstrated osteoblastic (depository) activity on the cranial surface and osteoclastic (resorptive) activity on the intraorbital surface. There was a net remodeling of the superior rim in a superior direction.

Lateral orbital rim (Figure 15B.10): The lateral or outer surface of the lateral orbital rim was actively osteoblastic, while the intraorbital surface was osteoclastic or resorptive. The lateral orbital rim was remodeling outward.

Inferior orbital rim (Figure 15B.11): Osteoblastic activity was evident on the intraorbital surface, while active resorption was seen on the maxillary sinus. Net remodeling was in a superior direction.

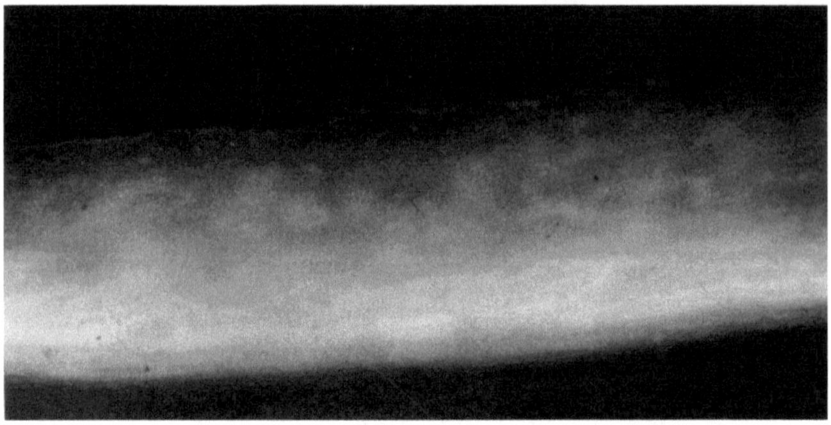

Figure 15B.9. Superior orbital rim. Note the osteoblastic activity on the cranial surface and osteoclastic activity on the intraorbital surface.

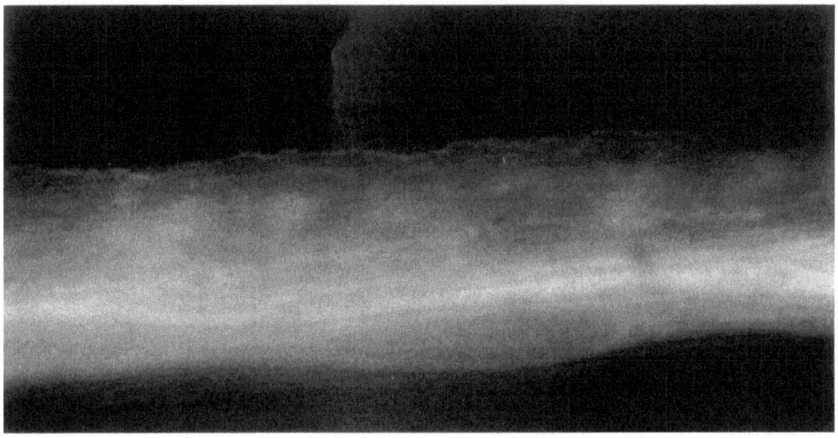

Figure 15B.10. Lateral orbital rim. Note the osteoblastic activity on the outer or temporal surface and the resorptive activity on the intraorbital surface.

Medial orbital rim (Figure 15B.12): Depository or osteoblastic activity was seen on the intraorbital surface, while the lateral nasal wall exhibited osteoclastic activity. The medial orbital wall was remodeling in a lateral direction.

Depository rates were calculated for all orbital rims and the groups compared. Because of the small sample size, only general conclusions can be made. In the enucleation-only group there was a trend toward a decrease in remodeling or growth in all dimensions, especially in the lateral portion of the orbit. The depository rate at the lateral orbital rim of the enucleated orbit was as low as 50% of the normal orbit. There was a decrease in the deposition rate of the superior rim, and this contributed to a net decrease in remodeling. At the medial and inferior orbital rims, the enucleated and the control orbits showed similar depository rates. Thus, the vertical orbital measurement was decreased in the enucleated orbit and the superior rim was lower than that of the contralateral side.

In the expansion group the depository rates of the superior and lateral rims were similar to those of the control orbits.

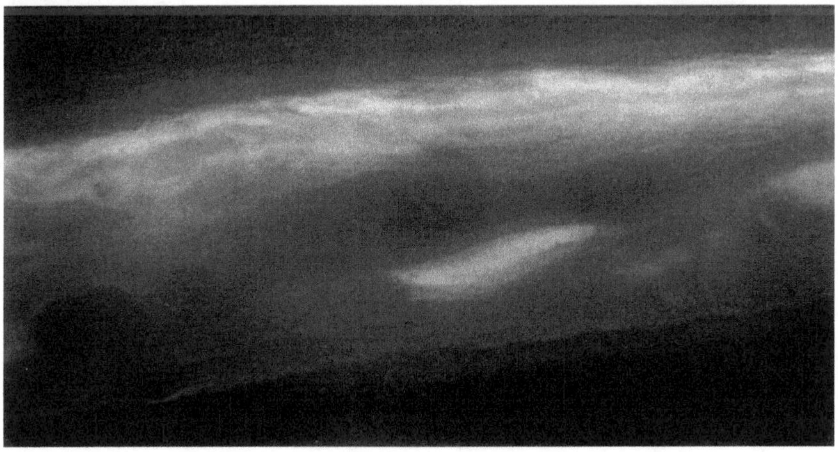

Figure 15B.11. Inferior orbital rim. Note the osteoblastic activity on the intraorbital surface and resorption on the maxillary sinus surface.

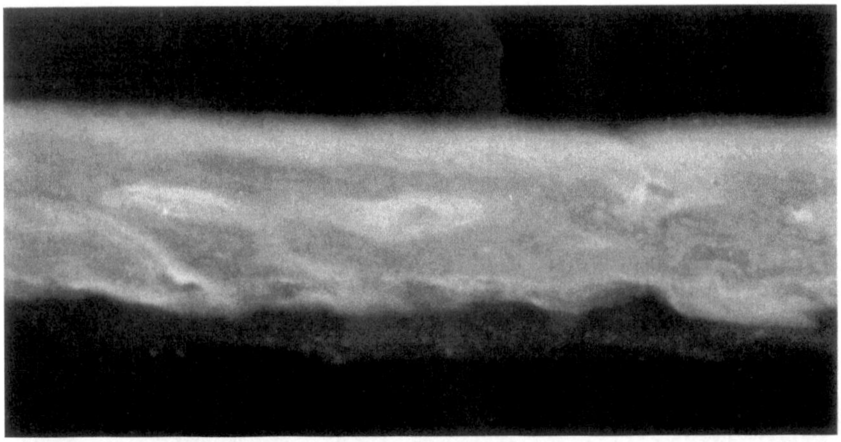

Figure 15B.12. Medial orbital rim. Note the osteoblastic activity on the intraorbital surface and the osteoclastic activity on the nasal side.

The main effect of the expander was to normalize the decreased growth of the lateral and superior orbital regions observed in the enucleation only orbits.

This study, therefore, helped to explain the mechanism of action that resulted in enlargement of the bony orbit. The device acts similarly to the normal growing eye by stimulating osteoblastic activity and bone remodeling. The major effect of the expander was on the lateral and superior orbital regions. Enucleation has little effect on the medial and inferior bony rims.

CLINICAL STUDIES

A 6-week-old male infant presented with right-sided microphthalmos associated with an orbitofacial cleft (Figure 15B.13). CT scan demonstrated severe bony hypoplasia. At 10 weeks of age the patient had an orbital expander device placed

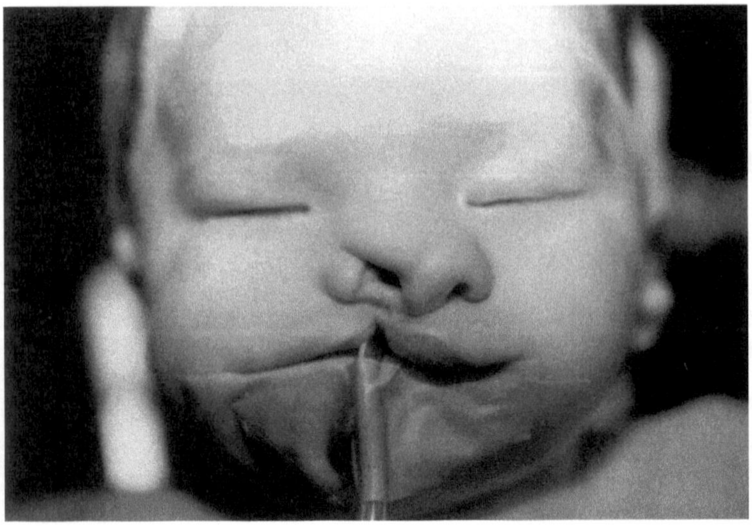

Figure 15B.13. A 6-week-old male infant with a right-sided naso-orbital cleft and microphthalmos.

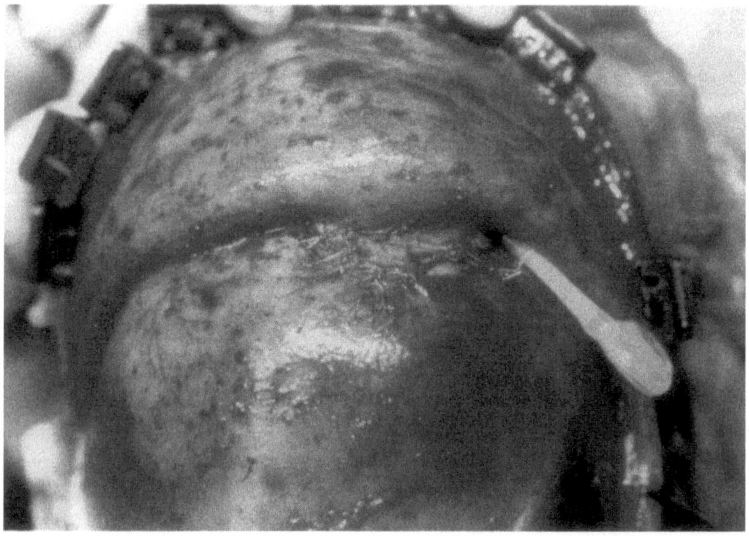

Figure 15B.14. Intraoperative view following the bicoronal approach. Note that the expander and port are in place (see Figure 15B.13).

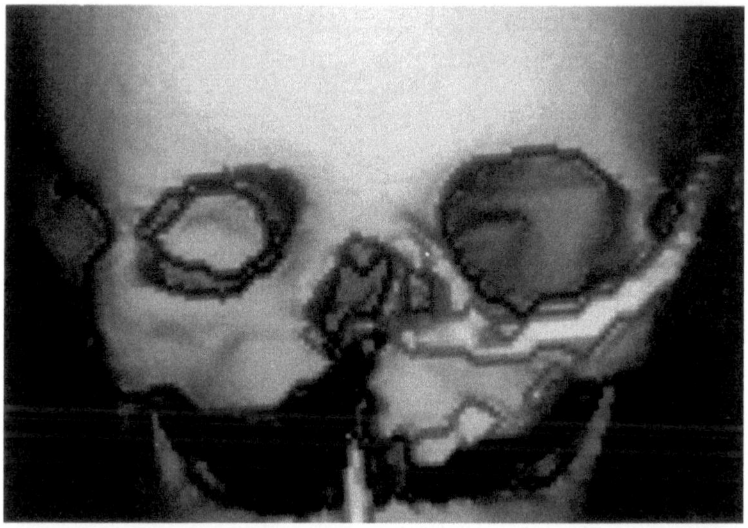

Figure 15B.15. Preoperative CT scan showing right-sided orbital hypoplasia. The naso-orbital cleft is also apparent (see Figure 15B.13).

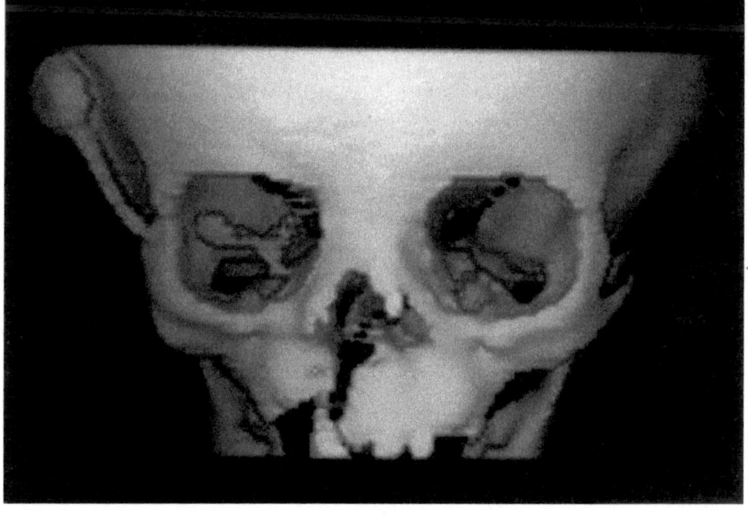

Figure 15B.16. Postoperative CT scan after expansion of the right orbit. Note that both orbits appear similar in size and configuration (see Figure 15B.13). The expander is also apparent.

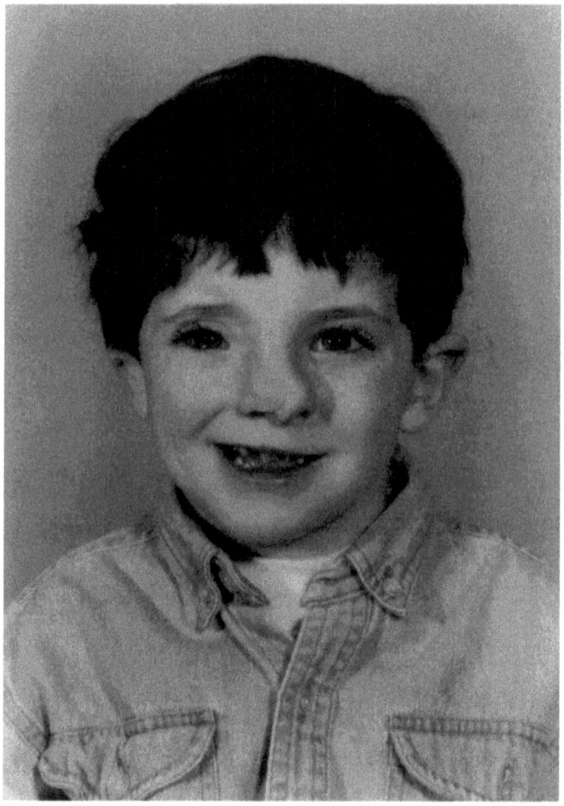

Figure 15B.19. The patient illustrated in Figure 15B.13 is shown 4 years after right orbital expansion. The cleft of the lip and nose has also been repaired.

Acknowledgments. The author wishes to acknowledge the assistance of the following: L. Allen, MBBCh, FRCS(C); A. Lo, MD, FRCS (C), C. Anderson, MD, FRCPath, FCAP, FRCP(C); M. Lacey, MD, FRCS (C); and S. Barr, MD, FRCS(C), all of London, Ontario Canada

References

1. Duke-Elder WS. *System of Ophthalmology, Vol. 3, Part 1: Embryology*, and *Part 3: Congenital Deformity*. London: Henry Kimpton, 1963.
2. Mann I. *Development Abnormalities of the Eye*. London: Cambridge University Press, 1985.
3. Kennedy RE. The effect of early enucleation on the orbit in animals and humans. *Trans Am Ophthalmol Soc* 62:459, 1964.
4. Barber AN. Embryology of the human eye. St. Louis: CV Mosby, 1955.
5. Van Limborgh J, Tonneyck-Muller I. Orbital growth pattern in experimental microphthalmia. *Mod Probl Ophthalmol* 14:1, 1975.
6. Guyuron B, Dagys PD, Munro IR, Ross RB. Effect of irradiation on facial growth: A 7- to 25-year follow-up. *Ann Plast Surg* 5:423, 1983.
7. Egawa S, Twukiyama I, Akine Y, Kajiura Y, Ogino T. Suppression of bony growth of the orbit after radiotherapy for retinoblastoma. *Radiat Med* 5:207, 1987.
8. Hartman DC. Anophthalmos and microphthalmos. In: Smith BC, Converse JM eds. *Proceedings of the Second International Symposium on Plastic and Reconstructive Surgery of the Eye and Adnexae*. St. Louis: CV Mosby, 1967.
9. Kiskadden WS, McDowell AJ, and Keiser T. Results of early treatment of congenital anophthalmos. *Plast Resonstr Surg* 4:426, 1949.
10. Steahly LP. Congenital anophthalmos: problems in management. *Trans Ophthalmos Soc UK* 98:28, 1978.
11. Lo AKM, Colcleugh RG, Allen L, Van Wyck L, Bite U. The role of tissue expanders in an anophthalmic animal model. *Plast Reconst Surg* 86:399, 1990.

Epilogue

Joseph G. McCarthy

> For I dipped into the future,
> far as the human eye could see,
> saw the vision of the world,
> and all the wonders that would be
> —Alfred Lord Tennyson

The future of craniofacial distraction lies in continued and vigorous clinical and laboratory research, involving not only surgeons, but other clinicians, bioengineers, and basic scientists. Such an interdisciplinary effort will ensure the refinement of the technique and its greater application.

I envision that there will be considerable innovation and improvement in the development and manufacture of distraction devices. For example, there will be commercial efforts at miniaturization that will permit intraoral distraction and therefore reduce the need for cutaneous scars. Multiplanar mechanisms will likewise be incorporated into the devices, and the surgeon will be able to control mandibular movement in a truly three-dimensional fashion. Miniaturized devices will also be developed for maxillary and mandibular distraction. Placed in a variety of anatomic positions and with sufficient strength to perform midface or maxillary movements, the devices will permit the surgeon to control large skeletal movements with the precision that the orthodontist currently employs in manipulating tooth position. Other anatomic areas that lend themselves to the distraction technique include the orbit for the correction of microphthalmos and the cranial vault for the correction of all of the abnormalities associated with craniosynostosis.

The bioengineer will develop motorized devices that permit remote control or activation of the devices by radio signals coordinated by a computer software program of the preoperative plan. Such a development will automate the period of activation and lessen the number of patient visits to the surgeon.

In the laboratory, the basic biomolecular mechanisms involved in membranous bone distraction will be elucidated. The critical cytokines and growth factors will be identified and their temporal interplay understood. The rewards will be enormous. For the first time, the surgeon will be able to manipulate the biology of bone distraction with a finesse unimaginable at the present time. Imagine what the application of various growth factors in proper sequence could do to permit acceleration of the distraction process at a rate exceeding 2mm per day. Likewise, this type of biologic manipulation would permit more rapid consolidation of the bony regenerate, thus shortening the entire treatment program to a period of less than one month. Similarly, the derived information could possibly allow distraction across sutures in the infant without even the need for osteotomies.

The information derived from the basic science laboratory could also allow the regeneration of onlay bone on hypoplastic portions of the craniofacial skeleton, thus replacing autogenous bone grafts or allografts and permitting, as an example, the augmentation of the zygoma in Treacher Collins syndrome.

As one looks to the future, the craniofacial surgeon will obviously be less interventive in the operating room. He will, however, be more involved in the postoperative manipulation of the bony regenerate. He will spend more time in the clinic than in the operating rooms. Bone graft harvesting will become a matter of surgical history and elaborate fixation systems will be displayed in museum exhibits. Blood banks will be necessary only for acute trauma cases.

The purpose of research is to reduce the amount of time spent by the surgeon in the operating room. The net result will be that the surgeon will have much more to offer the patient with craniofacial deformity, whether congenital, traumatic, or neoplastic in origin. It is the patient who will be the beneficiary of these efforts.

The Biomedical Research of Today Is the Clinical Medicine of Tomorrow; Without It, the Clinical Medicine of Tomorrow Will Be the Clinical Medicine of Today.

—James C. Thompson

BIBLIOGRAPHY

Craniofacial Distraction Osteogenesis

Altuna G, Walker DA, Freeman E: Surgically Assisted Rapid Orthodontic Lengthening of the Maxilla in Primates: A Pilot Study. *Am J Orthod Dentofac Orthops* 6:107, 1995.

Andrew JG, Hoyland JA, Freėmont AJ, Marsh DR: Platelet Derived Growth Factor Expression in Normally Healing Human Fractures. *Bone* 16:455, 1995.

Annino DJ Jr, Goguen LA, Karmody CS: Distraction Osteogenesis for Reconstruction of Mandibular Symphyseal Defects. *Arch Otolaryngol Head Neck Surg* 120:911, 1994.

Aronson J: Biology of Distraction Osteogenesis. In: Chapman, MW (ed). *Operative Orthopedics*. Philadelphia: JB Lippincott, 1993.

———: Experimental and Clinical Experience with Distraction Osteogenesis. *Cleft Palate Craniofac J* 31:473, 1994.

Barone CM, Ferder M, Jiminez DF, Grossman L, Hall C, Strauch B, Argamaso RV: Distraction of the Frontal Bone Outside the Cranial Plane: A Rabbit Model. *J Craniofac Surg* 4:177, 1993.

Bell WH, Harper RP, Gonzakz M, Cherkashin AM, Samchukov ML: Distraction Osteogenesis to Widen the Mandible. *Br J Oral Maxillofac Surg* 35:11, 1997.

Berry FD: A Modified Tissue Expander for Socket Enlargement in Clinical Anopthalmos. *Opthal Reconstr Surg* 7:41, 1991.

Block MS, Brister GD: Use of Distraction Osteogenesis for Maxillary Advancement: Preliminary Research. *J Oral Maxillofac Surg* 52:282, 1994.

Block MS, Cervini D, Chang A, Gottsegen GB: Anterior Maxillary Advancement Using Tooth Support Distraction Osteogenesis. *J Oral Maxillofac Surg* 53:561, 1995.

Block MS, Daire J, Stover J, Matthews M: Changes in the Inferior Alveolar Nerve Following Mandibular Lengthening in the Dog Using Distraction Osteogenesis. *J Oral Maxillofac Surg* 51:652, 1993.

Califano L, Cortese A, Zupi A, Tajana G: Mandibular Lengthening by External Distraction: Experimental Study in the Rabbit. *J Oral Maxillofac Surg* 52:1179, 1994.

Carls FR, Jackson IT, Topf JS: Distraction Osteogenesis for Lengthening of the Hard Palate: Part I. A Possible New Treatment Concept for Velopharyngeal Incompetence. Experimental Study in Dogs. *Plast Reconstr Surg* 100:1635, 1997.

Carls FR, Schupbach P, Sailer HF, Jackson IT: Distraction Osteogenesis for Lengthening of the Hard Palate: Part II. Histologic Study of the Hard and Soft Palate after Distraction. *Plast Reconstr Surg* 100:1648, 1997.

Chin M, Toth BA: Distraction Osteogenesis in Maxillofacial Surgery Using Internal Devices: Review of Five Cases. *J Oral Maxillofac Surg* 54:45, 1996.

Chin M, Toth BA: LeFort III Advancement with Gradual Distraction Using Internal Devices. *Plast Reconstr Surg* 100:819, 1997.

Cleall JF, Bayne DI, Posen JM, Subtelny JD: Expansion of the Midpalatal Suture in the Monkey. *Angle Orthod* 35:23, 1965.

Cohen SR, Boydston W, Burstein FD, Hudgins R: Monobloc Distraction Osteogenesis during Infancy. Report of a Case and Presentation of a New Device. *Plast Reconstr Surg* 101:1919, 1998.

Cohen SR, Burstein FD, Steward MB, Rathburn MA: Maxillary-Midface Distraction in Children with Cleft Lip and Palate: A Preliminary Report. *Plast Reconstr Surg* 99:1421, 1997.

Cohen SR, Rutrick RE, Burstein F: Distraction Osteogenesis of the Human Craniofacial Skeleton: Initial Experience with a New Distraction System. *J Craniofac Surg* 6:368, 1995.

Colcleugh RG, Allen L, Van Wyck L, Bite UL: Role of Tissue Expanders in an Anopthalmic Model. *Plast Reconstr Surg* 86:399, 1990.

Costantino PD, Friedman CD: Distraction Osteogenesis. Applications for Mandibular Regrowth. *Otolaryngol Clin North Am* 24:1433, 1991.

Costantino PD, Friedman CD, Shindo ML, Houston G, Sisson GA Sr: Experimental Mandibular Regrowth by Distraction Osteogenesis. Long-Term Results. *Arch Otolaryngol Head Neck Surg* 119:511, 1993.

Costantino PD, Shybut G, Friedman CD, Pelzer HJ, Masini M, Shindo ML, Sisson GA: Segmental Mandibular Regeneration by Distraction Osteogenesis. *Arch Otolaryngol Head Neck Surg* 116:535, 1990.

Corocoran J, Hubli EH, Salyer KE: Distraction Osteogenesis of Costochondral Neomandibles: A Clinical Experience. *Plast Reconstr Surg* 100:311, 1997.

Davidson MJ, Gullane PJ: Prosthetic Plate Mandibular Reconstruction. Management of Head and Neck Neoplasms. *Otolaryngol Clin North Am* 24:1419, 1991.

Diner PA, Kollar AEM, Martinez H, Vazquez MP: Submerged Intraoral Device for Mandibular Lengthening. *J Craniomaxillofac Surg* 25:116, 1997.

DoAmaral CM: Gradual Bone Distraction in Craniosynostosis. Preliminary Results in Seven Cases. *Scand J Plast Reconstr Surg Hand Surg* 31:2, 1997.

Ekstrom C, Henrikson CO, Jensen R: Mineralization in the Midpalatal Suture after Orthodontic Expansion. *Am J Orthod* 71:449, 1970.

Epply BL, Holley S, Sadove AM: Experimental Effects of Intraorbital Tissue Expansion on Orbital Growth in Anopthalmos. *Ann Plast Surg* 31:19, 1993.

Eydelshtein BM, Udalova F, Bochkarev GF: Dynamics of Reparative Regenerative Regeneration after Lengthening by the Method of Distraction Epiphysiolysis. *Acta Chir Plast* 15:149, 1973.

Fischer E, Staffenberg D, McCarthy JG, Miller DC, Zeng J: Histopathologic and Biochemical Changes in the Muscles Affected by Distraction Osteogenesis of the Mandible. *Plast Reconstr Surg* 99:366, 1997.

Friedrich RE, Hellner D, Plambeck K, Scmelzle R: Application of B-Scan Ultrasonography for Analysis of Callus Distraction in Vascularized Fibular Grafts of the Mandible: A Report of Three Patients. *J Oral Maxillofac Surg* 55:635, 1997.

Ganey TM, Klotch DW, Sasse J, Ogden JA: Basement Membrane of Blood Vessels During Distraction Osteogenesis. *Clin Orthop* 301:132, 1994.

Ganey TM, Klotch DW, Slater-Haase AS, Sasse J: Evaluation of Distraction Osteogenesis by Scanning Electron Microscopy. *Otolaryngol Head Neck Surg* 111:265, 1994.

Gantous A, Phillips JH, Catton P, Holmberg D: Distraction Osteogenesis in the Irradiated Canine Mandible. *Plast Reconstr Surg* 93:164, 1994.

Glat PM, Staffenberg DA, Karp NS, Holliday RA, Steiner G, McCarthy JG: Multidimentional Distraction Osteogenesis: The Canine Zygoma. *Plast Reconstr Surg* 94:753, 1994.

Guerrero C, Bell WH, Flores A, Modugno VL, Contasti G, Rodriguez AM, Meza L. Distraction Osteogenica Mandibular Intraoral. *Odontalal Dia* 10:116, 1995.

Guerrissi J, Ferrentino G, Margulies D, Fiz D: Lengthening of the Mandible by Distraction Osteogenesis: Experimental Work in Rabbits. *J Craniofac Surg* 5:314, 1994.

Guyette TW, Polley JW, Figueroa AA, Cohen MN: Mandibular Distraction Osteogenesis: Effects on Articulation and Velopharyngeal Function. *J Craniofac Surg* 7:186, 1996.

Haas AJ: Long-Term Posttreatment Evaluation of Rapid Palatal Expansion. *Angle Orthod* 50:189, 1980.

Habal MB: New Bone Formation by Biological Rhythmic Distraction. *J Craniofac Surg* 5:344, 1994.

Harper RP, Bell WH, Browne R, Cherkashin AM, Samchukov ML: Reactive Changes in the Temporomandibular Joint after Mandibular Midline Osteodistraction. *Br J Oral Maxillofac Surg* 35:20, 1997.

Havlik RJ, Bartlett SP: Mandibular Distraction Lengthening in the Severely Hypoplastic Mandible Problematic Case with Tongue Aplasia. *J Craniofac Surg* 5:305, 1994.

Hirakawa K, Hirota S, Ikeda T, Yamaguchi A, Takemura T, Nagoshi J, Yoshiki S, Suda T, Kitamura Nomura S: Localization of the mRNA for Bone Matrix Proteins During Fracture Healing as Determined in In Situ Hybridization. *J Bone Miner Res* 1551, 1994.

Ilizarov GA: The Principles of the Ilizarov Method. *Bull Hosp Joint Dis* 48:1, 1988.

Jonsson B, Siemssen SJ: Arced Segmental Mandibular Regeneration by Distraction Osteogenesis. *Plast Reconstr Surg* 101:1925, 1998.

Karaharju EO, Aalto K, Kahri A, Lindberg LA, Kallio T, Karaharju-Suvanto T, Vauhkonen M Pelton: Distraction Bone Healing. *Clin Orthop* 297:38, 1993.

Karaharju-Suvanto T: Cephalometric Changes after Gradual Lengthening of the Mandible: An Experimental Study in Sheep *Dento-Maxillo-Facial Radiology* 23:159, 1994.

Karaharju-Suvanto T, Karaharju EO, Ranta R: Mandibular Distraction. An Experimental Study on Sheep. *J Craniomaxillofac Surg* 18:280, 1990.

Karaharju-Suvanto T, Peltonen J, Kahri A, Karaharju EO: Distraction Osteogenesis of the Mandible. An Experimental Study on Sheep. *Int J Oral Maxillofac Surg* 21:118, 1992.

Karp NS, McCarthy JG, Schreiber JS, Sissons HA, Thorne CH: Membranous Bone Lengthening: A Serial Histological Study. *Ann Plast Surg* 29:2, 1992.

Karp NS, Thorne CH, McCarthy JG, Sissons HA: Bone Lengthening in the Craniofacial Skeleton. *Ann Plast Surg* 24:231, 1990.

Kim JW, Chin M, Cedars M: Distraction Osteogenesis and Its Application to the Midface and Bony Orbit in Craniosynostosis Syndromes. *J Craniofac Surg* 9:100, 1998.

Klein C, Howaldt HP: Lengthening of the Hypoplastic Mandible by Gradual Distraction in Children. A Preliminary Report. *J Craniomaxillofac Surg* 23:68, 1995.

———: Mandibular Distraction Osteogenesis as First Step in the Early Treatment of Severe Agnathia in Childhood. *Fortschr Kieferorthop* 57:46, 1996.

———: Correction of Mandibular Hypoplasia by Means of Bi-directional Craniofacial Distraction. *J Craniofac Surg* 7:258, 1996.

Klotch DW, Ganey TM, Slater-Haase A, Sasse J: Assessment of Bone Formation During Osteoneogenesis: A Canine Model. *Otolaryngol Head Neck Surg* 112:291, 1995.

Komuro Y, Takato T, Harii K, Yonemara Y: The Histologic Analysis of Distraction Osteogenesis of the Mandible in Rabbits. *Plast Reconstr Surg* 94:152, 1994.

Levine JP, Rowe NM, Bradley JP, Williams JK, Mackool RJ, Longaker MT, McCarthy JG: The Combination of Endoscopy and Distraction Osteogenesis in the Development of a Canine Midface Advancement Model. *J Craniofac Surg* 1998.

Lilakos JF, Tschakaloff A, Mooney MP, Losken HW, Siegel MI, Losken A, Reitz P, Wright M: Inter Calvarial Bone Distraction in Rabbits with Experimental Coronal Suture Immobilization

Effects of Overdistraction. *Plast Reconstr Surg* 96:689, 1995.

Liu SH, Yang RS, Al-Shaikh R, Lane JM: Collagen in Tendon, Ligament, and Bone Healing. *Clin Orthop* 318:265, 1995.

Losken A, Mooney MP, Siegal M: A Comparative Study of Mandibular Growth in Seven Animal Models. *J Oral Maxillofac Surg* 50:490, 1992.

Losken HW, Patterson GT, Lazarou SA, Whitney T: Planning Mandibular Distraction: Preliminary Report. *Cleft Palate Craniofac J* 32:71, 1995.

McCarthy JG: The Role of Distraction Osteogenesis in the Reconstruction of the Mandible in Unilateral Craniofacial Microsomia. *Clin Plast Surg* 21:31, 1994.

———: Mandibular Bone Lengthening. *Operative Tech Plastic Reconstr Surg* 1:99, 1994.

McCarthy JG, Schreiber J, Karp N, Thorne CH, Grayson BH: Lengthening of the Human Mandible by Gradual Distraction. *Plast Reconstr Surg* 89:1, 1992.

McCarthy JG, Staffenberg DA, Wood RJ, Cutting CB, Grayson BH, Thorne CH: Introduction of an Intraoral Lengthening Device. *Plast Reconstr Surg* 96:978, 1995.

McCarthy JG, Turk AE: Distraction Osteogenesis of the Cranial Skeleton: Mandibular Reconstruction. *Adv Plast Surg* 12:31, 1996.

McCarthy JG, Williams JK, Grayson BH: Controlled Multiplanar Distraction of the Mandible: Device Development and Clinical Application. *J Craniofac Surg* 1998.

McCormick SU: Reconstruction of the Mandibular Condyle Using Transport Distraction Osteogenesis. *J Craniofac Surg* 8:48, 1997.

McCormick SU, McCarthy JG, Grayson BH, Staffenberg D, McCormack SA: Effect of Mandibular Distraction on the Temporomandibular Joint: Part 1, Canine Study. *J Craniofac Surg* 6:358, 1995.

——: Effect of Mandibular Distraction on the Temporomandibular Joint: Part 2, Clinical Study. *J Craniofac Surg* 6:364, 1995.

Molina F, Ortiz-Monasterio F: Mandibular Elongation and Remodeling by Distraction: A Farewell to Major Osteotomies. *Plast Reconstr Surg* 96:825, 1995.

Movassaghi K, Altobelli DE, Zhou H: Frontonasal Suture Expansion in the Rabbit Using Titanium Screws. *J Oral Maxillofac Surg* 53:1033, 1995.

Murray J, Cleal JF: Early Tissue Response to Rapid Maxillary Expansion in the Midpalatal Suture of Rhesus Monkey. *J Dent Res* 50:1654, 1971.

Ortiz-Monasterio F, Molina F, Andrade L, Rodriguez C, Arregui JS: Simultaneous Mandibular and Maxillary Distraction in Hemifacial Microsomia in Adults: Avoiding Occlusal Disasters. *Plast Reconstr Surg* 100:852, 1997.

Pensler JM, Goldberg DP, Lindell B, Carroll NC: Skeletal Distraction of the Hypoplastic Mandible. *Ann Plast Surg* 34:6, discussion 136, 1995.

Perrott DH, Berger R, Vargervik K, Kaban LB: Use of a Skeletal Distraction Device to Widen the Mandible: A Report. *J Oral Maxillofac Surg* 51:435, 1993.

Persing JA, Babler WJ, Nagorsky MJ, Edgerton MT, Jane JA: Skull Expansion in Experimental Craniosynostosis. *Plast Reconstr Surg* 78:594, 1986.

Persing JA, Morgan EP, Cronin AJ, Wolcott WP: Skull Base Expansion: Craniofacial Effects. *Plast Reconstr Surg* 87:1028, 1991.

Polley JW, Figueroa AA: Management of Severe Maxillary Deficiency in Childhood and Adolescence Through Distraction Osteogenesis with an External, Adjustable, Rigid Distraction Device. *J Craniofac Surg* 8:181, 1997.

Prechter TK, Sarnat BG: Comparison of Direct and Indirect Determinations of Rabbit Orbital Volume. *Morphol Nether Scand* 11:151, 1973.

Rachmiel A, Jackson IT, Potparic Z, Laufer D: Midface Advancement in Sheep by Gradual Distraction. *J Oral Maxillofac Surg* 53:525, 1995.

Rachmiel A, Levy M, Laufer D: Lengthening of the Mandible by Distraction Osteogenesis: Report of Cases. *J Maxillofac Surg* 53:838, 1995.

Rachmiel A, Potparic Z, Jackson IT, Sugihara T, Clayman L, Topf JS: Midface Advancement by Gradual Distraction. *Br J Plast Surg* 46:201, 1993.

Remmler D, McCoy FJ, O'Neil D, Willoughby L, Patterson B, Gerald K, Morris DC: Osseous Expansion of the Cranial Vault by Craniostasis *Plast Reconstr Surg* 89:787, 1992.

Roth DA, Gosain AK, McCarthy JG, Strachor MA, Lefton DR, Graupon BH: A CT Scan Technique for Quantitative Volumetric Assessment of the Mandible after Distraction Osteogenesis. *Plast Reconstr Surg* 99:1237, 1997.

Sarnat BG, Shanedling PD: Increased Orbital Volume after Periodic Intrabulbar Injections of Silicon in Growing Rabbits *Am J Anat* 140:523, 1974.

Sawaki Y, Ohkubo H, Hibi HU: Mandibular Lengthening by Distraction Osteogenesis Using Osseointegrated Implants. An Intraoral Device: A Preliminary Report. *J Oral Maxillofac Surg* 54:594, 1996.

Schmelzeinsen R, Neumann G, von der Fecht R: Distraction Osteogenesis in the Mandible with a Motor-Driven Plate: A Preliminary Animal Study. *Br J Oral Maxillofac Surg* 34:375, 1996.

Snyder CC, Levine GA, Swanson HM, Browne EZ Jr: Mandibular Lengthening by Gradual Distraction. Preliminary Report. *Plast Reconstr Surg* 51:506, 1973.

Staffenberg DA, Wood RJ, McCarthy JG, Grayson BH, Glasberg SB: Midface Distraction Advancement in the Canine Without Osteotomies. *Ann Plast Surg* 34:512, 1995.

Stewart KJ, Lvoff GO, White SA, Bonar SF: Mandibular Distraction Osteogenesis: A Comparison of Distraction Rates in a Rabbit Model. *J Craniomaxillofac Surg* 26:43, 1998.

Sugawara Y, Hirabayashi S, Sakurai A, Haari K: Gradual Cranial Vault Expansion for the Treatment of Craniofacial Synostosis: A Preliminary Report. *Ann Plast Surg* 40:554, 1998.

Takato T, Harii K, Hirabayashi S, Komuro Y, Yonehara Y, Susami T: Mandibular Lengthening by Gradual Distraction: Analysis Using Accurate Skull Replicas. *Br J Plast Surg* 46:686, 1993.

Ten Cate AR, Freeman E, Dickinson JB: Sutural Development. Structure and Its Response to Rapid Expansion. *Am J Orthod* 71:622, 1977.

Tscakaloff A, Losken HW, Mooney MP, Siegel MI, Losken A, Swan J: Internal Calvarial Bone Distraction in Rabbits with Experimental Coronal Suture Immobilization *J Craniofac Surg* 5:318, 1994.

Weil TS, VanSickels JE, Payne CJ: Distraction Ostogenesis for Correction of Transverse Mandibular Deficiency: A Preliminary Report. *J Oral Maxillofac Surg* 55:953, 1997.

Yamamoto H, Sawaki Y, Ohkubo H, Ueda M: Maxillary Advancement by Distraction Osteogenesis Using Osseointegrated Implants. *J Cranio-Maxillo-Fac Surg* 25:186, 1997.

Endochondral Distraction Osteogenesis

Aaron AD, Eilert RE: Results of the Wagner and Ilizarov Methods of Limb Lengthening. *J Bone Joint Surg Am* 78:20, 1996.

Abbot LC: Operative Lengthening of the Tibia and Fibula. *J Bone Joint Surg* 9:128, 1927.

Ahmadi B, Akbarnia BA, Ghobadi F, Ganjavian MS, Nasseri D: Experience with 141 Tibial Lengthening in Poliomyelitis and Comparison of 3 Different Methods. *Clin Orthop* 145:150, 1979.

Aldegheri R, Renzi-Brivio L, Agostini S: Callotasis Method of Limb Lengthening. *Clin Orthop* 241:137, 1989.

Aldegheri R, Trivella G, Lavini F: Epiphyseal Distraction. Chondrodiastasis. *Clinical Orthop* 241:117, 1989.

Aldegheri R, Trivella G, Lavini F: Epiphyseal Distraction. Hemichondrodiastasis. *Clin Orthop* 241:128, 1989.

Aldegheri R, Trivella G, Renzi-Brivio L, Tessari G, Agostini S, Lavini F: Lengthening of the Lower Limbs in Achondroplastic Patients. A Comparative Study of Four Techniques. *J Bone Joint Surg Br* 70:69, 1988.

Alho A, Bang G, Karaharju E, Armond I: Filling of a Bone Defect During Experimental Osteotaxis Distraction. *Acta Orthop Scand* 53:29, 1982.

Amstutz HC, Sakai DN: Symposium. Equalization of Leg Length. *Clin Orthop* 136:1, 1978.

Anderson WV: Lengthening of the Lower Limb: Its Place in the Problem of Limb Length Discrepancy. *Mod Trends Orthop* 5:1, 1972.

Aronson J: Temporal and Spatial Increases in Blood Flow During Distraction Osteogenesis. *Clin Orthop* 301:124, 1994.

Aronson J, Good B, Stewart C, Harrison B, Harp J: Preliminary Studies of Mineralization During Distraction Osteogenesis. *Clin Orthop* 250:43, 1990.

Aronson J, Harp JH: Mechanical Forces as Predictors of Healing During Tibial Lengthening by Distraction Osteogenesis. *Clin Orthop* 301:73, 1994.

Aronson J, Harrison B, Boyd CM, Cannon DJ, Lubansky HJ: Mechanical Induction of Osteogenesis: The Importance of Pin Rigidity. *J Pediatr Orthop* 8:396, 1988.

Aronson J, Harrison BH, Stewart CL, Harp JH Jr: Histology of Distraction Osteogenesis Using Different External Fixators. *Clin Orthop* 241:106, 1989.

Aronson J, Johnson E, Harp JH, Local Bone Transportation for Treatment of Intercalary Defects by the Ilizarov Technique. *Clin Orthap* 243:71, 1989.

Aronson J, Shen X: Experimental Healing of Distraction Osteogenesis Comparing Metaphyseal with Diaphyseal Sites. *Clin Orthop* 301:25, 1994.

Ascani E, Giglio GC, Crostelli M, Gasbarra E: Biomechanical Problems, Axial Deviation and Functional Recovery in Extensive Limb Lengthening. *Basic Life Sci* 48:373, 1988.

Bell DF, Boyer MI, Armstrong PF: Use of the Ilizarov Technique in the Correction of Limb Deformities Associated with Skeletal Dysplasia. *J Pediatr Orthop* 12:283, 1992.

Bjerkreim I: Limb Lengthening by Physeal Distraction. *Acta Orthop Scand* 60:140, 1989.

Blackstone BG, Coleman SS: Treatment of Lower Limb Length Inequality. [Review] *Surg Annu* 16:259–296, 1984.

Bonnard C, Favard L, Sollogoub I, Glorion B: Limb Lengthening in Children Using the Ilizarov Method. *Clin Orthop* 293:83, 1993.

Bourque WT, Gross M, Hall BK: A Reproducible Method for Producing and Quantifying the Stages of Fracture Repair. *Lab Anim Sci* 42:369, 1992.

Bowen JR, Levy EJ, Donohue M: Comparison of Knee Motion and Callus Formation in Femoral Lengthening with the Wagner or Monolateral-Ring Device. *J Pediatr Orthop* 13:467, 1993.

Brutscher R, Rahn BA, Ruter A, Perren SM: Role of Corticotomy and Osteotomy in the Treatment of Bone Defects Using the Ilizarov Technique. *J Orthop Trauma* 7:261, 1993.

Canadell J, de Pablos J: Pamplona, Spain: Correction of Angular Deformities by Physeal Distraction. [Review] *Clin Orthop* 283:98, 1992.

Canadell J, Forriol F, Cara JA: Removal of Metaphyseal Bone Tumors with Preservation of the Epiphysis. Physeal Distraction Before Excision. *J Bone Joint Surg Br* 76:127, 1994.

Catagni MA: Management of Fibular Hemimelia Using the Ilizarov Method. *Instr Course Lect* 41:431, 1992.

Catagni MA, Bolano L, Cattaneo R: Management of Fibular Hemimelia Using the Ilizarov Method. *Orthop Clin North Am* 22:715, 1991.

Cattaneo R, Villa A, Catagni M, Tentori L: Limb Lengthening in Achondroplasia by Ilizarov's Method. *Int Orthop* 12:173, 1988.

———: Strategies for Limb Lengthening in Achondroplasia Using the Ilizarov Method—The Experience of the Hospital of Lecco, Italy. *Basic Life Sci* 48:381, 1988.

Chacha PB, Chong KC: Experience with Tibial Lengthening in Singapore. *Clin Orthop* (125):100, 1977.

Chadha DJ, Malde HM: Ultrasonography of Postosteotomy "Cysts." *Can Assoc Radiol J* 45:20, 1994.

Chandler D, King JD, Bernstein SM, Marrero G, Koh J, Hambrecht H: Results of 21 Wagner Limb Lengthenings in 20 Patients. *Clin Orthop* 230:214, 1988.

Chuang TY, Chan RC, Chin LS, Hsu TC: Neuromuscular Injury During Limb Lengthening: A Longitudinal Follow-Up by Rabbit Tibial Model. *Arch Phys Med Rehab* 76:467, 1995.

Codivilla A: On the Means of Lengthening in the Lower Limbs, the Muscles and Tissues Which Are Shortened Through Deformity. *Am J Orthop Surg* 2:353, 1905.

Coleman SS: Current Concepts of Tibial Lengthening. *Orthop Clin North Am* 3:201, 1972.

———: Simultaneous Femoral and Tibial Lengthening for Limb Length Discrepancies. *Arch Orthop Trauma Surg* 103:359, 1985.

———: Equalization of Lower-Limb Inequality by Lengthening. [Review] *Instr Course Lect* 38:317, 1989.

Coleman SS, Stevens PM: Tibial Lengthening. *Clin Orthop* 136:92, 1978.

Colville J, MacAuley P: Leg Lengthening: A Clinical Review of 45 Cases. *Ir Med J* 71:42, 1978.

Dahl MT, Fischer DA: Lower Extremity Lengthening by Wagner's Method and by Callus Distraction. *Orthop Clin North Am* 22:643, 1991.

Dal Monte A, Donzelli O: Tibial Lengthening According to Ilizarov in Congenital Hypoplasia of the Leg. *J Pediatr Orthop* 7:135, 1987.

———: Techniques and Complications in Extensive Limb Lengthening. *Basic Life Sci* 48:403, 1988.

Damsin JP, Pous JG, Ghanem I: Therapeutic Approach to Severe Congenital Lower Limb Length Discrepancies: Surgical Treatment versus Prosthetic Management. *J Pediatr Orthop* Part B. 4:164, 1995.

Daniel BL, Waanders NA, Zhang Y, Moskalik A, Fowlkes JB, Rubin JM, Goulet JA, Adler RS: Use of Ultrasound Mean Acoustic Attenuation to Quantify Bone Formation During Distraction Osteogenesis Performed by the Ilizarov Method. Preliminary Results in Five Dogs. *Investig Radiol* 29:933, 1994.

Datiashvili RO: Simultaneous Replantation of Both Lower Legs in a Child: A Long-Term Result. *Plast Reconstr Surg* 91:541, 1993.

De Bastiani G, Aldegheri R, Brivio LR, Trivella G: Chondrodiastasis—Controlled Symmetrical Distraction of the Epiphyseal Plate. *J Bone Jt Surg* 68:550, 1986.

———: Limb Lengthening by Distraction of the Epiphyseal Plate. *J Bone Joint Surg* 68:545, 1986.

De Bastiani G, Aldegheri R, Renzi-Brivio L, Trivella G: Limb Lengthening by Callus Distraction (Callotasis). *J Pediatr Orthop* 7:129, 1987.

De Bastiani G, Aldegheri R, Trivella G, Renzi-Brivio L, Agostini S, Lavini F: Lengthening of the Lower Limbs in Achondroplastics. *Basic Life Sci* 48:353, 1988.

De Pablos J, Canadell J: Experimental Physeal Distraction in Immature Sheep. *Clin Orthop* 250:73, 1990.

de Sanctis N, Razzano E, Scognamiglio R, Rega AN: Tibial Agenesis: A New Rationale In Management of Type II—Report of Three Cases with Long-Term Follow-Up. *J Pediatr Orthop* 10:198, 1990.

Delloye C, Delefortrie G, Coutelier L, Vincent A: Bone Regenerate Formation in Cortical Bone During Distraction Lengthening. An Experimental Study. *Clin Orthop* 250:34, 1990.

Dillaman RM, Wilbur KM, Crenshaw MA: Growth of Embryonic Chick Tibiae In Ovo and In Vitro: A Scanning Electron Microscope Study. *Calcif Tissue Int* 27:33, 1979.

Eckardt JJ, Safran MR, Eilber FR, Rosen G, Kabo JM: Expandable Endoprosthetic Reconstruction of the Skeletally Immature after Malignant Bone Tumor Resection. *Clin Orthop* 297:188, 1993.

Edwards DJ, Bickerstaff DB, Bell MJ: Periosteal Stripping in Achondroplastic Children. Little Effect on Limb Length in 10 Cases. *Acta Orthop Scand* 65:333, 1994.

Eldridge JC, Armstrong PF, Krajbich JI: Amputation Stump Lengthening with the Ilizarov Technique. A Case Report. *Clin Orthop* 256:76, 1990.

Elkins AD, Zembo M, Holmes R: Radiographic Analysis of Regenerate Formation Following Tibial Distraction Osteosynthesis by the Method of Ilizarov with a Cricular External Fixator in a Canine Model. *J Invest Surg* 4:295, 1991.

Eyres KS, Bell MJ, Kanis JA: Methods of Assessing New Bone Formation During Limb Lengthening. Ultrasonography, Dual Energy X-Ray Absorptiometry and Radiography Compared. *J Bone Joint Surg Br* 75:358, 1993.

———: New Bone Formation During Leg Lengthening. Evaluated by Dual Energy X-Ray Absorptiometry. *J Bone Joint Surg Br* 75:96, 1993.

Faber FW, Keessen W, Van Roermund PM: Complications of Leg Lengthening. 46 Procedures in 28 Patients. *Acta Orthop Scand* 62:327, 1991.

Fischgrund J, Paley D, Suter C: Variables Affecting Time to Bone Healing During Limb Lengthening. *Clin Orthop* 301:31, 1994.

Fishbane BM, Riley LH Jr: Continuous Transphyseal Traction: Experimental Observations. *Clin Orthop* 136:120, 1978.

Fjeld TO, Steen H: Limb Lengthening by Low Rate Epiphyseal Distraction. An Experimental Study in the Canine Tibia. *J Orthop Res* 6:360, 1988.

———: Growth Retardation after Experimental Limb Lengthening by Epiphyseal Distraction. *J Pediatr Orthop* 10:463, 1990.

Fjeld TO, Steen H: Limb Lengthening by Epiphyseal Distraction in Chondrodystrophic Bone: An Experimental Study in the Canine Femur. *J Orthop Res* 7:184, 1989.

Fontanesi G, Giancecchi F, Rotini R: Segmental Shortening and Equalization for Leg Length Discrepancies in Adults. *It J Orthop Traumat* 13:45, 1987.

Fowler JL, Gie GA, Maceachern AG: Upper Tibial Valgus Osteotomy Using a Dynamic External Fixator. *J Bone Joint Surg Br* 73:690, 1991.

Frierson M, Ibrahim K, Boles M, Bote H, Ganey T: Distraction Osteogenesis. A Comparison of Corticotomy Techniques. *Clin Orthop* 301:19, 1994.

Galardi G, Comi G, Lozza L, Marchettini P, Novarina M, Facchini R, Paronzini A: Peripheral Nerve Damage During Limb Lengthening. Neurophysiology in Five Cases of Bilateral Tibial Lengthening. *J Bone Joint Surg Br* 72:121, 1990.

Ganel A, Horoszowski H, Kamhin M, Farine I: Leg Lengthening in Achondroplastic Children. *Clin Orthop* 144:194, 1979.

Giglio GC, Pagnotta G, Caterini R: Neurological Complications Arising in Bilateral Lengthening of the Tibiae in an Achondroplastic Subject. *Basic Life Sci* 48:325, 1988.

Green SA: Ilizarov Method: Rancho Technique. *Orthop Clin North Am* 22:677, 1991.

Green SA, Harris NL, Wall DM, Ishkanian J, Marinow H: Racho Mounting Technique for the Ilizarov Method. A Preliminary Report. *Clin Orthop* 280:104, 1992.

Grundnes O, Reikeras O: Blood Flow and Mechanical Properties of Healing Bone. Femoral Osteotomies Studied in Rats. *Acta Orthop Scand* 63:487, 1992.

———: Role of Hematoma and Periosteal Sealing for Fracture Healing in Rats. *Acta Orthop Scand* 64:47, 1993.

Guichet JM, Spivak JM, Trouilloud P, Grammont PM: Lower Limb-Length Discrepancy. An Epidemiologic Study. *Clin Orthop* 272:235, 1991.

Hamanishi C, Yasuwaki Y, Kikuchi H, Tanaka S, Tamura K: Classification of the Callus in Limb Lengthening. Radiographic Study of 35 Limbs. *Acta Orthop Scand* 63:430, 1992.

Hamanishi C, Yoshii T, Tanaka S: Maturation of the Distracted Callus; Sonographic Observations in Rabbits Applied to Patients. *Acta Orthop Scand* 65:335, 1994.

Hamanishi C, Yoshii T, Totani Y, Tanaka S: Bone Miner Density of Lengthened Rabbit Tibia Is Enhanced by Transplantation of Fresh Autologous Bone Marrow Cells. An Experimental Study Using Dual X-Ray Absorptiometry *Clin Orthop* 303:250, 1994.

———: Lengthened Callus Activated by Axial Shortening. Histological and Cytomorphometrical Analysis. *Clin Orthop* 307:250, 1994.

Hamdy RC, Walsh W, Olmedo M, Wallach M, Ehrlich MG: Correlation Between Ultrasound Imaging and Mechanical and Physical Properties of Lengthened Bone: An Experimental Study in a Canine Model. *J Pediatr Orthop* 15:206, 1995.

Hang YS, Shih JS: Tibial Lengthening: A Preliminary Report. *Clin Orthop* 125:94, 1977.

Hardy JM, Tadlaoui A, Wirotius JM, Saleh M: Sequoia Circular Fixator for Limb Lengthening. *Orthop Clin North Am* 22:663, 1991.

Harp JH, Aronson J, Hollis M: Noninvasive Determination of Bone Stiffness for Distraction Osteogenesis by Quantitative Computed Tomography Scans. *Clin Orthop* 301:42, 1994.

Herring JA, Coleman SS: Femoral Lengthening. *J Pediatr Orthop* 2:432, 1982.

Herzenberg JE, Smith JD, Paley D: Correcting Torsional Deformities with Ilizarov's Apparatus. *Clin Orthop* 302:36, 1994.

Herzenberg JE, Waanders NA: Calculating Rate and Duration of Distraction for Deformity Correction with the Ilizarov Technique. *Orthop Clin North Am* 22:601, 1991.

Hood RW, Riseborough EJ: Lengthening of the Lower Extremity by the Wagner Method. A Review of the Boston Children's Hospital Experience. *J Bone Joint Surg Am* 63:1122, 1981.

Hootnick D, Boyd NA, Fixsen JA, Lloyd-Roberts GC: Natural History and Management of Congenital Short Tibia with Dysplasia or Absence of the Fibula. *J Bone Joint Surg Br* 59:267, 1977.

Hope PG, Crawfurd EJ, Catterall A: Bone Growth Following Lengthening for Congenital Shortening of the Lower Limb *J Pediatri Orthop* 14:339, 1994.

Hrutkay JM, Eilert RE: Operative Lengthening of the Lower Extremity and Associated Psychological Aspects: The Children's Hospital Experience. *J Pediatr Orthop* 10:373, 1990.

Hughes SS, Hicks DG, O'Keefe RJ, Hurwitz SR, Crabb ID, Krasinskas AM, Loveys L, Puzas JE, Rosier RN: Shared Phenotypic Expression of Osteoblasts and Chondrocytes in Fracture Callus. *J Bone Miner Res* 10:533, 1995.

Hughes TH, Maffulli N, Fixsen JA: Ultrasonographic Appearance of Regenerate Bone in Limb Lengthening. *J Royal Soc Med* 86:18, 1993.

Ilizarov GA: Principles of the Ilizarov Method. *Bull Hosp Joint Dis* 48:1, 1988.

———: Tension-Stress Effect on the Genesis and Growth of Tissues. *Clin Orthop* 238:241, 1989.

———: Tension-Stress Effect on the Genesis and Growth of Tissues. Part II. The Influence of the Rate and Frequency of Distraction. *Clin Othop* 239:263, 1989.

———: Clinical Application of the Tension-Stress Effect for Limb Lengthening. [Review Article] *Clin Orthop* 250:8, 1990.

Ilizarov GA, Devyatov AA, Kamerin VK: Plastic Reconstruction of Longitudinal Bone Defects by Means of Compression and Subsequent Distraction. *Acta Chir Plast* 22:32, 1980.

Kaljumae U, Martson A, Haviko T, Hanninen O: Effect of Lengthening of the Femur on the Extensors of the Knee. *J Bone Joint Surg* 77:247, 1995.

Karaharju EO, Aalto K, Kahri A, Lindberg LA, Kallio T, Karaharju-Suvanto T, Vauhkonen M, Peltonen J: Distraction Bone Healing. *Clin Orthop* 297:38, 1993.

Karger C, Guille JT, Bowen JR: Lengthening of Congenital Lower Limb Deficiencies. *Clin Orthop* 291:236, 1993.

Kawamura B: Limb Lengthening. *Orthop Clin North Am* 9:155, 1978.

Kawamura B, Hosono S, Takahashi T: Principles and Technique of Limb Lengthening. *Int Orthop* 5:69, 1981.

Kempf I, Grosse A, Abalo C: Locked Intramedullary Nailing. Its Application to Femoral and Tibial Axial, Rotational, Lengthening, and Shortening Osteotomies. *Clin Orthop* 212:165, 1986.

Kenwright J, Spriggins AJ, Cunningham JL: Response of the Growth Plate to Distraction Close to Skeletal Maturity. Is Fracture Necessary? *Clin Orthop* 250:61, 1990.

Kenwright J, White SH: A Historical Review of Limb Lengthening and Bone Transport. *Injury* 24 Suppl 2:S9, 1993.

Kirakawa K, Hirota S, Ikeda T, Yamaguchi A, Takemura T, Nagoshi J, Yoshiki S, Suda T, Kitamura Y, Nomura S: Localization of the mRNA for Bone Matrix Proteins During Fracture Healing as Determined by In Situ Hybridization. *J Bone Miner Res* 9:1551, 1994.

Kojimoto H, Yasui N, Goto T, Matsuda S, Shimomura Y: Bone Lengthening in Rabbits by Callus Distraction. The Role of Periosteum and Endosteum. *J Bone Joint Surg Br* 70:543, 1988.

Korkala O, Karaharju E, Gronblad M, Aalto K: Experimental Lengthening of Tibial Diaphysis: Gap Healing with or Without Gradual Distraction. *Arch Orthop Trauma Surg* 107:172, 1988.

Kossmann T, Giebel G, Glombitza A: Rat Model for Limb Lengthening by Callus Distraction. *Res Exp Med* 193:13, 1993.

Lee DY, Choi IH, Chung CY, Chung PH, Chi JG, Suh YL: Effect of Tibial Lengthening on the Gastrocnemius Muscle. A Histopathologic and Morphometric Study in Rabbits. *Acta Orthop Scand* 64:688, 1993.

Lee DY, Chung CY, Choi IH: Longitudinal Growth of the Rabbit Tibia after Callotasis. *J Bone Joint Surg Br* 75:898, 1993.

Lehman WB, Grant AD, Atar D: Preventing and Overcoming Equinus Contractures During Lengthening of the Tibia. *Orthop Clin North Am* 22:633, 1991.

Leung KS, Fung KP, Liu PEOPLE, Lee KM: Bone-Specific Alkaline Phosphatase Activities in Plasma and Callus During Callotasis in Rabbits. *Basic Life Sci* 57:637, 1995.

Liu SH, Yang RS, Al-Shaikh R, Lane JM: Collagen in Tendon, Ligament and Bone Healing. *Clin Orthop* 318:265, 1995.

Lynch MC, Taylor JF: Periosteal Division and Longitudinal Growth in the Tibia of the Rat. *J Bone Joint Surg Br* 69:812, 1987.

Ma RYP, Sykes JL, Cornish LS, Lau SH, Leung TM, Leung JCY: Tibial Lengthening Apparatus with Distractive Force Measurement System. *J Biomed Eng* 2:265, 1980.

Macnicol MF, Catto AM: Twenty-Year Review of Tibial Lengthening for Poliomyelitis. *J Bone Joint Surg Br* 64:607, 1982.

Maffulli N, Lombari C, Matarazzo L, Nele U, Pagnotta G, Fixsen JA: A Review of 240 Patients Undergoing Distraction Osteogenesis for Congenital Post-Traumatic or Postinfective Lower Limb Length Discrepancy. *J Am Coll Surg* 182:394, 1996.

Maffulli N, Pattinson RC, Fixsen JA, Hospital for Sick Children, London: Lengthening of Congenital Limb Length Discrepancy Using Callotasis: Early Experience of the Hospital for Sick Children. *Ann R Coll Surg Eng* 75:105, 1993.

Malhis TM, Bowen JR: Tibial and Femoral Lengthening: A Report of 54 Cases. *J Pediatr Orthop* 2:487, 1982.

Manning C: Leg Lengthening. *Clin Orthop* (136):105–10, 1978 Oct.

Martini Z, Castaman E: Tissue Regeneration in the Reconstruction of Lost Bone and Soft Tissue in the Lower Limbs: A Preliminary Report. *Br J Plast Surg* 40:142, 1987.

Mastragostino S, Bagliani GP, Boero S, Origo C: Techniques and Results in Extensive Limb Lengthening. *Basic Life Sci* 48:333, 1988.

Matev IB: Thumb Reconstruction Through Metacarpal Bone Lengthening. *J Hand Surg* 5:482, 1980.

McKellar CC: Congenital Pseudarthrosis of the Tibia—Treatment by Tibial Lengthening and Corrective Osteotomy Seven Years after Successful Bone Graft. A Case Report. *J Bone Joint Surg Am* 55:193, 1973.

Meehan PL: Longitudinal Growth of the Femur and Tibia after Diaphyseal Lengthening [Letter]. *J Bone Joint Surg Am* 70:951, 1988.

Mezhenina EP, Roulla EA, Pechersky AG, Babich VD, Shadrina EL, Mizhevich TV: Methods of Limb Elongation with Congenital Inequality in Children. *J Pediatr Orthop* 4:201, 1984.

Minty I, Maffulli N, Hughes TH, Shaw DG, Fixsen JA: Radiographic Features of Limb Lengthening in Children. *Acta Radiol* 35:555, 1994.

Miura Y, Fitzsimmons JS, Commisso CN, Gallay SH, O'Driscoll SW: Enhancement of Periosteal Chondrogenesis In Vitro. *Clin Orthop* 301:271; April.

Mizumoto Y, Mizuta H, Nakamura E, Takagi K: Tibial Nerve Function during Tibial Lengthening. Measurement of Nerve Conduction and Blood Flow in Rabbits. *Acta Orthop Scand* 66:275, 1995.

Monte AD, Donzelli O: Comparison of Different Methods of Leg Lengthening. *J Pediatr Orthop* 8:62, 1988.

Monticelli G, Spinelli R: Distraction Epiphysiolysis as a Method of Limb Lengthening. I. Experimental Study. *Clin Orthop* 154:254, 1981.

———: Distraction Epiphysiolysis as a Method of Limb Lengthening. III. Clinical Applications. *Clin Orthop* 154:274, 1981.

———: Limb Lengthening by Epiphyseal Distraction. *Int Orthop* 5:85, 1981.

———: Leg Lengthening by Closed Metaphyseal Corticotomy. *It J Orthop Trauma* 9:139, 1983.

Monticelli G, Spinelli R, Bonucci E: Distraction Epiphysiolysis as a Method of Limb Lengthening. II Morphologic Investigations. *Clin Orthop* 154:262, 1981.

Moseley CF: Leg Lengthening A Review of 30 Years. *Clin Orthop* 247:38, 1989.

———: Leg Lengthening: The Historical Perspective. *Orthop Clin of Am* 22:555, 1991.

Mosheiff R, Cordey J, Rahn BA, Perren SM, Stein H, Vascular Supply to Bone in Distraction Osteogenesis: An Experimental Study. *J Bone Joint Surg Br* 78-B:497, 1996.

Muir P, Markel MD, Bogdanske JJ, Johnson KA: Dual Energy X-Ray Absorptiometry and Force-Plate Analysis of Gait in Dogs with Healed Femora after Leg-Lengthening Plate Fixation. *Vet Surg* 24:15, 1995.

Mukhopadhyay D: Lower Limb Equalization in Dyschondroplasia. *Br J Surg* 54:701, 1967.

Nakamura E, Mizuta H, Otsuka Y, Mizumoto Y, Takagi K: Leg Lengthening and Glycosaminoglycans in the Rabbit Knee. *Acta Orthop Scand* 66:33, 1995.

Nakamura E, Mizuta H, Sei A, Takagi K: Knee Articular Cartilage Injury in Leg Lengthening. Histological Studies in Rabbits. *Acta Orthop Scand* 64:437, 1993.

Nakamura E, Mizuta H, Takagi K: Knee Cartilage Injury After Tibial Lengthening. Radiographic and Histological Studies in Rabbits after 3–6 Months. *Acta Orthop Scand* 66:313, 1995.

Nakamura K, Bell MJ, Saleh M, Smith TW: Results of Leg Lengthening Using Wagner's Technique. *Nippon Seikeigeka Gakkai Zasshi—Journal of the Japanese Orthopaedic Association*. 65:498, 1991.

Nakamura K, Nagano A, Tobimatsu H, Kurokawa T: Tibial Lengthening by Epiphyseal Distraction. *Nippon Seikeigeka Gakkai Zasshi—Journal of the Japanese Orthopaedic Association*. 62:37, 1988.

Noble J, Diamond R, Stirrat CR, Sledge CB: Breaking Force of the Rabbit Growth Plate and Its Aplication to Epiphyseal Distraction. *Acta Orthop Scand* 53:13, 1982.

O'Beirne J, Maher M, O'Flanagan S, McGuinness A: Early Experience with Leg Lengthening by Callostasis and Chondrodiastasis. *Ir J Med Sci* 162:301, 1993.

Ohyama M, Miyasaka Y, Sakurai M: Mechanical Behavior and Morphological Structure of Callus in Experimental Callostasis. *Med Mater Eng* 4:273, 1994.

Olerud C, Danckwardt-Lilliestrom G, Olerud S, Genu Recurvatum Caused by Partial Growth Arrest of the Proximal Tibial Physis: Simultaneous Correction and Lengthening with Physeal Distraction. A Report of Two Cases. *Arch Orthop Trauma Surg* 106:64, 1986.

Oni OOA: Protein Immunohistochemistry as a Means of Unraveling the Mysteries of Fracture Repair. *Injury* 26:523, 1995.

Onimus M, Laurain JM, Picard F: Congenital Diastasis of the Inferior Tibiofibular Joint. *J Pediatr Orthop* 10:172, 1990.

Orbay JL, Frankel VH, Finkle JE, Kummer FJ: Canine Leg Lengthening by the Ilizarov Technique. A Biomechanical, Radiologic, and Morphologic Study. *Clin Orthop* 278:265, 1992.

Osterman K, Merikanto J: Diaphyseal Bone Lengthening in Children Using Wagner Device: Long-Term Results. *J Pediatr Orthop* 11:449, 1991.

Ozonoff MB: Orthopedic Procedures in Neuromuscular Disease. *Radiol Clin North Am* 13:139, 1975.

Pablos J, Villas C, Canadell J: Bone Lengthening by Physeal Distraction; An Experimental Study. *Int Orthop* 10:163, 1986.

Paley D: Current Techniques of Limb Lengthening. [Review]. *J Pediatr Orthop* 8:73, 1988.

Paley D, Catagni MA, Argnani F, Villa A, Bendetti GB, Cattaneo R: Ilizarov Treatment of Tibial Nonunions with Bone Loss. *Clin Orthop* 241:146, Apr.

Paley D, Fleming B, Catagni M, Kristiansen T, Pope M: Mechanical Evaluation of External Fixators Used in Limb Lengthening. *Clin Orthop* 250:50, 1990.

Paley D, Tetsworth K: Percutaneous Osteotomies. Osteotome and Gigli Saw Techniques. *Orthop Clin North Am* 22:613, 1991.

Pandey R, White SH, Kenwright J: Callus Distraction in Ollier's Disease. *Acta Orthop Scand* 66:479, 1995.

Paterson D: Leg-Lengthening Procedures. A Historical Review. *Clin Orthop* 250:27, 1990.

Paterson JM, Waller CS, Catterall A: Lower Limb lengthening by a Modified Wagner Technique [Review]. *J Pediatr Orthop* 9:129, 1989.

Peltonen J: Bone Formation and Remodeling after Symmetric and Asymmetric Physeal Distraction. *J Pediatr Orthop* 9:191, 1989.

Peltonen J, Alitalo I, Karaharju E, Helio H: Distraction of the Growth Plate. *Acta Orthop Scand* 55:359, 1984.

Peltonen J, Karaharju E, Aalto K, Alitalo I, Hietaniemi K: Leg Lengthening by Osteotomy and Gradual Distraction: An Experimental Study. *J Pediatr Orthop* 8:509, 1988.

Peretti G, Memeo A, Paronzini A, Marzorati S: Staged Lengthening in the Prevention of Dwarfism in Achondroplastic Children: A Preliminary Report. *J Pediatr Orthop Part B* 4:58, 1995.

Price CT, Cole JD: Limb Lengthening by Callotasis for Children and Adolescents. Early Experience. *Clin Orthop* 250:105 1990.

Price CT, Matthews: Limb Lengthening for Achondroplasia: Early Experience [Published Erratum Appears in *J Pediatr Orthop* 1989 Nov-Dec; 9(6):733] *J Pediatr Orthop* 9:512, 1989.

Putti V: Operative Lengthening of the Femur. *Clin Orthop* 250:4, 1990.

Rajacich N, Bell DF, Armstrong PF: Pediatric Applications of the Ilizarov Method. *Clin Orthop* 280:72, 1992.

Raschke MJ, Mann JW, Oedekoven G, Claudi BF: Segmental Transport after Unreamed Intramedullary Nailing. Preliminary Report of a "Monorail" System. *Clin Orthop* 282:233, 1992.

Rezaian SM: Leg Lengthening with a New Type of External Fixator (A Preliminary Report on 24 Cases). *Pahlavi Med J* 7:233, 1976.

Rezaian SM, Abtahi M: A Simple and Safe Technique for Tibial Lengthening. *Clin Orthop* 207:216, 1986.

Saleh M, Goonatillake HD: Management of Congenital Leg Length Inequality: Value of Early Axis Correction. *J Pediatr Orthop.* Part B. 4:150, 1995.

Saleh M, Sharrard WJ: An Analysis of Referrals to a Regional Leg-Lengthening Service with Special Reference to Achondroplasia. *Basic Life Sci* 48:395, 1988.

Scheffer MM, Peterson HA: Opening-Wedge Osteotomy for Angular Deformities of Long Bones in Children. *J Bone Joint Surg Am* 76:325, 1994.

Schmelzeinsen R, Neumann G, von der Fecht R: Distraction Osteogenesis in the Mandible with a Motor-Driven Plate: A Preliminary Animal Study. *Br J Oral Maxillofac Surg* 34:375, 1996.

Schrodt MJ, Galante J, Shafer SJ, Gimbel J, Ray RD: Tibial Lengthening. A Review of 20 Cases. *Clin Orthop* 80:139, 1971.

Schumacher B, Keller J, Hvid I: Distraction Effects on Muscle. *Acta Orthop Scand* 65:647, 1994.

Seitz DG, Yancey HA: A Review of Tibial Lengthening Procedures. *South Med J* 69:1349, 1976.

Sferra J, Kambic HE, Schickendantz MS, Watson JT: Biomechanical Analysis of Canine Bone Lengthened by the Callotasis Method *Clin Orthop* 311:222, 1995.

Shapiro F: Longitudinal Growth of the Femur and Tibia after Diaphyseal Lengthening. *J Bone Joint Surg Am* 69:684, 1987.

Shatilov OE, Rozkov AV, Cheminova TV: Reconstructive Surgery for Fibular Deficiency. *Prosthet Orthot Int* 15:137, 1991.

Shearer JR, Roach HI, Parsons SW: Histology of a Lengthened Human Tibia. *J Bone Joint Surg Br* 74:39, 1992.

Simpson AH, Williams PE, Kyberd P, Goldspink G, Kenwright J: Response of Muscle to Leg Lengthening. *J Bone Joint Surg Br* 77:630, 1995.

Singer DI, McC O'Brien B, Angel MF, Gumley GJ: Digital Distraction Lengthening Followed by Free Vascularized Epiphyseal Joint Transfer. *J Hand Surg* 14A:508, 1989.

Spriggins AJ, Bader DL, Cunningham JL, Kenwright J: Distraction Physiolysis in the Rabbit. *Acta Orthop Scand* 60:154, 1989.

Steen H, Fjeld TO: Lengthening Osteotomy in the Metaphysis and Diaphysis. An Experimental Study in the Ovine Tibia. *Clin Orthop* 247:297, 1989.

Steen H, Fjeld TO, Bjerkreim I et al: Limb Lengthening by Diaphyseal Corticotomy, Callus Distraction, and Dynamic Axial Fixation. An Experimental Study in the Ovine Femur. *J Orthop Res* 6:730, 1988.

Steen H, Fjeld TO, Miller JA, Ludvigsen P: Biomechanical Factors in the Metaphyseal- and Diaphyseal-Lengthening Osteotomy. An Experimental and Theoretic Analysis in the Ovine Tibia. *Clin Orthop* 259:282, 1990.

Steiner GM, Sprigg A: Value of Ultrasound in the Assessment of Bone. *Br J Radiol* 65:589, 1992.

Stephens DC: Femoral and Tibial Lengthening. *J Pediatr Orthop* 3:424, 1983.

Sun JS, Hou SM, Liu TK, Lu KS: Analysis of Neogenesis in Rabbit Skeletal Muscles after Chronic Traction. *Histol Histopathol* 9:699, 1994.

Tajana GF, Morandi M, Zembo MM: Structure and Development of Osteogenetic Repair Tissue

According to Ilizarov Technique in Man. Characterization of Extracellular Matrix. *Orthopedics* 12:515, 1989.

Tanaka K, Kurokawa T, Nakamura K, Matsushita T, Horinaka S, Kusaba I, Okazaki H, Mamada K, Shiro R, Ou W, Hung SC: Callus Formation in Femur and Tibia during Leg Lengthening: 7 Patients Examined with DXA. *Acta Orthop Scand* 67:158, 1996.

Tjernstrom B, Olerud S, Rehnberg L: Limb Lengthening by Callus Distraction. Complications in 53 Cases Operated 1980–1991. *Acta Orthop Scand* 65:447, 1994.

Tjernstrom B, Thoumas KA, Pech P: Bone Remodeling after Leg Lengthening: Evaluation with Plain Radiographs, and Computed Tomography and Magnetic Resonance Imaging Scans. *J Pediatr Orthop* 12:751, 1992.

Torode IP, Gillespie R: Anterioposterior Instability of the Knee: A Sign of Congenital Limb Deficiency. *J Pediatr Orthop* 3:467, 1983.

Urist MR: A 37-Year Follow-Up Evaluation of Multiple-Stage Femur and Tibia Lengthening in Dyschondroplasia (Enchondromatosis) with a Net Gain of 23.3 Centimeters. *Clin Orthop* 242:137, 1989.

Utvag SE, Grundnes O, Reikeras O: Healing of Segmental and Simple Fractures in Rats. *Acta Orthop Scand* 65:559, 1994.

Vade A, Essenstat R: Radiographic Features of Bone Lengthening Procedures. *Radiology* 174:531, 1990.

Van Roermund PM, Hoekstra A, Visser WJ, Renooij W: Effect of Direct Current Stimulation on Bone Growth after Distraction Epiphysiolysis of the Rabbit Tibia. *J Orthop Res* 8:769, 1990.

Van Roermund PM, Hoekstra A, ter Haar Romeny BM, Renooij W: Bone Healing during Lower Limb Lengthening by Distraction Epiphysiolysis. *J Nucl Med* 29:1259, 1988.

Van Roermund PM, ter Haar Romeny BM, Hoekstra A, Schoonderwoert GJ, Brandt CJ, van der Steen SP, Roelofs JM, Scholten F, Visser WJ, Renooij W: Bone Growth and Remodeling after Distraction Epiphysiolysis of the Proximal Tibia of the Rabbit. Effect of Electromagnetic Stimulation. *Clin Orthop* 266:304, 1991.

Van Roermund PM, ter Haar Romeny BM, Schoonderwoert GJ, Brandt CJ, Sijbrandij S, Renooij W: Use of Computed Tomography to Quantitate Bone Formation after Distraction Epiphysiolysis in the Rabbit. *Skeletal Radiol* 16:52, 1987.

Van Roermund PM, Wijlens RA, Renooij W: Continuous Monitoring of Forces during Tibial Lengthening by Distraction Epiphysiolysis. *Acta Orthop Belg* 58:63, 1992.

Vauhkonen M, Peltonen J, Karaharju E, Aalto K, Alitalo I: Synthesis and Mineralization in the Early Phase of Distraction Bone Healing. *Bone Miner* 10:171, 1990.

Verkerke GJ, Schraffordt Koops H, Veth RP, Grootenboer HJ, De Boer LJ, Oldhoff J, Postma A: Development and Test of an Extendible Endoprosthesis for Bone Reconstruction in the Leg. *Int J Artif Organs* 17:155, 1994.

Vilarrubias JM, Cavaliere P, Ginebreda I: Lengthening of the Lower Limbs and Correction of Lumbar Hyperlorodosis in Achondroplasia. *Basic Life Sci* 48:357, 1988.

Vilarrubias JM, Ginebreda I, Jimeno E: Lengthening of the Lower Limbs and Correction of Lumbar Hyperlorodosis in Achondroplasia. *Clin Orthop* 250:143, 1990.

Vizkelety TL, Marschalko P: Limb Lengthening Operations. *Acta Chir Hung* 33:55, 1992–93.

Wallace AL, Draper ERC, Strachan RK, McCarthy ID, Hughes SPF: Vascular Response to Fracture Micromovement. *Clin Orthop* 301:281, 1994.

Walsh WR, Hamdy RC, Ehrlich MG: Biomechanical and Physical Properties of Lengthened Bone in a Canine Model. *Clin Orthop* 306:230, 1994.

Wasserstein I: Twenty-Five Years' Experience with Lengthening of Shortened Lower Extremities Using Cylindrical Allografts. *Clin Orthop* 250:150, 1990.

White SH, Kenwright J: Timing of Distraction of an Osteotomy. *J Bone Joint Surg Br* 72:356, 1990.

White SH, Sci BM, Kenwright: Importance of Delay in Distraction of Osteotomies. *Orthop Clin North Am* 22:569, 1991.

Wilde GP, Baker GC: Circumferential Periosteal Release in the Treatment of Children with Leg-Length Inequality. *J Bone Jt Surg Br* 69:817, 1987.

Wolfson N, Hearn TC, Thomason JJ, Armstrong PF: Force and Stiffness Changes during Ilizarov Leg Lengthening. *Clin Orthop* 250:58, 1990.

Yasui N, Kojimoto H, Sasaki K, Kitada A, Shimizu H, Shimomura Y: Factors Affecting Callus Distraction in Limb Lengthening. *Clin Orthop* 293:55, 1993.

Yasui N, Kojimoto H, Shimizu H, Shimomura Y: Effect of Distraction upon Bone, Muscle, and Periosteum. *Orthop Clin North Am* 22:563, 1991.

Young JW, Kostrubiak IS, Resnik CS, Paley D: Sonographic Evaluation of Bone Production at the Distraction Site in Ilizarov Limb-Lengthening Procedures. *Am Roentgenol* 154:125, 1990.

Young JW, Kovelman H, Resnik CS, Paley D: Radiologic Assessment of Bones after Ilizarov Procedures. *Radiology* 177:89, 1990.

Young NL, Davis RJ, Bell DF, Redmond DM: Electromyographic and Nerve Conduction Changes after Tibial Lengthening by the Ilizarov Method. *J Pediatr Orthop* 13:473, 1993.

Younge D, Dafniotis O: A Composite Bone Flap to Lengthen a Below-Knee Amputation Stump. *J Bone Joint Surg Br* 75:330, 1993.

INDEX

MIX
Papier aus verantwortungsvollen Quellen
Paper from responsible sources
FSC® C105338

If you have any concerns about our products,
you can contact us on
ProductSafety@springernature.com

In case Publisher is established outside the EU,
the EU authorized representative is:
Springer Nature Customer Service Center GmbH
Europaplatz 3, 69115 Heidelberg, Germany

Printed by Libri Plureos GmbH
in Hamburg, Germany